PHARMACEUTICAL MICROBIOLOGY

A COMPREHENSIVE APPROACH

SECOND EDITION

PHARMACEUTICAL MICROBIOLOGY

A COMPREHENSIVE APPROACH

SECOND EDITION

Dr. Ravi Kumar Maddali,
M.Pharm, Ph.D, PDF (USA)
Professor & Principal
Geethanjali College of Pharmacy,
Cheeryal(V), Keesara(M), Medchal District,
Hyderabad, Telangana State, India-501 301.

PharmaMed Press
An imprint of Pharma Book Syndicate
A Unit of BSP Books Pvt. Ltd.
4-4-309/316, Giriraj Lane,
Sultan Bazar, Hyderabad - 500 095.

Pharmaceutical Microbiology : A Comprehensive Approach
Second Edition* by *Ravi Kumar Maddali

Published by

PharmaMed Press
An imprint of Pharma Book Syndicate
A unit of BSP Books Pvt. Ltd.
4-4-309/316, Giriraj Lane, Sultan Bazar, Hyderabad - 500 095.
Phone: 040-23445600, 23445688; Fax: 91+40-23445611
e-mail: info@pharmamedpress.com
www.pharmamedpress.com/pharmamedpress.net

ISBN: 978-93-86819-66-6 (Hardback)

Dedicated to

My wife Sippora Maddali
Daughter Sravya Maddali
and
Son Sunit Wesley Maddali

Contents

Chapter 2

Diversity of Micro-organisms

Chapter 5

Immunology

Chapter 9

Applications of Microbes in Pharmacy

Chapter 10

Microbiological Assays

Chapter 11

Microbial Spoilage and Preservation of Pharmaceutical Products

Chapter 12

Miscellaneous Topics

Preface to Second Edition

Proper care has been taken to correct all minor errors like typographical errors, spelling mistakes, wrong heading numbers etc., that have been surfaced inadvertently in the first edition.

New topics like, Large scale sterilization equipments, Design of aseptic area, laminar flow equipments, and Different source of contamination and methods of prevention, Clean area classification have been included in Chapter 4 as per PCI syllabus for B.Pharmacy course.

Microbiological assays of Niacin (Vitamin B_3) and microbial assay of amino acids and assessment methods of new antibiotics topics have been included in chapter 10 titled microbiological assays.

In the Chapter 12 i.e. Miscellaneous Topics various biogeochemical cycles like carbon cycle, nitrogen cycle, phosphorus cycle and sulphur cycles have been redrafted with lucid explanation in this edition.

In the same chapter 12 a new topic on cell culture explaining procedure for cell culture, types of cell cultures and application of cell cultures in pharmaceutical industry and research have been added as per PCI syllabus.

In chapter 5 .i.e. Immunology examples of allergenic extracts have been added.

In chapter 6 i.e. Bacterial genetics, a figure for specialized transduction has been incorporated.

I sincerely acknowledge my heartfelt thanks to the principals, teachers and students of various pharmacy colleges across the nation for giving me encouraging and appreciating feed back of the first edition of this book "Pharmaceutical Microbiology: A Comprehensive Approach" authored by me.

I am also grateful to senior authors and my colleagues who gave their valuable suggestions in preparing this second edition of this text book. It's a matter of pride that there has been a good response for this book from the students across the country. I thank all the teachers for prescribing this book for their students.

-Author

Preface to First Edition

As a teacher of pharmaceutical microbiology for several years, I and my students faced difficulty to collect material from different textbooks for different topics, which is why I shouldered the responsibility of preparing a comprehensive textbook containing all prescribed topics in pharmaceutical microbiology syllabus. Moreover the syllabus of various Indian universities is very complex. To cater to the total needs of the students, I have tried to incorporate maximum & diverse topics in this book so as to fulfill the needs of all universities. Pharmaceutical microbiology topics and Pharmaceutical biotechnology topics are combined as a single subject in some of the universities where as other universities prescribed it with two separate titles.

Though some concepts of biotechnology are dealt to some extent in some of the chapters, this book is mainly dedicated to pharmaceutical microbiology syllabus. Recent advances resulted from the rapid progress of research in this subject area have also been dealt along with fundamentals in lucid language and logical sequence.

Introduction chapter introduces fundamentals of microbiology and scientists' contribution.

Second and third chapters are dedicated to deal different groups of microorganisms namely bacteria, fungi (i.e. yeasts and molds), viruses, rickettsias, algae, and protozoa etc., under the heading of microbial diversity and nutrition and growth respectively. Control of microorganism, disinfectants, antisepctics and sterilization procedures were thoroughly dealt in 6th chapter with necessary diagrams. Major diseases are discussed in detail in 7th chapter. Environmental effects on microbial growth are discussed in 8th chapter. Pharmaceutical applications of microorganisms are discussed in the 9th chapter. Microbiological assays, microbial limit tests and biosensors are discussed in 10th chapter. Subsequent chapters dealt the topic of microbial spoilage and preservation and miscellaneous topics. Valuable substantial information has been given on all topics and the text is supported by necessary photographs, ray diagrams, neat sketches, figures, and tables etc. Proper care has been taken to prepare the text in readable and interesting manner. I believe this book titled "Pharmaceutical Microbiology: A Comprehensive Approach" will be a book of choice for students and faculty in their academic pursuit.

Valued suggestions and comments are welcomed to refine the material and incorporate the suggestions in the future editions of this book.

-Author

Acknowledgement

My invocation to Omniscient, Omnipotent Almighty God for blessing me with knowledge and ability to author this book.

Gratitude to the management members especially beloved secretary Shri G. R. Ravinder Reddy, M.Tech (NIT Warangal) IPS. Chairman Geethanjali College of Engineering and Pharmacy for his continuous support and encouragement to complete this work.

Value additions to my teachers, friends and my colleagues who helped me in different ways to make my dream virtual.

Congratulation to Mr. Sabari Karthik Brahmanlapalli who spared no efforts to liaison with the publisher.

Special thanks to Mr. R. Naga Kishore for helping me in preparing the text.

Humble thanks to Anil Shah, Publisher of PharmaMed Press for giving me this opportunity to pendown my knowledge in the form of a book, inspite of various rigid restraints to comply with me for making this piece of work a note worthy one.

Special acknowledgements to all my family members who are with me to make this dream come true.

-Dr. Ravi Kumar Maddali

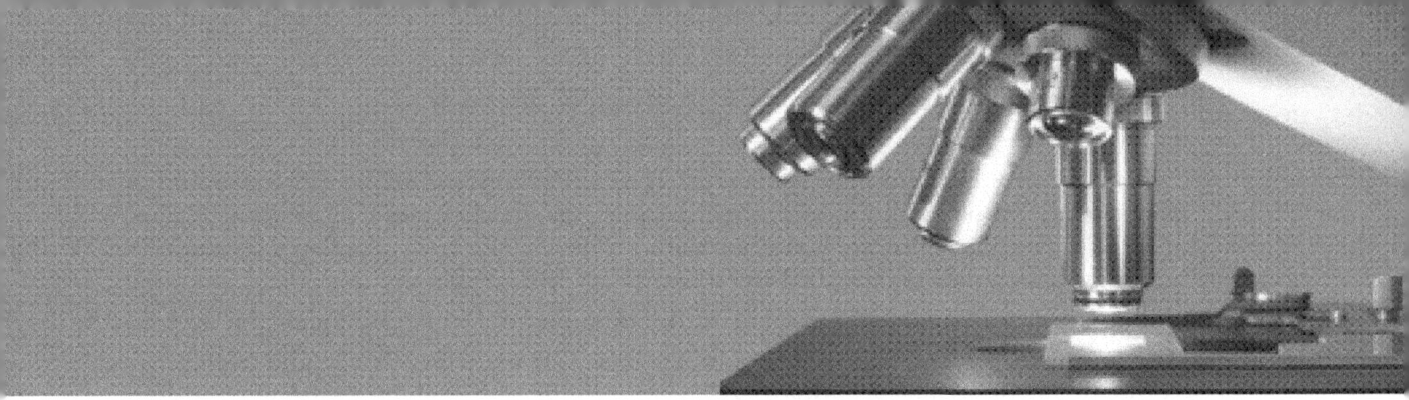

1 INTRODUCTION

LEARNING OBJECTIVES

After studying the chapter the students familiarize themselves with the following concepts:

- *Introducing the subject Microbiology and significance of micro-organisms*
- *Different varieties of microscopes their invention and constructions along with simplified ray diagrams*
- *Contribution of scientists for the development of microbiology*
- *Introducing various Branches of Microbiology*

The term Microbiology is coined with 3 Greek words (***Mikro*** – **small,** ***bios*** **- life,** ***logos*** **science**). In other words it is the study of organisms of microscopic size (micro-organisms) including their culture, economic importance, pathogenecity, etc. This study is concerned with their form, structure, reproduction, physiology, metabolism and classification. It includes the changes which micro-organisms bring about in other organisms and in nonliving matter and their distribution in nature, their effects on human beings and on other animals and plants, their abilities to make physical and chemical changes in our environment and their reactions to physical and chemical agents. This study revealed the fact that there are many a great number of very tiny life forms all about us everywhere too small to be seen usually by the naked eye. These organisms are usually invisible to naked eye because they are in micron size. Our eye fails to perceive any object that has a diameter less than 0.1 mm, so it is necessary to use microscope to see these tiny forms of life.

However, some micro-organisms, particularly some eukaryotic microbes, are visible without microscopes. For example, bread molds and filamentous algae are studied by microbiologists, yet are visible to the naked eye, as are the two bacteria ***Thiomargarita*** and ***Epulopiscioum***.

The difficulty in setting the boundaries of microbiology has led to the suggestion of other criteria for defining the field. For instance, an important characteristic of micro-organisms, even those that are large and multi cellular is that, they are relatively simple in their construction, lacking highly differentiated cells and distinct tissues.

Another definition for this field is based in terms of techniques employed such as sterilization and the use of culture media that are necessary for successful isolation and growth of micro-organisms. Micro-organisms include acellular entities (e.g., viruses), prokaryotic cells and eukaryotic cells. Cellular micro-organisms are found in all three domains of life *Bacteria, Archaea and Eucarya.*

It is estimated that microbes contain 50% of the biological carbon and 90% of the biological nitrogen on earth. They greatly exceed every group of organisms on the planet in number.

1.1 Significance of Micro-organisms

Micro-organisms are found in all places from geothermal vents in the oceans depths to the coldest arctic ice, to every person's skin. They are major contributors to the functioning of the biosphere, being indispensable for the cycling of the elements essential for life. They also are a source of nutrients at the base of all ecological food chains and webs. Most importantly, certain micro-organisms carryout photosynthesis, rivaling plants in their role of capturing Carbon dioxide and releasing oxygen into the atmosphere. Those microbes that inhabit humans also play important roles; including helping the body digests food and producing vitamins B and K. In addition society in general benefits from micro-organisms, as they are necessary for the production of bread, cheese, beer, antibiotics, vaccines, vitamins, enzymes and many other important products. Indeed modern biotechnology rests upon a microbiological foundation.

Although majority of micro-organisms play beneficial or benign roles, some harm humans and have disrupted society over the millennia. Microbial disease undoubtedly played a major role in historical events such as the decline of Roman Empire and the conquest of the new world. In 1347, plague or Black death, an arthropod – borne disease struck Europe with brutal force, killing 1/3 of the population (about 25 million people) within four years. Over the next 80 years, the disease struck again and again, eventually wiping out 75% of the European population. The plague's effect was so great that some historians believe, it changed European culture and prepared the way for the Renaissance. Today the struggle by microbiologists and others against killers like AIDS and malaria continue.

According to present knowledge we may put *Archaebacteria*, *Bacteria*, *Cyanobacteria*. *Microalgae*, *Protozoans*, *Microfungi*, *Viruses*, *Viroids*, *Prions* etc., under the domain of micro-organisms. Viruses are ultramicroscopic and have an obligate *parasitic* relationship but for particular purpose these still come under the domain of micro-organisms. Micro-organisms (Bacteria) were undoubtedly the first living inhabitants on the earth and they were anaerobic as molecular oxygen was either absent or present only in trace amounts. The oldest fossil records of plants and animals are only 0.6–0.7 million years old, but now there is credible evidence that microbial life existed more than 3.5 billion years ago, that is, just 1 billion years after the formation of the earth and almost 3 billion years before plants and animals appeared on Earth.

1.1.1 Endosymbiosis

The word Endosymbiosis was coined with three Greek words i.e., *endon "Within", Syn "Together" and Biosis "Living"* Endosymbiosis is the name given to processes wherein one cell lives inside another cell in a mutualist fashion.

- It is an evolutionary theory that explains the origin of eukaryotic cells from prokaryotes. It states that several key organelles of eukaryotes originated as a symbiosis between separate single-celled organisms. According to this theory, mitochondria, plastids (for example chloroplasts), and possibly other organelles representing formerly free-living bacteria, were taken inside by another cell as an endosymbiont around 1.5 billion years ago. Molecular and biochemical evidence suggest that mitochondria developed from proteobacteria (in particular, Rickettsiales, or close relatives) and chloroplasts from cyanobacteria (in particular, nitrogen-fixing filamentous cyanobacteria).
- They usually involve, a smaller prokaryotic cell living within the cytoplasm of eukaryotic cell.
- Endosymbiosis events between eukaryotic and prokaryotic cells have been taking place since the origin of the eukaryotic cell.
- About 1.5-2 billion years ago, oxygenic photosynthesis and aerobic respiration were predominant types of metabolism in bacteria.
- Cyanobacteria produced all of the earth's atmospheric (O_2) and oxygen respiratory bacteria had developed. Sophisticated membrane system allowing them to reduce O_2 and generate relatively large amounts of energy.
- The eukaryotic cell could provide nutrients and a protected habitat for its invader or prey. The prokaryotes invaded by primitive eukaryotic cells, hence, the two organisms were able to enter into a mutually beneficial and stable relationship.
- Eukaryotic organelles contain their own genome (DNA) and ribosomes both of which have a bacterial configuration and function.

- They synthesize their own proteins, chloroplasts and have the same type of chlorophyll, enzymes and metabolism as respiratory bacteria such as "*Pseudomonas*" and other proteobacteria.
- Based on their nutrition patterns, morphology, molecular arrangements these are evolved into distinct types.

1.2 Structure of Eukaryotic and Prokaryotic Cells

- Prokaryotic organisms (Archaea and Bacteria) and eukaryotic organisms (both unicellular and multi cellular forms) have evolved as two distinctive types of cells, differing fundamentally in their cell structure.
- Eukaryotes always contain a membrane enclosed nucleus, multiple chromosomes and various other membranous organelles, such as mitochondria, chloroplast, golgi apparatus, vacuoles etc.
- Prokaryotic cells are typically much smaller in size and never contain a nuclear membrane around their genetic material.
- The fundamental differences between eukaryotic and prokaryotic cells, as well as the similarities and differences between eukaryotes, bacteria and archaea, are evidenced by their nuclear organization, their cell wall, cell membrane and ribosome structure and their modes of protein synthesis.

1.3 Evolution of Micro-organisms on Earth

The earth was still in the process of developing and had a reduced atmosphere before life originated on it. It is thought that the reduced atmosphere of earth consisted largely of gaseous forms of nitrogen, hydrogen, carbon dioxide and water vapour, with smaller amounts of ammonia, carbon monoxide and hydrogen sulphide.

Oxygen was either absent or present only in trace amounts or therefore, the atmosphere was anaerobic (oxygen-free). Torrential rains poured over the developing Earth for centuries forming large masses of water in which the original gaseous raw materials of atmosphere gradually dissolved forming "ocean".

The oceans were like a 'broth' and with the aid of energy from ultraviolet rays and electrical discharges (lightening), variety of organic compounds were synthesized progressively in them abiotic (nonliving) reactions and these organic compounds slowly evolved into larger and more complex organic molecules (macromolecules). The macromolecules had inherent tendency to aggregate in various combinations and appeared as distinct bodies (the microspheres) in the surrounding water medium.

These microspheres are postulated to be the first step toward cellular organization and referred to as progenotes or protobionts. Acquisition and use of nucleic acids, development of enzymatic capabilities and membrane organization further led the progenotes or protobionts to create eugenotes or primitive version of prokaryotic cell (bacterial cell).

The micro-organisms are almost Omni present and are characterized with a very high degree of adaptability. They constitute a world of their own; full of uniqueness from different biological standpoints. The microbial world is spread over the entire biosphere-the lithosphere (rocky substances), the hydrosphere (liquid components) and the atmosphere (gaseous mantle envelopes the litho and hydrosphere); the latter being their temporary abode. The micro-organisms are also found in the living as well as dead bodies of the organisms.

1.4 Microscopy

Microscope is the instrument used to provide magnification that enables us to see micro-organisms and their structures which are invisible to the naked eye shown in Fig. 1.1.

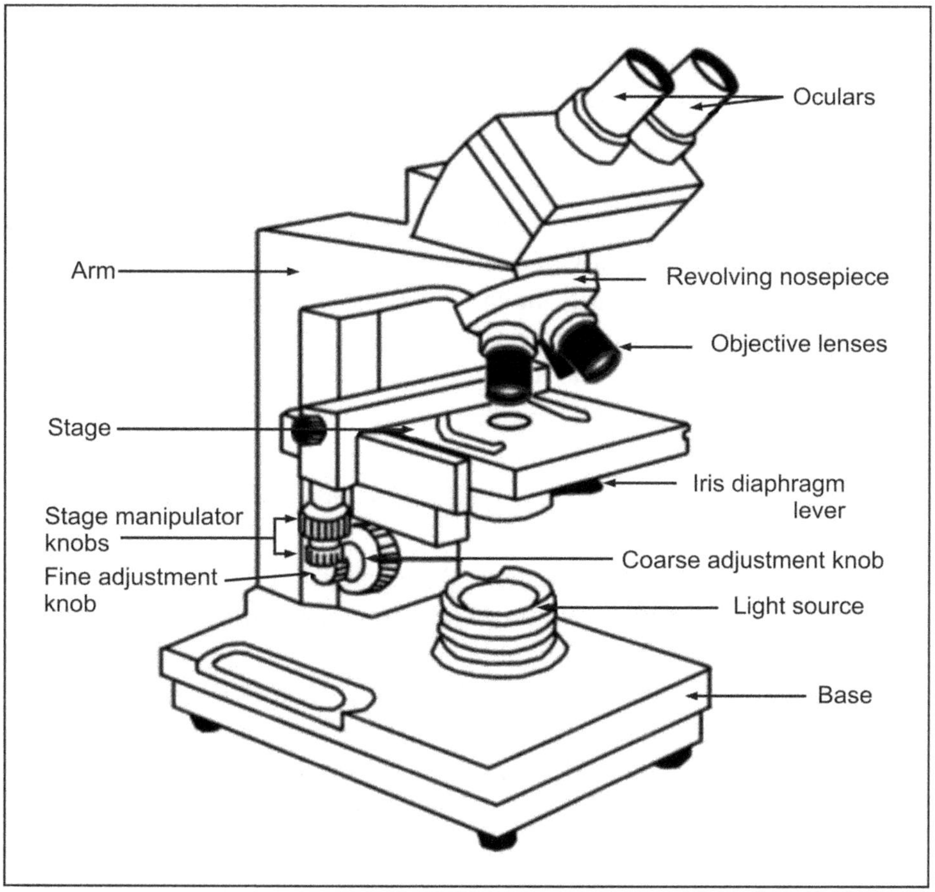

Fig. 1.1 Microscope

The magnification attained by microscopes range from 100 to 400,000.

Microscopes are of two categories:

1. Light or Optical microscopes
2. Electron microscopes

1.4.1 Light or Optical Microscopes

In this microscopes magnification is obtained by a system of optical lenses using light waves. These include:

1. Bright-field Microscope
2. Dark–field Microscope
3. Fluorescence Microscope
4. Phase-contrast Microscope

1. **Bright–Field Microscope:** In this microscopy the microscopic field is brightly lighted and the micro-organisms appear dark because they absorb some of the light. Ordinarily, micro-organisms do not absorb much light, but staining them with a dye greatly increases their light-absorbing ability, resulting in greater contrast and color differentiation shown in Fig. 1.2.

   These microscopes are useful in providing magnification of about 1000 × to 1200 x.

   Resolving power: It is the ability of a microscope to distinguish two adjacent points as distinct and separate. The basic limitation of Bright-Field microscope is resolving power. The largest magnification produced by a microscope may not be useful because the image may be unclear and fuzzy.

   The more lines or dots per unit area that can be seen distinctly as separate lines or dots, the greater the resolving power of microscope.

   This resolving power of a microscope is a function of wavelength of light used and the numerical aperture (NA) of the lens system.

   Numerical Aperture (NA): The angle θ subtended by the optical axis and the outermost rays still covered by the objective is the measure of aperture of the objective. It is the half aperture angle.

   The magnitude of this angle is expressed as a Sin value. The sine value of the half-aperture angle multiplied by the refractive index "n" of the medium filling the space between front lens and the cover slip gives the numerical aperture (NA): NA = n Sin θ. With dry objectives the value of "n" is 1, since refractive index (R_I) of air is 1.

   When oil immersion is used as the medium, n is 1.56 and if θ = 58 degrees, then NA = n Sin θ = 1.56 × 58 degree = 1.56 × 0.85 = 1.33.

   Limit of Resolution: It is the smallest distance by which two objects can be separated.

The greatest resolution in light microscopy is obtained with shorter wavelength of visible light and an objective with the maximum Numerical Aperture.

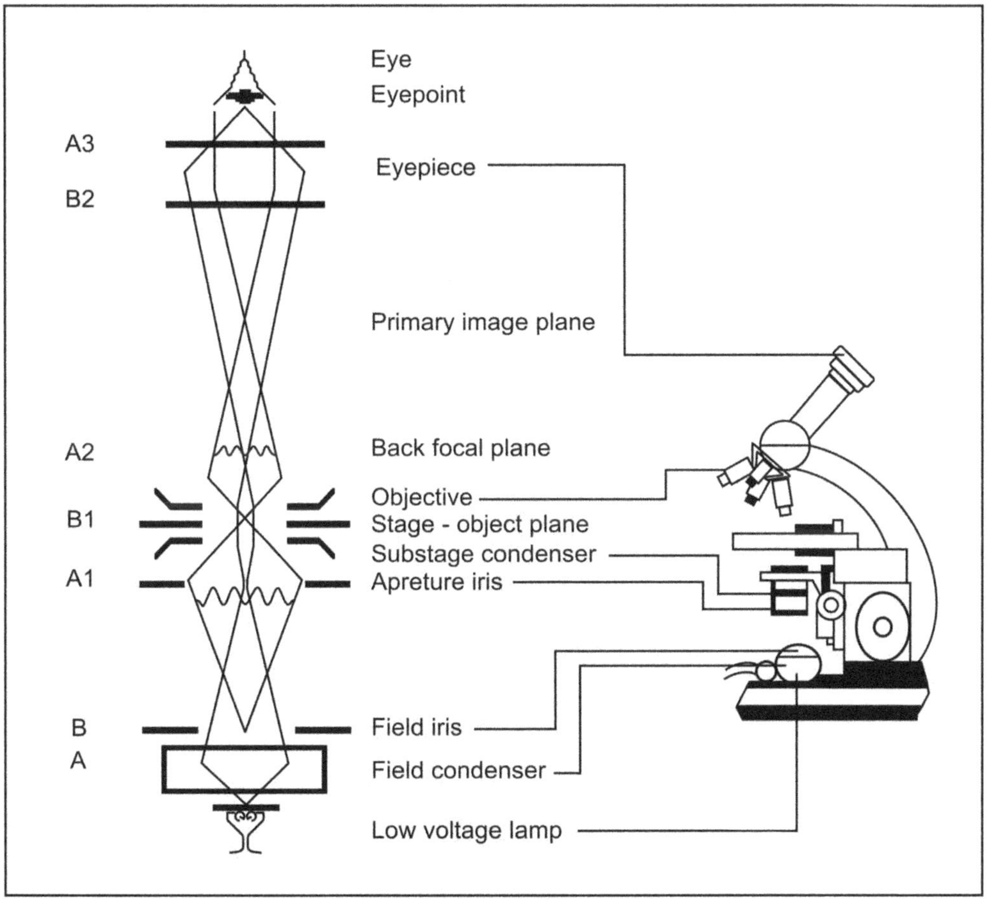

Fig. 1.2 Bright field microscope pathways

The relationship between NA and resolution can be expressed as

$$d = \text{lambda } (\lambda)/2NA$$

Where d = resolution, λ = wavelength.

***Magnification*:** magnification beyond the resolving power is of no value since larger image will be less distinct and fuzzy in appearance.

Microscopes are equipped with 3 objectives each capable of a different degree of magnification and they are oil-immersion, high-dry and low-power objectives.

The total magnification is determined by multiplying the magnifying power of objective and that of the eye-piece.

An eye- piece of a magnification of 10 is used. Objectives used are 10x;40x and 100x (oil immersion objective).

2. **Dark–Field Microscopy:** The effect produced by this microscope is that of a dark background against which objects are brightly illuminated.

   It contains equipment with a special kind of condenser that transmits a hollow cone of light from source of illumination.

   Most of the light directed through the condenser does not enter the objective, so field is essentially dark. And some of the light rays will be scattered if transparent medium contains objects such as microbial cells shown in Fig. 1.3 and 1.4. This ray will enter the objective and reach the eye, thus the object will appear bright.

   This microscopy is valuable for examining of unstained micro-organisms suspended in fluid - wet - mount and hanging drop preparation.

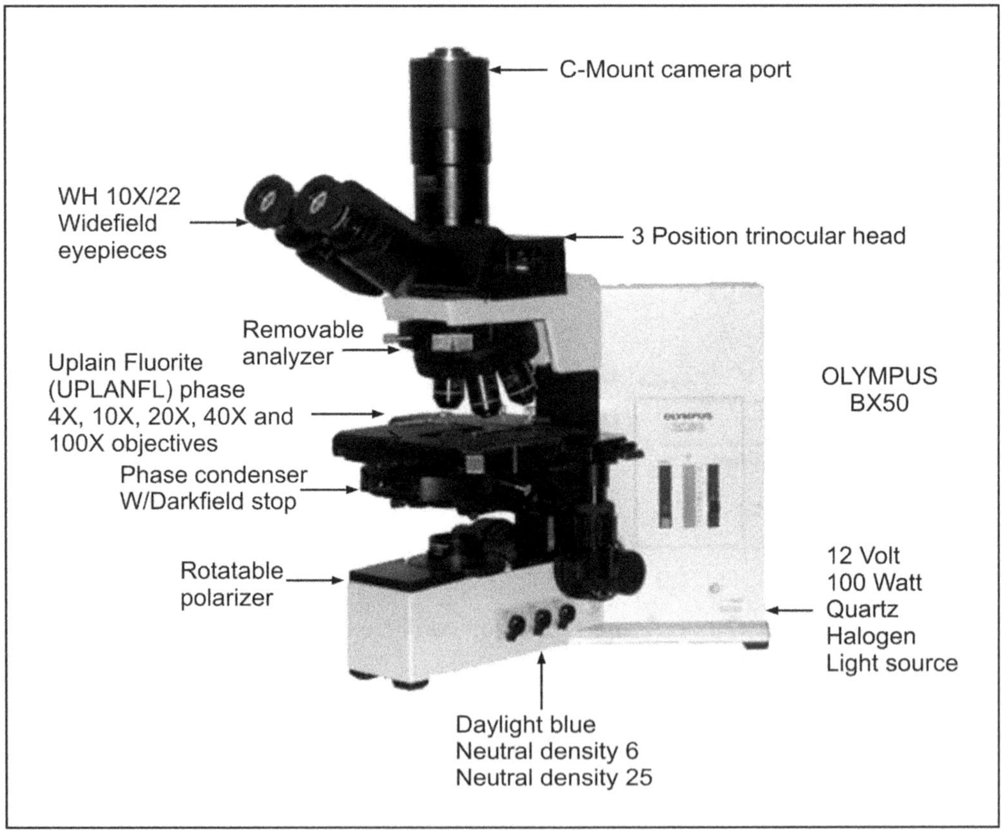

Fig. 1.3 Dark field microscopy

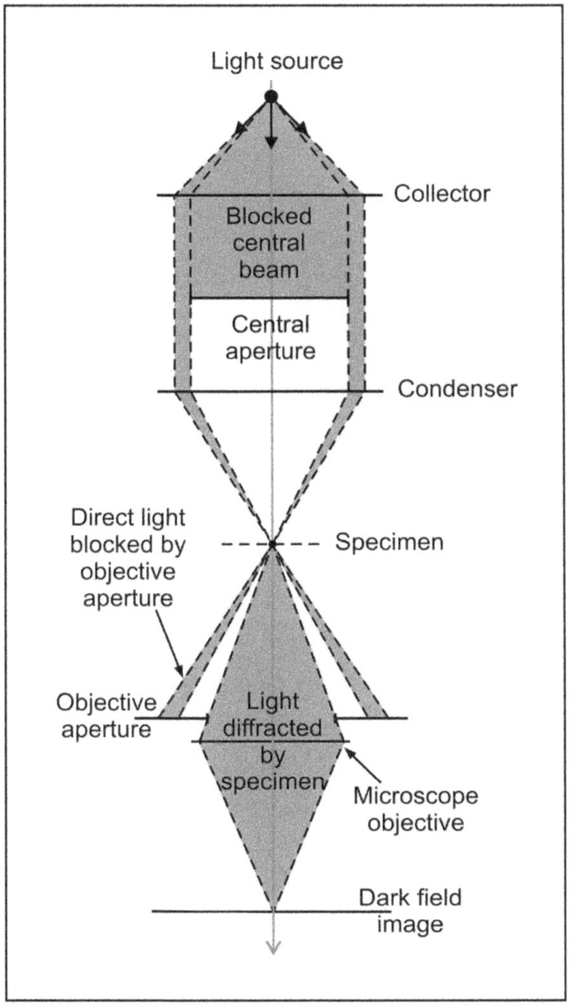

Fig. 1.4 Light path through dark field microscope

3. **Fluorescence Microscope:** Many chemical substances absorb light of a particular wavelength and energy and some substances will emit light of longer wave length and less energy content. Such substances are called fluorescent and the phenomenon is termed as fluorescence. In this micro-organisms are stained with a fluorescent dye and then illuminated with blue light, the blue light is absorbed and green light is emitted shown in Fig. 1.5.

   The function of exciter-filter is to remove all but blue light. Barrier filter block out blue light and allows green light to pass through.

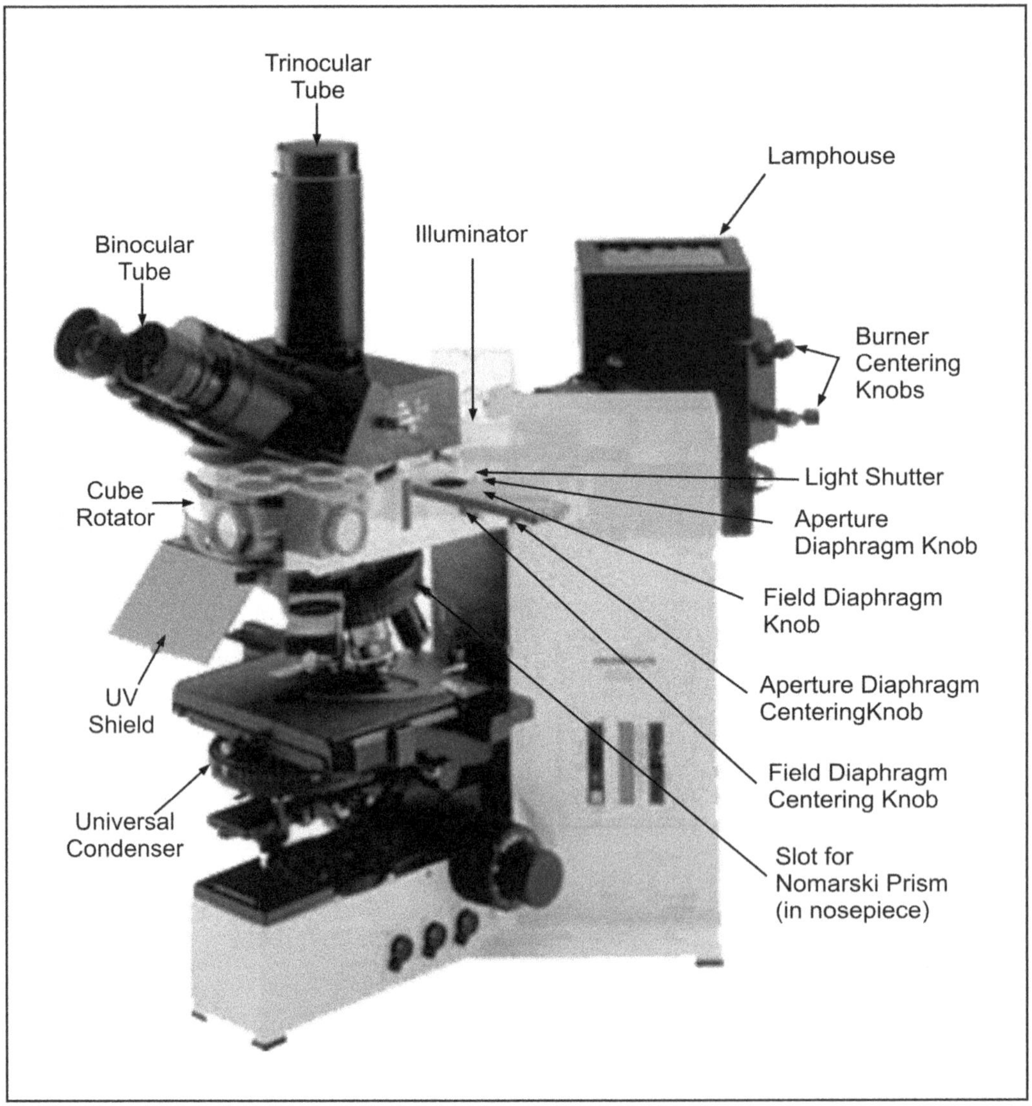

Fig. 1.5 Fluroscence microscope

4. **Phase–Contrast Microscopy:** The principle is based on the fact that light passing through one material and into another material of a slightly different refractive index and thickness will undergo a change in phase. These differences in phase are translated into variations in brightness of the structures and hence are detectable by the eye shown in Fig. 1.6, 1.7 and 1.8.

   With phase–contrast microscopy it is possible to reveal differences in cell and their structures.

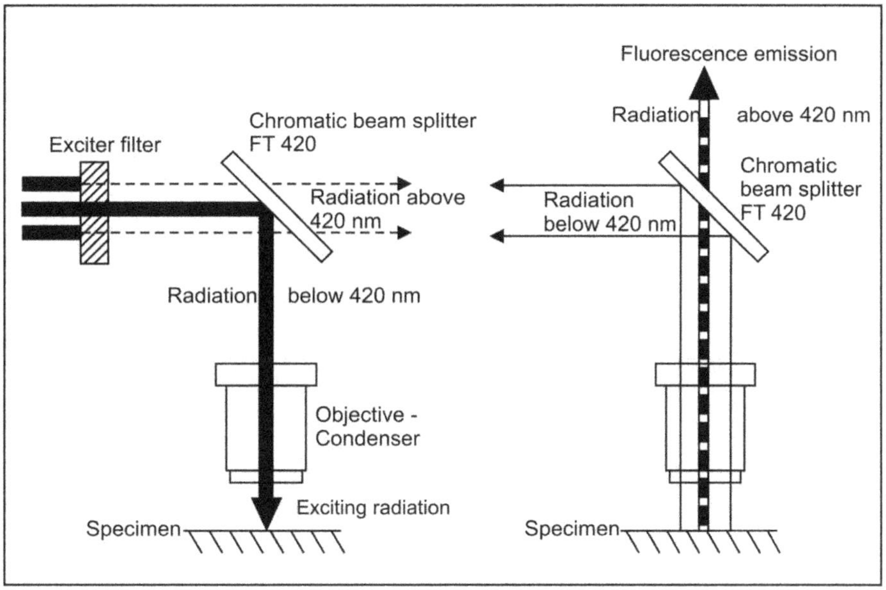

Fig. 1.6 Flourescence microscope pathways

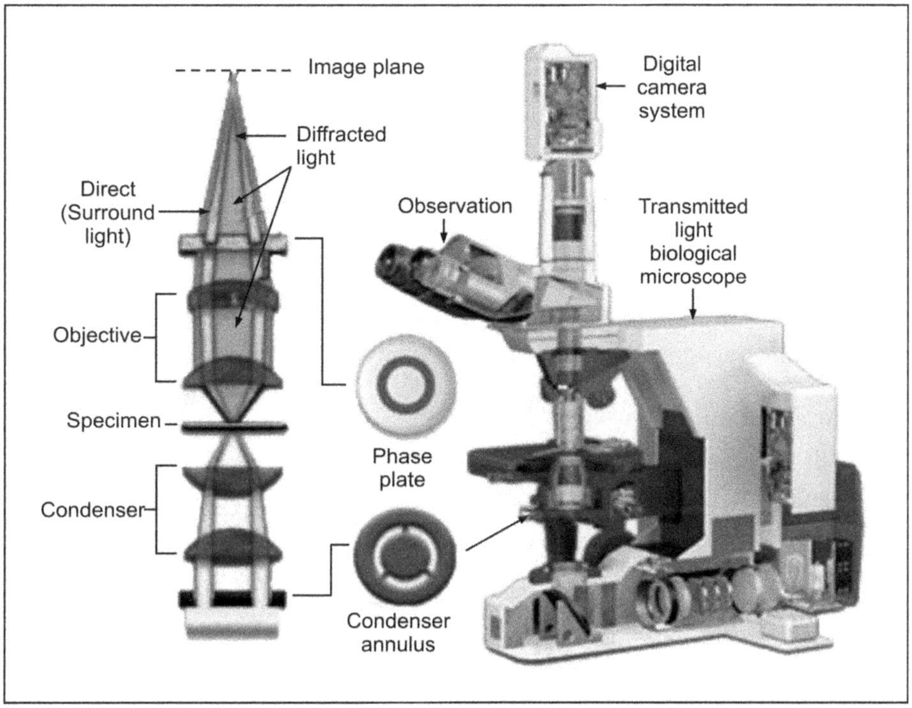

Fig. 1.7 Phase contrast microscope configuration

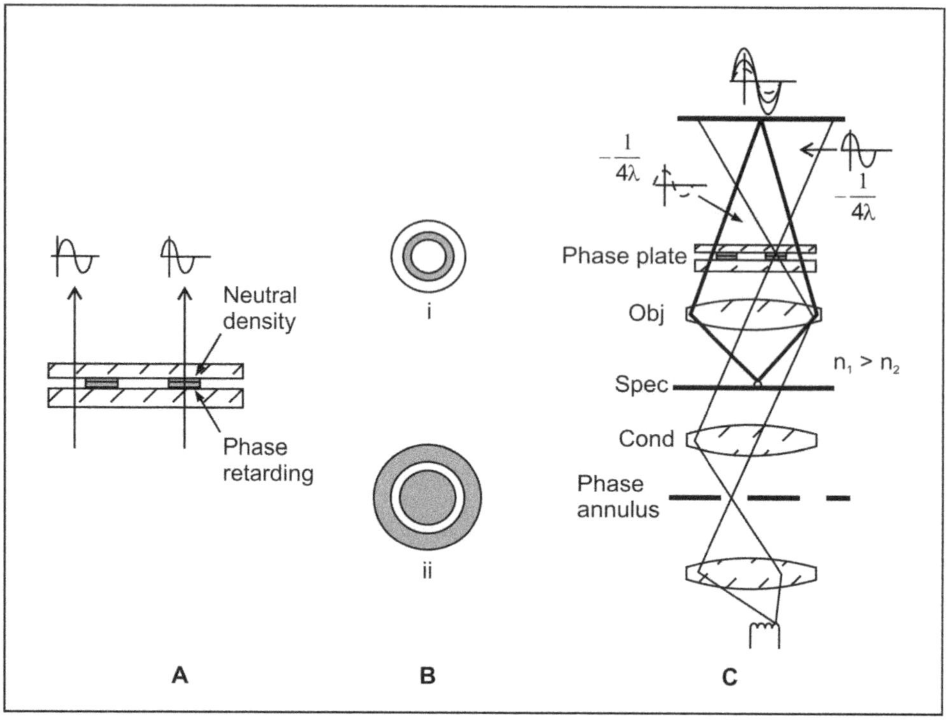

Fig. 1.8 Zernike negative phase contrast. **A:** Construction of the phase plate showing the relative phase shifts induced by the phase rings. **B:** Face view of the phase annulus (ii) and phase plate (i) **C:** The optical path for phase contrast illumination. Cond: condenser lens; Spec: specimen plane; Obj: objective lens; n_1, n_2: refractive index of the sample and background, respectively, (Figure C redrawn from Francon, 1968.)

1.4.2 Electron Microscope

It uses a beam of electron in place of light waves to produce the image, Specimens can be examined by either transmission electron microscopy or scanning electron microscopy.

Transmission Electron Microscopy (TEM)

TEM (Fig. 1.9) was developed in 1931by Max Knoll and Ernst Ruska at Berlin. It gives 2-D image and having resolution of 0.5 angstroms and gives up to 50 million magnification level. This microscope provides tremendous useful magnification, because of much higher resolution obtained with extremely short wave length. The electron microscope uses electron beams and magnetic fields to produce the image. Electrons replace light as the illuminating beam. They can be focused, much as light in a light microscope, but their wavelength is around 0.005 nm, approximately 100,000 times shorter than that of visible light. Therefore electron microscope have a practical resolution roughly, 1,000 times better than the light microscope; with many electron microscopes, points closer than 0.5 nm can be distinguished, and the useful magnification is well over 100,000x.

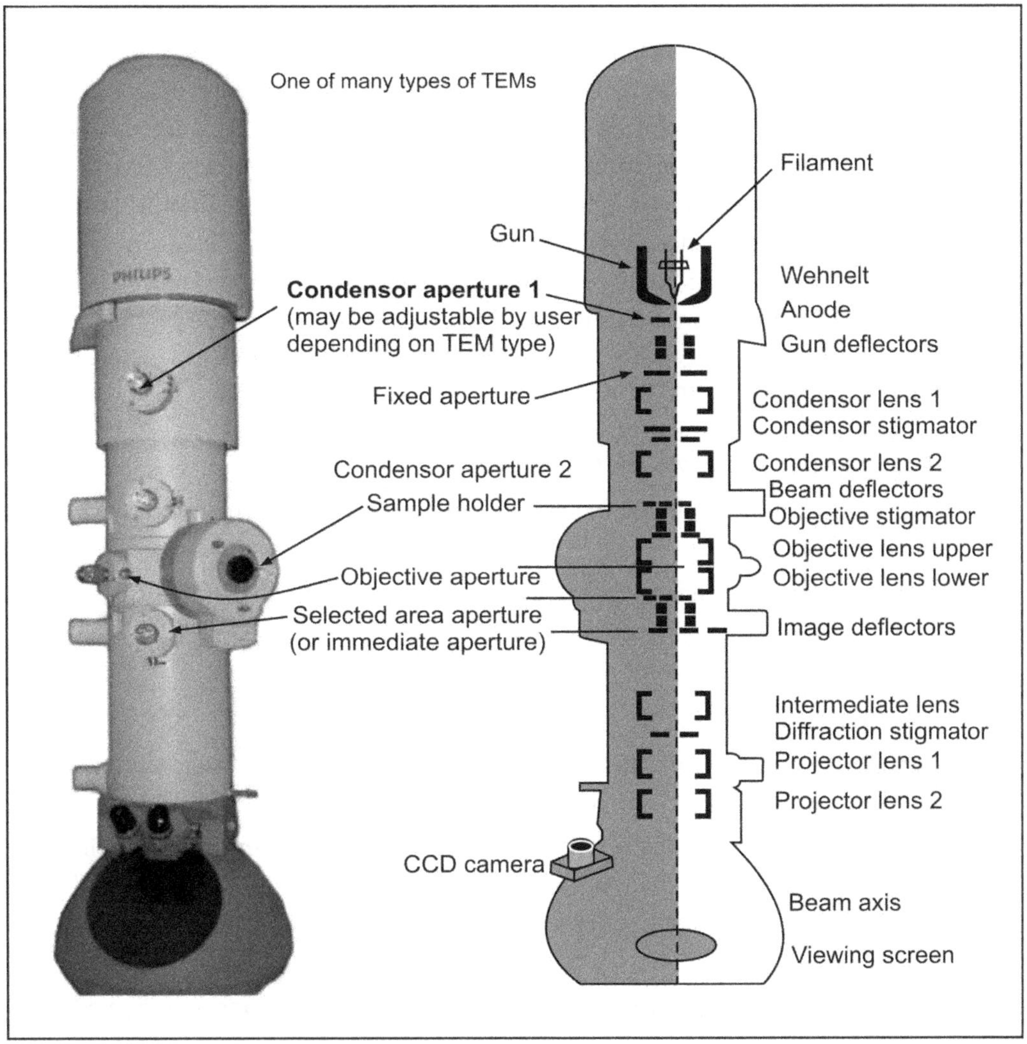

Fig. 1.9 Transmission electron microscopy (TEM)

Working: A modern transmission electron microscope (TEM) shown in Fig 1.9 is complex and sophisticated, but the basic principles behind its operation can be readily understood. A heated tungsten filament in the electron gun generates a beam of electrons that is then focused on the specimen by the condenser. Since electrons cannot pass through a glass lens, doughnut shaped electromagnets called magnetic lenses and specimen must be under high vacuum to obtain a clear image because electrons are deflected by collisions with air molecules. For this microscope, the specimen to be examined is prepared as an extremely thin dry film on small screens and is introduced into the instrument at a point between the magnetic condenser and the magnetic objective. The specimen scatters some electrons, but those that pass through are used to form an enlarged image of the specimen on a fluorescent screen. A denser region in the specimen scatters more electrons and therefore appears darker in the image since fewer electrons strike that area of the screen; these regions are said to be "electron dense". In contrast, electron-transparent regions are brighter. The image can also be captured on photographic film as a permanent record. Extremely thin slices (20 to 100 nm) of a microbial specimen can be viewed in the average TEM.

Steps in Transmission Electron Microscopy:

1. Fixing the specimen with chemicals like glutaraldehyde or Orosmium tetra oxide to stabilize cell structure.
2. The specimen is dehydrated with organic solvents (acetone or ethanol).
3. The specimen is soaked in unpolymerized, liquid epoxy plastic until it is completely permeated,
4. The plastic is hardened to form a solid block.
5. Thin sections are cut from this block with a glass or diamond knife using a special instrument called an ultra microtone.
6. Specimens are prepared for observation by soaking thin sections with solutions of heavy metal salts like lead citrate and uranyl acetate these ions bind to cell structures and make them more electron opaque, thus increases contrast in the material).
7. The stained thin sections are then mounted on tiny copper grids and viewed.

Negative staining technique: Specimen is spread out in a thin film with either phosphor tungstic acid or uranyl acetate, (these do not penetrate the specimen but render the background, whereas the specimen appears bright in photographs).

Uses: To study the structure of viruses, bacterial gas vacuoles and other similar objects.

Shadowing: A specimen is coated with a thin film of platinum or other heavy metal by evaporation at an angle of about 45 degrees from horizontal so that the metal strikes the micro-organism on only one side.

The area coated with metal appears dark in photographs, whereas the uncoated side and the shadow region created by the object is light.

***Uses*:** Useful in studying virus morphology, prokaryotic flagella and DNA.

Freeze–Etching Electron Microscopy Method

The introduction of the Balzers freeze-fracture machine by Hans Moor in 1961 had a much greater impact on the advancement of electron microscopy. Freeze-fracturing proved to be crucial for developing modern concepts of how biological membranes are organized, with this method within millisecond time-scale membrane cynamics can be captured. When freeze-fracturing was combined with methods for freezing cells that allowed microscopists to avoid even the aldehyde-prefixation and cryoprotection steps.

It is devised originally to find the solution

For the dangers of dehydration

For plastic embedding required for classical thin-section techniques

To provide unique en face views of cell membranes that could not be obtained by classical thin section techniques,

1. Cells are rapidly frozen in liquid nitrogen
2. Warmed to -100 °C in a vacuum chamber.
3. A knife that has been pre cooled with liquid nitrogen fractures the frozen cells
4. Specimen is left in the high vacuum for a minute or more
5. The exposed surfaces shadowed and coated with layers of platinum and carbon to form a replica of the surface.
6. After the specimen has been removed chemically, this replica is studied in the TEM.

***Uses*:** This provides three -dimensional view of intracellular structures. It minimizes the danger of artifacts.

Scanning Electron Microscope (SEM)

In 1942, the first scanning electron microscope with a sub-micron probe was developed by Von Ardenne, a private consultant who had his own laboratory in Berlin, over the very short period of about 2 years. It gives 3-D image having up to 2 million magnification levels and 0.4 nanometers resolution.

In this microscopy, the specimen is subjected to a narrow electron beam which rapidly moves over the surface of the specimen, as a result causes the release of shower of secondary electrons and other types of radiation from the specimen surface. The SEM has been used to examine the surfaces of micro-organisms in great detail, many SEMs will have a resolution of 7 nm or less.

The secondary electrons are trapped by a special detector shown in Fig. 1.10 and 1.11. Secondary electrons entering the detector strike a scintillator causing it to emit light flashes that a photomultiplier converts to an electrical current and amplifies. These signals are scanned in a manner of a television system to produce an image on a cathode ray tube. It has the advantage of revealing a striking 3-dimentional picture. The surface topography of a specimen can be revealed with a clarity and depth of field not possible by any method. The disadvantage is that it lacks the resolving power.

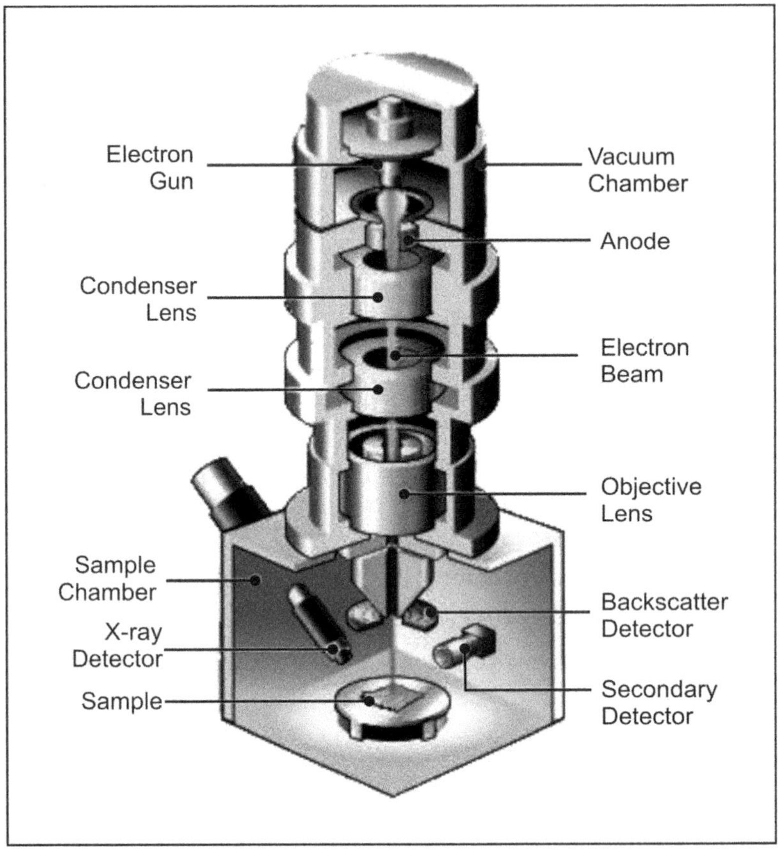

Fig. 1.10 How scanning electron microscopes work

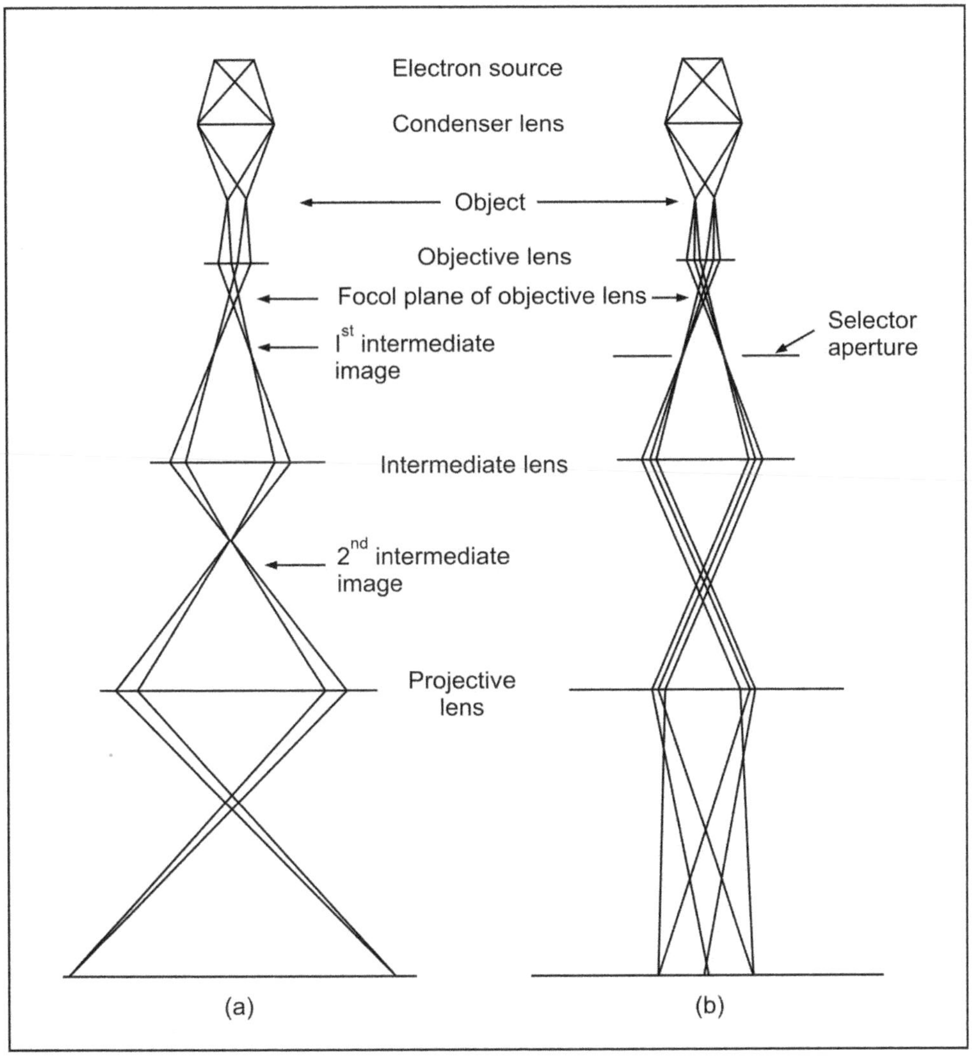

Fig. 1.11 The Electron Microscope **(a)** Cometrical optics representation of the TEM in imaging mode and **(b)** diffraction mode

Very simple Block Diagram of Electron vs Light Micrscope

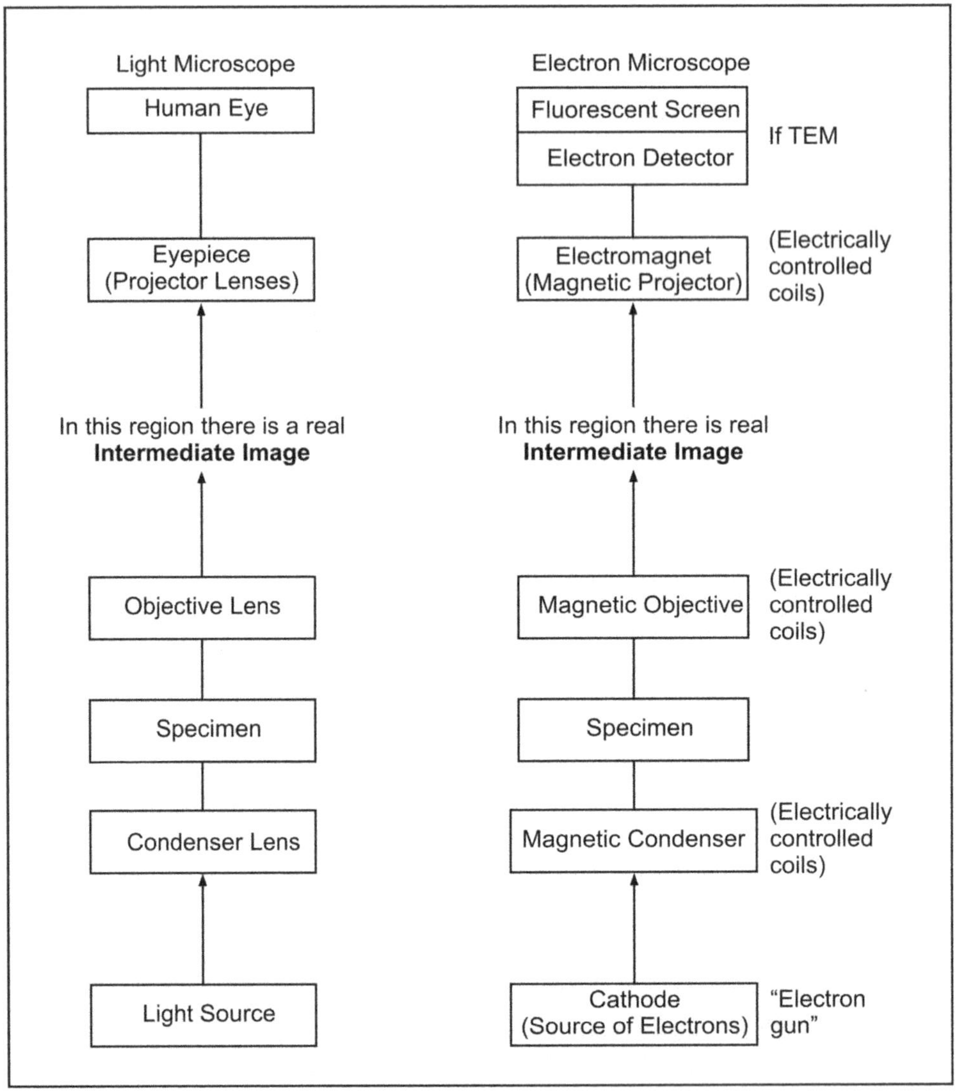

1.5 Contribution of Scientists

1.5.1 Antony Van Leeuwenhoek (October 24-26 August 1632-1723)

Leeuwenhoek succeeded in making some of the most important discoveries in the history of biology. He set himself up in business as a draper (a fabric merchant), a wine assayer.

At sometime before 1668, Leeuwenhoek learned to grind lenses, made simple microscopes and began observing with them. He seems to have been inspired to take up microscopy by having seen a copy of Robert Hooke's illustrated book *Micrographia*, which depicted Hooke's own observations with the microscope and was a very popular.

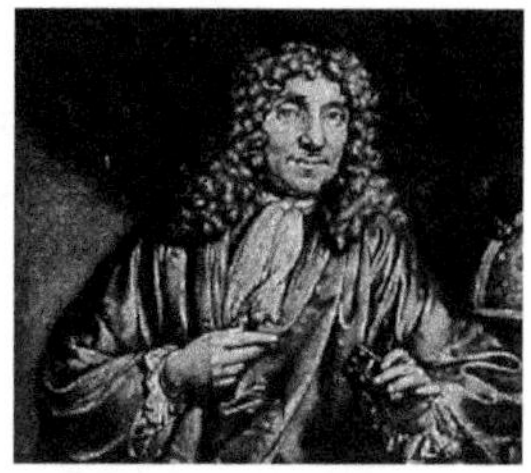

Antony Van Leeuwenhoek

Leeuwenhoek is known to have made over 500 "microscopes" of which fewer than ten have survived to the present day. In basic design,– were simply powerful magnifying glasses, not compound microscopes of the type used today.

Construction of Microscope (Fig. 1.12)

It is a simple device, using only one lens, mounted in a tiny hole in the brass plate that makes up the body of the instrument. The specimen was mounted on the sharp point that sticks up in front of the lens and its position and focus could be adjusted by turning the two screws. The entire instrument was only 3-4 inches long and had to be held up close to the eye; it required good lighting and great patience to use.

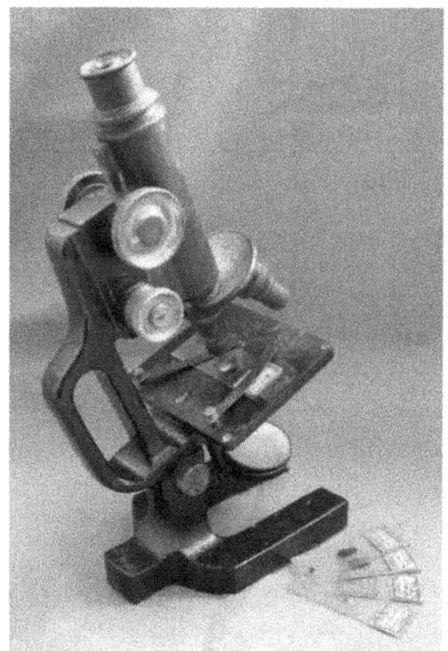

Fig. 1.12 Microscope

Compound microscopes (i.e., microscopes using more than one lens) had been invented by Robert Hooke (England) and Jan Swammerdam (Netherland) around 1595, nearly forty years before Leeuwenhoek was born. These were much more similar to the microscopes in use today. However, because of various technical difficulties in building them, early compound microscopes were not practical for magnifying objects more than about 20 or 30 times natural size.

Leeuwenhoek's skill at grinding lenses, together with his naturally acute eyesight and great care in adjusting the lighting where he worked, enabled him to build microscopes that magnified over 200 times, with clearer and brighter images than any of his colleagues could achieve. He was curious to observe almost anything that could be placed under his lenses and his care in describing what he saw which were instantly recognizable.

In 1673, Leeuwenhoek began writing letters to the newly – formed Royal Society of London, describing what he had seen with his microscopes –

His first letter contained some observations on the stings of bees.

For the next fifty years he corresponded with the Royal Society; his letters, written in Dutch, were translated into English or Latin and printed in the Philosophical Transactions of the Royal Society and often reprinted separately.

He described observations on lake water, including green chlorophyte algae *Spirogyra*. He gave descriptions of many protists, including this ciliate, *Vorticella*.

He wrote about his observations on the plaque between his own teeth. Leeuwenhoek found an unbelievably great company of living animalcules.

He looked at animal and plant tissues, at mineral crystals and at fossils. He was the first to see microscopic foraminifera, which described as "little cockles – no bigger than coarse sand–grain."

He discovered blood cells and was the first to see living sperm cells of animals.

He discovered microscopic animals such as nematodes and rotifers.

In 1680 he was elected a full member of the Royal Society, joining other luminaries of his day – although he never attended a meeting.

In 1698 he demonstrated circulation in the capillaries of an eel; He continued his observations until the last days of his life finally he breathed his last on August 30th 1723.

Leeuwenhoek who was famous throughout the whole philosophical world was praised as remarkably good scientist and craftsman who worked with diligence and tireless to discover many secrets of Nature.

1.5.2 Alexander Fleming (6 August 1881-11 March 1955)

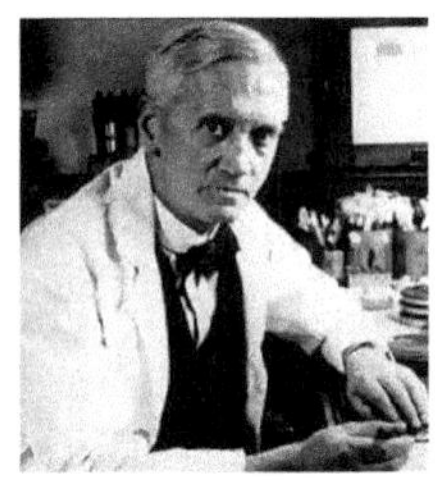

He was a Scottish biologist and pharmacologist. Fleming published many articles on bacteriology, immunology and chemotherapy. His best known achievements are the discovery of the enzyme lysozyme in 1923 and the antibiotic substance penicillin from the fungus *Penicillium notatum* in 1928, for which he shared Noble prize in physiology or Medicine in 1945 with H.W. Florey and E.B. Chain.

Fleming was born on 6 August 1881 Scotland. After his schooling, Fleming enrolled at St Mary's Hospital, Paddington, London. He qualified for the school with distinction in 1906 and had the option of becoming surgeon. Fleming joined research department at St. Mary's where he became assistant bacteriologist to Sir Almroth Wright, a pioneer in vaccine therapy and immunology. He gained M.B. and then B.Sc. with Gold Medal in 1908 and became a lecturer at St. Mary's teaching hospital until 1914. He worked in battle field hospitals at the Western Front in France. In 1918 he returned to St. Mary's Hospital, and was elected a Professor of Bacteriology in 1928.

After the war, Fleming actively searched for anti-bacterial agents, having witnessed the death of many soldiers from septicemia resulting from infected wounds. Unfortunately antiseptics killed the patients' immunological defenses more effectively than they killed the invading bacteria because they were effective on the surface only.

By 1928, Fleming was investigating the properties of *staphylococci.* He was already well-known from his earlier work and had developed a reputation as a brilliant researcher. After returning from a long holiday, Fleming noticed that many of his culture dishes were contaminated with fungus and he threw the dishes in disinfectant. But subsequently, he had to show a visitor what he had been researching and so he retrieved some of the submerged dishes that he would have otherwise discarded. He then noticed a zone around an invading fungus where the bacteria could not seem to grow. Fleming proceeded to isolate an extract from the mold, correctly identified it as being from the *Penicillium* genus, and therefore named the agent penicillin.

He investigated its positive anti-bacterial effect on many organisms and noticed that it affected bacteria such as *staphylococci* and indeed all Gram-positive pathogens (scarlet fever, pneumonia, meningitis, diphtheria causing bacteria). It also affected gonorrhea, causing microbes, although this condition is caused by Gram-negative pathogen.

Fleming found cultivating *penicillium* was quite difficult, it was even more difficult to isolate the antibiotic agent and its action appeared to be rather slow. Fleming also became convinced that penicillin would not last long enough in the human body to kill bacteria effectively.

So Fleming soon abandoned penicillin and not long after Florey and Chain took up researching and mass producing it with funds from the U.S. and British governments. The mass production and mass distribution was done in 1945 after several clinical trials. Fleming was the first to discover the properties of the active substance. He also kept, grew and distributed the original mold for twelve years, and continued until 1940 to try to get help from any chemist that had enough skill to make penicillin.

Fleming's accidental discovery and isolation of penicillin in September 1928 marks the start of modern antibiotics. Fleming also discovered very early that bacteria develop antibiotic resistance whenever too little penicillin was used or when it was used for too short a period.

1.5.3 Louis Pasteur (December 27, 1822 – September 28, 1895)

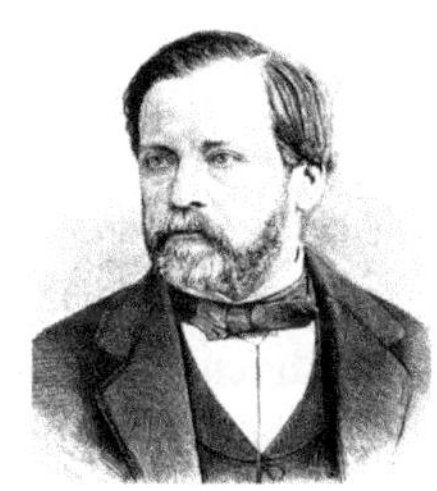

He was a French chemist and microbiologist best known for his remarkable breakthroughs in the causes and prevention of disease. His experiments supported the germ theory of disease, also reducing mortality from puerperal fever (childbed) and he created the first vaccine for rabies. He was best known to general public for inventing a method to stop milk and wine from causing sickness – this process came to be *Pasteurization.* He is regarded as one of the three main founders of microbiology, together Ferdinand Cohn and Robert Koch. He also made many discoveries in the field of chemistry, most notably the asymmetry of crystals.

Louis Pasteur was born on December 27, 1822 in Dole in France and grew up in the town of Arbios. There he later has his house and laboratory, which is a Pasteur museum today. After serving briefly as professor of physics at Dijon Lycee in 1848, he became professor of chemistry at University of Strasbourg.

Pasteur found the concept of light rotation in crystals: in solution one form rotated light to the left, the other to the right, while an equal mixture of the two forms cancelled each other's rotation. Hence the mixture does not rotate polarized light.

He resolved a problem concerning the nature of tartaric acid. For the first time he demonstrated chiral molecule.

Spontaneous Generation (Abiogenesis) versus Biogenesis

Pasteur performed experiments to demonstrate that the growth of micro-organisms in nutrient broths is not due to spontaneous generation but rather to biogenesis. Pasteur showed that growth did not occur in infusions which had been heated but exposed to air provided the incoming air was treated to remove the micro-organisms.

Fermentation

Pasteur demonstrated that the fermentation process is caused by the growth of micro-organisms. He found that fermentation of fruits and grains', resulting in alcohol, was brought by microbes. By proper selection of the microbe, the manufacturer might be assured of a consistently good and uniform product. Pasteur suggested that the undesirable types of microbes might be removed by heating - not enough to hurt the flavor of the fruit juice, but enough to destroy very high percentage of the microbial population. He found that holding the juices at a temperature of 62.8 °C (145 °F) for 30 minutes did the job pasteurization. Today Pasteurization is widely used in fermentation industries, but we are most familiar with it in the dairy industry.

Germ Theory of Disease

Micro-organisms are the causative agents of some diseases; many observant students had expressed strong arguments for the germ theory of disease. Fracastro, Von Plenciz, Jonathan Swift and Oliver Wendell Holmes are some of them. Pasteur's success in solving the problem of fermentation led the French government to request that he investigate perbine, a silkworm disease that was ruining an important French industry. For several years Pasteur struggled with this problem. Eventually he isolated the parasite (protozoan) causing the disease. He also showed that silkworm farmers could eliminate the disease by using only healthy, disease-free caterpillars for breeding stock. Pasteur next tackled the problem of anthrax, a disease of cattle, sheep, and sometimes human beings. He grew the microbes in laboratory flasks after isolating them from the blood of animals that had died of the disease. Robert Koch, German physician also identified *Anthrax bacilli* in the blood of cattle that had died of anthrax.Koch's series of observations led to the establishment of Koch's postulates.

Immunology and Vaccination

Pasteur continued to make discoveries concerning the cause and prevention of infectious diseases. About 1880 he isolated the bacterium responsible for chicken cholera and grew it in pure culture. Pasteur made use of the Robert Koch's postulates in this work.

Experiment: To prove that he really had isolated the organisms responsible for chicken cholera; he inoculated healthy chickens with his pure culture. But to his dismay, the chickens failed to get sick and die! Reviewing each step of the experiment, Pasteur found that he had accidentally used cultures several weeks old instead of the fresh ones grown especially for the demonstration. Some weeks later he repeated the experiment, using two groups of chickens. One of these groups had been inoculated at the first demonstration with the old cultures that had proved ineffective, and the second had not been previously, exposed. Both groups received bacteria from fresh young cultures.

Result

Chickens in the second group (which were not previously exposed to old culture) got sick and died.

Chickens in the first group (which were previously exposed to old culture) remained hale and healthy

Explanation

In some way bacteria could lose their ability to produce disease, i.e., their virulence, after standing and growing old.

But these attenuated (having decreased virulence) bacteria still retained their capacity for stimulating the host to produce substances, i.e., antibodies, that protect against subsequent exposure to virulent organisms.

This experiment of Pasteur explained the principle involved in Edward Jenner's successful use of cowpox virus, in 1798, to immunize people against smallpox.

Pasteur next applied this principle to the prevention of anthrax and again it worked.

He called the attenuated cultures vaccines, a term derived from the Latin ***vacca***, meaning **"cow"** to honor Jenner who for the first time used cowpox material to immunize against smallpox

Pasteur produced the first vaccine for rabies by inoculating rabbits with saliva from mad dogs. Then the brain and spinal cord could be removed from the infected rabbits, dried for several days, pulverized and mixed with glycerin. Injecting this mixture into dogs protected them against rabies. Emile Roux, a French doctor and a colleague of Pasteur helped Pasteur to prepare rabies vaccine. This vaccine was first used on 9 year old boy Joseph Meister on July 6, 1885, after the boy was badly mauled by a rabid dog. After consulting with colleagues, Pasteur decided to go ahead with the treatment. Pasteur was as surprised as anyone else when after the crucial trial, which took several weeks, Joseph Meister did not die.

1.5.4 Robert Koch (11 December 1843 – 27 May 1910)

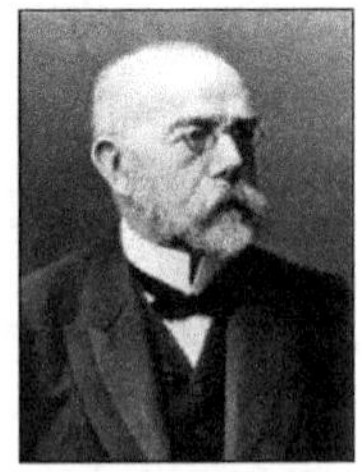

He was a German physician. He became famous for isolating anthrax causing *Bacillus anthracis*, the tuberculosis causing *Mycobacterium tuberculosis* and Cholera causing *Vibrio cholera* and for his series of observations led to the establishment of Koch's Postulates. He was awarded the Noble Prize in physiology or Medicine for his tuberculosis findings in 1905. He is considered one of the founders of microbiology.

Heinrich Hermann Robert Koch was born in Clusthal, Germany as the son of a mining official. He studied medicine at the University of Gottingen and graduated in 1866. He then served in the Franco-Prussian War and later became district medical officer in Wollstein, working with very limited resources.

After Casimir Davaine showed the direct transmission of the *Anthrax bacilli* between cows, Koch studied anthrax more closely; He invented methods to purify the bacillus from blood samples and grew pure cultures. He found that, while it could not survive outside a host for long, anthrax built persisting endospores that could last a long time.

These endospores, embedded in soil, were the cause of unexplained "spontaneous" outbreaks of anthrax. In 1881, he urged the sterilization of surgical instruments using heat.

In Berlin, he improved the methods he used in Wollstein, including staining and purification techniques and bacterial growth media, including agar plates i.e. Petri dishes (invented by Julius Richard Petri an assistant of Koch). Angelina wife of Walther Hesse student of Koch, suggested using agar as solidifying agent. These devices are still used today. With these techniques he was able to discover the bacterium causing tuberculosis in 1882.

In 1883, Koch worked with a French research team in Alexandria, Egypt, studying cholera. Koch identified the vibrio bacterium that caused cholera, though he never managed to prove it in experiments. The bacterium had been previously isolated by Italian anatomist Filippo Pacini in 1854, but his work had been ignored due to the predominance of the miasma (stinking miasma in the air) theory of disease. Koch was unaware of Pacini's work and made an independent discovery and his greater preeminence allowed the discovery to be widely spread for the benefit of others. In 1965, however, the bacterium was formerly renamed *Vibrio cholera Pacini* 1854. The series of observations led to the establishment of Koch's postulates, which provided guidelines to identify the causative agent of an infectious disease.

Koch's postulates are

1. A specific organism can always be found in association with a given disease.
2. The organism can be isolated and grown in pure culture in the laboratory.
3. The pure culture will produce the disease when inoculated into a susceptible animal.
4. It is possible to recover the organism in pure culture form the experimentally infected animal.

1.5.5 Joseph Lister (5 April 1827 – 10 February 1912)

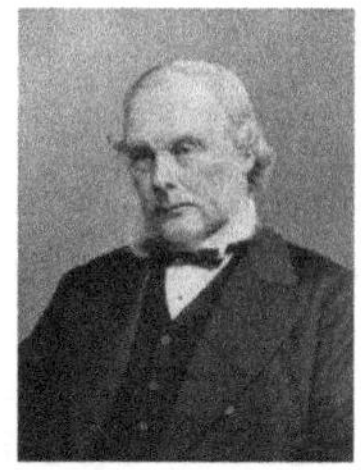

He was an English surgeon who promoted the idea of sterile surgery while working at the Glasgow Royal Infirmary. He successfully introduced carbolic acid (phenol) to sterilize surgical instruments and to clean wounds.

Joseph Lister came from a prosperous family, son of Joseph Jackson Lister, the pioneer of the compound microscope. He graduated with honours as Bachelor of Medicine and entered the Royal College of Surgeons. In 1867 Joseph discovered the use of carbolic acid as an antiseptic, such that it became the first widely used antiseptic in surgery. At University of Glasgow he was studying wound infection, at the time the usual explanation for wound infection was that the exposed tissues were damaged by chemicals in the air or via a stinking "miasma" in the air. The sick wards actually smelled bad, not due to a "miasma' but due to the rotting of wounds. Hospital wards were occasionally aired out at midday, but Florence Nightingale's doctrine of fresh air was still seen as science fiction. Facilities for washing hands or the patient's wounds did not exist and it was even considered unnecessary for the surgeon to wash his hands before he saw a patient.

Lister became aware of a paper published (in French) by Louis Pasteur that rotting and fermentation could occur without any oxygen if micro-organisms were present. Lister confirmed this with his own experiments. If micro-organisms were causing gangrene, the problem was how to get rid of them. Pasteur suggested three methods: filter, heat, or expose them to chemical solutions. The first two were inappropriate in a human wound, so Lister experimented with the third.

Carbolic acid (phenol) had been in use as a means of deodorizing sewage, so Lister tested the results of spraying instruments, the surgical incisions and dressings with a solution of it. Lister found that carbolic acid solution swabbed on wounds markedly reduced the incidence of gangrene and subsequently published a series of articles in 1867.

He also made surgeons wear clean gloves and wash their hand before and after operations with 5% carbolic acid solutions. Instruments were also washed in the same solution and assistants sprayed the solution in the operating theatre. One of his conclusions was to stop using porous natural material in manufacturing the handles of medical instruments.

Lister in 1869, returning to Edinburgh continued to develop improved methods of antisepsis and asepsis.

As germ theory of disease became more widely accepted, it was realized that infection could be better avoided by preventing bacteria from getting into wounds in the first place. This led to the rise of sterile surgery. Some consider Lister "the father of modern antisepsis."

In 1879 Listerine mouthwash was named after him for his work in antisepsis. Also named in his honour is the bacterial genus *Listeria*, typified by the food-borne pathogen *Listeria monocytogenes*.

Lister in King's College Hospital in London, became the second man in England to operate on a brain tumor. He also developed a method of repairing kneecaps with metal wire and improved the technique of mastectomy. His discoveries were greatly praised.

1.5.6 Spontaneous Generation Theory

This theory has been referred as doctrine of spontaneous generation theory /Abiogenesis (Gr. ***a*** = not; ***bios*** = life; ***genesis*** = origin). According to this theory all living organisms could spring forth spontaneously from nonliving matter. As far as human beings were concerned, the Greek explanation that Goddess Gaea was able to create people from stones. Men of ancient times do not know about micro-organisms and evolution theory. Even astute Aristotle (384-322 BC) taught that animals might originate spontaneously from the soil, plants or other unlike animals. They believed that frogs, snakes and mice could be born of moist soil, that flies could emerge from manure and that maggots could arise from decaying corpses.

Virgil (70-19 BC) gave directions for the artificial propagation of bees.

Van Helmont (1577-1644) devised a method for manufacturing mice from a mixture of wheat grains with soiled linen and cheese.

Felix Archimede Pouchet (1800-1872) revived for the last time and published an extensive report proving the occurrence of spontaneous generation Fig. 1.13.

There was a great opposition against spontaneous generation theory.

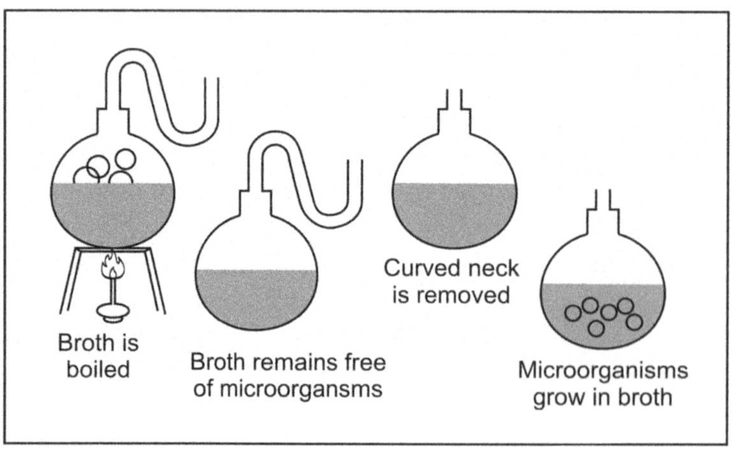

Fig. 1.13 Pasteur's test of spontaneous generation

Biogenesis

This fact was lately realized that **"Only living things could beget living things."** After the discovery of micro-organisms and improvements in microscopy that enabled scientists to think seriously about original life. Francesco Redi (1626-1679) an Italian physician demonstrated by simple experiments that spontaneous generation does not exist. The following series of experiments were conducted by the scientists who supported and opposed spontaneous generation theory. Finally spontaneous generation or abiogenesis theory was proved wrong.

First Experiment by Redi*:* Rotting meat pieces were placed in jars.

Some of the jars were sealed tightly and other jars were left open

After few days both sealed and open jars were observed.

Observation 1: Maggots appeared in open jars

***Reason* 1:** Flies were freely in and out and laid eggs on meat present in the open jars that resulted development of maggots.

Observation 2: Maggots did not appear in sealed jars.

***Reason* 2:** Flies could not enter into sealed jars.

Conclusion

Maggots arise from the eggs laid down by the parent flies but not appear spontaneously.

Criticism by the Supporters of Abiogenesis

Free air is the vital force necessary for spontaneous origin of life. That free air was not allowed to reach the meat placed in sealed jars by Redi.

Second Experiment by Redi**:** Rotting meat pieces were placed in jars.

Jars were covered with fine muslin cloth or gauge instead of sealing them tightly. This provision allowed free air to go in and out of the jars, few jars were left open.

Result

Maggots appeared only in those jars in which flies were allowed free to go in and lay their eggs on the meat.

Maggots did not appear in jars covered with fine muslin cloth.

Third Experiment by Lazaro Spallanzani (1729-1799). He Boiled beef broth for an hour and then sealed flasks. No micro-organisms appeared following incubation.

Contd...

Criticism by the Supporters of Abiogenesis

John Needham insisted that air was essential to the spontaneous production of microscopic beings and it had been excluded from the flasks by sealing them in Lazzaro Splallanjani experiments.

Fourth Experiment by Franz Schulz (1815–1873) and The Odor Schwan (1810-1882) conducted the following experiments to give answer to John Needham's criticism

Schulz passed air through strong acid solutions and boiled infusions, whereas Schwann passed air into his flasks through red hot tubes.

Result

In neither case did microbes appear.

Criticism by the Supporters of Abiogenesis

Acid and heat altered the air so that it would not support growth.

Fifth Experiment by H. Schroder and T. Von Dusch (1850) performed a more convincing experiment by passing air through cotton into flasks containing heated broth.

Result

The microbes were filtered out of the air by the cotton fibers so that growth did not occur.

Opposition by the Supporters of Abiogenesis

Again Archimede Pouchet (1859) published an extensive report proving occurrence of spontaneous growth.

Sixth Experiment by Louis Pasteur prepared flasks with a long, narrow gooseneck opening. The nutrient solutions were heated in the flask and air, untreated and unfiltered could pass in or out. In his swan-necked flask experiments, he took various types of broths (Yeast water, Sugared yeast water, Urine sugar beet juice etc.).

Result: The germs settled in the gooseneck and no microbes appeared in the solution.

Setbacks

Despite Pasteur's successful demonstrations against spontaneous generation, attempts to repeat his experiments occasionally failed because, after some time, existence of microbes was evident in some broths of Swan-necked flasks. This created doubt in the minds of many.

Seventh Experiment by John Tyndall an English physicist, in the year 1877 explained that bacteria exist in two forms. Heat labile forms (Thermo-labile) which could be killed by exposure to high temperatures and heat-resistant (Thermo-

Contd...

stable) forms which could not be killed by continuous boiling of the broth and after the broth has cooled, they resulted in microbial growth in such broths. If such broths are subjected to intermittent boiling (discontinuous boiling) on successive occasions the heat-resistant forms of bacteria will be killed and the broths became completely free of them and do not show any microbial growth. This process is called as Tyndallization.

- The first boiling kills vegetative cells of bacteria but endospores remain as such.
- In cooled broth the endospores germinate into new bacteria cells which are killed during further boiling and so on.

Eighth (Final) Experiment: Tyndall conducted experiments in a specially developed box to prove that dust carried the germs. He demonstrated that if no dust was present sterile broth remained free of microbial growth for indefinite periods.

In this manner Tyndall validated Pasteur's results and helped ending the debate of spontaneous generation or Abiogenesis verses Biogenesis.

Chronology of Scientists and their Contributions

Name of Scientist	Area of Research	Year
Zacharias Janssen	Invention of microscope	1590
Robert Hooke	Discovered plant cells while observing thin slices of ark in a microscope	1665
Antony Van Leeuwenhoek	Described the structure of red blood cells, protozoa and bacteria using his homemade microscope	1676
Spallanzani	Disputed the theory of spontaneous generation	1767
Edward Jenner	Introduced vaccination against smallpox	1796
M.J. Schleiden and T. Schwan	Proposed cell theory, an important landmark in biological research	1838 & 1839
Joseph Lister	Father of antiseptic surgery	1867
Louis Pasteur	Demonstrated that yeast can degrade sugar to ethanol and carbondioxide and multiply in the process	1857
Louis Pasteur	Published experiments that refuse the theory of spontaneous generation	1861
Louis Pasteur	Developed Pasteurization technique	1864
Gregor Mendel	Considered as father of genetics and published results of experiments on the laws of inheritance	1866
Koch	Demonstrated that anthrax is caused by *Bacillus anthracis*	1876 & 1877
Laveran	Discovered *Plasmodium*, that causes malaria	1880

Contd...

Name of Scientist	Area of Research	Year
Koch	Discovered Cultures bacteria on gelatins, Pasteur develops anthrax vaccine	1881
Elie Metchnikoff	Discoverd phagocytic cells and thus begins the study of immunology	1884
Koch	Proposed Postulates for determining the cause of a disease	1884
Christian Gram	Developed the staining techniques for identification	1884
Chamberland	Developed autoclave	1884
Louis Pasteur	Developed rabies vaccine	1885
Theodor Excherich	Identified *Escherichia* Coli as a natural inhabitant of the human gut	1885
Richard Julius Petri	Developed Petri dish	1887
Winogradsky	Studied sulphur and nitrifying bacteria	1887 – 1890
Beijerinck	Isolatedc root nodule bacteria	1889.
Weisman	Demonstrated the role of nucleus in heredity	1892
Paul Ehrlich	Formulated sidechain theory of antibody formation	1897
Sir Ronald Ross	Received the Nobel prize for the discovery of the lifecycle of malarial parasite in humans and mosquitoes	1902
Karl Landsteiner	Discoverd blood groups	1902
Robert Koch	Received Nobel prize for founding scientific bacteriology and proving the cause of tuberculosis	1905
Wasserman	Developed complement fixation test for syphilis	1906
Paul Ehrlich	Started the use of chemotherapy to treat diseases. Receives Nobel Prize	1908
Paul Ehrich	Synthesized a “magic bullet” for syphilis	1912
Frederick Griffith	Discoverd genetic transformation in bacteria	1928
Alexander Flemming	Discoverd Penicillin, the first antibiotic	1929
Karl Landsteiner	Received the Nobel prize for the discovery of the ABO human blood groups	1930
Gerhardt Komagk	Discovered sulfur drug for chemotherapy	1935
Waksman	Received Nobel prize for the discovery of streptomycin	1952
George Beadle and Edward Tatum	Produced evidence of genetic mutants	1941
Oswald Avery, Colin Mac Leod and Maclyn Mc carty	Demonstrated that Griffith’s transforming principle in DNA	1944

Contd...

Name of Scientist	Area of Research	Year
Alexander Felming	Received the Nobel prize for discovering Penicillin, the first antibiotic	1945
Max Theiler	Received the Nobel prize for development of vaccine against yellow fever	1951
F.H.C Crick, J.D. Watson, M. Wilkins	Determined the structure of DNA	1953
Jonas Salk	Developed the first polio vaccine	1954
D. Bovet	Received the Nobel prize for the discovery of the first antihistamine	1957
S.Ochoa, A.Kornberg	Received Nobel Prize for the discovery of enzyme catalyzing Nucleic acid synthesis	1959
F. Jacob, J. Monod	Made discoveries about the regulation of genes	1965
Max Delbruck, Alfred Hershey and salvadore E.Luria	Received Nobel prize for describing the mechanism of viral infection of bacterial cell	1969
Hamilton Smith	Reported the discovery of the first restriction enzyme	1970
Herbert Boyer and Stanley cohen	The first Biotechnologists to clone DNA using plasmids	1973
Cesar Milsein, Georges Kohler, Niels Kai Jerne	Developed the technique for making monoclonal antibodies	1975
J.M. Bishop and H.E. Varmus	Discovered the cancer causing genes called Oncogenes	1989
R. Yalow	Received the Nobel prize for the development of the radio immuno assay technique	1977
H.D. Smith, D. Nathans, W. Arber	Received the Nobel prize for the discovery of restriction enzymes and their applications to solve the problem in molecular genetics	1978
E. Ruska	Developed the Electron Microscope	1986

1.6 Branches in Microbiology

Since the field of microbiology is a vast area, classification of this subject will help us to thoroughly understand this subject. The branches of microbiology can be classified into pure microbiology and applied microbiology. Microbiology can be also classified based on taxonomy, which are Bacteriology, Mycology, Protozoology and Phycology etc. But there is considerable overlap between the specific branches of microbiology with each other and with other disciplines.

1.6.1 Branches of Pure Microbiology

Taxonomic Arrangement of Micro-organisms

- ***Bacteriology***: The study of bacteria
- ***Mycology***: The study of fungi
- ***Protozoology***: The study of protozoa
- ***Phycology (or algology)***: The study of algae
- ***Parasitology***: The study of parasites
- ***Immunology***: The study of the immune system

Integrative Arrangement of Micro-organisms

Microbial cytology: The study of microscopic and submicroscopic details of micro-organisms.

Microbial physiology: The study of how the microbial cell functions biochemically. It includes the study of microbial growth, microbial metabolism and microbial cell structure.

Microbial ecology: The relationship between micro-organisms and their environment.

Microbial genetics: The study of how genes are organized and regulated in microbes in relation to their cellular functions. It is closely related to the field of molecular biology.

Cellular microbiology: A discipline bridging microbiology and cell biology.

Evolutionary microbiology: The study of the evolution of microbes. This field can be subdivided into:

Microbial taxonomy: The naming and classification of micro-organisms.

Microbial systematic: The study of the diversity and genetic relationship of micro-organisms.

Generation microbiology: The study of those micro-organisms that have the same characters as their parents.

Other Arrangement of Micro-organisms

Nano microbiology: The study of those micro-organisms at nano level.

Exo microbiology (or Astro microbiology): The study of micro-organisms in outer space.

1.6.2 Branches of Applied Microbiology

Medical Microbiology: The study of the pathogenic microbes and the role of microbes in human illness include the study of microbial pathogenesis and epidemiology and is related to the study of disease pathology and immunology.

***Pharmaceutical Microbiology*:** The study of micro-organisms that are related to the production of antibiotics, enzymes, vitamins, vaccines, and other pharmaceutical products and that cause pharmaceutical contamination and spoil.

***Industrial Microbiology*:** The exploitation of microbes for use in industrial processes. Examples include industrial fermentation and wastewater treatment. This branch is closely linked to the biotechnology industry. This field also includes brewing, an important application of microbiology.

***Microbial Biotechnology*:** The manipulation of micro-organisms at the genetic and molecular level to generate useful products.

***Food Microbiology and Dairy Microbiology*:** The study of micro-organisms causing food spoilage and food borne illness. It also includes using micro-organisms to produce foods, for example by fermentation.

***Agricultural Microbiology*:** The study of agriculturally relevant micro-organisms. This field can be further classified into the following:

***Plant microbiology and Plant pathology*:** The study of the interactions between micro-organisms and plants and plant pathogens.

***Soil microbiology*:** The study of those micro-organisms that are found in soil.

***Veterinary microbiology*:** The study of the role in microbes in veterinary medicine or animal taxonomy.

***Environmental microbiology*:** The study of the function and diversity of microbes in their natural environments. This involves the characterization of key bacterial habitats such as the rhizosphere and phyllosphere, soil and groundwater ecosystems, open oceans or extreme environments (extremphiles). This field includes other branches of microbiology such as:

(a) Microbial Ecology
(b) Microbial-mediated Nutrient Cycling
(c) Geomicrobiology
(d) Microbial Diversity
(e) Bioremediation

***Water microbiology (or Aquatic microbiology)*:** The study of those micro-organisms that are found in water.

***Aeromicrobiology (or Air microbiology)*:** The study of airborne micro-organisms.

***Epidemiology*:** The study of the incidence spread and control of disease.

Essay Questions

1. Explain in detail the detailed structure of micro-organisms.
2. Write a note on initial microscopes and their constructions along with a simplified ray diagrams.
3. Explain the developments and discoveries of scientists in microbiology.

Multiple Choice Questions

1. Spontaneous generation theory is also known as
   (a) Biogenesis
   (b) Abiogenesis
   (c) Neobiogenesis
   (d) Microbiogenesis
2. Bright field microscope provides magnification of about
   (a) 1000x to 1200x
   (b) 500x to 1000x
   (c) 2000x to 4000x
   (d) 5000x to 10000x
3. Main disadvantage of Scanning Electron Microscope is
   (a) Lacking projection power
   (b) Lacking focal power
   (c) Lacking resolving power
   (d) Lacking diffracting power
4. Scientist who made more than 500 microscopes
   (a) Max Theiler
   (b) Frederick grifth
   (c) Leeuwenhoek
   (d) Robert Koch
5. Fleming was investigating the properties
   (a) Staphylococci
   (b) Anthrax bacilli
   (c) Listeria monocytogenes
   (d) Eschereschia coli
6. Manipulation of micro-organisms at genetic and molecular level to generate useful products is known as
   (a) Pharmaceutical Microbiology
   (b) Industrial Microbiology
   (c) Microbial biotechnology
   (d) Food microbiology & Diary microbiology
7. The study of incidence, spread and control of disease is called as
   (a) Geo microbiology
   (b) Microbial diversity
   (c) Epidemiology
   (d) Bioremediation

Answers

1. (b)	2. (a)	3. (c)
4. (c)	5. (a)	6. (c)
7. (c)		

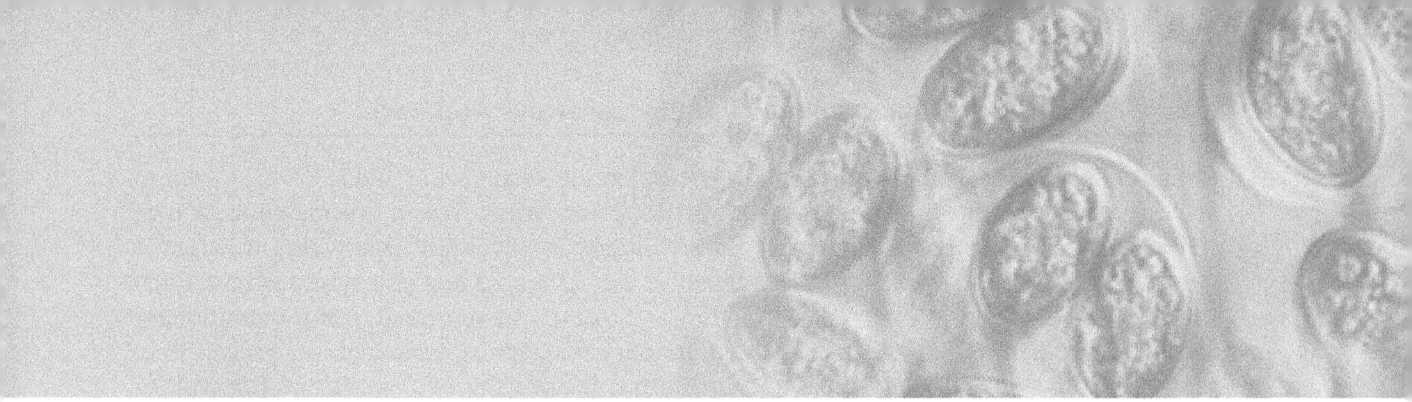

2 DIVERSITY OF MICRO-ORGANISMS

LEARNING OBJECTIVES

After studying the chapter the students familiarize themselves with concepts in:

- *Understanding Microbial Taxonomy*
- *Understanding types of Micro-organisms*
- *Reproduction in bacteria*
- *Insight into Replication of virus*
- *Classification of virus*
- *Identify special groups of bacteria along with distinguishing features*
- *View of Taxonomy and classification of microbes*
- *Understanding techniques of staining*
- *Performing and identifying biochemical tests for unknowns*
- *Understanding Fungal Growth and Metabolism*

2.1 Introduction to Microbial Classification and Taxonomy

About 1.4 million different species have been described as living organisms in the world today, but this is only a fraction of the actual number of species that exist. In all groups of organisms new species are described every day and in some habitats we are woefully ignorant of the true extent of the biological diversity that exists. A high estimate of the number of species that could exist on earth would be around 100 million species. A low estimate is 2 million. The best estimate might be around 10 million. Whichever estimate is favoured, all estimates are large numbers and they indicate the scale of the taxonomic and systematic problem faced by biologists because these organisms must be sorted into groups to aid our study of them. In dealing with diversity, classification is essential for efficient thought. To sort out these species into groups, several approaches were adopted and several new methods have been invented.

Among different methods, the most important sequence-based investigation was initiated was by Carl Woese. In 1977, Woese and his collaborator George Fox used the nucleotide sequence of the small sub unit ribosomal RNAs (SSU rRNAs) from a variety of organisms to determine that all living organisms belong to one of three domains. The three domains of life Bacteria, Archaea and Eukarya are represented in universal phylogenetic tree. Nucleotide sequence of SSUr RNA is used to measure the relatedness of organisms. 16S rRNA sequences from a diverse collection of prokaryotes and 18S rRNA sequences from a diverse collection of eukaryotes are aligned from the 5′ to 3′ end and homologous residues are compared in a pair-wise fashion. Each nucleotide sequence is differently counted and serves to represent some evolutionary distance between the organisms. The evolutionary distance is measured along each line: the longer the line, the more evolutionarily diverged are the two organisms (or type of organisms) at each end.

2.1.1 Features of Phylogenetic Tree

The phylogenetic tree is a tree diagram to show the evolutionary histories and relationships among taxonomic groups. It is used in phylogenetics, which is a branch of biology that is concerned mainly in the study of evolutionary relatedness among various groups of organisms through molecular sequencing data and morphological data matrices. The relatedness between taxa is usually demonstrated through molecular sequencing data and morphological data matrices. The relatedness between taxa is usually demonstrated through molecular sequencing data and morphological data matrices. The phylogenetic tree is essential in phylogenetics since it has been used to understand biodiversity, genetics, evolutions, and ecology among groups of organisms.

Close to the center is a line labeled "Root", this is where the data indicates the last common ancestor to all three domains should be placed

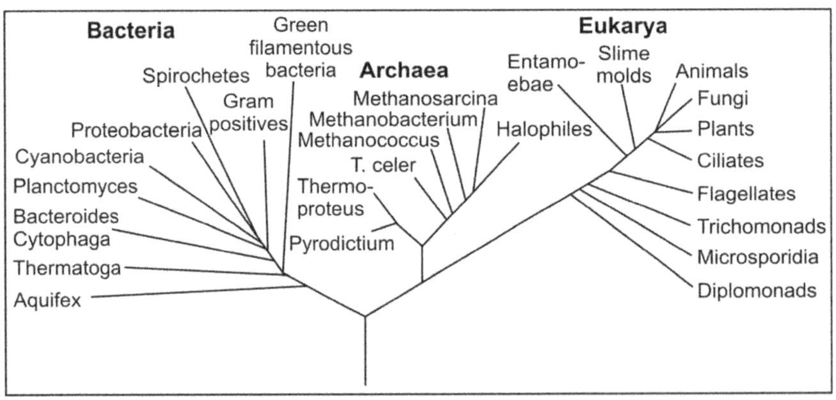

Fig. 2.1 Phylogenetic tree

1. The root, or origin of modern life, is on the bacterial branch; it appears that the Archaea and the Eukarya are evolved independently, separate from the Bacterial branch.
2. Line of descent is away from the root; toward the Archaea and the Eukarya, it is evident that they shared common evolution of these two forms of life.
3. Thus the universal phylogenetic tree presents a picture whereby all life, regardless of eventual domain, arose from a single, common ancestor shown in Fig. 2.1.

2.1.2 Assessing Microbial Phylogeny

Microbial taxonomy is changing rapidly. This is caused by ever-increasing knowledge of the biology of microorganisms, remarkable advances in computer technology and the use of molecular characteristics to determine phylogenetic relationships between micro-organisms.

Molecular chronometers: The sequence of nucleic acids and proteins change with time and are considered to be molecular chronometers. Zuckerkandi and Pauling (1965) suggested this concept (molecular chronometers) in determining phylogenetic relationships and is based on the assumption that there is an evolutionary clock. According to this idea, the sequences of many rRNAs and proteins gradually change over time without destroying or severely altering functions. Such changes are selectively neutral, occur fairly randomly, and increase linearly without time when the sequences of similar molecules are quite different in two groups of organisms, the groups diverged from one another long time ago. Phylogenetic analysis using molecular chronometers is somewhat complex and controversial because the rate of sequence change can vary.

Phylogentic trees: Phylogenetic trees are developed by comparing nucleotide or amino acid sequence. To compare two molecules, their sequences must first be aligned so that similar parts match up. The object is to align and compare homologous sequences, ones that are similar because they had a common origin in the past. This is not an easy task, and computers and fairly complex mathematics must be employed to minimize the number of gaps and mismatches in the sequences being compared. Evolutionary distance a quantitative indication of the number of positions that differ between two aligned macromolecules is used to express the difference.

Parsimony analysis is an another method used in phylogentic relations. Estimation of the minimum number of sequence changes required to give the final sequence are being compared in this method.

Phylogenetic relationships are illustrated in the form of branched diagram or trees

A phylogenetic tree is a graph made of branches that connect the nodes

The nodes represent taxonomic units such as species or genes; the external nodes at the end of the branches represent living (extant) organisms.

Living (extant) organisms are denoted by external nodes.

The numbers of molecular changes that have taken place are represented by the length of the branches between two nodes.

Phylogentic trees are of two types, one is un-rooted tree and the other is rooted tree

Un- rooted tree does not provide an evolutionary path.

The rooted tree gives a node that serve as the common ancestor and shows the development of the species from this root.

2.2 Archaea Resembles Eucarya in many Ways

1. Both Archaea and Eucarya lack muramic acid in their cell walls.
2. Both Archaea and Eucarya possess membrane lipids with ether linked branched aliphatic chains.
3. Both Archaea and Eucarya possess transfer RNAs without thymidine in the T or TC arm.
4. Both Archaea and Eucarya possess distinctive RNA polymerase enzymes.
5. Both Archaea and Eucarya possess ribosomes of different composition and shape.

2.2.1 Relation and Difference between Three Domains

1. Bacteria and the Archaea share some biochemical properties with Eukarya.
   For example Bacteria and eucaryotes have ester-linked membrane lipids.
2. Archaea and Eukaryotes are similar with respect to some components of the RNA and protein synthetic system.
3. Archaea and Bacteria have similar cell architecture, they vary considerably at the molecular level.
4. Archaea and Bacteria differ from eucaryotes in their cell ultra-structure and many other properties.

Table 2.1 Comparision of Bacteria, Archaea and Eukarya

Property	Bacteria	Archaea	Eukarya
Biochemical property	Similar to eukarya with ester linked membrane lipids	-	Similar to bacteria
RNA and protein synthetic system	-	Similar to eukarya	Similar to archaea
Cell architecture	Similar to archaea	Similar to bacteria	-
Cell ultra structure	Bacteria and archaea differ from eukarya	Bacteria and archaea differ from eukarya	-

Microbiologists are faced with the daunting task of understanding diversity of life forms that cannot be seen with the naked eye but can live seemingly anywhere on earth. One of the first tools needed to survey this level diversity is a reliable classification (shown in 2.1.3). Taxonomy (Greek *taxia*:, arrangement or order and *nomos*: law) is defined as the science of biological classification. In a boarder sense it consists of three separate but interrelated parts: classification, nomenclature and identification. Once classification scheme is selected, it is used to arrange organisms into groups called taxa based on mutual similarity. Nomenclature is the branch of taxonomy concerned with the assignment of names to taxonomic groups in agreement with the published rules. Identification is the practical side of taxonomy, the process of determining if a particular isolate belongs to a recognized taxon. The term systematic is often used for taxonomy.

Carolus Linnaeus in middle of the eighteenth century developed one of the oldest classification systems, called a natural classification, based on anatomical characteristics, i.e., arranges organisms into groups whose members share many characteristics and reflects as much as possible to the biological nature of organisms. However, the taxonomic assignment of microbes is not necessarily rooted in evolutionary relatedness. For instance bacterial pathogens and microbes of industrial importance were historically given names that described the diseases they cause or the process they perform. This will do little to guide taxonomists. Our recent understanding of the evolutionary relationships among microbes now serves as the theoretical underpinning of taxonomic classification.

Polyphasic taxonomy: This approach includes phenotypic, phylogenetic and genotypic features.

Numerical taxonomy: The grouping by numerical methods of taxonomic units into taxa on the basis of their character states.

Taxonomic ranks: Placing microbes within hierarchical taxonomic levels (ranks) is involved in this approach. Each rank shares a common set of specific features. The ranks are arranged in a non-overlapping hierarchy so that each level includes not only the traits that define the rank above it, but new set of more restrictive traits. The highest rank is the domain and all prokaryotes belong to either the *Bacteria* or the *Archaea* within each domain, each microbe is assigned (in descending order) to a phylum, class order, family, genus, and species. Some prokaryotes are also given a subspecies designation. Microbial groups at each level have a special suffix indicative of that rank or level. A prokaryotic species is a collection of strains that share many stable properties and differ significantly from other groups of strains. A strain consists of the descendents of a single, pure microbial culture. The revised definition of species is a species should be the collection of organisms that share the same sequences in their core house keeping genes (genes coding for products that are required by all cells and which are usually continually expressed). Each species is assigned to a genus, the next rank in the taxonomic hierarchy. A genus is well defined group of one or more species that is clearly separate from other genera.

Domain	Bacteria
Phylum	Proteobacteria
Class	γ - proteobacteria
Order	Enterobacteriales
Family	Enterobacteriaceae
Genus	Shigella
Species	*S.dysenteriae*

2.2.2 Techniques for Determining Microbial Taxonomy and Phylogeny

Many different approaches are used in classifying and identifying micro-organisms. Two clear approaches are classical and molecular.

2.2.3 Classical Approaches

In this approach taxonomy make use of morphological, physiological, biochemical, ecological and genetic characteristics. These techniques are old and quite useful in routine identification and may provide the phylogenetic information as well.

1. **Morphological characteristics:** Morphological features are important in microbial taxonomy for many reasons. Morphology is easy to study and analyze, particularly in eukaryotic micro-organisms and the more complex prokaryotes.

   Some morphological features used in classification and identification

   - Cell shape
   - Cell size
   - Colonial morphology
   - Ultra-structural morphology
   - Staining behavior
   - Cilia and flagella
   - Mechanism of motility
   - Endo-spore shape and location
   - Spore morphology and location
   - Cellular inclusion
   - Color

2. **Physiological and metabolic characteristics:** Physiological and metabolic characteristics are very useful because they are directly related to the nature and activity of microbial enzymes and transport proteins.

   Characteristics used in classification and identification: Carbon and nitrogen sources, Cell wall constituents, Energy sources, fermentation products, General nutritional type, Growth temperature optimum and range, Luminescence, mechanisms of energy conversion, motility, osmotic tolerance, oxygen relationships, pH optimum and growth range, Photosynthetic Pigments, salt requirements and tolerance, Secondary metabolites formed, sensitivity to metabolic inhibitors, antibiotics and storage inclusions.

3. **Ecological characteristics:** The ability of a micro-organism to colonize a specific environment is of taxonomic value. Some examples of taxonomically important ecological properties are life cycle patterns; the nature of symbiotic relationships; the ability to cause disease in a particular host; and habitat preferences such as requirements for temperature, pH, oxygen and osmotic concentration.

4. **Genetic analysis:** Classification of eucaryotes is possible with genetic analysis, because eucaryotes reproduce sexually. The study of chromosomal gene exchange through transformation, conjugation and transduction is sometime useful in their classification.

2.2.4 Molecular Characteristics

Molecular analysis is the feasible means of collecting a large and accurate data set from a number of micro-organisms. When scientists are careful to make only valid comparisons, phylogenetic inferences based on molecular approaches provided the most robust analysis of microbial evolution.

1. **Nucleic acid base composition:** In double stranded DNA, A pairs with T, and G pairs with C, thus the (G + C)/(A + T) ratio or G + C content, the percent of G + C in DNA, reflects the base sequence and varies with sequences changes as follows:

$$\text{Mole\% (G + C)} = \frac{(G+C)}{(G+C)+(A+T)} \times 100$$

   The G + C content of DNA from animals and higher plants average around 40% and ranges between 30% and 50%.

   For example *Staphylococcus* has G + C content of 30% to 38%, whereas *Micrococcus* DNA has 64% to 75% G + C; yet these two genera of Gram-positive cocci have many other features in common.

2. **Nucleic acid hybridization:** The similarity between genomes can be compared more directly by use of nucleic acid hybridization studies.

   Double stranded DNA is heated at temperature above T_m. Mixture of single – standard DNA (ssDNA) are formed. It is cooled and held at about 25 °C below. T_m. Strand with complementary base sequence will reassociate to form stable dsDNA, whereas non-complementary strands will remain unpaired. If DNA molecules are very different in sequences, they will not form a stable, detectable hybrid. Therefore DNA hybridization is used to study only closely related micro-organisms.

3. **Nucleic acid sequencing:** The rRNA s from small ribosomal subunits (16S and 18S r RNA from prokaryotes and eucaryotes, respectively) have become the molecules of choice for inferring microbial phylogenies and making taxonomic assignments at the genus level.

   The small subunit rRNA s are almost ideal for studies of microbial evolution and relatedness because:

   1. They play the same role in all micro-organisms
   2. The ribosome is absolutely necessary for survival
   3. They are part of the complex ribosomal structure
   4. The genus encoding SSU rRNAs cannot tolerate large mutations

   The utility of SSU rRNAs is extended by the presence of certain sequences that are variable among organisms and other regions that are quite stable. The variable regions enable comparison between closely related microbes while the stable sequences allow the comparison of distantly related micro-organisms.

4. **Genomic fingerprinting:** It employs the capacity of restriction endonucleases to recognize specific nucleotide sequences. Thus the pattern of DNA fragments generated by endonuclease cleavage (restriction fragments) is a direct representation of nucleotide sequence. The comparison of restriction fragments between species and strains is a direct representation of nucleotide sequence. The comparison of restriction fragments between species and strains is the basis of restriction fragment length polymorphism (RELP) analysis.
5. **Amino acid sequencing:** The amino acid sequence of proteins directly reflect mRNA sequences and therefore represent the genes coding for their synthesis. The sequence of a protein with the same function are similar, the organisms possessing them may be closely related.

2.3 Kingdoms

2.3.1 Taxonomy and Classification of Microbes

Three kingdom system: [1866]

- Haeckel was the first to create a natural kingdom for the microbes, which had been discovered nearly two centuries before by Antony van Leeuwenhoek.
- Haeckel placed all unicellular organisms in a new kingdom "protista", on the level with the existing kingdoms for plants (plantae) and animal (Animalis), which are multicellular organisms
- All of the microscopic forms of life are landed in the protista
- Haeckel separated life into three kingdoms and rooted them as a "Tree of Life" most primitive forms of life are closed to the main trunk of the tree, most advanced form are at the tips of the branches.

Five kingdom system by Robert Whittakar in 1969: The first classification system to have gained popularity is the five-kingdom system first suggested by Robert Whittakar in 1969.

This system of classification is based on three levels of cellular organization which evolved to accommodate three principal modes of nutrition; photosynthesis, absorption, and ingestion. The prokaryotes are included in the kingdom *Monera*; they lack the ingestive mode of nutrition. Unicellular eukaryotic micro-organisms are placed in the kingdom *Protista*; The multicellular and multinucleate eukaryotic organisms are found in the kingdoms *Plantae* (multicellular green plants and higher algae), *Animalia* (multicellar animals), and *Fungi* (multinucleate higher fungi). Micro-organisms are found in three of the five kingdoms: Monera (bacteria and cyanobacteria), Protista (microalgae and protozoa), and Fungi (yeasts and molds) shown in Fig. 2.2.

The five kingdom system is no longer accepted by most biologists. A major problem is its lack of distinction between *Archaea* and *Bacteria*. Additionally the kingdom *Protista* is too diverse to be taxonomically useful. Finally the boundaries between the kingdoms *Protista*, *Plantae*, and *Fungi* are ill-defined. For example, the brown algae are probably not closely related to the plants even though the five kingdom system places them in the *Plantae*.

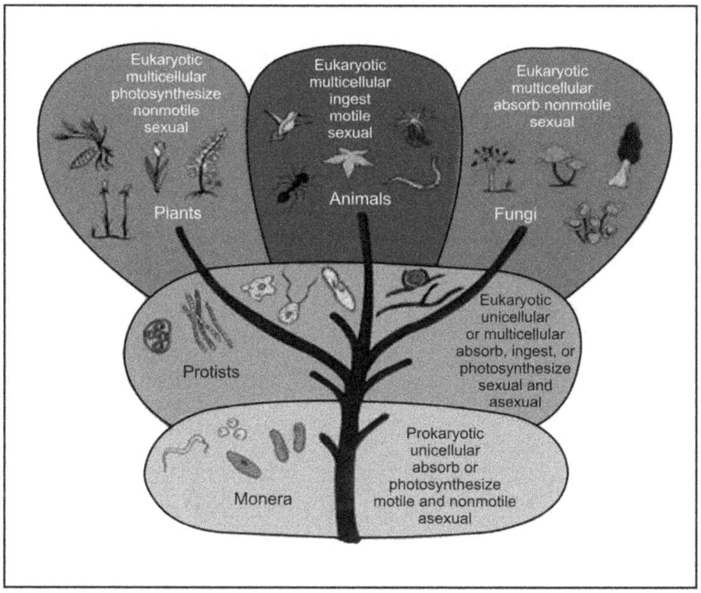

Fig. 2.2 Five kingdom system

2.3.2 Alternatives

The six-kingdom system is the simplest option; it divides the kingdom *Monera* into two kingdoms, The *Eubacteria* and *Archaebacteria*. The following are the kingdoms

Kingdom ***Eubacteria***. Kingdom ***Archaebacteria***, kingdom ***Protista***, kingdom ***Plantae***, kingdom ***Fungi*** and kingdom ***Animalia***.

The eight-kingdom system of Thomas Cavalier- Smith: He believes that the difference in cellular structure and genetic organization are exceptionally important in determining phylogeny; thus he has used ultra structural characteristics as well as rRNA sequences and other molecular data in developing his classification. These are two empires and eight kingdoms.

Empire Bacteria contains 1. Eubacteria and 2. Archaebacteria kingdoms Empire Eucaryota – containes kingdom 3. Archezoa, kingdom 4. Protozoa, kingdom 5. Plantae kingdom 6. Chromista, kingdom 7. Fungi, kingdom 8. Animalia.

The kingdom *Archezoa* are primitive eukaryotic unicellular organisms such as Giardia that have 70S ribosomes and lack Golgi apparatuses, mitochondria, chloroplasts, and peroxisomes

The kingdom *Chromista* contains mainly photosynthetic organisms that have their chloroplasts within the lumen of the rough endoplasmic reticulum rather than in the cytoplasmic matrix. *E.g.*, Diatoms, brown algae, crytomonads and oomycetes.

2.3.3 Higher Level-Classification of Eucarya

In 2005, the International society of Protistologists, in collaboration with parasitologists, mycologists, and phycologists, proposed a classification scheme based on morphological biochemical and molecular phylogenetic analyses of eukaryotic microoraganisms. Six phylogentically coherent clusters were established but not placed in hierarchical order shown in Fig. 2.3.

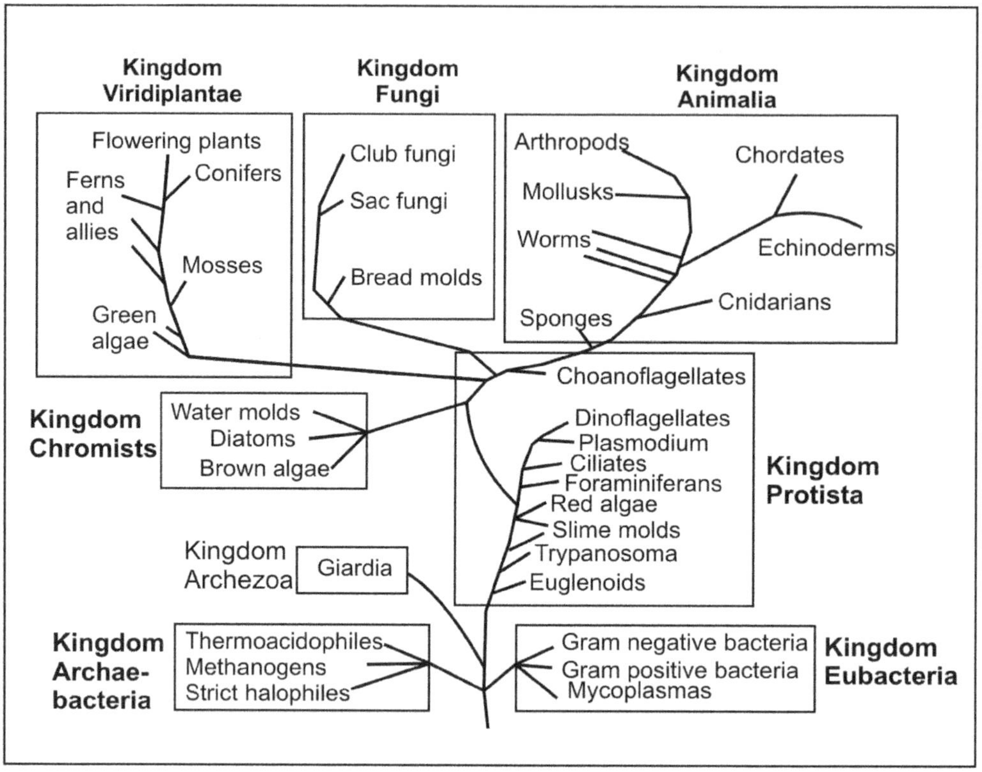

Fig. 2.3 An eight kingdom system classification

Opisthokonta: Animals and fungi share a line of descent

E.g., Fungi, Mesomycetoza, Metazoa, Choanomonada.

Uni-or multicellular: During at least one stage of life cycle, cells have single posterior cilium without mastigonemes (hair like projections on the flagella); possess kinetosomes (basal bodies) or centrioles; when unicellular, mitochondria have flat cristae. It includes yeast, fungi, and *Animalia.*

Archaplastids: Higher plants (plantae) arose from the green algae

E.g., Glaucophyta, Rhodophyceae, Chloroplastida.

Ancestral cyanobacterial endosymboint has given rise to photosynthetic plastid with chlorophyll a, plastid later lost in starch as a storage product; usually with cell wall made of cellulose mitochondria with flattened cristae. It includes the *Charophyta* (green algae) and higher plants.

Amoebozoa: Amoeba without shells

Amoeboid motility usually based on actin-myosin cytoskeleton with rounded pseudopodia (lobopodia); cells either naked or testate (having a shell); mitochondria usually have tubular cristae; usually uninucleate but sometimes multinucleate; cysts common; some lack mitochondria, peroxisomes, and hydrogenosomes (*Entamoeba*). It includes cellular and acellular slime molds.

E.g., Tubulinea, Flabellinea, Sterromyxida, Acanthamabidae, Entamiebida, Mastigamiebidae, Pelomyxa, Eumycetozoa.

Rhizaria: Species-rich super group of unicellular eukaryotes Amoeboids with frils, retieulos.

Possess thin pseudopodia (filopodia) that can be simple, branching, or supported by microtubules; biciliate or amoeboid. Include plasmodial endoparasites of marine and fresh water animals.

E.g., Cercozoa, Haplosporidia, Foraminifera, Gramia, Radiolaria.

Chromalveolate:

Auto-mixo-, and heterotrophic forms; some bear ejectosomes(trichocysts – dartlike structures used for defense); plastid form secondary endosymbiosis with an ancestral archaplastid; plastid then lost or reduced in some, or re-acquired in others. Includes diatoms, dinoflagellates, coccolinths, *Apixcomplexa* (eg., *Plasmidium*), seaweeds/kelps and Ciliophora (eg. *Paramacium, Stentor*).

E.g., Cryptophycae, Haptophyta, Stramenopiles, Alveolata.

Excavata:

- Suspension feeding groove (cytostome) present or thought to have been lost in some;
- Feed by capturing particles from a flageliar-generated current.
- Includes *Giardia*, *Trichomonas*, and *Euglend.*

E.g., Fornicata, Malawimonas, parabasalia, Jakobida, Heterolobosea, Euglenozoa

2.3.4 Bergy's Manual of Systematic Bacteriology (BMSB)

In 1923, David Bergy, professor of bacteriology at the University of Pennsylvania, and four colleagues published a classification of bacteria that could be used for identification of bacterial species, named as the Bergy's Manual of Determinative Bacteriology. This manual is now in its ninth edition. In 1984, the first edition of BMSB was published. It contained descriptions of all prokaryotic species then identified. The second edition will consist of five volumes; the first volume was published in 2001 and the second in 2005. Three additional volumes were published in 2007.

Division-I (Gram negative included) GRAEILICUTES

- The Spirochetes
- Aerobic/Microaerophilic, Motile, Helical/Vibroid, Gram–negative Bacteria
- Nonmotile (or rarely motile), Gram-negative curved Bacteria.
- Aerobic Gram-negative Rods and Cocci,
- Facultatively Anaerobic Gram-negative Rods,
- Anaerobic Gram-negative straight, curved and helical Rods,
- Dissimilatory Sulphate or Suphur reducing Bacteria,
- Anaerobic Gram-negative Cocci,
- The Rickettsias and Chlamydias
- The Mycoplasmas,
- Endosymbionts.

Division-II FERMICUTES

- Gram-positive Cocci,
- Endospore – forming Gram-positive Bacteria,
- Non spore forming Gram-positive Rods or regular shape,
- Non spore forming Gram-positive Rods of irregular shape,
- Mycobacteria,
- Nocardioforms.

Division-III TENERICUTES

- Anoxygenic Phototrophic Bacteria,
- Oxygenic Phototropic Bacteria,
- Glinding, Fruiting Bacteria,
- Glinding, Nonfruiting Bacteria,
- The Sheathed Bacteria,
- Budding and/or Appendaged Bacteria,
- Chemolithotrophic Bacteria,
- Archaebacteria.

Division-IV MENDOSICUTES

- Filamentous Bacteria that divide in more than one plane,
- Filamentous Bacteria that form true sporangia,,
- Streptomyces and Similar Genera,
- This division includes additional filamentous bacteria, having uncertain taxonomic placement.

2.4 Types of Micro-organisms

Classification of micro-organisms: All organisms can be broadly classified into two classes:

1. ***Prokaryotes*:** Bacteria, Cyanobacteria
2. ***Eukaryotes*:** Protozoa, Fungi, Algae, animals and plants

Bacteria and Cyanobacteria represent Prokaryotes. Fungi, Algae, Protozoa higher Plants and Animals represent Eukaryotes. Eukaryotic cells have a variety of membrane bound components lacking in prokaryotes and those are organelles, which include endoplasmic reticulum, Golgi complex, lysosome, mitochondria, chloroplast and cyto skeleton. Both possess ribosomes, ultra-microscopic bodies of RNA where protein synthesis takes place in cell.

Table 2.2 Differences between prokaryotic cells and eukaryotic cells

Prokaryotic cells	Eukaryotic cells
1. Group: Bacterial cells Blue green algae and Mycoplasma cells	1. Group: Algae,fungi,protozoa,Plant cells Animal cells
2. Size range of organisms: 1-2 by 1-4 μm or less	2. Size range of organisms: Greater than 5 μm in width or diameter
3. Cell wall is thin and consists of mucopeptides i.e., peptidoglycan	3. In plant cells usually cellulose cell wall is formed.peptidoglycan is absent
4. Nucleus is absent but nucleoid, chromatin body or nuclear material is present.	4. Nucleus with nuclear envelope, nucleoplasm, chromatin reticulum and nucleolus is found.
5. Circular naked DNA molecule is the genetic material	5. Store house of genetic material is nucleus
6. Membrane bound cell organells like mitochondria, endoplasmic reticulum, golgic complex, lysosomes are absent	6. Membrane bound cell organells are present
7. Ribosomes are of 70S type	7. 80S types of Ribosomes are present in cytoplasm. The cell organelles like plastids of Ribosomes
8. Indirect cell divisions like mitosis, and a reduction division meiosis are absent. Amitosis or direct cell division occur	8. Mitosis and meiosis occur.
9. Cytoplasmic streaming is absent and vacuoles are absent	9. Cytoplasmic streaming is observed in plant cells in addition to vacuoles
10. Microbodies are absent	10. Microbodies are present
11. Respiratory enzymes are found in plasma membrane	11. Respiratory enzymes are confined to mitochondria
12. DNA base ratios as moles% og guanine +cytosine (G+C)% is 28-73	12. DNA base ratios as moles% og guanine +cytosine (G+C)% is about 40

2.5 Bacteria

Bacteria are Single-celled prokaryotic micro-organisms that can exist either as independent (free-living) organisms or as parasites (dependent on another organism for life). Bacteria are the plural of bacterium and they are very small, most being approximately 0.5 to 1.0 μm (micrometer) in diameter. Their reproduction is by binary fission. The shape of bacterium is governed by its rigid cell wall. Bacterial cells are spherical (cocci), straight rods or rods (bacilli) and helically curved (spirilla). Bacterial cells are usually arranged in a manner characteristic of their particular species. Cocci appear in several characteristic arrangements depending on the plane of cellular division. Bacilli are arranged, mostly occur singly or in pairs but bacillus reduce the space subtilis forms chains, others such as Beggiatoa and saprospira species form trichomes. *Corynebacterium diphtheria* cells are lined side by side like match sticks and to one another.

Streptomyces species form long branched, multi nucleate filaments called hyphae which collectively form a mycelium.

Bacteria with less than one complete twist or turn have a vibriod shape, spirilla are rigid helical bacteria, and Spirochetes are highly flexible.

2.5.1 Morphology of Bacteria

Size: Bacteria are very small, most being approximately 0.5-1.0 μm in diameter. An important consequence of small size of micro-organisms is that the surface area/volume ratio of bacteria is exceedingly high compared to the same ratio for larger organisms. Moreover, because of the high surface area volume ratio, the mass of cell substance to be nourished is very close to the surface; therefore, no circulatory mechanism is required to distribute the nutrients that are taken in, and there is thought to be little or no cytoplasmic movement within a bacterial cell.

E. coli, a bacillus of about average size is 1.1 to 1.5 μm wide by 2.0 to 6.0 μm long.

Spirochaetes occasionally reach 500 μm in length and the *Cyanobacterium oscillatoria* is about 7 μm in diameter.

The bacterium, *Epulosiscium fishelsoni*, can be seen with the naked eye (600 mm long by 80 mm in diameter).

One group of bacteria called the *Mycoplasmas*, have individual with size much smaller than these dimensions. They measure about 0.25 μ and are the smallest cells known as far. They were formerly known as pleurophneumonia-like organism (PPLO).

Mycoplasma gallicepticum, with a size of approximately 200 to 300 nm are thought to be the world smallest bacteria.

Thiomargarita namibiensis is world's largest bacteria, a gram-negative proteobacterium found in the ocean sediments off the coast of Namibia. Usually it is 0.1 -0.3 mm (100-300 μm across, but bigger cells have been observed upto 0.75 mm 750 μm.

Shape and Arrangement:

The shape of a bacterium is governed by its rigid cell wall. Typical bacterial cells are: Spherical (Cocci)

Straight rods (Bacilli)

Rods that are helically curved (Spirilla) most bacterial species have cells that are of a fairly constant and characteristic shape, some have cells that are pleomorphic i.e that can exhibit a variety of shapes.

Bacterial species are differentiated by morphology, chemical composition, nutritional requirements, biochemical activities and source of energy.

The Size, Shape, and Arrangement of Bacterial Cells:

Most bacteria are 0.2 μm in diameter and 2-8 μm in length.

The three basic bacterial shapes are coccus (spherical), bacillus (rod-shaped), and spiral (twisted), however pleomorphic bacteria can assume several shapes.

Arrangement of Cocci:

Cocci may be oval, elongated, or flattened on one side.

Cocci may remain attached after cell division. These group characteristics are often used to help identify certain cocci.

- Cocci appear in several characteristic arrangements, depending on the plane of cellular division.
- Cocci bacteria can exist singly, in pairs (as diplococcic), in groups of four (as tetrads), in chains(as streptococci), in clusters (as staphylococci), or in cubes consisting of eitht cells (as sarcinae). Cocci may be oval, elongated, or flattened on one side. Cocci may remain attached after cell division. These group characteristics are often used to help identify certain cocci.
    1. ***Diplococci***: The cocci are arranged in pairs. Examples: *Streptococcus pneumonia, Morzxella catarrhalis, Neisseria gonorrhoeae*, etc.
    2. ***Streptococci*:** The cocci are arranged in chains, as the cells divide in one plane. Examples: *Streptococcus pyogenes, Streptococcus agalactiae.*
    3. ***Tetrads*:** The cocci are arranged in packets of four cells, as the cells divide in two plains. Examples: *Aerococcus, Pediococcus and Tetragenococcus.*
    4. ***Sarcinae*:** The cocci are arranged in a cuboidal manner, as the cells are formed by regular cell divisions in three planes. Cocci that divide in three planes and remain in groups cube like groups of eight.

       Examples: *Sarcina ventriculi, Sarcina ureae,* etc.

5. ***Staphylococci*:** The cocci are arranged in grape-like clusters formed by irregular cell divisions in three plains. Examples: *Staphylococcus aureus.*

Arrangement of Bacilli:

The cylindrical or rod-shaped bacteria are called "bacillus" (plural: bacilli).

1. ***Diplobacilli*:** Most bacilli appear as single rods. Diplobacilli appear in pairs after division. Example of single rod: *Bacillus cereus*. Examples of Diplobacilli: *Coxiella burnetii, Moraxella bovis, Klebssiella rhinoscleromatis*, etc.
2. ***Streptobacilli*:** The bacilli are arranged in chains, as the cells divide in one plane. Examples: *Streptobacillus maniliformis*.
3. ***Coccobacilli*:** These are so short and stumpy that they appear ovoid. They look like coccus and bacillus. Examples: *Haemophilus influenza, Gardnerella vaginalis*, and *Chlamydia trachomatis*.
4. ***Palisades*:** The bacilli bend at the points of division following the cell divisions, resulting in a palisade arrangement resembling a picket fence and angular patterns that look like Chinese letters. Example: *Corynebacterium diphtheria,* the cells are lined side by side like matchsticks.

   Since bacilli only divide across their short axis there are fewer groupings.

Bacilli are not arranged in patterns as complex as those of cocci, and most occur singly or in pairs (diplobacilli) chains (streptobacilli).

Arrangement in Spiral Bacteria:

Spirilla (or spirillum for a single cell) are curved bacteria which can range from a gently curved shape to a corkscrew-like spiral. Many spirilla are rigid and capable of movement. A special group of spirilla known as spirochetes are long, slender and flexible.

1. ***Vibrio*:** They are comma-shaped bacteria with less than one complete turn or twist in the cell. Example: *Vibrio Cholerae.*
2. ***Spirilla*:** They have rigid spiral structure. Spirillum with many turns can superficially resemble spirochetes. They do not have outer sheath and endoflagella, but have typical bacterial flagella.

   Example: *Campylobacter jejuni, Helicobacter pylori, Spirillum wingogradskyi*, etc.
3. ***Spirochetes*:** Spirochetes have a helical shape and flexible bodies. Spirochetes move by means of axial filaments, which look like flagella contained beneath a flexible external sheath but lack typical bacterial flagella.

   Examples: *Leptospira species (Leptospira interrogans), Treponema palladium, Borrelia recurrentis, etc.*

Other Shapes and Arrangements of Bacteria (Fig. 2.4)

1. ***Filamentous bacteria*:** They are very long thin filament-shaped bacteria. Some of them form branching filaments resulting in a network of filaments called "mycelium".
   Example: *Candidatus savagella.*
2. ***Star shaped bacteria*:** Examples: *Haloarcula spp (H.vallismortis, H.marismortui)*
3. ***Pleomorphic bacteria*:** These bacteria do not have any characteristic shape unlike all others described above. They can change their shape. In pure cultures, they can be observed to have different shapes.
   Examples: *Mycoplasma pneumonia, M.genitalium,* etc.

Cocci

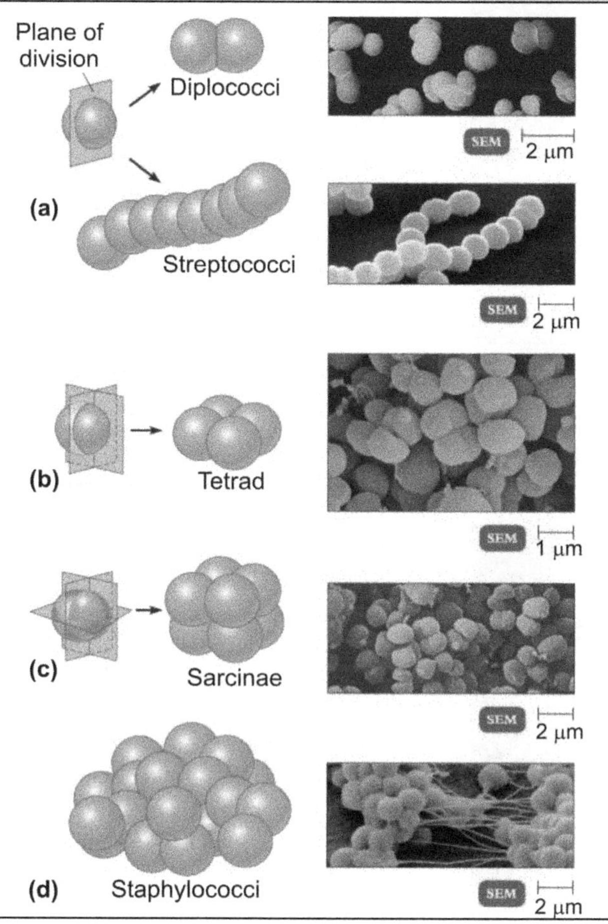

Cocci that remain in pairs after dividing are called diplococci.

Cocci that remain in chains after dividing are called streptococci.

Cocci that divide in two planes and remain in groups of four are called tetrads.

Cocci that divide in three planes and remain in groups cube like groups of eight are called sarcinae.

Cocci that divide in multiple planes and form grape like clusters or sheets are called staphylococci.

Bacilli

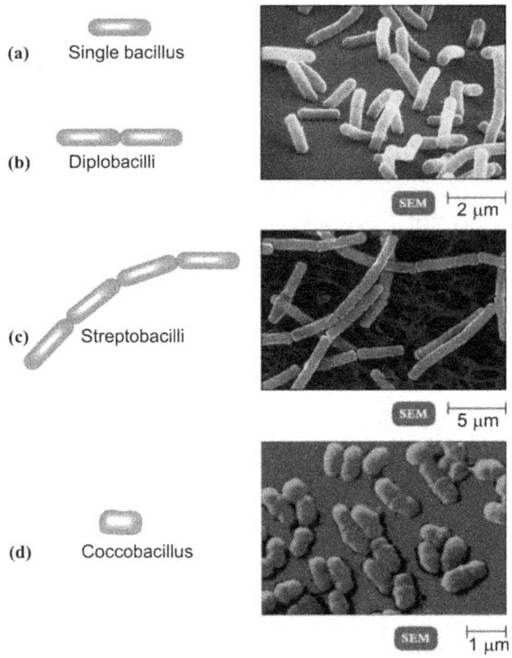

Most bacilli appear as single rods. Diplobacilli appear in pairs after division.

Streptobacilli appear in chains after division.

Some bacilli are so short and fat that they look like cocci and are referred to as coccobacilli.

Spiral bacteria

Spiral bacteria have one or more twists.

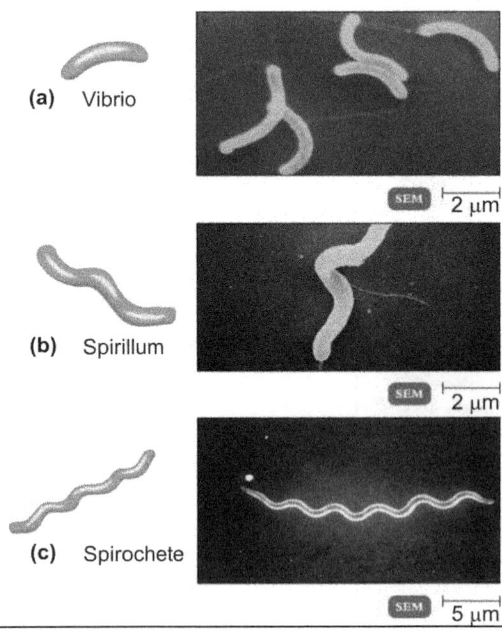

Vibrios look like curved rods.

Spirilla have a helical shape and fairly rigid bodies.

Spirochetes have a helical shape and flexible bodies. Spirochetes move by means of axial filaments, which look like flagella contained beneath a flexible external sheath.

Other shapes	
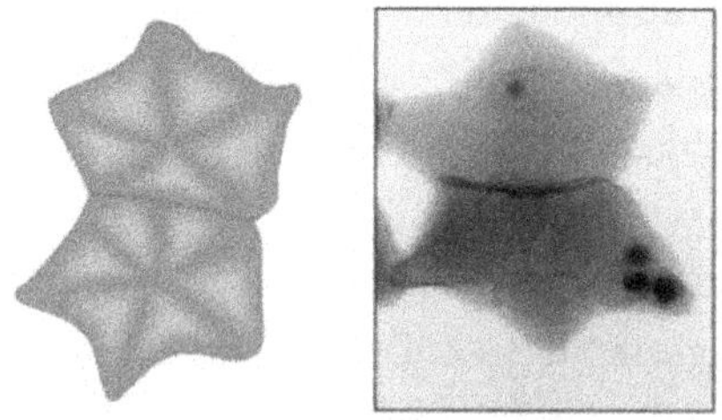 **(a)** Star-shaped bacteria LM 0.5 μm	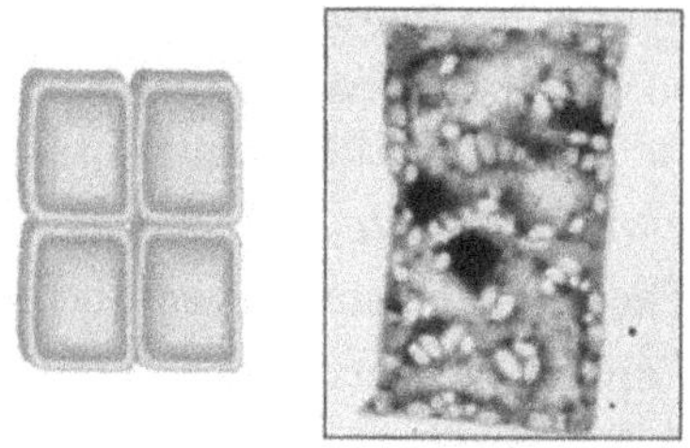 **(b)** Rectangular bacteria LM 0.5 μm
Stella are star-shaped.	*Haloarcula*, a genus of halophilic archaea, are rectangular.

Fig. 2.4 Morphology of bacteria (size, shape and arrangement)

2.5.2 Structure of Bacterial Cell

1. **Capsule:** Some of the bacterial cells are surrounded by extracellular polymeric substances which are commonly called capsule glycocalyx, structure of bacterial cell shown in Fig. 2.5.
   - The presence of capsule may be detected by negative staining such as Indianink method.
   - The capsule is gelatinous polymer made up of either polysaccharide or polypeptide or both (*Klebsiella pneumoniae*) (*B. anthracis*)

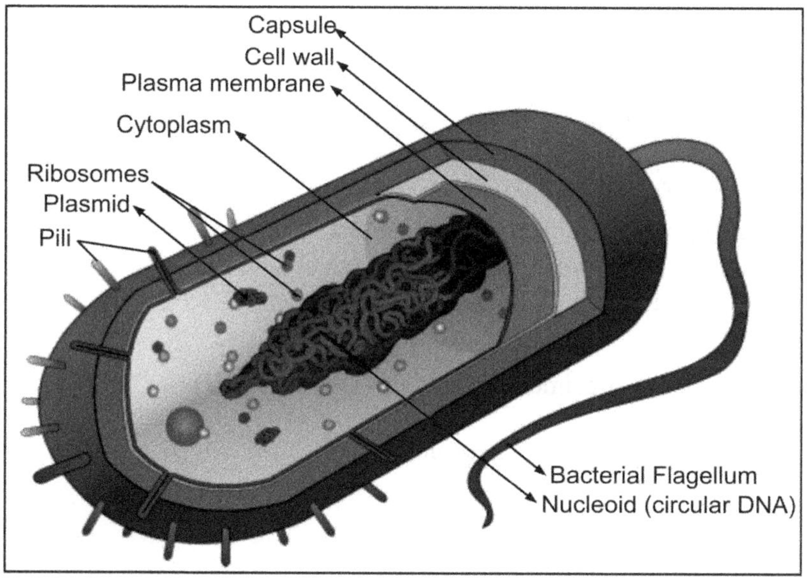

Fig. 2.5 Bacterial cell and its parts

- The capsule of pneumococci is made of hexoses, uronic acids and amino sugars and that of streptococci consists of L – aminoacids
- The bacterial capsule is species specific and, therefore can be used for immunological differentiation of related species.

Function of capsule

(i) The capsule may prevent the attachment of bacteriophages
(ii) Capsule protects the bacterial cells against desiccation
(iii) It may survive in natural environment due to its sticky property.

2. Flagella

- Bacterial flagellum is a helical filament.
- The hook and filament are composed of protein sub-units arranged in a helical fashion.
- The protein of filament is known as flagellin.
- Unlike a hair, flagellin grows at its tip rather than at the base.
- Flagellin monomers synthesized in cell are believed to pass along the hollow center of the flagellum and are added to the distal end of the filament.

Flagella and motility: Bacterial flagella are hair like, helical appendages that protrude through the cell wall and are responsible for swimming motility. They are much thinner than the flagella of eukaryotes. Their location varies depending on the bacterial species and may be polar or lateral.

- The motile bacterium may possess a flagellum
- The flagellum is hair like, helical and surface appendages emerging from the cell wall.
- It is of 20-30 nm in diameter and 15 μm long
- It provides various types of motility to the bacterial cell.

Arrangement of flagella (Fig. 2.6)

The arrangement may be:

Monotrichous – a single polar flagellum e.g.: *Vibrio cholera*

Lophotrichous – a cluster of polar flagellum e.g.: Spirillum

Amphitrichous – flagella at both the ends either singly or in clusture.

Cephalotrichous – two or more flagella at one end of bacterial cell
e.g., *Pseudomonas*

Peritrichous – cell surface evenly surrounded by several lateral flagella
e.g.: *Proteous vulgaris*

Atrichous – cells devoid of flagella e.g: *Lactobacillus*

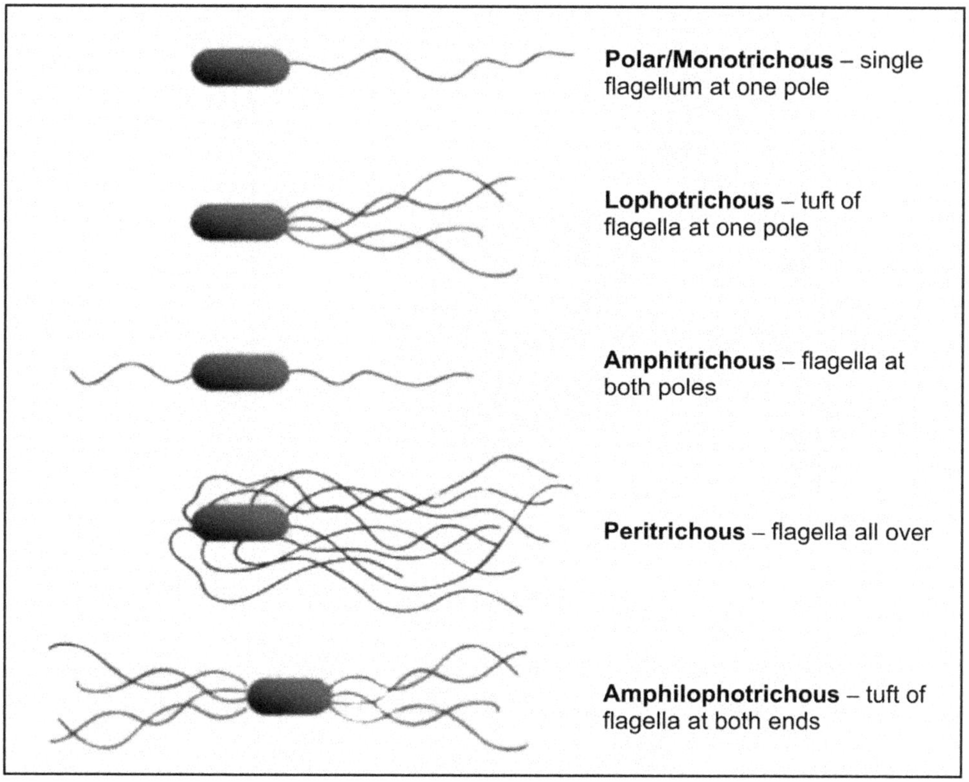

Fig. 2.6 Types of flagellar arrangement

Structure of flagella: A flagellum consists of three basic parts, the basal body, hook and filament shown in Fig. 2.7.

(a) ***Basal body:*** The basal body attaches the flagellum to the cell wall and plasma membrane. It is composed of a small central rod inserted into a series of rings.

- In Gram-negative bacteria two pairs of rings, the proximal ring and the distal ring, are connected by a central rod.
- In Gram-positive bacteria only the distal pair of rings is present.

(b) ***Hook:*** The hook is present outside the cell wall and connects filament to the basal body.

- It consists of different proteins
- The hook in Gram positive bacteria is slightly longer than the Gram negative bacteria.

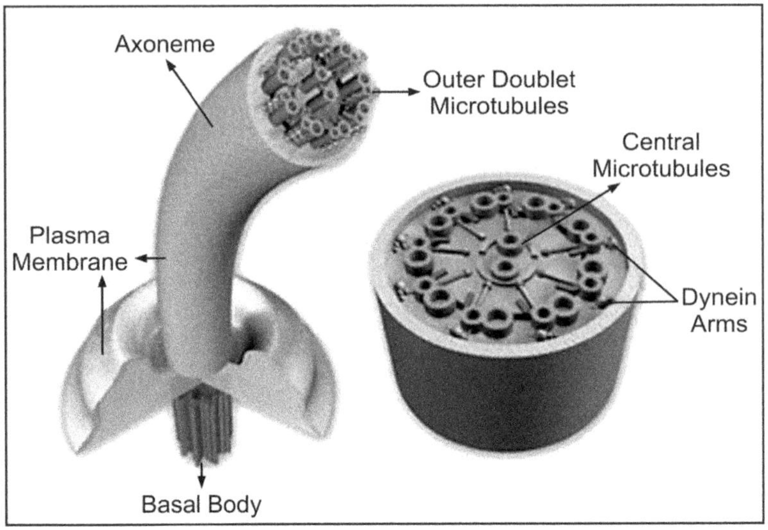

Fig. 2.7 Ultrastructure of cilia and flagella

(c) ***Filament or shaft*:** The outermost long region of the flagellum is called filament or shaft.

- It has a constant diameter and is made up of globular proteins, the flagellin.
- The flagellins are arranged in several chains that interwine and form a helix around a hollow core.
- The proteins of flagella act to identify certain pathogenic bacteria. Unlike eukaryotes, the filaments are not covered by a membrane or sheath

Locomotion: There are three types of movement in bacteria

(i) ***Flagellar movement:*** Bacterial flagella are motile and help in locomotion of bacterial cells

- Prokaryotic flagellum is semi rigid, helical rotor that moves the cell by rotating from the basal body either clockwise or counter clockwise around its axis
- The helical waves are generated from the base to the tip of flagellum. The rotating flagellum forms a bundle that pushes against water and propel the bacterium
- The basal body acts as motor and causes rotation.

Mechanism of prokaryotic flagellar movement

- The polar flagellum rotates anticlockwise but the cell rotates clockwise when moving normally
- Rotation of flagellum in anticlockwise direction results in movement of bacterial cell in opposite direction
- Energy is required for the movement of flagella. In eukaryotes, energy is generated by ATP.

- The mechanism of energy generation for the movement of prokaryotic flagella is not known

(ii) ***Spirochaetial movement:*** The spirochaetes show several types of movements such as flexing, spinning, free swimming and creeping as they are flexible within the cell envelope they have flagella like structure which are known as periplasmic flagella or axial fibrils. The rotation of axial fibrils causes the movement in the opposite direction

(iii) ***Gliding movement*:** Some bacteria such as species like *Cyanobacteria* and *Mycoplasma* show gliding movement when they come in contact with a solid surface. No organelles are associated with their movement but the slime, they secrete help them to get attached to the substratum.

Hanging drop preparation (Fig. 2.8) is a special type of wet mount (in which a drop of medium containing the organisms is placed on a microscope slide), often is used in dark illumination to observe the motility of bacteria. In this method a drop of culture is placed on a coverslip that is encircled with petroleum jelly (or any other sticky material). The coverslip and drop are then inverted over the well of a depression slide. The drop hangs from the coverslip, and the petroleum jelly forms a seal that prevents evaporation. This preparation gives good views of microbial motility. Actively motile organisms (*Pseudomonas aeruginosa*) give true motility that can be observed clearly through this method.

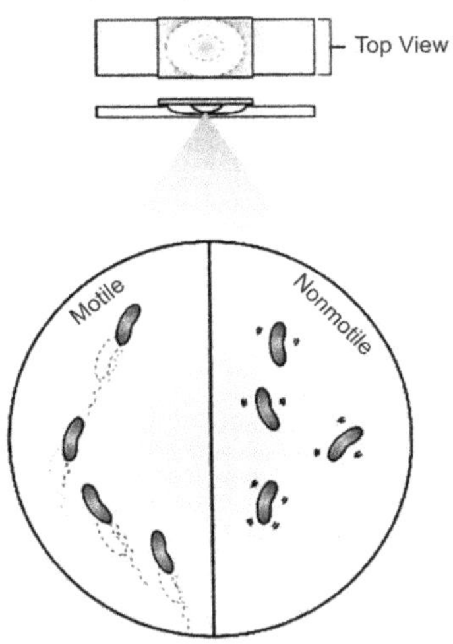

Fig. 2.8 Hanging drop slide

3. **Pili and fimbriae:** Pili and fimbriae are hair like appendages found on surface of cell wall, in Gram–negative bacteria.

- Eukaryotic cells lack pili.
- The term fimbriae is used for all hair like structure covering the surface of the cell.
- Pili are genetically governed by plasmids, the number of which varies from 3 to 5.
- The number of fimbriae is around 1000.

- Pili differ from flagella in being shorter and thinner, sight and less rigid. But they are in large number.
- The pili are 0.2-20 μm long.

Classes of pili: According to the function pili are of two types

(a) Common pili – Act by adhering the cell to surfaces.

(b) Sex pili – Act by joining the outer bacterial cell for transfer of genome.

Structure of pili: Both fimbria and pili are like flagella as both are the appendages on bacterial cell wall. They originate from cytoplasm that protrudes outside after penetrating the peptidoglycan layer of cell wall. Fimbriae are made up of 100% protein called fimbrilin or pilin which consists of about 163 amino acids.

Function of pili and fimbriae

- Fimbriae have the adhesion properties.
- Fimbriae agglutinate the blood cells such as erythrocytes, leucocytes, epithelial cells.
- Fimbriae are equipped with antigenic properties as they act as thermolabile nonspecific agglutinogen.
- The sexpili make contact between two cells. Since they posses hollow core, they act as conjugation tube.

4. **The cell wall (outer membrane):** The basic bacterial cell structure are shown in Fig. 2.9. The cell wall of bacteria is a semirigid and complex structure present beneath capsule and external to the plasma membrane. It is responsible for characteristic shape of the cell. The cell wall protects the plasma membrane and the outer cytoplasmic inclusions from adverse environments.

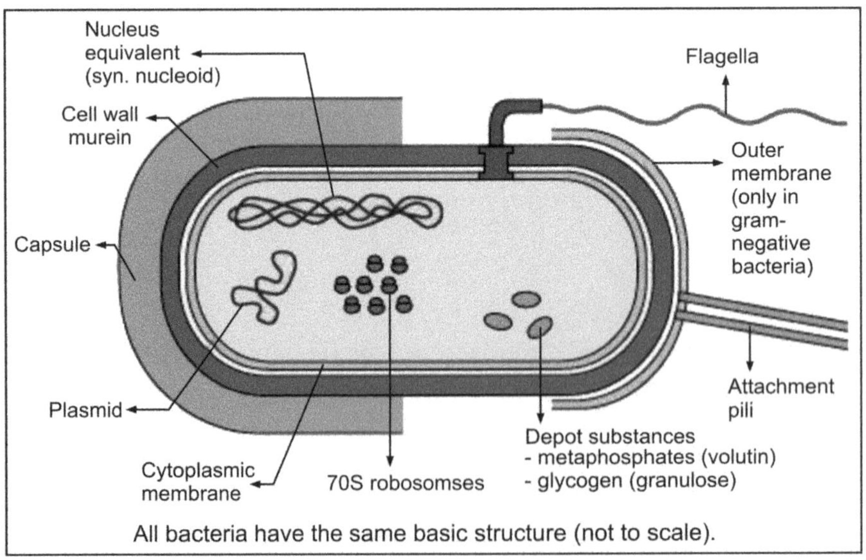

Fig. 2.9 Basic bacterial cell structure

- It also protects the bacterial cell from bursting when the osmotic pressure of cytoplasm is higher than that of out side of the cell wall.
- It provides support for the attachment to the flagella.

Chemical composition of cell wall: The cell wall of bacteria is made up of network of peptidoglycan (murein, murus = wall). It was present almost on all bacterial cell wall except *Halobacterium* and *Halococcus,* because these bacteria live in marine water which contains high salt concentration.

- Peptidoglycon determines the shape of a cell. It accounts for 40-80% of total dry weight of cell. Its thickness is about 30-80 nm. It is insoluble and porous polymer that provides rigidity. It is a mucopolysaccharide.
- However, its chemical composition differs from species to species. It consists of repeating disaccharides attached to chains of four or five amino acids.
- The monosaccharides, N - acetylglucosamine (NAG) and N - acetylmuramic acid (NAM) are linked by $\beta - 1, 4 -$ glycosidic bond
- A tetrapeptide side chain containing four amino acids, (L - alanine, D - glutamate, L - lysine and D - alanine) is attached to each NAM.
- The third amino acid varies with different bacteria and may be lysine, diamino pametic acid or threonine.

For example in *E.coil* instead of L-lysine (the third amino acid) there is mesodiaminopimelic acid.

L - Alanine

D - Glutamate

L - lysine - third amino acid which varies

D - Alanine

The D and L forms of amino acids alternate to each other.

- Except peptidoglycan, the amino acids found in protein are L - forms
- The parallel tetrapeptide side chains are linked by a pentaglycine peptide cross bridge that contains five amino acid.
- The parallel tetrapeptide cross bridge links L - lysine of one tetrapeptide with D - alanine at the terminal end.

Gram-negative bacteria

Gram-negative bacteria contain pepti doglycan but in very low amount. They totally lack teichoic acids. Due to the low amount of peptidoglycon the cell wall of Gram-negative bacteria can easily be disintegrated. The cell envelope of Gram- negative bacteria is a bi layered structure consisting of mainly Lipoproteins, lipopolysaccharides and phospholipids.

Table 2.3 Difference between gram positive and gram negative bacteria

Gram Positive Bacteria	Gram Negative Bacteria
1. Cell wall contains several layers of peptidoglycan 40-90% of total dry weight thickness may vary from 30 nm to 8 nm. 2. Teichoic acid is present. 3. Lipopolysaccharides are absent. 4. Lipid and lipoprotein are in low amount. 5. Produce exotoxin. 6. Periplasmic space is absent. 7. Flagella contain 2 rings in basal body. 8. Susceptibility to penicillin and sulfonamide is high 9. Pores are absent.	1. Single layer of peptidoglycan. Thickness may vary from 2-7 nm. 2. Teichoic acid is absent 3. Lipopolysaccharides are present in high amount. 4. Lipid and lipoprotein are present in high amount. 5. Produces endotoxin. 6. Periplasmic space is present. 7. Flagella contains 4 ring in basal body. 8. Susceptibility to penicillin and sulfonamide is low. 9. Pores are present.

Table 2.4 Differences between gram-positive and gram-negative cell wall

Property	Gram positive cell wall	Gram negative cell wall
Thickness of wall	Thick (20 to 80 nm)	Thin (10nm)
Number of layers	1	2
Peptidoglycan(murein) content	Greater than 50%	Between 10%to 20%
Teichoic acids in wall	Present	Absent
Lipid and Lipoprotein content	0 to 3%	58%
Protein content	0	9%
Lipopolysaccharide content	0	13%

Chemical constituents of gram negative bacterial cell wall

(a) ***Lipoproteins*:** Lipoproteins occur freely and in bound forms as well lipoproteins together with matrix proteins form a complex which contains diffusion channels. Lipoproteins have a molecular weight of about 7000 daltons and consist of about 58 aminoacids.

(b) ***Lipopolysaccharides*:** The outer membrane of Gram-negative bacteria is covered by lipopolysaccharides which are made up of polysaccharides covalently linked to lipid A.

Lipid A: It consists of glucosamine, phosphate and fatty acids. The $\beta -1, 6 - D -$ glucosamine disaccharide units constitute the carbohydrate component of lipid A.

The esterified group of lipid A is referred to as endotoxin which is toxin when present in blood lipid A of lipopolysaccharide is responsible to induce fever and shocks.

(c) ***Polysaccharide***: The polysaccharide portion of lipopolysaccharide of *Salmonella* cell wall is composed outer core and the o – Antigen side chain. The polysaccharide of lipopolysaccharide is also known as o – polysaccharide. These chains have antigenic property and, therefore, can be distinguished serologically.

(d) ***Matrix proteins***: The outer membrane of cell envelope does not warrant the entry of all substances since the nutrients are passed across the membrane. It is impermeable only to macromolecules such as proteins, lipids etc. The permeability of outer membrane is due to the presence of proteins called porins that form channels. Porins also act as receptor sites for bacteriophages and bacteriocins

Functions of cell wall

- Peptidoglycan provides structure integrity of cell by forming a rigid layer in outer membrane
- Matrix protein act as receptor sites for bactriophages and bacteriocins
- O – Antigen side chain determines the antigen specificity of Gram-negative bacteria.

5. **Plasma membrane** is also called as cell membrane or cytoplasmic membrane. It is a structure internal to the cell wall. It is situated just beneath the cell wall and is 7.5 nm thick. The plasma membrane consists of a continuous bi layer of phospholipid molecules in which globular proteins are embedded.

(i) ***Fluid mosaic model:*** This is shown in Fig. 2.10. Singer and Nicolson have given the fluid masaic model of plasma membrane to explain its major features. This model is well accepted which states that the cell membrane is a semisolid layer and shows elasticity and differential permeability. The property of selective permeability is facilitated by the arrangement of lipid molecules in a liquid matrix state accommodating protein molecules as floating masses in a mosaic pattern. As the icebergs float in an ocean, similarly the protein molecules appear to be floating in the ocean of lipid molecules. This arrangement of proteins and lipid molecules help the membrane to regulate the entry and exit of substance through it and hence it plays an important role in the osmoregulatory processes of cells.

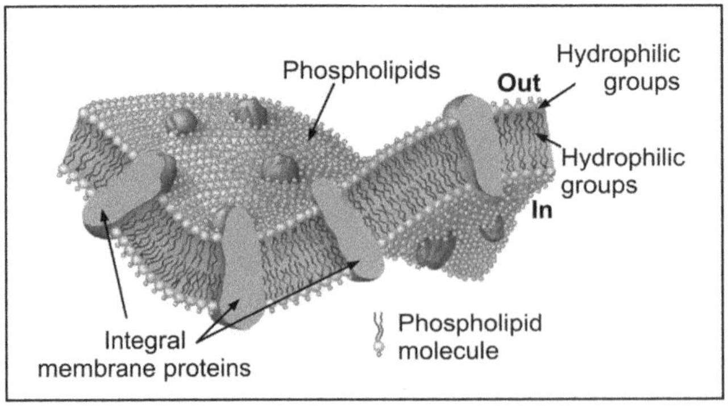

Fig. 2.10 Bacterial cell membrane fluid mosaic model

In some micro-organisms such as mycoplasma and fungi, sterols and found to be associated within the plasma membrane.

Functions of plasma membrane

- The organic and inorganic nutrients are transported
- It consists of enzymes of bio synthetic pathways that synthesize different components of the cell wall such as peptidoglycan, teichoic acid, polysaccharides, lipopolysaccharides and phospholipids
- It provides permeability barrier and thus prevents the escape of cellular materials outside the cell, and facilitate the selective entry of organic and inorganic substances inside.
- It possesses the attachment sites for bacterial chromosomes and plasmid DNA.

6. **Mesosomes:** Mesosomes are the invaginated structures formed by the localized infoldings of the plasma membrane. The invaginated structures comprise of vesicles, tubules. Generally mesosomes are found in association with nuclear area or near the site of cell division. They are absent in eukaryotes.
   - The vesicles are formed probably by invagination and tubular accretion of the plasma membrane.
   - Mesosomes are supposed to take part in respiration but they are not analogous to mitochondria because they lack outer membrane.
   - In the vesicle of mesosomes the respiratory enzymes and the components of electron transport such as ATP ase, dehydrogenase, cytochrome are either absent or present in low amount.
   - Infoldings of mesosomes increase the surface area of plasma membrane that in turn increases the absorption of nutrients.
7. **Cytoplasm:** Cytoplasm is thick and semitransparent. The DNA molecules, ribosomes and the other inclusions are the structure of cytoplasm.
   - In certain cyanobacteria gas vacuoles are found.

- The prokaryotic cytoplasm differs from the eukaryotic cytoplasm. Prokaryotic cytoplasm lacks cytoskeleton and cytoplasmic streaming.
- Compartmentation of organelles are absent in prokaryotes and present in eukaryotes
- Cytoplasm consists of water (80%), proteins, carbohydrates, lipids, inorganic ions and certain low molecular compounds.

8. **Ribosomes:** All living cells contain ribosomes which act as site of protein synthesis.
   - High number of ribosomes represents high rate of protein synthesis.
   - Presence of ribosomes in high number gives the cytoplasm a granular appearance
   - The eukaryotic ribosomes are found attached to cell membrane, where as the prokaryotic ribosomes are free in cytoplasm.
   - Prokaryotic ribosomes are smaller and less dense than eukaryotic ribosomes.
   - Ribosomes of prokaryotes are often called 70s ribosomes and that of eukaryotes as 80s ribosomes. The letter'S' refers to Svedberg unit which indicates the relative rate of sedimentation during ultra centrifugation sedimentation rate depends on size, shape and weight of particles.

   Ultra structure of ribosomes

   Subunits: In general the ultra structure of ribosomes reveals that these are composed of two subunits, a large 50 s subunit and a smaller 30s subunit.
   - Each subunit is composed of protein and ribosomal RNA (r RNA).
   - Their association and dissociation depends on the concentration of Mg^{++} ions.

9. **Molecular Chaperones:** It was thought for many years that polypeptide after synthesis fold into native stage and this folding is not determined by its amino acids. It is now clear that there are certain helper proteins called molecular chaperones (or) chaperones which recognize the newly formed polypeptides and fold to its proper shape.

10. **Nucleoids:** The nucleoid is a single long circular double stranded DNA molecule devoid of highly conserved histone protein. The histone is present in eukaryotes, therefore, results the eukaryotic DNA converted into the beaded structures i.e nucleosomes. The eukaryotes contain a well organized nucleus in which genetic material is enclosed by a nuclear membrane. Therefore, the DNA material is not enclosed by any covering. Hence the bacterial chromosome is known as chromatin bodies (or) nucleiods.

11. **Plasmids:** Plasmid may be defined as small circular self replicating and double stranded DNA molecule present in bacterial cell, in addition to the bacterial chromosome.
    - The number of plasmids ranges from one to hundreds or more per bacterial cell.

Type of plasmids

On the basis of function, plasmids are divided into several types

(i) ***Sex factor or fertility (F) factor:*** The plasmids of male cells that confer on their host cells have capability to transmit chromosomal markers but not having other properties are called sex factor of F factor. For the first time F factor was discovered in *E.coli.*

(ii) ***R (resistance) plasmids:*** The resistance genes are associated in various combinations as parts of transmissible plasmids known as R factor.

- In pBR 322 plasmid there are two antibiotic resistance genes. One is Ampicillin resistant gene and the other is Tetracycline resistant gene.
- These antibiotic resistant genes act as markers
- An R factor consists of two segments of DNA, one is the resistance transfer gene and the second is resistant determinants.

(iii) ***Heavy- metal resistance plasmids:*** There are several bacterial strains that contain genetic determinant of resistance to heavy metals. These determinants for resistance are often found on plasmids and transponsons

(iv) ***Col Plasmids:*** These plasmids associated with colicin production are called colicingeny (col) factor.

- Toxins secreted by the strains of *E.coil* are called colicins

(v) ***Degradative Plasmids:*** Special genes present on different plasmids confer degradation capacity to the species of *Pseudomonas*.

For example, the camphor (cam) plasmid of *Pseudomonas putida* encodes enzymes for degradation of camphor.

(vi) ***Penicillinase Plasmid*** of *Staphylococcus aureus*

Staphylococcus aureus is a Gram–positive bacterial pathogen causing infection of skin and wound of humans. After treatment with penicillin antibiotic, several penicillin–resistant staphylococci developed high level resistance to penicillin due to secretion of an enzyme, penicillinase which degrade penicillin by hydrolyzing its, β–lactum ring. Penicillinase plasmids also confer resistance against kanamycin, neomycin, tetracycline, chloramphenicol.

(vii) ***Cryptic Plasmids:*** They do not carry any gene; therefore, they are non–functional. These plasmids have been called as cryptic plasmid.

(viii) ***Ti – Plasmids*** of *Agrobacterium tumifaciens*

It consists of T – DNA that encodes enzymes for the synthesis of avxin and cytosine which interfere plant metabolism, and develop tumour and enable the infected plant to produce a nitrogenous compound called opines. Ti plasmid also contains several genes such as vir (for virulence), ori (for origin of replication), tra (for transfer).

(ix) ***Ri – Plasmids:*** The Ri (Root inducing) plasmids are found in *Agrobacterium rhizogenes* which cause hairy root disease in plants. Ri – Plasmids are closely related to Ti plasmids.

12. **Cytoplasmic Inclusion:** The cytoplasm of prokaryotic and eukaryotic cells contains several reserve deposits which are called inclusions. These inclusions serve as the basis for identification of bacteria. The inclusion bodies are of two types

   (i) Free inclusion bodies (eg. Polyphosphate granules and cyanophycean granules)

   (ii) Single–layered non–unit membrane enclosed inclusion bodies (such as poly b–hydroxybutyrate granules, glycogen granules, sulphur granules, carboxysomes and gas vacuoles)

   Some of the Cytoplasmic Inclusion

   (a) ***Volutin Granules*:** The volutin granules are also known as polyphosphate granules. These granules are found in algae, fungi, protozoa and bacteria. The volutin granules are composed of polyphosphate i.e inoraganic phosphates which are used in synthesis of ATP. The phosphate incorporated into nucleic acid. These are generally formed when the cells grow in phosphate rich environment.

   (b) ***Polysaccharide Granules*:** They are found in protozoa, yeasts, fungi and algae. These can be identified by using iodine solution.

   (c) ***Lipid Inclusions*:** Lipids are found in high amount in several species of *Bacillus, Azotobacter, Mycobacterium, Spirillum* etc. these are present as storage material and is polymer of poly β–hydroxybutyric acid. The collective term poly β–hydroxybutyrate represents the all classes of carbon storage reservoir polymer acting as source of energy and biosynthesis. These are found naturally in Archaea but not in Eukarya. The presence of lipid inclusions can be demonstrated by using fat soluble dyes, for example Sudan dye.

   (d) ***Glycogen*:** Glycogen is another storage product of prokaryotes. It is polymer of glucose sub – units looking like starch. The glucose units are linked by α (1–4) glycosolic bonds. The branching chains are connected by α (1–6) glycosidic bonds. Glycogen is also a storage reservoir for carbon and energy.

   (e) ***Carboxysomes*:** Carboxysomes are found in photosynthetic bacteria, nitrifying bacteria, cyanobacteria and thermobacilli. These are polyhedral or hexagonal inclusion containing ribulose –1, 5 – biphosphate carboxylase. This enzyme is required in CO_2 fixation during photosynthesis.

   (f) ***Sulphur Granules*:** They are temporarily stored by some bacteria which are also called a second type of inorganic inclusion body. It is exemplified by photosynthetic purple sulphur bacteria (eg: *Thiobacillus, Thiospirillum*) which are found in anaerobic, sulphide–rich zones of lake. They oxidize H_2O to S and internally deposit as sulphur granules within invaginated structures of plasma membrane.

(g) ***Magnetosomes***: Magnetosomes are the intracellular chains of magnetite (Fe O_4) particles of about 40–100 nm diameter found in magnetotactic bacteria. Magnetsomes are surrounded by membrane containing phospholipids, proteins and glycoproteins. Each iron particle is a tiny magnet. Hence, the bacteria employ their magnetosomes to determine northward and downward direction. With the help of magnetosomes they swim to nutrient-rich sediments or locate the optimum depth in fresh water and marine habitats.

(h) ***Gas Vesicles***: Gas vesicles are gas-filled structures which contain the same gas in which the organisms are suspended. Gas vesicles provide buoyancy and keep the cells in floating form (gas vesicles cannot resists high hydrostatic pressure and can be collapsed resulting in loss of buoyancy. Gas vesicles attain a density of about 5 – 20% of the cell.

2.5.3 Reproduction in Bacteria

When bacteria are inoculated into a suitable medium and incubated under appropriate conditions, a tremendous increase in the number of cells occurs within a relatively short time. This phase is known as reproduction phase.

The ways in which bacteria reproduces are:

1. ***Binary Fission***: The most common and the most important mode of cell division in the usual growth cycle of bacterial populations is transverse binary fission.

   In transverse binary fission a single cell divides after developing a transverse septum.

   It is an asexual reproduction process. In transverse binary fission, septum formation does not begin until the chromosome content of the cell has been doubled i.e., cell division is triggered by completion of DNA replication.

   The first step is an inward growth of cytoplasmic membrane at the middle of the cell and usually a mesosome is attached to the cytoplasmic membrane.

   New cell formation (Macromolecular synthesis): A bacterial cell inoculated into a fresh medium selectively takes up nutrients from its environment.

   The nutrients are converted into cell substance – RNA, DNA, proteins, enzymes and other macromolecules shown in Fig. 2.11.

   Cell mass and cell size increase and new cell wall building blocks are synthesized, and then the process of binary fission is initiated resulting in the formation of two new cells.

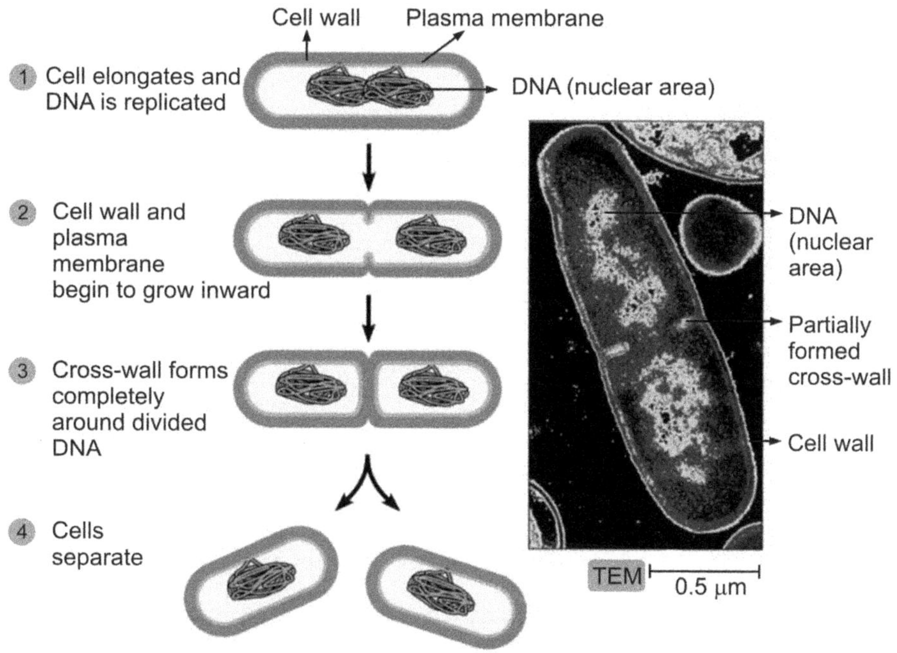

(a) A diagram of the sequence of cell division. **(b) A thin section of a cell of *Bacillus licheniformis* starting to divide.**

Fig. 2.11 Reproduction in bacteria by binary fission

2. ***Budding***: It is a process in which protuberance develops at one end of the cell, this enlarges and eventually develops into a new cell which separates from the parent Fig. 2.12.

   E.g. Rhodopseudomonas acidophila

   In *Hyphomicrobium* species the bud may develop at the end of a prostheca.

3. ***Fragmentation:*** Bacteria that produce extensive filamentous growth reproduce by fragmentation of the filaments into small bacillary or Coccoid cells. Each gives rise to a new growth (Fig. 2.13).

   E.g., *Nocardia* species

4. ***Formation of conidiospores and spragiospores***: Bacteria produce many spores/ organism by developing crosswalls at the hyphal tips each spore gives rise to a new organism shown in Fig. (2.14).

   E.g., Streptomyces species

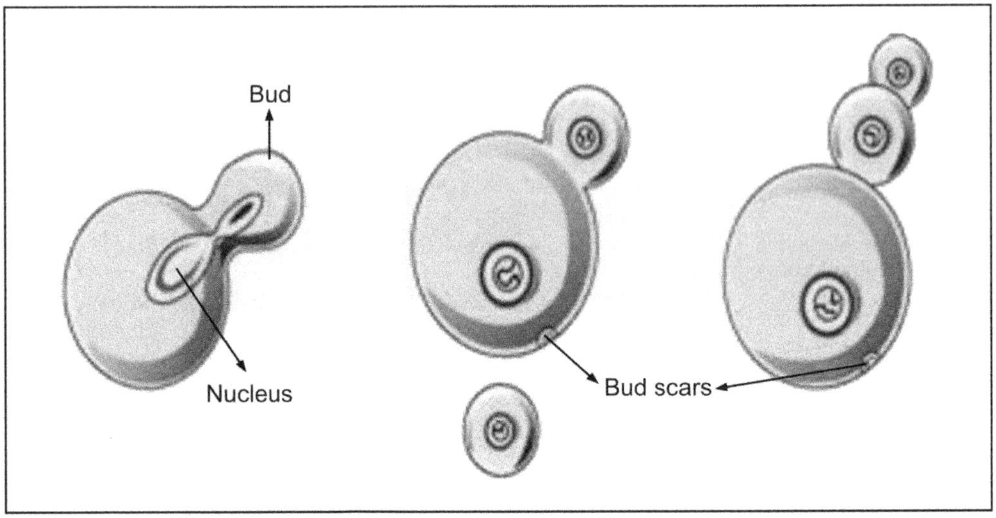

Fig. 2.12 Reproduction by budding in yeasts

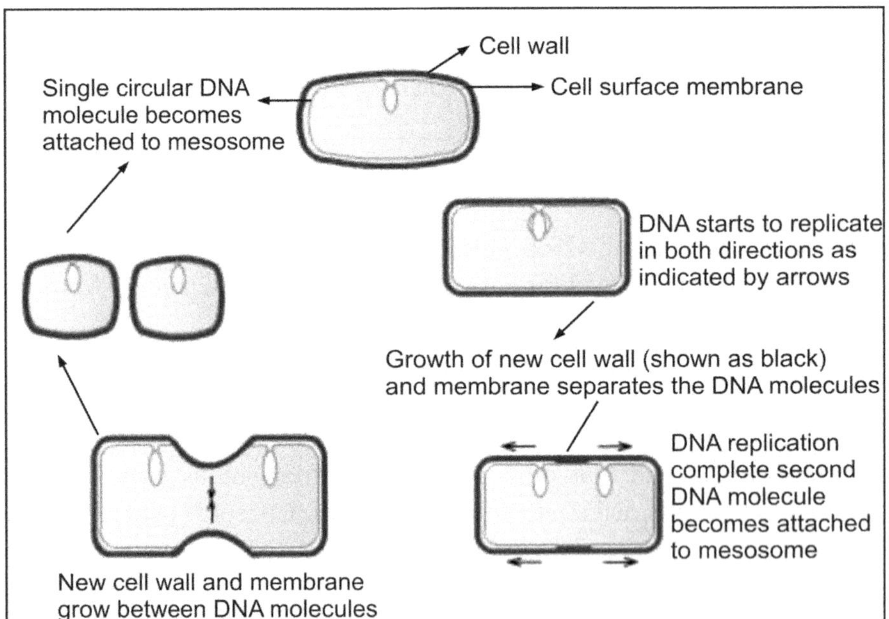

Fig. 2.13 Fragmentation in bacteria

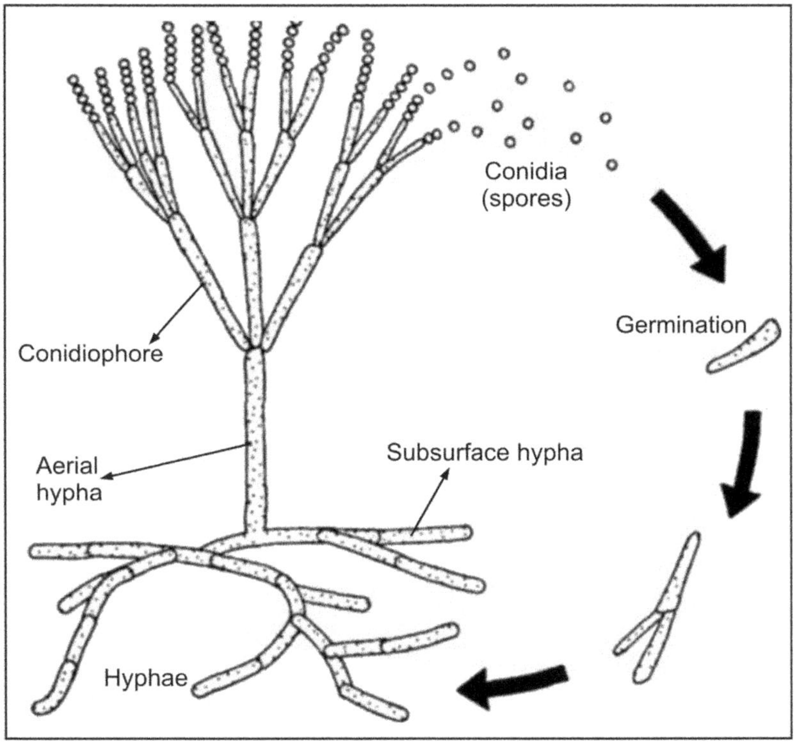

Fig. 2.14 Penicillium species life cycle showing conidiospores

2.5.4 Some Special Groups of Bacteria

1. Spirochaetes

The phylum spirochaetes (*Greek Spira* = a coil, and *chaete* = hair) contains Gram-negative, chemoheterotrophic bacteria.

- The exterior boundary is a special outer membrane that surrounds the protoplasmic cylinder, which contains the cytoplasm and nucleoid.
- Periplasmic Flagella lie between the protoplasmic cylinder and the outer membrane.
- The Flagella rotate and move the cell even though they donot directly contact the external environment.
- These chemoheterotrophs can be free living, symbiotic or parasitic.

The distinguishing features of spirochetes are:

1. A helical shape
2. An ability to twist or control their shape
3. The occurence of a special kind of flagella termed periplasmic flagella

- Spirochetes swim best in media of high viscosity, where as bacteria with ordinary flagella swim best in media of low viscosity.
- Most spirochetes are so thin that they cannot be seen easily by light microscopy, even when gram – stained
- **Order:** Spirochaetales, this order is divided into two families
- **Family:** Spirochaetaceae
- They are stringent anaerobes, facultative anaerobes or microaerophiles
- Carbohydrates or aminoacids are used as carbon and energy sources.
- **Family:** Leptospiraceae
- They are aerobes
- Long–chain fatty acids are used as the carbon and energy source.

Family: Spirochaetaceae

Order: Spirochaetales

Phylum: Spirochaetes

Genus: Spirochaeta

- Spirochetes shown in (Fig. 2.15) differ greatly from other bacteria with respect to motility and can move through very viscous solutions though they lack external rotating flagella.
- Their unique pattern of motility is due to an unusual morphological structure called the axial filament.

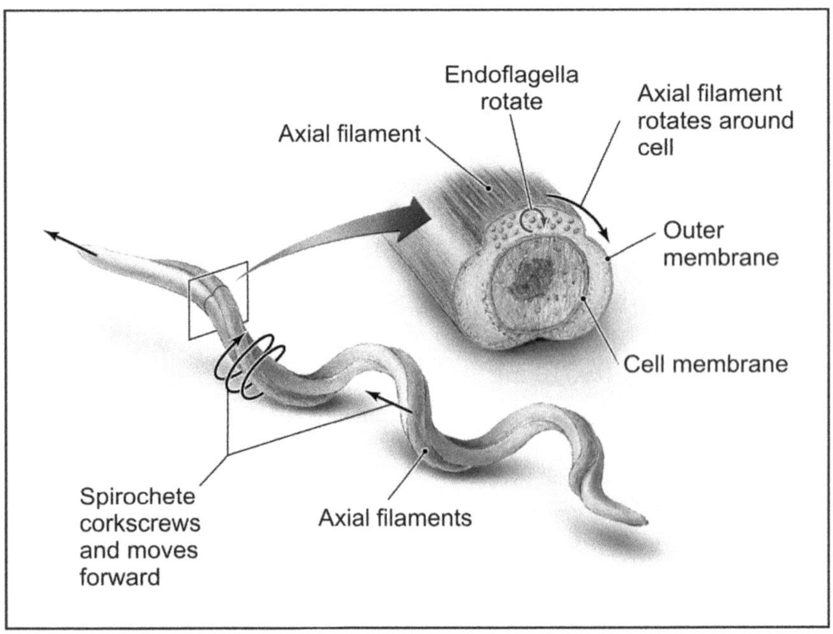

Fig. 2.15
Spirochetes

- When in contact with a solid surface, they exhibit creeping or crawling movements
- Two to more than a hundred flagella, called axial fibrils, periplasmic flagella or endoflagella, extend from both ends of the cylinder and often overlap one another in the center of the cell.
- The whole complex of periplasmic Flagella, the axial filament, lies inside a flexible outer sheath.
- The outer sheath contains lipid, protein and carbohydrate and varies in structure between different genera. Its precise function is unknown, but the sheath is essential because spirochetes die if it is damaged or removed
- The outer sheath of *Treponema pallidum* has few proteins exposed on its surface. This allows the syphilis spirochete to avoid attack by host antibodies.
- The way in which periplasmic Flagella propel the cell has not been fully established
- Mutants with straight rather than curved flagella are Nonmotile
- The periplasmic flagella rotate like the external Plagella of other sheath to rotate and move the cell through the surrounding liquid.
- Flagellar rotation may also flex or bend the cell and account for the crawling movement seen on solid surfaces.
- Spirochetes can be anaerobic, facultatively anaerobic, or aerobic.
- Carbohydrates, amino acids, long chain fatty acids, and long chain fatty alcohols may serve as carbon and energy sources.
- Members of the genus spirochaeta are free-living and often grow in anoxic and sulfide-rich freshwater and marine environments.
- Some spirochetes form symbiotic associations with other organisms and are found in a variety of locations
    1. The hindguts of termites
    2. wood – eating cockroaches
    3. the digestive tracts of mollusks (*cristespia*) and mammals
    4. the oral cavities of animals (*Treponema denticola, T. oralis*)

Spirochetes from termite hindguts and freshwater sediments have nitrogenase and can fix nitrogen. They contribute significantly to the nitrogen nutrition of termites. Spirochaetes coat the surfaces of many protozoa from termite and wood – eating cockroach hindguts.

Bergey's Manual divides the phylum spirochaetes into one class, one order (spirochaetales), and three families (spirochaetaceae, serpulinaceae, leptospiraceae). At present, there are 13 genera in the phylum.

Table 2.5 Characteristics of Spirochete Genera

Genus	Oxygen relationship	Carbon source + energy	Habitates
Spirochaeta	Facultatively anaerobic or anaerobic	Carbohydrates	Aquatic and free – living
Cristispira	Facultatively anaerobic anaerobic or microaerophilic	N.A	Mollusk digestive track
Treponema	Anaerobic or microaerophilic	Carbohydrates or amino acids	Mouth, intestianal track , and genital areas of animals, some are pathogenic (syphilis, yaws)
Borrelia	Anaerobic or microaerophilic	Carbohydrates	Mammals and arthropods pathogens (rlapsing fever, lyme disease)
Leptospira	Aerobic	Fatty acids and alcohol	Free – living or pathogens of mammals, usually located in the kidney (leptospirosis)
Leptonema	Aerobic	Fatty acids	Mammals
Brachyspira	Anaerobic	N.A	Mammalian intestinal tract
Serpulina	Anaerobic	Carbohydrates and amino acids	Mammalian intestinal tract.

2. Rickettsias

Most of these tiny, non motile, Gram-negative bacteria are obligate parasites, able to grow only within host cells.

Table 2.6 Characteristics of Rickettsias

Property	Rickettsias
Nucleic acid, DNA or RNA	Both
Multiplication by binary fission	Yes
Cell wall contain muramic acid	Yes
Ribosomes are present	Yes
Contain metabolically active enzymes	Yes
Inhibited by antibacterial drugs	Yes
Synthesize ATP as a source of energy	Yes

Rickettsia

Genus: Rickettsia

Order: Rickettsiales

Family: Rickettsiaceae

- These bacteria are rod shaped, coccoid or pleomorphic with typical Gram – negative walls and no flagella.
- Although their size varies, they tend to be very small

For example

Rickettsia is 0.3 to 0.5 μm in diameter and 0.8 to 2.0 μm long.

- All species are parasitic or mutualistic.
- The parasitic forms grow in vertebrate erythrocytes,
- The parasitic forms grow in vertebrate erythrocytes, macrophages and vascular endothelial cells. Often they live in macrophages and vascular endothelial cells. Often they also live in blood-sucking arthropods such as fleas, ticks, mites or lice, which serve as vector or as primary hosts.
- Rickettsias enter the host cell by inducing phagocytosis.
- Members of the genus Rickettsia immediately escape the phagosome and reproduce by binary fission in the cytoplasm.
- Rickettsias are very different from most other bacteria in physiology and metabolism.
- They lack glycolytic pathways and donot use glucose as an energy source, but rather oxidize glutamate and tricaboxylic acid cycle intermediates such as succinate.
- The rickettsial plasma membrane has carrier mediated transport systems, and host cell nutrients and coenzymes are absorbed and directly used.
- For example, rickettsias take up both NAD^+ and vridine diphosphate glucose.
- Their membrane also has an adenylate exchange carrier that exchanges ADP for external ATP. Thus host ATP may provide much of the energy needed for growth.
- This metabolic dependence explains why many of these organisms must be cultivated in the yolksacs of chick embryos or in tissue culture cells.
- Genome sequencing shows that *Rickettsia prowazekii* is similar in many ways to mitochondria.
- Possibly mitochondria arose from an endosymbiotic association with an ancestor of Rickettsia.

Rickettsia prowazekii – typhus fever

Rickettsia typhi – typhus fever

Rickettsia rickettsii – Rocky mountain spotted fever.

Rickettsia rickettsii – Rocky mountain spotted fever.

- Rickettsias are also important pathogens of domestic animals such as dogs, horses, sheep and cattle.

The order Rickettsiales (Fig. 2.16)

This order contains rickettsias which have a more complex metabolism that allows them to synthesize ATP.

- Lacking a complex development cycle.

Rickettsias are associated with various arthropods which may serve as major hosts or which can act as vectors for transmission of the rickettsias to vertebrates. Those rickettsias which are capable of multiplying within vertebrates grow within the reticuloendothelial cells, vascular endothelial cells, or erythrocytes of these animals.

The Family Rickettsiaceas

This family consists of small rod-shaped or coccoid rickettsias which are often pleomorphic. The family is subdivided into three tribes on the following basis

The tribe Rickettsieae – pathogenic for humans

The tribe Ehrlichieae – pathogenic for vertebrate hosts other than humans.

The tribe wolbachieae – Not pathogenic for vertebrates, infect arthropods only.

Rickettsieae contains three genera, which are described as follows

- Rickettsia
- Rochalimaea
- Coxiella

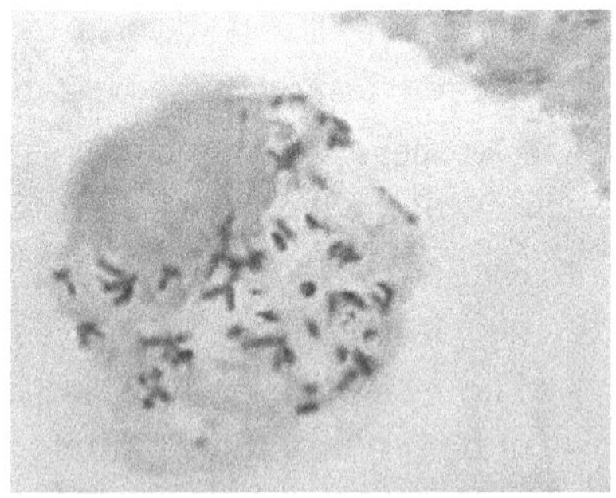

Fig. 2.16 Rickettsia rickettsii

3. Actinobacteria

- The phylum Actinobacteria is large and very complex, it contains one class (Actinobacteria), five subclasses, six orders, 14 sub orders and 44 families.
- Actinobacteria or Actinomycetes are a group of Gram – bacteria with high G + C ratio.
- The actinomycetes are a fascinating group of microoraganisms
- They are the source of most of the antibiotics used in medicine today.
- They also produce metabolites that are used as anticancer drugs, antihelminthics and drugs that suppress the immune system in patients who have received organ transplants.

Life Cycle of Actinobacteria

- The life cycle of many actinomycetes includes the development of filamentous cells, called hyphae, and spores.
- When growing on a solid substratum such as soil or agar, the actionomycetes develop a branching network of hyphae.
- The hyphae grow both on the surface of the substratum and into it to form a dense mat of hyphae termed as substrate mycelium.

Septae usually divide the hyphae into long cells (20 μm and longer) containing several nucleoids.

In many actinomycetes, substrate hyphae differentiate into upwardly growing hyphae to form an aerial mycelium that extends above the substratum. It is at this stage medically useful compounds are formed.

The aerial hyphae form thin-walled spores upon septation. These spores are considered exospores because they do not develop within a mother cell like the endospores of bacillus and clostridium.

If the spores are located in a sporangium, they may be called sporangiospores.

Actinomycete sporulation is usually in response to nutrient deprivation.

Most actinomycete spores are not particularly heat resistant but can withstand desiccation.

Cell Wall Composition of Actinobacteria

Four major cell wall types can be distinguished according to three features of peptidoglycan composition and structure are shown in Table 2.7.

1. The amino acid in tetrapeptide side chain
2. The presence of glycine in interpeptide bridges
3. Preptidoglycan sugar content

Table 2.7 Actinomycete cell wall types

Cell wall type	Diaminopimelic acid isomer	Glycine in Interpeptide bridges	Characteristic Sugars	Representative Genera
I	L, L	+	NA	Nocardioides Streptomyces
II	Meso	+	NA	Micromonospora, Pilimelia, Actinoplanes
III	Meso	–	NA	Actinomadura, Frankia
IV	Meso	–	Arabinose, galactose	Saccharomonosp ora, Nocardia

Importance of Actinobacteria

They are primarily soil inhabitants and are very widely distributed.

They can degrade an enormous number and variety of organic compounds and are extremely important in the mineralization of organic matter.

Phylum = Actinobacteria

Class = Actinobacteria

Actinobacteria or actinomycetes are a group of Gram-positive bacteria with high G+C ratio.

Characteristics

They include some of the most common soil life, playing an important role in decomposition of organic materials, such as cellulose and chitin and thereby playing a vital part in organic matter turnover and carbon cycle. This replenishes the supply of nutrients in the soil and is an important part of humus formation. Other Actinobacteria inhabit plants and animals, including a few pathogens, such as *Mycobacterium, Corynebacterium, Nocardia, Rhodococcus and a few species of Streptomyces.*

Actinobacteria are well known as secondary metabolite producers and hence of high pharmacological and commercial interest. In 1940 Selman Waksman discovered that the soil bacteria he was studying made actinomycin, a discovery which granted him a Nobel Prize. Since then hundreds of naturally occurring antibiotics have been discovered in these terrestrial micro-organisms, especially from the genus Streptomyces shown in Fig. 2.17.

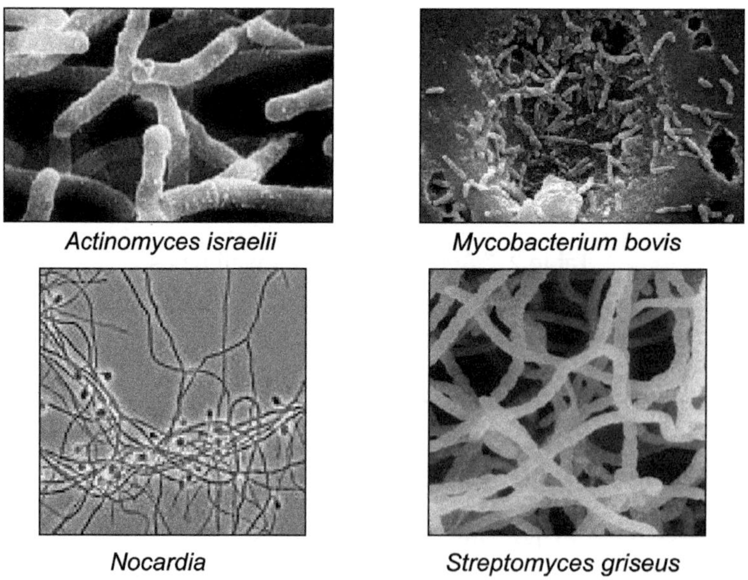

Fig. 2.17 Actinomeyetes

Some Actinobacteria form branching filaments, which somewhat resemble the mycelia of the unrelated fungi, among which they were originally classified under the older name Actinomycetes. Most members are aerobic, but a few, such as *Actinomyces israelii*, can grow under anaerobic conditions. Unlike the Firmicutes, the other main group of Gram-positive bacteria, have DNA with a high GC – content and some Actinomycetes species produce external spores.

Some types of Actinobacteria are responsible for the peculiar odor emanating from the soil after rain, mainly on warmer climates.

Genera

Most Actinobacteria of medical or economic significance are in subclass Actinobacteridae, order Actinomycetales. While many of these cause disease in humans, *Streptomyces* is notable as a source of antibiotics. Examples of organisms in this order include:

- Suborder Actinomycineae
- Family Actinomycetaceae
- Actinomyces
- Family Propionibacteriaceae
- Propionibacterium
- Family Frankiaceae
- Frankia
- Family Micrococcaceae
- Arthrobacter
- Micrococcus
- Family Micromonosporaceae
- Micromonospora
- Family Streptomycetaceae
- Streptomyces
- Suborder Corynebacterineae
- Family Mycobacteriaceae
- Mycobacterium
- Family Corynebacteriaceae
- Corynebacterium
- Family Nocardiaceae
- Nocardia

Of those Actinobacteria not in Actinomycetales, *Gardnerella* is one of the most researched. Classification of *Gardnerella* is controversial, and MeSH catalogues it as both a gram-positive and gram-negative organism.

Genomes of 44 different strains of Actinobacteria from different genera are either already sequenced or underway right now. The Actinobacteria of medical and economic importance are in the subclass Actinobacteridae, order Actinomycetales. These bacteria are identified in damp indoor environments.

4. Archaeobacteria

Archaea are prokaryotic cells

Unlike the bacteria and the eukarya, the archaea have membranes composed of branched hydrocarbon chains attached to glycerol by ether linkages.

The cell wall of Archaea contains no peptidoglycan.

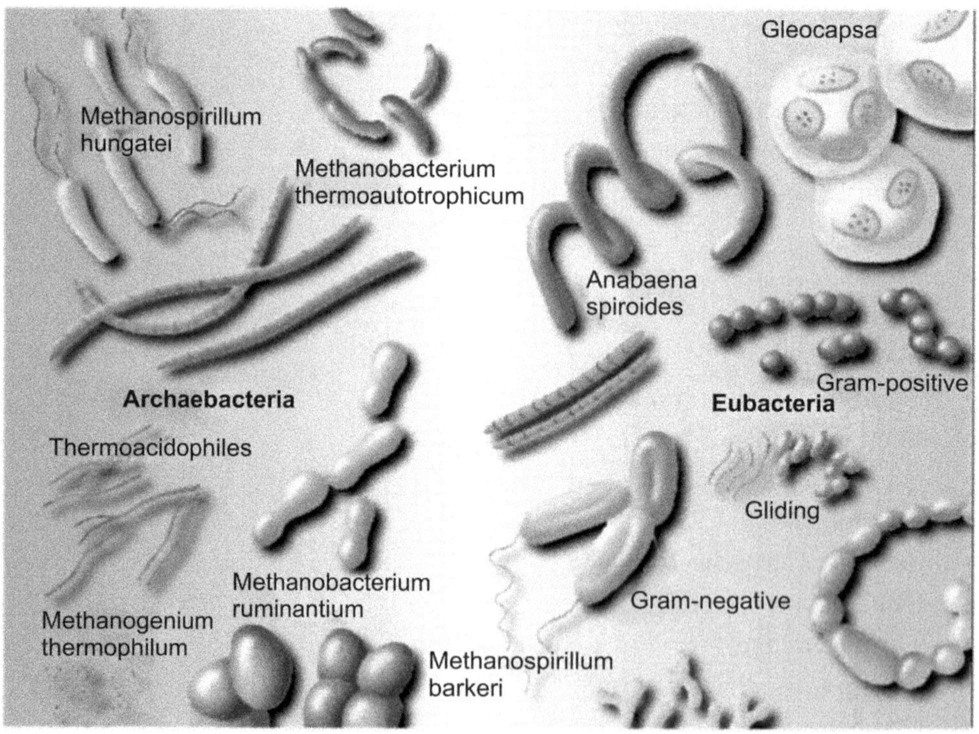

Fig. 2.18 Archaebacteria figures

Archaea are not sensitive to some antibiotics that affect bacteria but are sensitive to some antibiotics that affect eukarya.

Archaea contain r-RNA that is unique to the archaea as indicated by the presence of molecular regions distinctly different from r-RNA of bacteria and eukarya shown in Fig. 2.18.

Archaea more closely related to eukarya than bacteria.

Archaea are a major group of bacteria that include methanogens, the red extreme halophiles and the thermoacidophiles and which diverged from other bacteria at a very early stage in evolution. They are also called as archaebacteria.

Ether containing linkages in the Archaea membrane is more stable than ester containing linkages in the bacteria and eukarya.

Methanogenic bacteria: They are anaerobic and they obtain energy by oxidizing H_2 or formate and utilize the electrons generated to reduce CO_2 with the formation of methane gas.

Some grow as autotrophs using H_2 and CO_2 as sources of carbon and energy, where as others require substances like vitamins, acetate, Aminoacids or organic sulphur compounds.

- Most of them grow in complex media
- They contain two coenzymes
  1. Co-enzyme M: involved in methyl transfer reactions
  2. Co-enzyme F_{420}: involved in anaerobic electron transport system of these bacteria.
- They can be observed by flrorescence microscope
- They occur in anaerobic habits rich in organic matter

E.g., Marshes, swamps, ponds, marine sediments, the intestinal tract of humans and animals.

Extreme Halophiles: They are aerobic and require NaCl for good growth. They are rod shaped cells.

- They occurs in salt lakes, industrial plants that produce salt and salted fish
- Their colonies are red to orange color due to carotenoids
- At high NaCl concentrations they resist dehydration by maintaining high intracellular osmotic concentration of KCl.
- Cytoplasmic membrane and ribosomes are stable only at high concentrations of KCl where as enzymes are active only high levels of KCl or NaCl.
- Halobacterium cell wall is composed of protein subunits that are held together only in presence of salt and if the salt level is less than 10% cell lyses.

Halobacteria are aerobic and synthesize ATP by 3 methods:

1. By electron transport chain
2. By fermenting aminoacid arginine
3. By bleaching bacteriorhodopsin pigment formed in cell membrane at low oxygen levels.

Table 2.8 Phenotypic properties of Bacteria and Archaea compared with Eucarya

	Property	Eucarya	Bacteria	Archaea
1.	Cell configuration	eucaryotic	procaryotic	prokaryotic
2.	Nuclear membrane	present	absent	absent
3.	Number of chromosomes	>1	1	1
4.	Chromosome topology	linear	circular	circulat
5.	Murein in cell wall	–	+	–
6.	Cell membrane lipids	Ester. Linked Glycerides, unbranched; polyunsaturated	Ester- linked glycerides; unbranched; saturated (or) monounsaturated	ether – linked, branched; saturated
7.	Cell membrane sterols	present	absent	absent
8.	Organells (mitochondria of chloroplast)	present	absent	absent
9.	Ribosome size	80s (cytoplasmic)	70s	70s
10.	Cytoplasmic streaming	+	–	–
11.	Meiosis and mitosis	present	absent	absent
12.	Transcription and translation coupled	–	+	+
13.	Amino acid initiating protein synthesis	methionine	N. formyl methionine	Methionine
14.	Protein synthesis inhibited by Streptomycin or chloramphenicol	–	+	–
15.	Protein synthesis inhibited by diphtheria toxin	+	–	

2.6 Fungi

Diversity in Kingdom Fungi

There are an extremely large number of fungi that dwell in the world today. Hawksworth (1997) conducted an investigation in which he compared fungal species figures with other groups obtained from ecological regions that had been deeply researched for their biodiversity. These studies led to the conclusion that there were near 1.5 million species of fungi worldwide (Hawksworth, 2001).

As per the literature available approximately 98,000 fungal species have been described, and the majority being members of the Ascomycota (about 64,000 known species) and the Basidiomycota (about 32,000 known species), meaning there is still around 95% of the fungi population that remain undescribed.

Fungi: The fungi are a group of eukaryotic organisms; they are of microscopic cellular dimensions. Fungus is singular form for Fungi which lack chlorophyll and are usually filamentous. They contain a mold or yeast.

Fungi are eukaryotic spore bearing protists that lack chlorophyll. These are of great practical and scientific interest to microbiologists. Fungi consists of yeasts and molds.

Molds: Molds consist of long, branching filaments of cells called hyphae. A tragled mass of hyphae among cells of the hyphae are interrupted by cross walls. These fungi are said to be coemocytic fungi. These fungi that have cross walls are called septate fungi, since the cross walls are called septa.

Examples of common molds are *Acremonium*, *Alternaria*, *Aspergillus*, *Cladosporium*, *Fusarium*, *Mucor*, *Penicillium*, *Rhizopus*, *Stachybotrys,* and *Trichoderma*.

Yeasts are a kind of fungi that are unicellular and lack typical mycelia. Yeasts producing daughter cells either by budding (the **budding yeasts**) or by binary fission (the **fission yeasts**). They differ from most fungi, which grow as thread-like hyphae. But this distinction is not a fundamental one, because some fungi can alternate between a yeast phase and a hyphal phase, depending on environmental conditions. Such fungi are termed **dimorphic** (with two shapes) and they include several (Pathogens) that cause disease of humans.

The common baker's yeast, ***Saccharomyces cerevisiae*** the genus ***Cryptococcus***, which includes *C. neoformans*, a pathogen of humans the dimorphic fungus ***Candida albicans*** which can be a significant pathogen of humans some of the common leaf surface yeasts. The yeast cell or mold filament is surrounded by a true cell wall.

2.6.1 Characteristics of Fungi

Fungi are eukaryotic chemo organotrophic organisms that have no chlorophyll.

The thallus or body of a fungus may consist of a single cell as in the yeasts; more importantly the thallus consists of filaments, 5-10 μm across, which are commonly branched.

The fungi are placed in the kingdom called Myceteae. The subdivisions of this kingdom have endings as:

Division	:	mycota
Sub Division	:	mycotina
Class	:	mycetes
Sub class	:	mycetidae
Order	:	ales
Family	:	aceae

Slime molds: Slime molds have morphological similarity of both fungi and protozoa. They are of two types:

1. Cellular slime molds 2. Acellular slime molds

Cellular slime molds are composed of single amoeba – like cells, while acellular slime molds are naked masses of protoplasm of indefinite size and shape called plasmodia. They live on decaying plant matter and soil and take their food by engulfing bacteria (phagocytosis). The cellular slime mold is *Dictyostelin*, while acellular is *plasmodium*.

When they feed on dead organic matter, they are known as saprophytes and decompose complex plant and animal remains, breaking them down into simpler chemical substances that are returned to soil for increasing fertility.

Saprophytic fungi are also important in industrial fermentation for e.g: brewing of beer, making of wine and production of antibiotics such as penicillin.

As parasites, fungi cause disease in plants, humans and other animals.

Morphology: Yeast cells are larger than most bacteria, and vary size considerably from

1-5 μm in width and 5-30 μm or more in length.

They are commonly egg-shaped but some are elongated and some spherical.

Yeasts have no flagella or other organelles of locomotion.

The thallus of a mold consists essentially of two parts – the mycelium and the spores

The mycelium is a complex of several filaments called hyphae.

New hyphae generally arise from a spore which on germination puts out a germ tube.

Each hyphae is about 5–10 μm wide.

The yeast cell or mold filament is surrounded by a true cell wall.

Some fungi are dimorphic i.e. they exists in two forms.

The fungi are heterotrophic organisms they require organic compounds for nutrition.

When they feed on dead organic matter, they are Saprophytes which decompose complex plant and animal remains, breaking them down into simpler chemical substances that are returned to the soil, thereby increasing soil fertility shown in Fig. 2.19.

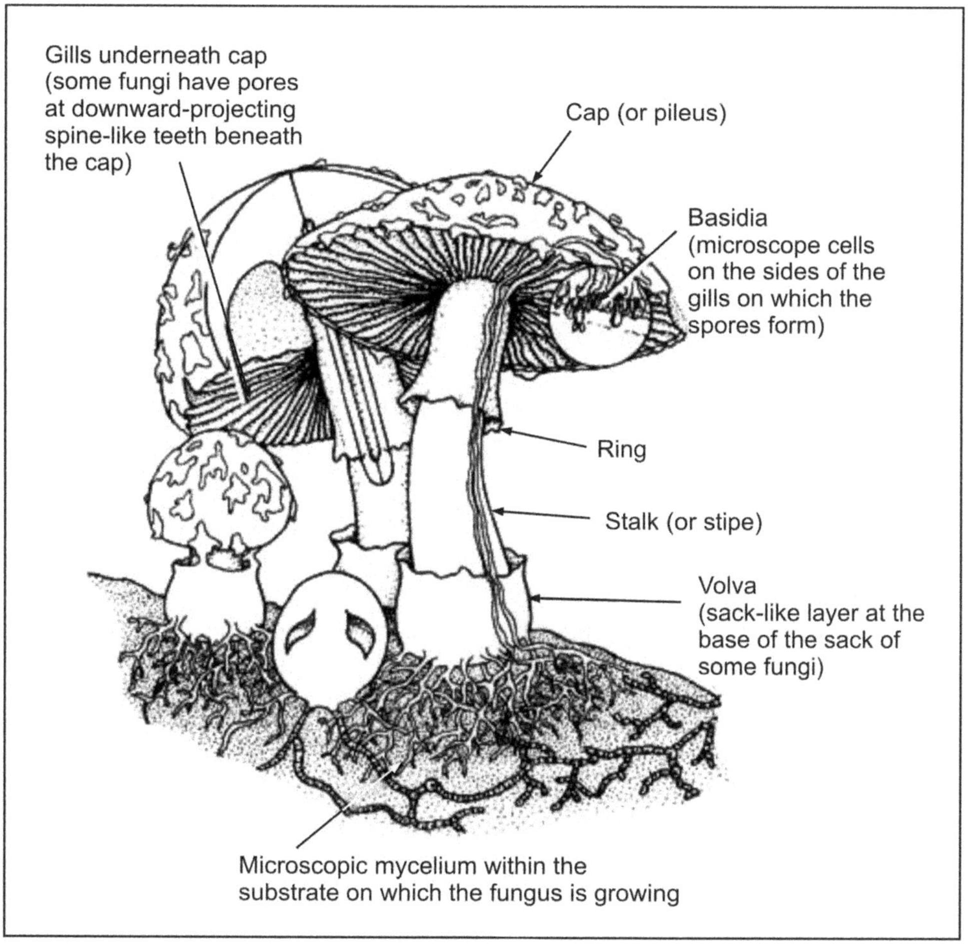

Fig. 2.19 Fungi of basidiomycetes group (Mushrooms)

Saprophytic fungi are also important in industrial fermentations: for example, the brewing of beer, the making of wine, and the production of antibiotics such as pencillin etc.

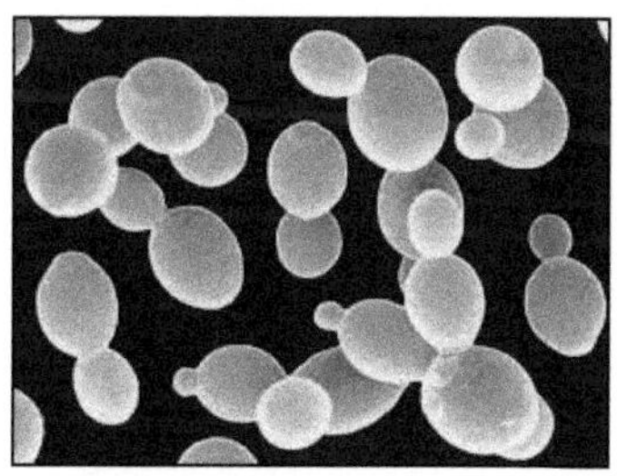

Fig. 2.20 Yeasts

2.6.2 Cell Biology of the Fungi (Hyphal Tip Structure)

Septate Hypae

Their basic cellular unit is described as hypha. This is usually a tubular cell which is surrounded by a rigid, chitin –containing cell wall. The hypha extends by tip growth, and multiplies by branching, creating a fine network called a mycelium. Hyphae contain nuclei, mitochondria, ribosomes, golgi and membrane-bound vesicles within a plasma-membrane bound cytoplasm. The sub-cellular structures are supported, and organized, by micro-tubules and endoplasmic retitulum shown in Fig. 2.20.

Not all fungi are multicellular; some are uni cellular and are termed yeast ; these grow by binary fission or budding creating new individuals from the parent cell.

2.6.3 Structure and Physiology of Fungi

There is considerable variation in the structures, size, and complexity of various fungae species. For example, fungi include the microscopic yeasts; the molds grow on contaminated bread, and the common mushrooms.

Nutrition: Fungi grow best where there is a rich supply of organic matter. Most fungi are saprobic. Since they lack photosynthetic pigments, fungi cannot perform photosynthesis and must obtain their nutrients from performed organic matter. They are chemoheter tropic organisms. Fungi store glycogen for their energy needs and glucose and maltose for immeadiate energy metabolism.

Most fungi grow at an acidic pH of about 5.6. Although some species grow at lower and higher pH, most fungi grow at about 25 °C except for pathogens, which grow at 37 °C.

Most yeast and molds can grow in high concentrations of sugar that inhibit most bacteria. Maida spoil jellies and jams because of high sugar concentrations withstanding property. Molds and many types of yeast are usually aerobic but some yeast can grow under both aerobic and anaerobic conditions.

Saprophytic fungi grow at 22-30 °C and grow slowly than bacteria

Pathogenic fungi grow at 30-37 °C

Fungi which spoil foods in the cold storage grow at °C

Fungi are heterotrophic, the carbon must come from an organic source, such as glucose and nitrogen from inorganic and organic nitrogen source can be utilized. All fungi can use organic nitrogen that is why the culture media for fungi usually contain peptone.

Sabouraud's media is the best-known fungal media which contains Per liter of medium:

Peptone, 10 g Glucose, 40 g Agar, 15 g.

2.6.4 Fungal Metabolism

Fungi prefer moist habitats and they are largely mesophyllic, preferring temperature between 15 °C and 35 °C. The carbon needs of fungi for energy metabolism and biosynthesis has to be met heterotrophically by one of three life styles:

(a) Parasitism of plants or animals (causing disease)

(b) Saprophytism, growing on dead animal, plant or microbial biomass

(c) Saprophytism, growing together with algae, plants or insects soluble carbohydrates must enter hyphae by diffusion, and this is followed by active up take across the fungal membrane. For the saprophytic fungi most carbon in the environment is present as a complex polymer like cellulose, chitin or lignin. These materials must be broken down enzymically before they can be utilized. Therefore fungi release degradative enzymes into their environments in including cellulases, chitinases, proteases and multi- component lignin degrading enzymes, depending on the type of substrate the fungus is growing on. Regulation of these enzymes is by substance-induction and end-product inhibition. Most fungal carbohydrate metabolism is via glycolysis and the tricarboxylic acid cycle, although both fermentative pathways and anaerobic pathways have been found in specialized fungi.

Fungi cannot fix gaseous nitrogen. They can however utilize nitrate, ammonia and some amino acids by direct uptake across the hyphal membrane. More complex nitrogen sources, such as proteins and peptides, can be utilized, once extracellular proteases have degraded them into amino acids. Fungi require both macro and micronutrients, but these are usually available to excess in their environments, and some fungi may have other requirements, for example thiamin and biotin, sterols, riboflavin, nicotinic acid and folic acid.

Fungi are capable of the formation and secretion of many types of secondary metabolities. These compounds can be produce by many different metabolic pathways.

2.6.5 Classification Taxonomic Groups in Fungi

Organisms formerly classified as fungi

Several interesting points can be brought up to clarify the identity of the 'true' fungi:

(i) ***Hyphochytriomycota, Labyrinthulomycota*** and ***Oomycota***, three groups of organisms traditionally studied by mycologists have been placed in an entirely new kingdom, the kingdom **Chromista** (or kingdom **Stramenopiles**), because the structural, biochemical, physiological and molecular data, has contributed to the knowledge that, they are so phylogenetically far from the kingdom fungi.

(ii) The ***Oomycota*** group e.g, *Saprolegniales* (water molds) and *Peronosporales*, have been placed in the family Xanthophyceae, a group of algae in which the hyphal form is common. Though Oomycota contains many serious plant pathogens, resemble fungi, being composed of hyphae and in their absorptive nutrition but differ in fundamental and biochemical features including cellulose-based walls and biochemical features resembling those of plants. So it is likely that they arose in the Precambrian era from the ***Xanthophyceae***, a group of algae in which the hyphal form is common.

(iii) The ***Acrasid*** and ***Dictyostelid*** slime molds (**cellular slime molds**) and the ***Myxomycota*** (**plasmodial slime molds**) are classified within the "Kingdom" of protists (Protoctista) that includes all the small organisms those posess nuclei - the amoebae, protozoa, algae, slime molds, etc. Since both groups form fungus-like fruiting bodies to release air-borne spores, indicating this is the reason why they were once treated as fungi.

Little information is known on the ***Plasmodiophoromycota***, possibly intracellular parasites of fungi, algae and some higher plants. They can form highly persistent thick-walled resting spores, maybe a reason for the confusion with fungi.

The origin of the fungi appears to be very ancient. They first appear in the fossil record coincidentally with the appearance of the land plants. This was in the Devonian period 400 million years ago.

Fungi are more closely related to animals than to plants and are placed with the animals in the monophyletic group of opisthokonts analyses using molecular phylogentics support a monophyletic origin of the fungi. The taxonomy of the fungi is in a state of constant flux, especially due to recent research based on DNA comparisions.

These current phylogenetic analyses often overturn classifications based on older and sometimes less discriminative methods based on morphological features and biological species concepts obtained from experimental matings

The 2007 classification of kingdom fungi is the result of a large-scale collaborative research effort involving dozens of mycologists and other scientists working on fungus taxonomy. It recognizes seven phyla, two of which – A the Ascomycota and the Basidiomycota are contained within a branch representing sub kingdom dikarya. The below cladogram depicts the major fungal taxa and their relationship to opisthokont and unikont organisms. The lengths of the branches in this tree are not proportional to evolutionary distances.

(i) ***Zygomycota*:** Members of the division zygomycota are known as zygomyctes. Zygomycetes produce sexual spores known as zygospores as well as asexual sporangiospores. A familiar member of the division is rhizopus stolonifer, a fungus found on fruits, vegetables, and breads. It is the familiar bread mold. It anchors itself to the substraction with special hyphae known as rhizoids. Rhizopus is used in the industrial production of steroids, meat tenderizers, industrial chemicals, and certain coloning agents. Some e.g. of this class – mucor, schizo saccharomyes, saccharomyces.

(ii) ***Ascomycota*:** The *Ascomycota*, commonly known as sac fungi or ascomycetis constitute the largest taxonomic group within the eumycota. These fungi form meiotic spores called ascospores, which are enclosed in a special sac-like structure called an ascus. This phulum includes morels, a few mushrooms and truffles, single-celled yeasts (e.g. of the genera saccharomyces, kluyveromyces, pichia, and candiada), and many filamentous fungi living as saprotrophs, parasites, and mutualistic symbionts. Prominent and important genera of filamentous ascomyctes include aspergullus, penicillium, fusarium and claviceps. members of the division ascomycota are referred to as ascomycetes. After sexual fusion of cells has taken place, these organisms form their sexual spores within a sac called an ascus. Therefore, they are called sac fungi. E.g. of this class – *neurospora*

(iii) ***Basidiomycota*:** The *Blastoladiomycota* were previously considered a taxonomic clade within the chytridiomycota. Recent molecular data and ultra structural characteristics, however, place the *Blastocladiomycota* as a sister clade to the zygomycota, glomermycata, and *Dikarya* (*Ascomycota* and *Basidiomycota*). The blastocladiomycetes are saprotrophus feeding on decomposing organic matter, and they are parasites of all eukaryotic groups.

(iv) Members of the division basidiomycota referred to **abasidiomycetes** and are called club fungi. After the sexual cells have united, they under go division and produce a club shipped structure called a basidium. Sexually produced basidiospores form at the tips of the basidia. Basidia are often found on huge visible fruiting bodies called basidiocarps. The typical mushroom is basidiocarp. e.g. *Agaricus, Filobasidiella neoformans*.

(v) ***Deuteromycota*:** Members of the deuteromycota division are called deuteromycotes. These fungi lack a known sexual cycle in reproduction and are said to be "imperfect" when its sexual cycle is discovered. A fungus from this division is usually reclassified in one of the other divisions. Among the imperfect fungi are the organisms of athlete's foot and ringworm.

E.g.: Aspergillus, Penicillium, Candida

(vi) ***Oomycota and Hyphochytriomycota*:** The phylum Oomycota comprises approximately 700 species. Cellulose and β-glucan are the main components of their cell walls. Some of them are virulent plant pathogens, while others are aquatic species and fish pathogens. Only a few members of this phylum, particularly species of *Phythophthora* and *Pythium*, have been the focus of molecular studies aimed at species level and below. *ythium insidiosum*, is an opportunistic pathogen in warm-blooded animals, it rarely causes infection in humans. *Rhinosporidium* *seeberi*, which belongs to the phylum Hyphochytriomycota, causes rhinosporidiosis in humans and is characterized by the formation of cysts in the subepithelial tissue of nasal mucosa.

(vii) ***Chytridiomycota*:** The chytridiomycota are commonly knowm as chytrids. These fungi are distributed world wide. Chytrids produce 300 spores that are capable of active movement through aqueous phages with a single flagellum, leading early taxonomists to classify them as protists. Molecular phylogenics, suggests that the chytrids are a basal group divergent from the other fungal phyla, consisting of four major clades with suggestive evidence for paraphyly, a possible polyphyly.

2.6.6 Reproduction in Fungi

Classification of Fungi is based more on morphological than physiological criteria.

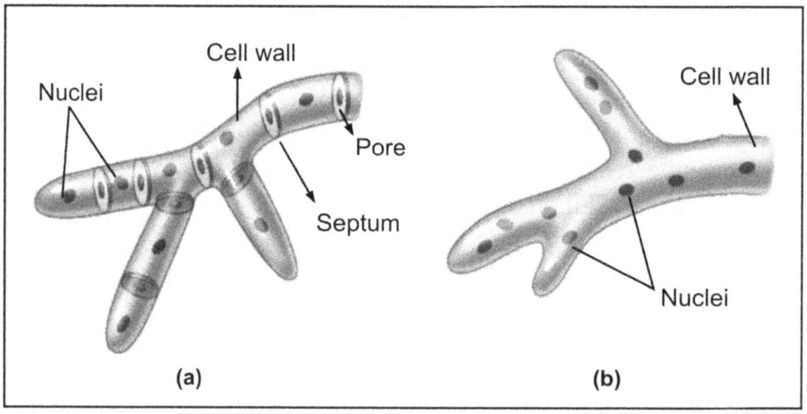

Fig. 2.21 **(a)** Septate hypha **(b)** Coenocytic hypha

For broader classification, the nature of sexual spores is important.

There are some fungi which do not produce sexual spores and exhibit a para sexual life cycles where there is no regular diploidization or meiosis.

Plasmogamy, karyogamy and haploidazation take place but not at specified points in the thallus.

When sexual life cycle is absent, the fungus perpetuate in its asexual state, i.e., anomorph.

Under some environmental conditions an occasional fungus belonging to this category may produce its perfect state or sexual life cycle (telemorph) and then occupies its correct place in the sexual cycle based classification.

An assemblage of unrelated fungi existing in their anamorphic state are now placed in the special class or form-class Deuteromycetes.

They are composed of an outer tube like wall surrounding a cavity, the lumen, which is filled by protoplasm.

The hyphal wall consists of micro fibrils composed for the most part of hemicelluloses or chitin.

Hyphae occur in three forms (Fig. 2.21)

1. Non-septate or coenocytic have no septa.
2. Septate with uni-nucleate cells.
3. Septate with multinucleate cells: Each cell has more than one nucleus in each compartment.

Reproduction in yeasts usually involves spores. Spores are produced by either sexual or asexual means.Fungi reproduce naturally by a variety of means.

Asexual Spores (Fig. 2.22)

Asexual spores occur in the fungi when spores form by mitosis. These spores can be conidia, sporangiospores, arthrosphores (fragments of hyphae) or chlamypdospores (spores with thick walls).

(i) ***Sporangiospores*****:** Sporangiospores are spores formed within the sporangium by formation of cheavage planes. They develop on the ends of branches or hyphae called sporangiophores. Aplanospores are nonmotile sporangiospores. Zoospores are motile sporangiospores, their motility being due to the presence of flagella.These are characteristic of lower fungi of the class zygomycetes, such as Rhizapus microsporus.

(ii) ***Conidiospores*** or conidia borne extremely on sides are naked spores. These are found in aspergillus, penicillium and the dermatophytes when the spores are small and single, they are called microconidia. Where as macroconidia are large and septate and are often multicellular.

(iii) ***Oidia*** (singular oidium) or arthrospores. These single-celled spores are formed by disjoining of hyphal cells.

(iv) ***Chlamydospores:*** These thick-walled, single-celled spores are highly resistant to adverse conditions. They are formed from cells of the vegetative hypha.

(v) ***Blastopsores:*** These are spores formed by budding.

(vi) ***Sexual Reproduction in Fungi*****:** It is carried out by fusion of the compatible nuclei of two parent cells.

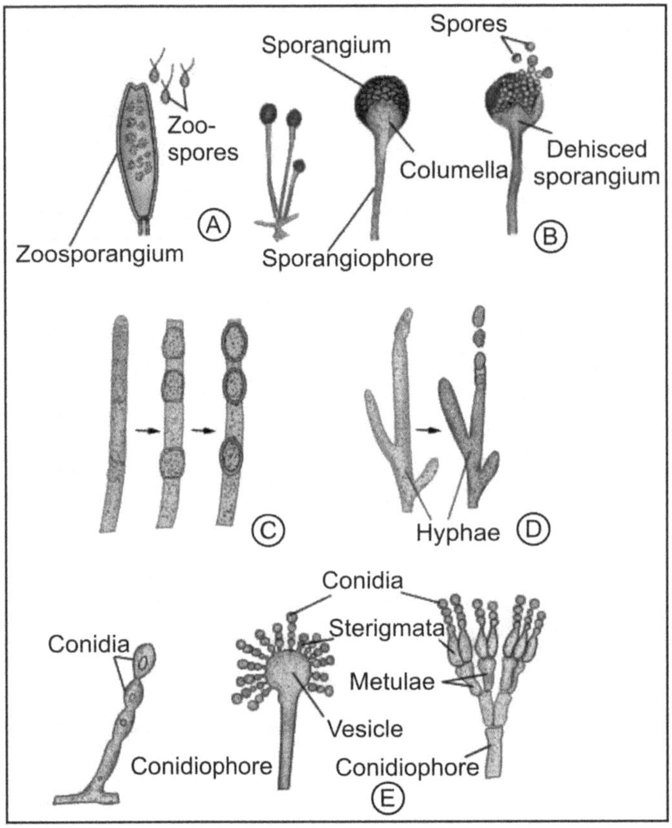

Fig. 2.22 Asexual spores in Fungi
(A) Zoospores
(B) Sporangiospores
(C) Chlamydospores (D) Oidia
(E) Conidia

This process begins with the joining of two cells and fusion of their protoplasts, thus enabling the two haploid nuclei of two mating types to fuse together to form a diploid nucleus.

This is followed by meiosis, which again reduces the number of chromosomes to the haploid number.

The sex organelles of fungi if present are called gametangia.

If the male and female gametangia are different morphologically, the male gametangia are called as antheridium and the female gametangium is called oogonium.

Various methods of sexual reproduction

1. ***Gametic copulation***: Fusion of naked gametes, one or both which are motile.
2. ***Gamete–gametangial copulation***: Two gametes come into contact but do not fuse.
   The male nucleus migrates through pore or fertilization tube into the female gametangium.

3. ***Gametangial copulation***: Two gametangia or their protoplasts fuse and give rise to a zygote that develops into a resting spore.
4. ***Somatic copulation***: Fusion of somatic vegetative cells.
5. ***Spermatization:*** Union of a special male structure called a spermatium with a female receptive structure.

The spermatium empties its contents into the latter during plasmogamy.

Sexual Spores (Fig. 2.23): Sexual spore are formed by fusion of protoplasm of two cells followed by the fusion of two nuclei (karyogamy) and meiosis as in all forms of higher life. The development of zygote and formation of sexual spores varies in different group of fungi. Sexual spores are of four types – Oospores, zygospores, ascospores and basidiospores.

(i) ***Ascospores***: These single-celled spores are produced in a sac called an ascus (plural, asci). There are usually eight ascospores in each ascus.

(ii) ***Basidiospores***: These single-celled spores are borne on a club-shaped structure called a basidium (plural, basidia).

(iii) ***Zygospores***: Zygospores are large, thick-walled spores formed when the tips of two sexually compatible hyphae, are gametangia, of certain fungi fuse together.

(iv) ***Oospores***: These are formed within a special female structure, the oogonium. Fertilization of the eggs, or oopheres, by male gamets formed in an antheridium gives rise to oospores. There are one or more oospheres in each oogonium.

A single fungus may produce **both asexual and sexual spores** by different methods at different times and under different conditions. The spores produced are constant in their structures and in the method by which they are produced. These constant structures are used to identification and classification.

There are one or more oospheres in each organism.

Asexual and sexual spores may be surrounded by highly organised protective structures called fruiting bodies.

Asexual fruiting bodies have names as acervulus and pycnidium.

Sexual fruiting bodies have names as perithecium and apothecium.

Any of numerous eukaryotic organisms of the kingdom fungi which lack chlorophyll and vascular tissue and range in form a single cell to a body mass of branched filamentous hyphae that often produce specialized fruiting bodies. The cells have their shape defined by a thick wall around the membrane, just like any plant, but the cell wall is not made of cellulosis, but of chitin the same substance found on insects exoskeleons. The kingdom includes the yeasts, molds, and mushrooms.

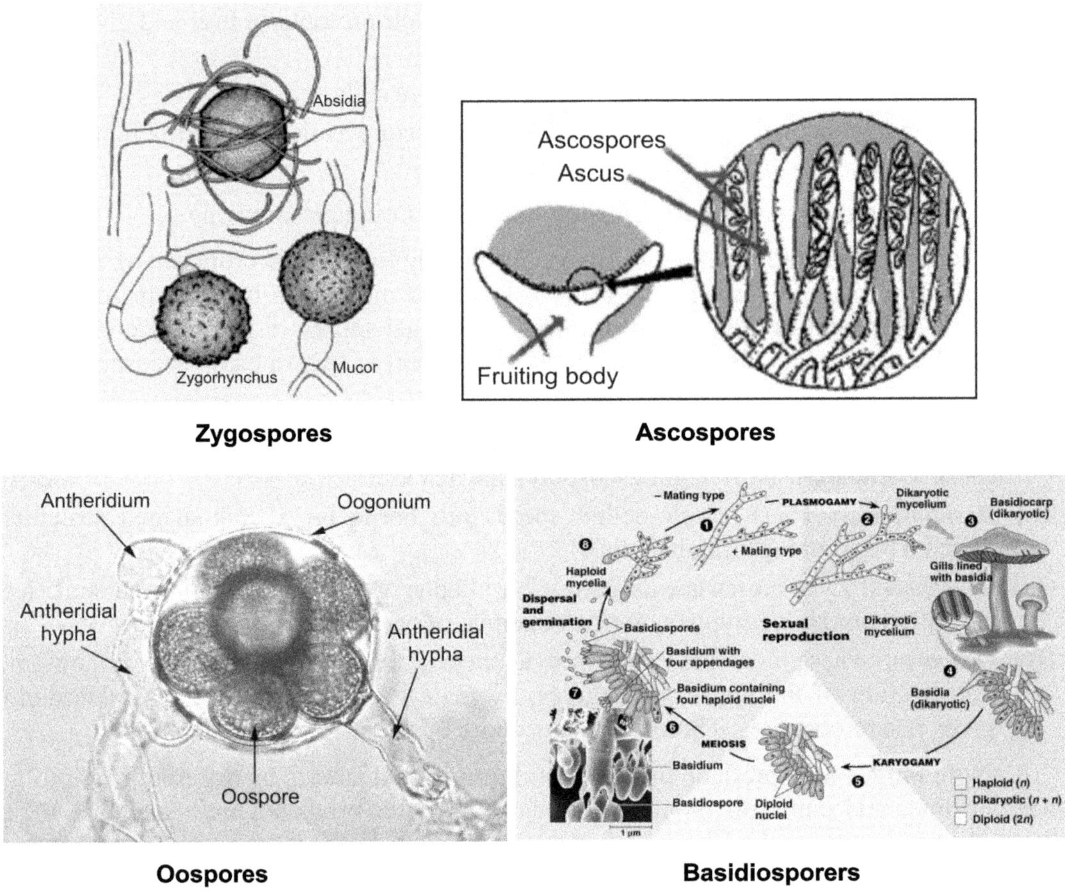

Fig. 2.23 Sexual spores in fungi

2.6.7 Economic Importance of Fungi

Hardly a day passes when we are not benefitted or harmed directly or indirectly by fungi. Fungi include hundreds of species which are of tremendous economic importance to mass. In fact our lives are intimately linked with those of fungi. They play an important role in medicine yielding antibiotics. In agriculture by maintaining the fertility of the soil and causing crop and fruit diseases, some of the fungi particularly molds and yeasts play a negative role by causing spoilage and stored goods such as foods stuffes, timber, textiles, leather and rubber. Various roles of fungi have mentioned below.

Role of Fungi as Food and as Food Producers

About 2000 species of edible fungi have been reported from all over the world of these about 250 species are said to occur in the western Himalayas. The fructification of some fungi such as the field mushroom (*Agaricus campestris*), podascon padaxis, the puff balls (*Lycoperdon* and *Claviata excipulformis*), *morels* (*morchellia*) and *truffles* are edible. Bakers yeast or *Saccharomyces cerevisiae,* a single-celled fungus is used to make bread and other wheat-based products, such as pizza dough and dumplings. Yeast species of the genus *Saccharomyces* are also used to produce alcoholic beverages through fermentaion.

Role of Fungi in Medicines

Certain fungi produce biochemical substances which help to cure diseases caused by the pathogenic micro-organisms. The substances are called antibiotics. The most important antibiotic is produced by the bacteria, moulds and actinomycotes. They are used to combat evil effects of pathogenic bacteria and viruses.

The role of fungi in producing antibiotic substances was first established by sir Alexander Fleming in 1929 extracted the great antibiotic drug penicillin from *Penicillium notatum*. Penicillin was the first antibiotic to be widely used. It has no adverse effect on human protoplasm but kills bacteria especially Gram-positive type. Penicillium is now produced on a commercial scale from the improved stains of *Penicillium notatum &.P. chrysogenum.*

Streptomycin is obtained from *Streptomyces griseus*. This antibiotic is of great value in medicine. It destroys many organisms which are not killed by penicillium particularly the Gram-negative organisms.

Certain mushrooms enjoy usage as therapeutics in folk-medicines, such as traditional Chinese medicine. Notable medicinal mushrooms with a well-documented history of use include *Agaricus subrufescens*, *Granoderma bucidum* and *Ophiocordyceps sinensis.* Research has identified compounds produced by these and other fungi that have inhibitory biological effects against viruses and cancer cells.

Bioremediation

Certain fungi in particular 'which rot' fungi, can degrade insecticides, herbicides, pentachlirphenol, creosote, cool tars, and heavy fuels and turn them into CO_2, water, and basic elements. Fungi have been shown to biomineralize uranium oxides, suggesting they may have application in the bioremediation of radio activity polluted sites.

Pest control

In agriculture, fungi may be useful if they actively competete for nutrients and space with pathogenic molds such as bacteria or other fungi via the competitive exclusion priniciple, or if they are parasites of those pathogens. For example certain species may be used to eliminate or suppress the growth of harmful plant pathogens, such as insect, mites, weeds, nematodes and other fungi that cause disease of important crop plants. This has generated strong interest in practical applications that use fungi in the biological control of these agricultural pests. Entomopathogenic can be used as biopesticides, as they actively kill insects. Examples that have been used as biological insectiecides are '*Beauveria bassiana*, *Metarhizium* spp. *Hirsutella* spp, *Paecilomyces* (*Isaria*) spp., and *Lecamicillium lecanic*'. Endophytic fungi of grasses of the genus *Neotyphodium*, such as *N. coenophialum*, produce alkaloids that are toxic to a range of invertebrates and vertebrate herbivores. These alkaloids protect gross plant from herbivores, but several endophyte alkaloids can poison grazing animals, such as cattle and sheep, infecting cultivators of pastiive or forage grasses with *Neotyphodium endophytes* is one approach being used in gross breeding programs. The fungal strains are selected for producing only alkaloids that increase resistance to herbivores such as insects, which being non-toxic to livestock.

Enzyme Preparations

Takaminc on the basis of his intensive study of enzymes produced by the aspergillus *flavus* – oryzae series has introduced a few products of high enzymatic activity in the worlds market. These are taka diastase, digestion etc., they are used for dextrinization of desizing of textiles. Cultures of *Aspergillus niger* and A. oryzae on troys of moist, sterile bran produce a well known enzyme amylase which contains two starch splitting components.

Enzymes invertase is extracted from saccharomyces cericisvae. It has various industrial uses. It hydrolyses sucrose to a mixture of glucose and fructose.

Cheese Industry

Certain fungi popularly known as 'cheese molds' play an important role in the refining of cheese. They give cheese a characteristic texture and flavour examples include the blue colour in cheeses such as stallion or Roguefort, which are made by inoculation with panicillium roguefortic. Molds used in cheese production are non-toxic and are thus safe for human consumption.

Vitamins

The yeasts are the best source of vitamins B – complex. A number of preparations of high potency have been made from the dried yeast or yeast extracts and sold in market at commercial level. A number of moulds and yeasst are utilized in the synthesis of ergosterol which contains vitamin – D. Riboflauin, another vitamin useful in human and animal's food is obtained from a filamentous yeast *Ashby gossypii*.

Production of Protein

Some fungi particularly the yeasts are employed to synthesize proteins as a supplement to the normal diet. The yeasts; *Candida utilis* and *Saccharomyces cerevisiae*, contain high percentage of protein of great nutritive value. They are grown with ammonia as the source of nitrogen and molasses as the sources of carbon.

The manufactured product is called food yeast. It contains 10-15% protein and vitamin B-complex.

Organic Acid Preparation

The important organic acids produced commercially as the result of biochemical activites of molds are feumaric acid, citric acid, Onalic acid, gallic acid, gluconic acid, etc. Oxalic acid is the fermentation product of *Aspergillus niger*. Citric acid is made by mould fermentation, species of *periculllium* are used for that purpose.

Alcoholic Fermentation

Bakers' Yeast, brewers' yeast: *Saccharomyces cerevisiae* used in brewing beer, making alcoholic liquors, and baking bread. Alcoholic fermentation is the basis of two important industries of all over the world. These are brewing and baking. Both are dependent on the fact that the fermentation of sugar solutions by yeasts produces ethyl alcohol (C_2H_5OH) and CO_2. In brewing or wine making industry alcohol is the important product. The other by-product which is CO_2 was formerly allowed to escape as a useless thing. Now CO_2 is also considered a valuable by-product. It is collected, solidified and sold as 'dry ice' in the baking (bread making) industry. CO_2 is the useful product because it serves important purpose such as causes the dough to rise and makes the bread light.

The other by–product which is alcohol is incidental. The yeasts secrete the enzymes complex called zymase which brings about conversion of sugar into alcohol.

Uses of Molds

- Molds are used for the fermentation of rice to produce a variety of oriental foods and food additives
- Molds also produce several enzymes like proteases, anylases and pectinases.
- Some industrial products other than Antibiotics derived from molds are:
  1. Citric acid
  2. Fumaric acid
  3. Gluconic acid
  4. Itaconic acid
  5. Lactic acid
  6. Gibberellic acid (a simple gibberellin, a pentacyclic diterpene acid promoting growth and elongation of cells).

2.7 Algae

Algae are a large and diverse group of simple, typically autotrophic organisms, ranging from unicellular forms, such as the gient kelps that grow to 65 meters in length they are photosynthetic like plants, and "simple" because their tissues are not organized into the many distinct organs found in land plants. The largest and most complex marine forms are called seaweeds.

Algae are found in the fossil record dating back to approximately 3 billion years in the Precambrian. They exhibit a wide range of reproduction strategies, from simple asexual cell division to complex forms of sexual reproduction.

Algae cell

The cells containing a true nucleus are called eukaryotic cells. Algae is a eukaryotic cell. The algae cell has definite of cytoplasm and a nucleus. The nucleus is surrounded by a nuclear membrane which separates the nuclear materials from the cytoplasm.

The algae cells are larger in size. In algae cells there is a cell wall containing cellulose (glucan), a polysaccharide.

The cell is filled with a jelly-like fluid called cytoplasm. The cytoplasm is in constant motion called cytoplasmic streaming.

The algae cells contain membrane-bound bodies called organelles. The organelles include mitochondria, plastids, endoplasmic reticulum, ribosomes etc.

Ribosomes are spherical bodies lying in the cytoplasm. The ribosomes of eukaryotic cells are larger in size and are called 80S.

The photosynthetic apparatus is in the form of plastids. They contain chlorophyll – a, chlorophyll – b and β – carotene. It is a characteristic feature of plant cell.

The eukaryotic cell contains a well-defined nucleus. The nucleus is filled with nucleplasm and chromosomes. It is bounded by a nuclear membrane. It separates the nuclear materials from the cytoplasmic material.

Nucleolus is a small body lying inside the nucleus. It is involved in RNA synthesis. The nucleus of algae cells contains thread like structure called chromosomes. The chromosomes are composed of RNA. The characters are transmitted by DNA.

Algae Cell Walls

Like plant, algae have cell wall. Algae cell walls contain either polysaccharide (such as cellulose (aglucan) or a variety of glycoproteins or both. The inclusion of additional polysaccharides in algae cell wall is used as a feature for algae taxonomy.

Mannanes

In a number of manic green algae (*codium, dasyclades, acetabularia* etc) as well as in the walls of some red algae (*Poryphyria, Bangic*) constitute mannanes the main structural elements. They are linear and mannosyl residuces are (1 – 4) glycosidically linked. Hydrogen bonds that are (just like in cellulose) the cause of the partially crystalline organization of microfibrids may develop. In codium the carbohydrates are tightly associated with protein.

Xytanes

Xytanes are polymers where β – D – xylosyl residues are linked via, (1 – 3) and (1 – 4) glycosidic bonds.

Alginic Acid

Alginic acid and its salt, the alginates are important components of the walls of *phaeophyta* (brown algae). They are singuer in many respects. They consist exclusively of uronic acids, mannuronic acid β – L – glucuronic acid in changing ratios and of small amounts of β – D – glucuronic acid.

Sulfated Polysaccharides

Polysaccharides whose monomers are esterized to sulfuric acid residues and are moreover partially methylated have been detected in nearly all marine algae. The major sulfated polysaccharides synthesized by seaweeds including the galactans (e.g., agarans and carrageenans), ulvans, and fucans. They occur partially in the cell wall itself and partially in the intercellular substance. Sulfated galocatanes are typical for many red algae, depending on their origin are they called agarose, carrageenan, porphyran, furcelleran and funoran.

L – and D – galactose, which are linked by β – (1 – 3) or a (1 – 4) glucosidic bonds form the basic pattern of aganose and porphyran, it the latter alternate L – and – D – galactosyi residues. Carrageenan and furecelleran contain exclusively D – compounds.

Other compounds that may accumulate in algal cell walls include sporaopollenin and calcium ions. Red seaweed galactans are of great commercial importance as they are used widely in the food industry because of their rheological properties as jelling and thickening agents. The ability of sulfated polysaccharides from seaweeds to inhibit the replication of enveloped viruses including herpes simplex virus (HSV), human immunodeficiency virus (HIV), human cytomegalovirus, dengue virus and respiratory syncytial virus is well established. The original observations on antiviral activities of seaweed constituents go back more than 50 years to the observation that seaweed extracts protected chicken embryos against influenza B and mumps.

2.7.1 Major Classification of Algae

The basis of classification of algae is its nature i.e. cellular characteristic and form and size.

- *Bacillariophyta (diatoms)*
- *Charophyta (stoneworts)*
- *Chlorophyta (green algae)*
- *Chrysophyta (golden algae)*

- *Cyanobacteria (blue-green algae)*
- *Dinophyta (dinoflagellates)*
- *Phaeophyta (brown algae)*
- *Rhodophyta (red algae*)

Bacillariophyta (diatoms)

Bacillariophyta are unicellular organisms that are important components of phytoplankton as primary sources of food for zooplankton in both marine and freshwater habitats. Most diatoms are planktonic, but some are bottom dwellers or grow on other algae or plants.

Except for their male gametes, diatoms lack flagella. Instead many diatoms achieve locomotion from controlled secretions in response to outside physical and chemical stimuli. Diatoms have unique shells, which serve as their cell wall. The overlapping shells, or frustules that surround the diatom protoplasm are made of polymerized, opaline silica. Identification of diatom species is based on the delicate markings on their frustules, comprising a large number of tiny, intricately-shaped depressions, pores and passageways that bring the diatom's cell membrane in contact with the environment. Diatom frustules have accumulated over millions of years to form the fine, crumbly substance known as diatomaceous earth, which has a variety of uses (e.g. for filtration and insulation). Diatom remains in both marine and freshwater sediments are also important as indicators of paleo-environmental conditions at the time the sediments were formed.

Bacillariophytes have brownish plastids containing chlorophylls a and c and fucoxanthin. The primary means of reproduction is asexual, by cell division. Most diatoms are autotrophic, but a few are obligate heterotrophs (they must absorb organic carbon) because they lack chlorophyll altogether. Some diatoms even lack their distinctive frustules and live symbiotically in large marine protozoa, providing organic carbon for their hosts.

Charophyta (stoneworts)

Charophyta are freshwater plants and generally grow anchored to the substratum by rhizoids with a shoot extending upward. The shoot then divides and forms nodes from which a whorl of side filaments projects. Charophyta reproductive structures develop at these nodes and are, along with the biflagellate sperm produced in the male gametangium, quite similar to those of mosses. These similarities have led some scientists to identify the charophytes as ancestors of the mosses. Their green color comes from chlorphylls A and B.

Chlorophyta (green algae)

Most chlorophytes are aquatic, but some green algae can live on the surface of snow, on tree trunks, in soils, or symbiotically with protozoans, hydras or lichen-forming fungi. *Chlorophyta* numbering about 8,000 species, the chlorophytes range in size from microscopic to quite large. The typical color of plants in the *Chlorophyta*, resulting from the dominant chlorophyll pigments, is some shade of apple or grass green, although certain species may appear yellow-green or blackish-green due to the presence of carotenoid pigments or high concentrations of chlorophyll. Chlorophytes appear more than a billion years ago in the fossil record.

Calcified green algae, particularly *Halimeda* spp., are especially important as major contributors of marine sediments. The sparkling white sand beaches of the Caribbean and many other areas in the world are largely the sun-bleached and eroded calcium-carbonate remains of green algae. The deepest occurring, fleshy, erect alga Johnson-sea-linkia profunda, (Littler et al., 1985) was found attached to bedrock at a depth of 157 meters off the Bahamas and is a member of this group.

Green algae have chlorophylls a and b and store starch as a food reserve inside their plastids. Most green algae have firm cell walls composed of cellulose along with other polysaccharides and proteins.

Chrysophyta (golden algae)

Chrysophytes are photosynthetic, unicellular organisms that are abundant in freshwater and marine environments shown in Fig. (2.24). *Chrysophytes* contain chlorophylls a and c, which are masked by the accessory pigment fucoxanthin, a carotenoid. In many ways, golden algae are, biochemically and structurally similar to brown algae. Both golden algae and brown algae store food outside of the chloroplast in the form of polysaccharide laminarin, or chrysolaminarin. In both groups, motile cells have unequal flagella of similar structure.

Cyanobacteria (blue-green algae)

Even though the *Cyanobacteria* are classified as bacteria (lacking a membrane-bounded nucleus) they are photosynthetic and are included among our algal collections. *Cyanobacteria* played a decisive role in elevating the level of free oxygen in the atmosphere of the early Earth. *Cyanobacteria* can change remarkably in appearance, depending on the environmental conditions. Blue-green algae are common in soil, in both salt and fresh water, and can grow over a wide range of temperatures. They have been found to form mats in Antarctic lakes under several meters of ice and are responsible for the beautiful colors of the hot springs at Yellowstone and elsewhere. *Cyanobacteria* can also occur as symbionts of protozoans, diatoms and lichen-forming fungi, and vascular plants. Some blue-greens can fix nitrogen as well as photosynthesize, allowing them to grow with only light, water, a few minerals, and the nitrogen and carbon dioxide in the atmosphere.

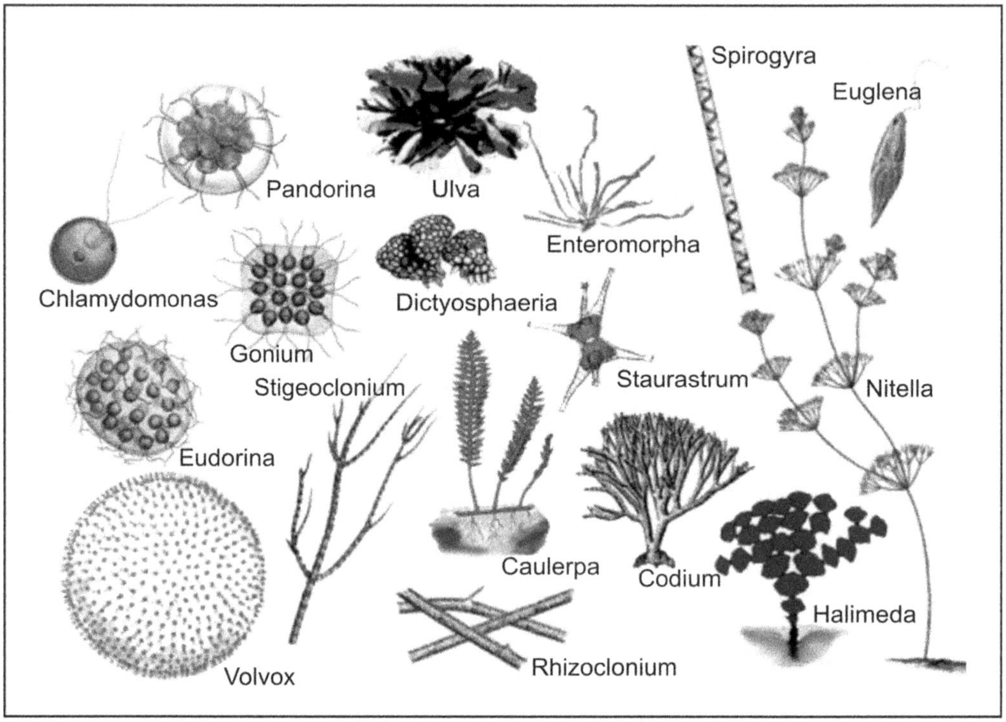

Fig. 2.24 Chrysophyta (Golden algae)

Cyanobacteria are different in many important ways from other photosynthetic prokaryotes. Instead of the bacteriochlorophylls found in purple and green bacteria, blue-greens contain chlorophyll a, as in eukaryotic phototrophs, and, produce free oxygen as a byproduct of photosynthesis. *Cyanobacteria*, however, lack the organized chloroplasts of eukaryotes and have their photosynthetic apparatus distributed peripherally in the cytoplasm.

The variety of striking colors exhibited by *Cyanobacteria* are a result of their major light-gathering pigments, the phycobilins, that are bound to protein granules, (phycobilisomes), that are attached to the photosynthetic membranes.

Large blooms of freshwater *Cyanobacteria* may produce toxins that can kill livestock. Other forms (Spirulina) are grown commercially and marketed as a high-protein dietary supplement.

Dinophyta (dinoflagellates) (Fig. 2.25)

The division Pyrrophyta (from the Greek "pyrrhos" meaning flame-colored) comprises a large number of unusual algal species of many shapes and sizes. There are about 130 genera in this group of unicellular microorganims, with about 2000 living and 2000 fossil species described so far. These are important members of the phytoplankton in marine and freshwater ecosystems.

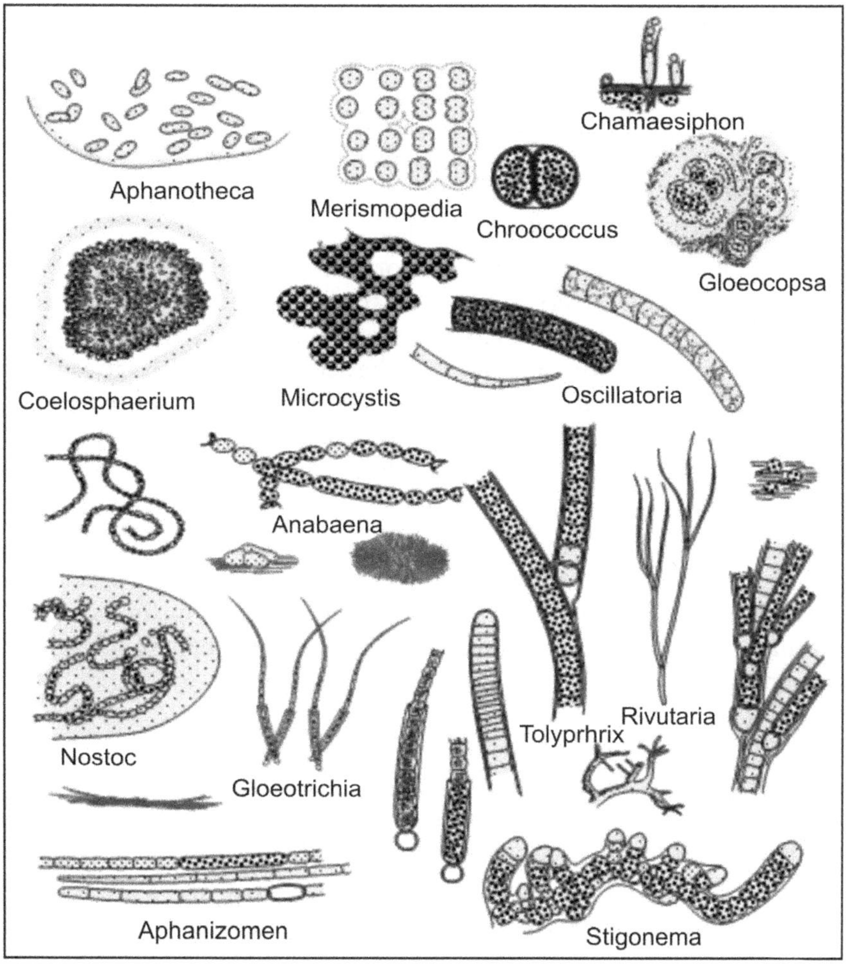

Fig. 2.25 Pyrrophyta/dinophyta (Dinoflagellates)

[Dinoflagellata - Pyrrophyta - Pyrrhophyta] * (Current names in use by various authorities)

The name "*dinoflagellate*" refers to the forward- spiraling swimming motion of these organisms. They are free-swimming protists (unicellular eukaryotic micro-organisms) with two flagella, a nucleus with condensed chromosomes, chloroplasts, mitochondria, and Golgi bodies. Biochemically, photosynthetic species possess green pigments, chlorophylls a and c, and golden brown pigments, including peridinin. *Dinoflagellates* primarily exhibit asexual cell division, some species reproduce sexually, while others have unusual life cycles. Their nutrition varies from autotrophy (photosynthesis; in-nearly 50% of the known species) to heterotrophy (absorption of organic matter) to mixotrophy (autotrophic cells engulf other organisms, including other *dinoflagellates*).

Free-living *dinoflagellates* are an ancient and successful group of aquatic organisms.

They have adapted to pelagic (free-floating) and benthic (attached) habitats from arctic to tropical seas, and to salinities ranging from freshwater, to estuaries, to hypersaline waters. Many species are found in numerous habitats, living in the plankton or attached to sediments, sand, corals, or to macroalgal surfaces or to other aquatic plants. Some species are present as parasites in marine invertebrates and fish. Some even serve as symbionts, known as zooxanthellae, providing organic carbon to their hosts: reef-building corals, sponges, clams, jellyfish, anemones and squid.

Dinoflagellates exhibit a wide variety in morphology and size (from 0.01 to 2.0 mm). They commonly have a cell covering structure (theca) that differentiates them from other algal groups. Cells are either armored or unarmored. Armored species have thecae divided into plates composed of cellulose or polysaccharides which are key features used in their identification. The cell covering of unarmored species is comprised of a membrane complex. The theca can be smooth and simple or laced with spines, pores and/or grooves and can be highly ornamented shown in Fig. (2.23).

In systematics, *dinoflagellates* have been claimed by both botanists and zoologists. *Dinoflagellates* share features common to both plants and animals: they can swim, many have cell walls, and both photosynthetic and nonphotosynthetic species are known. Botanists have grouped them with the "microalgae" and zoologists have grouped them with the protozoa, and both have produced classification schemes for this diverse and confusing group.

Dinoflagellates negative attention

1. Blooms (population explosions) of *dinoflagellates* can cause the water to turn a reddish-brown color known as "red tide". Red tides can have harmful effects on the surrounding sea-life and their consumers.
2. Certain species of *dinoflagellates* produce neurotoxins which are toxins are carried up the food chain, ultimately to humans and can, sometimes result in permanent neurological damage or even death.

Phaeophyta (brown algae)

The *Phaeophyta* are almost entirely marine, frequently dominating rocky shores in cold and temperate waters throughout the world. The giant kelp, *Macrocystis pyrifera,* forms expansive seaweed forests off the west coast of North America and provides habitat and shelter for many other organisms. Tropical waters have fewer species of brown algae, although genera such as Sargassum and Turbinaria can dominate in some areas to form small-scale forests. Sargassum is also unique among macroalgal genera in that it contains totally free-floating species with no requirement for attachment to the bottom, as in the Sargasso Sea.

The colors of brown algae (predominantly due to the brown accessory pigment fucoxanthin) cover a spectrum from pale beige to yellow-brown to almost black. In tropical seas, they range in size from microscopic filaments to several meters in length.

The large kelps are harvested for use as an emulsion stabilizer, in products such as ice cream. They are also used as fertilizer and as a vitamin rich food source.

Rhodophyta (red algae)

Of the approximately 6000 species, most red algae are marine, only a few occur in freshwater. Rhodophytes are usually multicellular and grow attached to rocks or other algae, but there are some unicellular or colonial forms. They do not have flagellated cells, are structurally complex, and have complex life cycles divided into three phases. Many red algae feature pit connections between the cells, and their cell walls include a rigid component composed of microfibrils and a mucilaginous matrix. Agar and carrageenin are two red algal mucilages that are widely used for jelling and thickening purposes in the food and pharmaceutical industries.

Rhodophytes contain *chlorophyll* a which is masked by phycobilin pigments bound to proteins. The chloroplasts in red algae resemble *Cyanobacteria* both biochemically and structurally. Food reserves are stored outside of the chloroplasts as Floridean starch.

The coralline red algae deposit calcium carbonate in their cell walls, making them particularly tough and stony. They are often abundant, ecologically important, and widespread from the arctic regions to the tropics and play an important role in building tropical reef communities. Coralline red algae can form an algal ridge that absorbs wave energy and thereby protects the more delicate organisms that inhabit the sheltered lagoons and back-reef habitats.

Some red algae are of economic importance, either as food (Porphyra) or as producers of secondary products (*Gelidium, Gracilaria, Chondrus*, etc.) used in the food and drug industries. The basis of classification of algae is its nature i.e. cellular characteristic and form and size.

Miscellaneous Groups of Algae

***Glaucophytes (Red algae & brown algae)*:** The glaucophytes, also known as glaucocystophytes or glaucocystids, are a small group of freshwater microscopic algae. Together with the red algae (*Rhodophyta*) and green algae plus land plants (Viridiplantae or Chloroplastida), they form the Archaeplastida. However, the relationships among the red algae, green algae and glaucophytes are unclear, in large part due to limited study of the glaucophytes.

Heterokonts (golden algae, brown algae & diatoms): Heterokonts are a group of closely related phyla with flagella in pairs, one long and one short. They include oomycetes, chrysophytes, diatoms, and brown algae. The term "heterokont" refers either to the flagellar arrangement of biflagellate cells in which the two flagella differ in length (as in anisokonts), type of motion, or ornamentation, or to those organisms (and organisms evolutionarily derived from such lineages) in which biflagellate cells with heterokont flagella are produced at some point during their life cycle.

***Euglenophytes*:** Euglenophytes are plantlike protists that have two flagella and no cell wall. They are eukaryotic Organisms from phylum Euglenophyta. They are closely related to animal like flagellates (zooflagellates). Typical size is 50 micrometers. Euglenophytes typically live in freshwater all throughout the world. They are Capable of photosynthesis, for this they use their eyespot and chloroplasts. When there is lack of sunlight, they eat bacteria or other material through their cytostome. They can store carbohydrates in small storage bodies

Chlorarachmiophyte (mixotrophic): Chlorarachniophytes are marine unicellular algae that live widely in the coastal and oceanic waters of temperate to tropical zone. They possess green plastids (chloroplasts) that have originated from a green algal endosymbiont via a secondary endosymbiosis. The plastid is accompanied by a reduced nucleus of the endosymbiont, called a nucleomorph, which still contains a highly reduced and compacted eukaryotic genome.

2.7.2 Identification of Algae

Algae are the photo autotrophic, eukaryotic micro-organism. There are different types of algae belonging to different classes found in sample. They can be isolated and identified in laboratory. Most of the algae are microscopic, so need close examination to identify, so a good compound microscope is essential.

Sample Collections

A water sample of known volume can be taken and allowed to settle, to concentrate it. This will take long time, and preservative will need to be added. Samples can also be filtered through membrane filters which are than examined directly under the microscope soft sediments can be scraped with a spoon or other implement to sample the growth, while racks can be scraped with a blade, or more conveniently a fingernail, and stones can be lifted from the water and brushed into a container using an old paint brush or tooth brush collected from a paddy field soil samples.

Preservation

For best results, one need to look at the samples while they are still fresh, as all preservatives have their disadvantages. Lugol's lodine is widely used and appears to work well with diatoms and some green algae, so long as it is not used in excess (enough is added to turn the sample a "pale straw color", about 0.3 ml per 100 ml sample, but the amount needed varies with the amount of algae material in the sample). 4% formalin Glutaraldehyde are alternate pereservatives used to avoid Zygnemataccean algae break up problems but they are toxic in nature.

Beneck's Broth

KNO_3	0.2 g
Mg SO_4	0.2 g
K2HPO_4	0.2 g
$CaCO_3$	0.1 g
$FeCl_3$ (1%)	2 drops
Distilled water	1 litre
PH	7.5
Agar	20 g (in Beneck's agar medium only)

Procedure

1. Prepare Beneck's broth medium, transfer 250 ml in 500 ml Erlenmeyer flasks, plug and autoclave them.
2. When the broth is cold, add 1g of soil in each flask, shake well and incubate the flask at 35 °C for 15 days in illuminated growth chamber.
3. After incubation, algal colonies appear in flasks in broth.
4. Prepare Beneck's agar medium by adding 2% agar in Beneck's broth and autoclaving as described above.
5. To get pure cultures, transfer a few cells of algal calonies with the help of the platinum loop on the Beneck's agar medium in Petri dishes.
6. Incubate the plates at 37 °C for a week in illumination chamber.

Isolation of *Cyanobacteria* from Samples

Cyanobacteria blue–green algae are the members of cyanophyceae. They are photo autotrophic, nitrogen fixing prokaryotes occurring throughout the world and growing in a diversified habitat. *Cyanobacteria* fix atomospheric N_2 and result in nitrogen –rich– environment in their surroundings. Now–a–days, some of the members are being grown on a large scale and used as biofertiliser.

Cyanobacteria which are commonly found in rich field /soil are the species of *Anabaena, Anabaenophsis, Aulosira, Cylindrospermum, Nostic, Scytonema, Fishcheralla, Stigonema, Tolyphthrix,* etc.

Fhu's medium

Ca $(NO_3)_2$	0.004%
Mg $SO_4 . 7 H_2O$	0.0025%
K_2HPO_4	0.0005% – 0.001%
NO_2CO_3	0.002%
NO_2 SiO_3	0.0025%
$FeCl_3$	0.008%

Pringsheim's broth

KNO_3	0.02%
$MgSO_4$	$7H_2O$-0.001%
(NH_4) . HPO_4	0.002%
$CaCl_2$. $6H_2O$	0.0005%
$Fecl_3$	0.00005%

Procedure

1. Collect soil sample in a polythene or colonies of blue – green algae floating on water surface in rice field in a glass bottle and bring it to the laboratory.
2. Prepare Fhu's medium No.10 or Pringsheim's broth, transfer 20 ml into 100 Erlenmeyer flasks and autoclave at 121 °C for 30 minutes.
3. Serially dilute the soil / algal sample (10^{-2} – 10^{-7}) in sterile distilled water
4. Pour aliquots of 1 ml of various dilutions of soil / algal sample into 20 ml of sterilllised medium in flasks.
5. Incubate the flasks at 30 $\pm$ 1 °C for 2–3 weeks in an alternate light and dark regime of 12 hours. Algal colonies appear in broth medium.
6. Soon pick up individual colonies and transfer onto fresh agar slants and incubate as above

Examination

Spread your sample thinly on a slide and place a cover slip on top. Soon using the 10x, objective, then switch to a higher power when you find something interesting. Focus up and down to view the object's upper surface, circumference, and (sometimes) lower surface. The 3 – Dimensional nature of algal cells can make them difficult to view (and photograph successfully), but shutting down the condenser iris a tilt can help by giving a greater depth of field.

2.7.3 Economic Importance of Algae

The algae are of importance in the fields of agriculture and industry. In addition they are used as manure, food and folder.

Role of algae in industry: Algae are useful for the source of many commercial products. Commercially major products are:

(a) ***Alginic Acid:*** The chief sources of Alginic acid are *Ascophyllum, Eisenia, Laminaria, and Lessonia and Ecklonics macrocystis*. Algin is a carbohydrate which occurs in the middle lamellae and primary walls of the above mentioned sea weeds. Algin is a colloidal material having formula (C_6 H_8 O_6) n. The soluble calcium salt of alginic acid is called algin. The alginic acid is an insoluble extract. The alginates are used in food industry, in textile industry as printing paster and in cosmetics. Alginates are of great use in the production of plastic and artificial fibers. They are also used in the leather production and rubber industry.

(b) ***Carrageenin***: The chief source if carrageenin is red algae – *Chordus crispus* and *gigartina*. Carrageenin is acell wall polysaccharide and is mucilaginous extranct. It is used in food, textile, leather and brewing industries, pharmaceuticals.

(c) ***Iodine***: Japan alone produces about 100-120 tons of Iodine annually from the kelps (brown sea weeds). The main genera employed for this purpose are *Laminaria, Eisenia, Ececklomia k and fucus*. The kelp algae are the source sodium and potassium.

(d) ***Bromine***: The red algae *Polysephonia and Rhodomeba* are the source of bromine.

(e) ***Glue manufacturing***: Glue manufacturing is another important algal industry in Japan. Red algae *Gloeopeltis furcata* is used for the manufacture of glue. This glue is known as "**Funori**" which is used for sizing paper and cloth. It is also used as an adhesive.

Agar – agar

The main sources of Agar agar are the Thalli of *Gracilaria, Gigarina and Gelidium, Hypnea, Compylaephora, Ahnfettia, Eucheuma and Furcellaria.*

Agar – agar is mucilage produced by the above mentioned red algae and stored along with the cellulose in the cell – walls, gelatinous clear and nitrogen free extract. The extract is a gel containing galactose and sulphate, its melting point ranges between 85 °C. It changes into a solid at lower temperature. Agar – Agar is insoluble in cold water but soluble in the hot water.

It is used in the preparation of certain medicines and in cosmetics, baked goods, meat industry and as emulsifier in dairy products and also used in culture media.

Role of Algae in Agriculture

For centuries seaweed has been used as fertilizers, the algae occupy a volume three times that of the soil algae the blue greens are the most important.

According to recent reports the blue green algae are the chief agents for nitrogen fixation in rice fields. They increase the fertility rate of the soil by fixing transpheric nitrogen.

According to recent reports the blue – green algae are used in reclamination of barren alkaline soils such soils have been reclaimed and brought to a productive state by inducing a proper growth of certain cyanophyceae. Successive crops of these neutralize the alkalinity and increase fertility of the rest.

The algae are also used as fertilizers particularly the sea weeds. Large brown and red algae are used as organic fertilizers. They are richer in potassium but poorer in nitrogen and phosphorous than the farm manure.

In many countries there is a productive to grind up lithothamnion and lichophyllum and use it in a place of lime. Species of chara are encrusted with calcium carbonate are used in the same for the purpose.

In India Turbinaria is used as fertilizers around palem trees. *Anabaena and spirulina* are produced in enormous quantities in sambhar salt lake (Rajasthan) are employed as green manure by farmers. The sea – weeds are also used as compost. Concentrated liquid extracts of sea weeds are used as fertilizer and also as insecticides.

Some of the important nitrogen fixing blue green algae are *osuilloitoria princeps, oscillatoria formose, cylindrospermum, n stoe spiruline and species of Anabaena.*

Ornamental Uses of Algae

Certain algae like *sptrogipra* and *Botvydium* are grown in the garden ponds for their good looking habit.

Role of Algae for Manufacturing Light Weight Building

Germany and France have developed a new technique in which the sea weeds are mixed with cement to make buildings light in weight and good heat resistant.

Nutrition

Naturally growing seaweeds are an important source of food especially is Asia. They provide many vitamins including A, B_1, B_2, B_6 Niacin and C and are rich in iodine, potassium, iron, magnesium and calcium. In addition commercially cultivated microalgae, including both algae and cyanobacteria, are marketed as nutritional supplements, such as spiruline, chlorella and the vit – c supplement, Dimaliella, high in beta – carotene.

Algae are national foods of many nations. China consume more than 70 species, including **Fat choy**, a cyanobacterium considered a vegetable. Several algae called as **Dulse**; **Chite, Cochayuyo, Laver, Gim, Nori Aonori**, are being used as nutritional foods in countries like Japan, Ireland, and Korea.

2.8 Protozoa

The sub kingdom protozoa which was originally included in the kingdom protista includes unicellular, non photosynthetic, eukaryotic micro-organisms that are considered single celled animals. (***protos***: primitive, ***zoan***: animal) shown in Fig.(2.26).

All protozoans are not related to each other but are grouped together only for convenience.

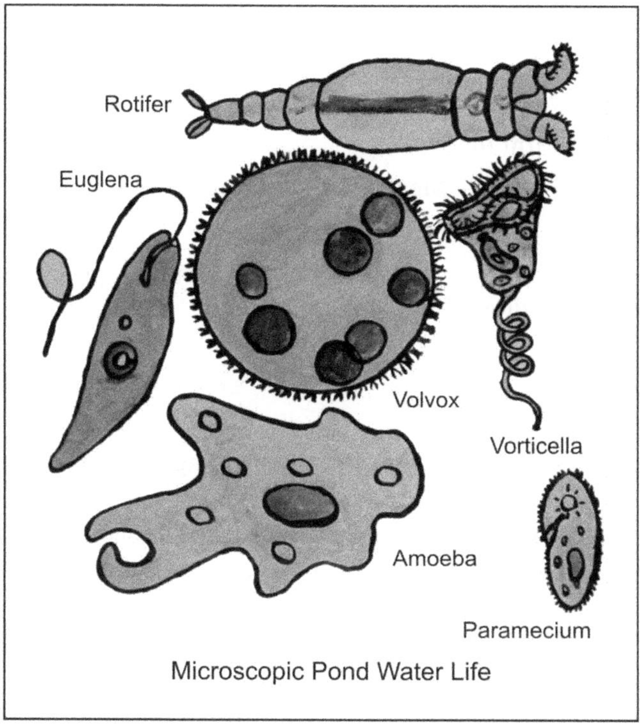

Fig. 2.26 Various protozoa

There are counter parts of some of the protozoans in the photosynthetic algae i.e, Euglena, polystona, chlamydomonas, diatoms and dinoflagellates

Many of the living protozoans are parasitic causing disease to humans such as amoebiasis, giardiasis, trichomoniasis and malaria.

Importance

1. The free living protozoans play an important role in maintaining the ecological balance in nature as many of them feed on fungi and bacteria.
2. Many protozoans help in purification of polluted waters as they utilize the inorganic nitrates and phosphates for their metabolism
3. Protozoans such as paramecium, tetrahymena and euplotes have been used as research materials by biologists.
4. Protozoa serve as an important link in food chain in aquatic environments.

   e.g., In marine waters, zooplankton are protozoa that feed on the photosynthetic phytoplankton. They are in turn become food for larger marine organisms.

   Light energy → phytoplankton → Zooplankton → Carnivores
   (Primary producers) (Primary consumers) (Secondary consumers)

2.8.1 Morphology of Protozoa

The size and shape of these organisms show considerable variation.

E.g.: *Leishmania donovani* measures 1-4 μm in length.

– cause **Kala azar** diseases Ameoba proteus – Measures 600 μm or more

Ciliated *protozoans* – measures 2000 μm or 2 mm

Foraminifera a class of ameoboid protists, & the present –day marine protozon *Nummulites* (a large lenticular fossile) – measures 15 cm in diameter

2.8.2 Intracellular Structures

Protozoan cell also consists of cytoplasm, separated from the surrounding medium by a special cell envelope, the nucleus.

1. **Cytoplasm:** Cytoplasm is a more or less homogeneous substance consisting of globular protein molecules loosely linked together to form a three dimensional molecular frame work.

   The ectoplasm is a more gel – like and the endoplasm is more voluminous and fluid, structures are predominantly found in endoplasm.

   Protozoa have membrane systems in the cytoplasm which form a more or less continuous network of canals and lacunae giving rise to endoplasmic reticulum.

   Other structures in the cytoplasm include ribosomes, golgi complex, mitochondria, kinetosomes, food vacuoles, contractile vacuoles and nuclei.

2. **Nucleus:** The protozoan cell has atleast one eukaryotic nucleus.

   Many protozoa have multiple nuclei throughout the greater part of the life cycle.

   In several species each individual organism has two similar nuclei.

   In the ciliates, two dissimilar nuclei, one large (macro) and one small (micro) are present.

   The macro nucleus controls the metabolic activities and regeneration processes.

   The micronucleus is concerned with reproductive activity.

   The essential structural elements of the nucleus are chromosomes, the nuclear substances, the nuclear membrane, karyoplasms.

3. **Plasmalemma and other cell organelles:** The cytoplasm with its various structures is separated from the external environment by a cell unit membrane called plasmalemma.

   The plasmalemma not only provides protection but also controls exchange of substances.

   It is the site of perception of chemical and mechanical stimulti as well as the establishment of contact with other cells.

Many protozoa have a compound coverings of membranes modified for protection, support and movement. Such combinations of membrane are referred to as pellicle.

In its simplest form, the pellicle is plasmalemma itself. E.g. amoebas are surrounded by a plasmalemma only.

The pellicle of a ciliate is thick and often variously ridged and sculptured. There may be even rows of elevated platelets and nodular thickening.

e.g., Pellicle of paramecium consists of three membranes, the outer one sculptured in a series of evenly distributed polygons. The contact between adjacent polygons results in a series of ridges giving latticed pattern.

Additional protective coverings external to the pellicle have also evolved for some protozoa. These coverings are known variously as theca, shells, tests or lorica.

The theca is a secreted layer directly opposed to the coil surface.

Tests, shells, lorica are coverings that are loose fittings.

4. **Feeding structures:** Food gatherings structures in protozoa are diverse and range from the pseudopodia of amoebas through the tentacular feeding tubes of suctorians to the well-developed "mouths" of many ciliates.

   Amoebas gather food by means of pseudopodial engulfment.

   In ciliates the cytosome is the actual opening through which food is ingested.

   An oral groove is an indentation in the pellicle of certain ciliates. It guides food toward the cytosome and acts as a concentrating device.

   The cytopharynx is a region through which nutrients must pass to be enclosed in food vacuole.

Cysts: Cysts are typically resting, dormant and/or resistant stages in the full life cycle of many protozoan species, sometimes playing a role in dispersal of the organism. The cysts survive adverse environmental conditions such as desiccation, low nutrient supply, and anaerobiosis.

In parasitic protozoa the development stages are often transmitted from host to host within a cyst.

The cysts enter the alimentary tract as resting cysts, hatch in a suitable region, and then leave the host again as dormant cysts. By this means, they can survive for large periods outside the host.

Asexual reproduction in some ciliates and flagellets is associated with cyst formation.

The cyst wall is secreted as a closely fitting extra cellular coat or structures.

Locomotor Organelles

Pseudopodia: A pseudopodium is a temporary projection of part of the cytoplasm of those protozoa which do not have a rigid pellicle.

Flagella and Cilia: A flagellum, also called undulipodium, is a whip-like structure used for locomotion, for feeding or other purposes. The flagellum is an extremely fine filamentous extension of the cell. A flagellum is composed of two parts: an elastic filament called axoneme and contractile cytoplasmic sheath that surrounds axoneme. An interested flagellated protist is Euglena.

The **cilia** of Ciliates are just shorter versions that act different. A cilium beats like a small pedal and generates a sideways motion. Most undulipodia act more like a propellor, wavy motions push or pull an organism in a forward direction.

2.8.3 Classification of Protozoa

The classification of protozoa recognized four phyla based basically on their means of locomotion.

1. Sarcodina : Amoeboid forms moving by pseudopodiasis
2. Mastigophora : Flagellates
3. Ciliaphora : Ciliates
4. Sporozoa : Spore formers

Classification of Protozoa (modified Sleigh's system by A. Pechenik, 2002) shown in Fig. 2.27.

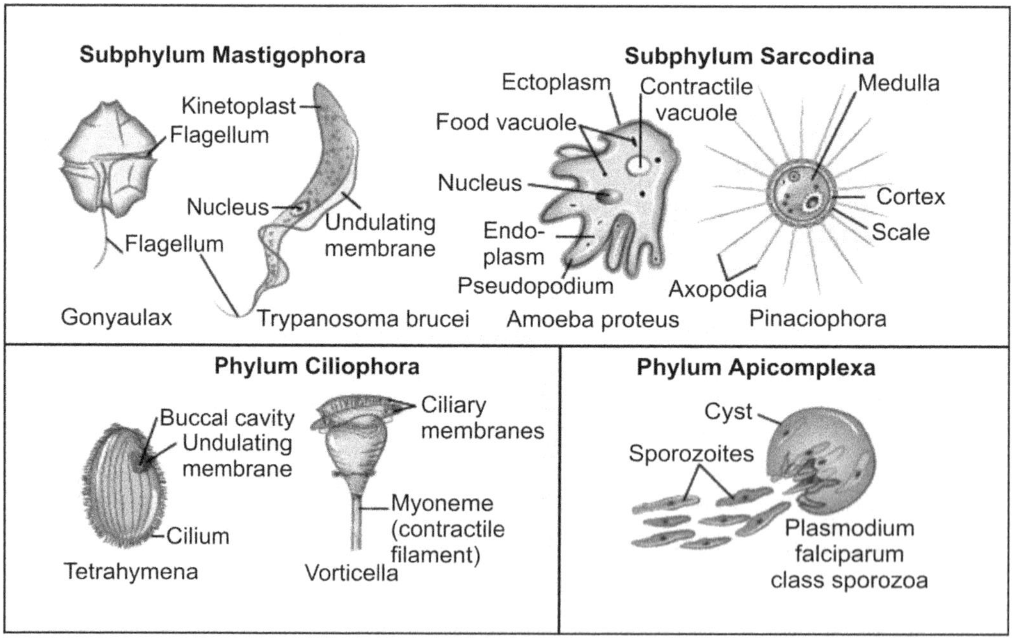

Fig. 2.27 Phylum sarcomastigophora

Kingdom PROTOZOA (14 phyla)

1. **Phylum CILIOPHORA** (ciliates).
2. **Phylum AMOEBOZOA** (Amoebas).
3. **Phylum RADIOZOA** (radiolarians).
4. **Phylum HELIOZOA** (sun animalcules).

FLAGELLATED PROTOZOA

5. **Phylum TRICHOZOA** *(Trichomonas).*
6. **Phylum EUGLENOZOA** *(Euglena).*
7. **Phylum DINOZOA** (Dinoflagellates).
8. **Phylum CHOANOZOA** (Choanoflagellates).
9. **Phylum METAMONADA** *(Giardia).*

SPORE-FORMING PROTOZOA

10. **Phylum APICOMPLEXA (=SPOROZA),** includes three subphyla.

HONORARY PROTOZOA

11. **Phylum LABYRINTHOMORPHA** (Slime-nets).
12. **Phylum OPALOZOA** *(Opalina).*
13. **Phylum MICROSPORIDEA** (now transferred to fungi).
14. **Phylum MYXOZOA** (now shifted to kingdom Animalia).

2.8.4 Protozoan Diseases

Protozoa are one-celled organisms that can cause diseases ranging in severity from mild to deadly. These organisms can be classified as parasitic or free-living. Parasitic protozoa are found in organisms such as ticks, flies and mosquitoes. Free-living protozoa are found in water that is contaminated with fecal matter and other wastes.

***Amoebiasis*:** Amoebiasis is a protozoan disease caused by *Entamoeba histolytica*, which secretes enzymes that dissolve the host's tissues. Amoebiasis infection is spread by contact with feces, which can occur if water or foods are contaminated, or if someone has oral contact with fecal matter. This condition can occur without symptoms, but some of the common signs and symptoms of amoebiasis include bloody diarrhea and inflammation of the colon.

***Giardiasis*:** Giardiasis is caused by the parasite known as *Giardia intestinalis*. This parasite is found in fecal matter, so it can be contracted through oral contact with feces. This can occur if proper hand washing is not done after using the bathroom, changing a baby's diaper or cleaning bathroom fixtures. Drinking water from contaminated sources and accidentally swallowing contaminated swimming water can also cause giardiasis infection. The symptoms of giardiasis include greasy stools, upset stomach, diarrhea, nausea, flatulence and abdominal cramps.

African sleeping sickness: African sleeping sickness is caused by protozoa in the Trypanosoma genus. These organisms are carried by the tsetse fly and transmitted to humans via tsetse fly bites. According to the World Health Organization, *Trypanosoma brucei gambiense* causes more than 90 percent of African sleeping sickness cases. Trypanosoma *brucei rhodesiense* is responsible for less than 10 percent of reported cases of the disease. Signs and symptoms of African sleeping sickness can include insomnia, progressive confusion, seizures, irritability, personality changes, weight loss, and loss of concentration, slurred speech and difficulty talking and walking.

Leishmaniasis: Leishmaniasis is caused by the Leishmania parasite, which is found in southern Europe, the subtropics and the tropics. This disease is spread by the bites of sand flies that are infected with the parasite. Cutaneous leishmaniasis affects the skin, while visceral leishmaniasis affects the spleen, liver and other organs. Cutaneous leishmaniasis causes skin sores that can change in size and shape as the disease progresses. Visceral leishmaniasis symptoms include weight loss, fever, liver enlargement, spleen enlargement and abnormal blood counts.

Toxoplasmosis: Toxoplasmosis is caused by an organism known as *Toxoplasma gondii,* which is one of the most common parasites in the world. While most people with this disease do not have any symptoms, serious complications can occur when toxoplasmosis develops in people with compromised immune systems. Infants born to mothers infected with the disease can also experience serious complications. Toxoplasmosis signs and symptoms are flu-like in nature and include bodyaches, headache, fatigue, fever, swollen lymph nodes and sore throat.

Malaria: Malaria is spread by mosquitoes that are infected by the parasites *Plasmodium falciparum, P. ovale, P. vivax and P. malariae.* Malaria signs and symptoms include shaking, headache, chills, fatigue and muscle aches.

Babesiosis: Babesiosis is caused by the Babesia parasite, which is carried by ticks. This disease can also be spread through blood transfusions if a donor has a Babesia infection that has not been diagnosed. Babesiosis caused by tick bites usually occurs in USA (New England). This condition may not cause any signs or symptoms, but some common symptoms of babesiosis include fatigue, nausea, bodyaches, headache, loss of appetite, chills, fever and sweats. This disease can be life-threatening in people who have weakened immune systems, serious health problems or spleens that do not function properly.

2.9 Viruses

Introduction

The name virus was coined from the Latin word meaning *slimy liquid* or *poison*. It was originally used to describe any infectious agent, including the agent of tobacco mosaic disease, tobacco mosaic virus. In the early years of discovery, viruses were referred to as filterable agents. Only later was the term virus restricted to filterable agents that require a living host for propagation.

Important Developments and Inventions in Branch of Virology

There is a evidence that viral infections were existing from ancient times as Egyptian hieroglyph depicted its priest as polio effected person. But it took thousands of years to identify and discover virus.

1798- Experiments on virology began with the experiments of Jenner. Jenner did not know the cause but found that that individuals exposed to cow pox did not suffer from small pox.

1881-1885 Louis Pasteur first used animals as model for growing and studying viruses. He found that the rabies virus could be cultured in rabbit brains and discovered the rabies vaccine. However, Pasteur did not try to identify the infectious agent

1898 – Marcus Beijerinck makes the same observation; concludes that the pathogen must be a distinctive agent

1898 – Friedrich Loeffler and Paul Frosch (former students of Koch), find that causative agent of foot-and-mouth disease is filterable (the first animal virus)

1901 – Yellow fever virus – Walter Reed (the first human virus)

1903 – Rabies virus (Remlinger, Riffat-Bay)

1906 – Variola virus (Negri)

1908 – Poliovirus (Karl Landsteiner and E. Popper); chicken leukemia virus (Ellerman, Bang)

1911 – Rous sarcoma virus (Peyton Rous)

1915 – Bacteriophages -Frederik Twort, Felix D'Herelle

1931 – Swine influenza virus (Shope)

1933 – Human influenza virus (Smith)

1935 – Image of Viruses observed.(Wendell Stanley examined the tobacco mosaic virus in Electron Microscope)

Between 1938 and 1970 virology developed by leaps and bounds into Molecular biology.

The 1940's and 1950's was the era of the Bacteriophage and the animal virus.

Delbruck considered father of modern molecular biology. He developed the concepts of virology in the science.

In 1952 Hershey and Chase showed that it was the nucleic acid portion that was responsible for the infectivity and carried the genetic material.

In 1954 Watson and Crick found the exact structure of DNA. Lwoff in 1949 found that virus could behave like a bacterial gene on the chromosome and also found the operon model for gene induction and repression.

Lwoff in 1957 defined viruses as potentially pathogenic entities with an infectious phase and having only one type of nucleic acid, multiplying with their genetic material and unable to undergo binary fission.

In 1931, American pathologist Ernest William Goodpasture grew influenza and several other viruses in fertilised chickens' eggs.

In 1949, John F. Enders, Thomas Weller, and Frederick Robbins grew polio virus in cultured human embryo cells, the first virus to be grown without using solid animal tissue or eggs. This enabled Jonas Salk to make an effective polio vaccine.

Era of polio research was next and was very important as in 1953 the Salk vaccine was introduced and by 1955 poliovirus had been crystallized. Later Sabin introduced attenuated polio vaccine.

In the 1980's cloning of viral genes developed, sequencing of the viral genomes was successful and production of hybridomas was a reality.

The AIDS virus HIV came next in the 1980's. Further uses of viruses in gene therapy developed over the next two decades.

Viruses are small obligate intracellular parasites, which by definition contain either a RNA or DNA genome surrounded by a protective, virus-coded protein coat. The largest among them measuring about 300 nm where as the smallest virus measuring 20 nm. Hence they were known as 'Filterable viruses'. Viruses vary widely in size.The method of estimating the size of virus particle was by passing them through collodion membrane filters of graded porosity. The average pore diameter of the finest filter that permitted passage of the virion gave an estimate of its size. Ultra centrifuge was the second method used to find out the size of virus.

The rate of sedimentation of virus in the ultra centrifuge, the particle size could be calculated using stokes law.

The third and the most direct method of measuring virus size is electron microscopy.

Purified preparation of virions may be examined under the electron microscope either stained or unstained. By this method both shape and size of virions can be studied.

Viruses are infectious acellular agents *i.e.* devoid of cell components like nucleus, organelles, cytoplasm, or plasma membrane

- Replicate or multiply only inside living host cell
- Possesses only one type of nucleic acids- either DNA or RNA but never both (exception is cytomegalovirus)
- Virion – a complete single viral particle
- Obligatory intracellular parasites
- Do not undergo binary fission

- Sensitive to interferon
- Contain a protein coat
- Some are enclosed by an envelope
- Some viruses have spikes
- Most viruses infect only specific types of cells in one host
- Host range is determined by specific host attachment sites and cellular factors (receptors)
- Viruses replicate through replication of their nucleic acid and synthesis of the viral protein.
- Viruses do not multiply in chemically defined media
- All ss-RNA viruses with negative polarity have the enzyme transcriptase (RNA dependent RNA polymerase) inside virions.
- Retroviruses and hepatitis B virus contain the enzyme reverse transcriptase.

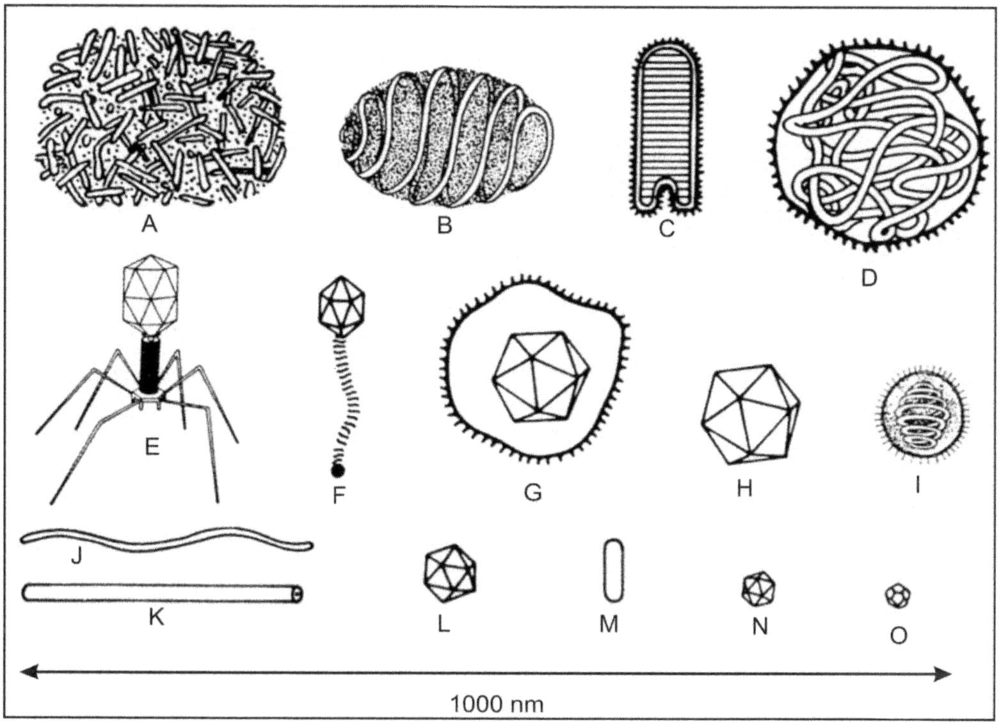

Fig. 2.28 A-*Vaccinia* (pox)virus; B-ORF virus; C-Rhabdo virus; D-paramyxo virus; E-T-even coliphage; F-flexous tailed phage; G-Herpes virus; H-Polyoma virus; I- Influenza virus; J-Label; K-Tubro virus; L-Picorno virus; M-Rabies virus. N-Adeno virus; O- parvo virus

Structure and Shape: The virion consists essentially of a nucleic acid surrounded by a protein coat, the capsid.

The capsid with the enclosed nucleic acid is known as the nucleocapsid.

The function of the capsid is to protect the nucleic acid from inactivation by nuclease.

Cilia, in addition to their loco motor function also aid in the ingestion of food and serve often as a tactile organelle.

Cilia are arranged in longitudinal, oblique, or spiral row, inserted either on the ridges or in the furrows.

Viruses are called acellular microbes as they lack cytoplasmic membrane to separate them from their surroundings.

The acellular microbes are obligate intracellular inhabitants that totally depend on compatible host cells for their replication.

Viruses contain only one type of nucleic acid either DNA or RNA but never both.

2.9.1 Morphology of Viruses

Size

Virus size is determined by electron microscopy, ranges from 28 to 750 nm in length.

Viruses are of variable sizes. Initially their sizes were estimated by passing them through membranes of known pore diameter. In recent years, their size is determined by ultracentrifugation and electron microscopy. Size varies from 20 nm to 300 nm in diameter. They are smaller than bacteria; some are slightly larger than protein and nucleic acid molecules and some are about of the small size (small pox virus) as the smallest bacterium and some virus (virus of lymphogranuloma, 300-400 nm) are slightly larger than the smallest bacterium.

Viral Structure

Typical viral components are shown in Fig. 2.29. These components are a **nucleic acid core** and a surrounding protein coat called a **capsid**. In addition some viruses have a surrounding lipid bilayer membrane called an **envelope**. Protein submits may be seen as projecting spikes on the surface of the envelope. These structures are called Peplomers.A virus may have more than one type of peplomer.e.g., Influenza virus carries two kinds of peplomers – the hemagglutinin which is a triangular spike and the neuraminidase which is a mushroom shaped structure.

Enveloped viruses are susceptible to the action of lipid solvents like ether, $CHCl_3$ and bile salts. In some animal viruses the nucleocapsid (the nucleic acid and capsid) is covered by an outer membrane like structure called the envelope. Chemically the envelope is made up of proteins and glycoproteins. Virions may be enveloped or non-enveloped.

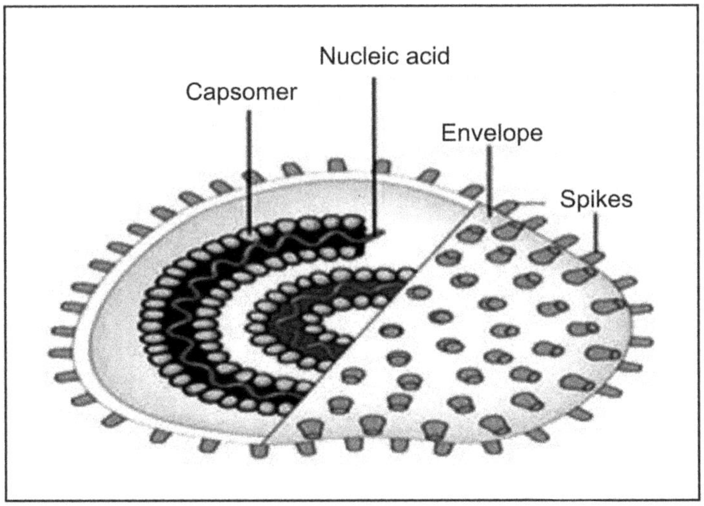

Fig. 2.29 The components of helical virus

The overall shape of the virus particle varies in different groups of viruses.

Most animal viruses are roughly spherical.

Some are irregular and pleomorphic.

The rabies virus is bullet shaped, ebola virus filamentous and pox viruses are brick shaped, tobacco mosaic virus is rod shaped and other deleterious agents in the environment.

Capsid: Capsid is a protein coat which provides protection for nucleic acid and also provides specificity for attachment; capsomeres are subunits of the capsid. This is shown in Fig. 2.30. The capsid is composed of a large number of capsomers which form its morphological units. The chemical units of capsid are polypeptide molecules which are arranged symmetrically to form an impenetrable shell around the nucleic acid core. The major function of capsid is to introduce adsorbing viral genome into host cell by adsorbing to cell surface.

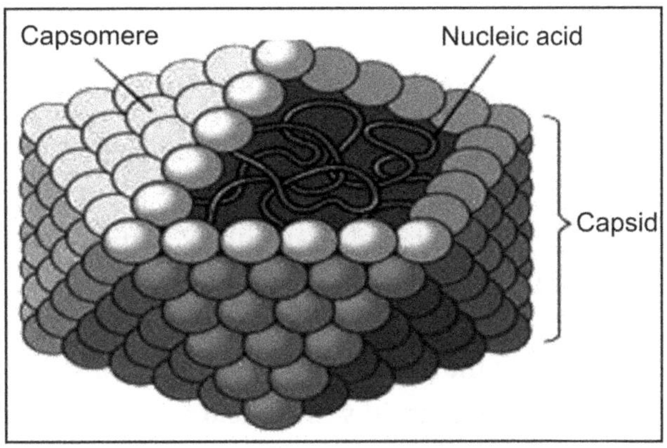

Fig. 2.30 Capsid structure

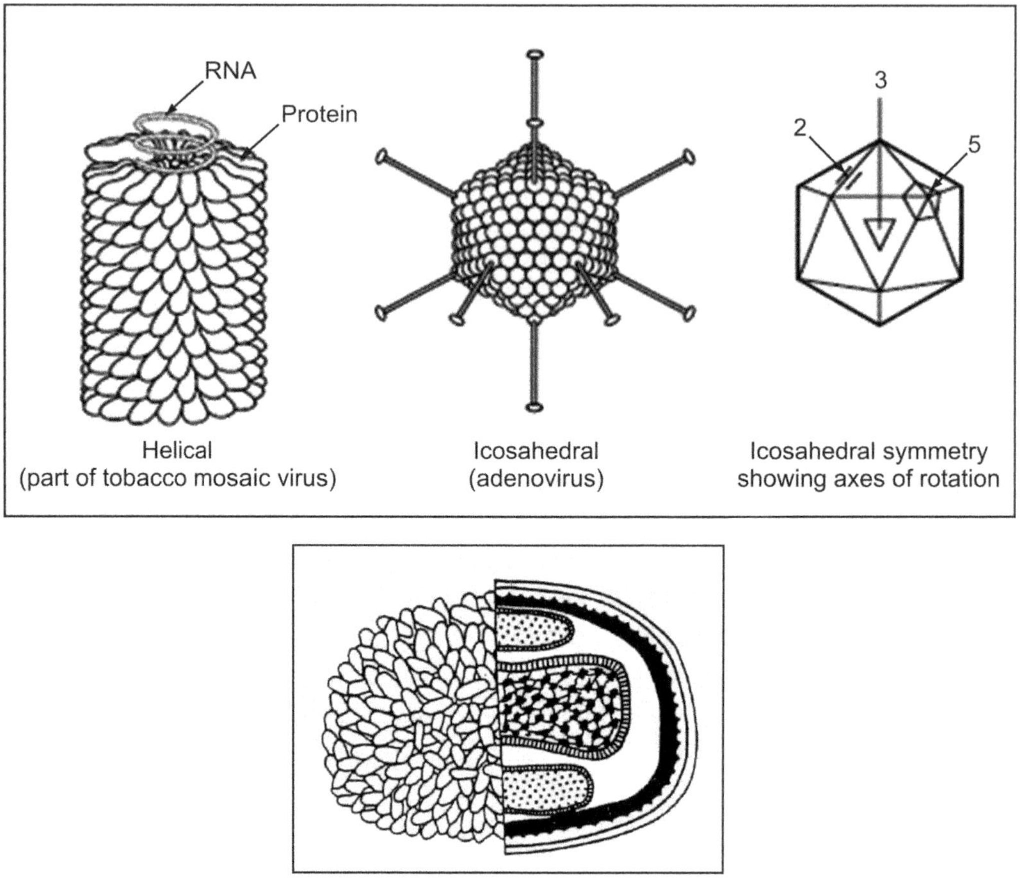

Fig. 2.31 Viral capsid structures of Helical, Icosahedral and complex symmetry

Two kinds of symmetry are encountered in the capsid – icosahedral (cubical) and helical.

Icosahedrons are polygon with 12 vertices or corners and 20 facets or sides.

Each facet is in the shape of an equilateral triangle.

Two types of capsomers constitute the icosahedral capsid. They are the pentagonal capsomers at the vertices and hexagonal capsomers making up the facets.

In the nucleocapsid with helical symmetry, the capsomers and nucleic acid are wound together to form a helical or spiral tube.

Shape of Viruses: Four basic morphologies shown in Fig. 2.31 and Fig. 2.32.

- ***Icosahedral:*** efficient means to conserve and enclose space; form capsomers (planar faces formed by association of proteins)
- ***Helical:*** capsid is shaped like a hollow protein tube

- ***Icosahedral Enveloped/Helical Enveloped*:** outer covering derived from the host cell's nuclear or plasma membrane and often possessing spikes or peplomer projections involved in attachment and entry into a host cell sometimes via their enzymatic activity
- ***Complex symmetry:*** viruses that fit neither of the above categories or which may employ portions in combination, e.g., bacteriophage

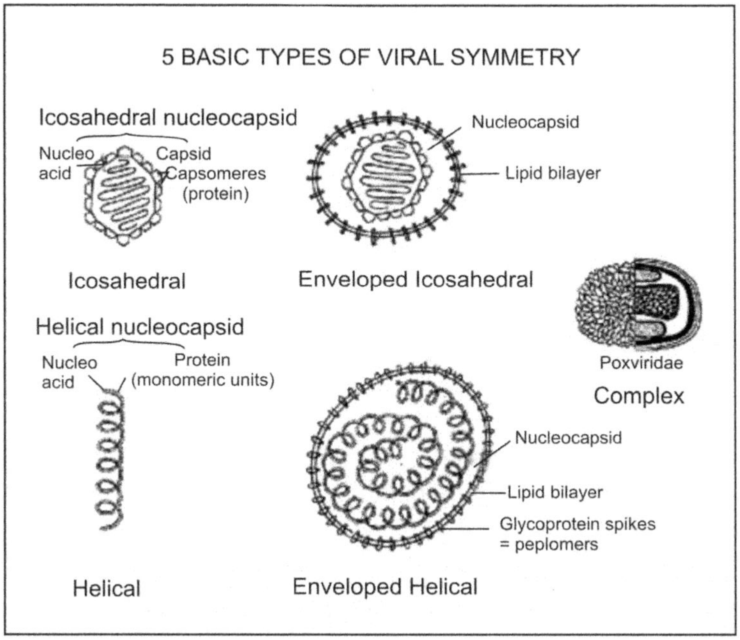

Fig. 2.32 Viral symmetry

Viruses are of different shapes such as:

- Spheroid or cuboid (adenoviruses)
- Elongated (potato viruses)
- Flexuous or coiled (beet yellows virus)
- Bullet shaped (rabies virus)
- Filamentous (bacteriophage M13)
- Pleomorphic (alfalfa mosaic virus AMV)

Viral Nucleic Acid

The viral genome is composed of either DNA or RNA. It can be double stranded (ds) or single-stranded (ss), linear (e.g.poliovirus) or circular (e.g. hepatitis B virus), containing several segments (e.g. influenza-8 segments of minus-sense ss RNA) or one molecule (e.g., poliovirus).

The nature of the viral nucleic acid is important for the effectiveness of antiviral treatements.For example, retroviridae such as HIV require a specific virus-encoded enzyme, a reverse transcriptase, to convert their ssRNA into ssDNA to be able to replicate within the host cell. This enzyme is a primary target site of many antiviral drugs.

On some occasions, the viral genome has been shown to be infectious, i.e. to cause an infection.

Drugs should damage not only viral capsid or viral envelop but viral nucleic acid also. Viral nucleic acid after damaging may be reconstruct by hybridization of the gene pool of inactivate particles and become infectious, so viral nucleic acid should be rendered non-infectious following a verucidal treatment.

Structural Arrangement of Different Parts of Virion

Nucleic Acid
Capsid symmetry
Number of capsomeres
Virion
Envelope

ENVELOPE

- The envelope or outer covering of viruses (Fig. 2.33) is derived from the host cell membrane when the progeny virus is released by budding.
- The envelope is lipoprotein in nature.
- The lipid is largely of host cell origin while the protein is virus coded.
- Some enveloped viruses have spikes, which are viral glycoproteins that project from the envelope. Non enveloped viruses are referred to as naked virions. Such viruses are not affected by lipid solvents. Naked (non-enveloped) viruses are protected by their capsid alone.
- Biological properties such as attachment to host cell surface or hemaglutination depend on the envelope.

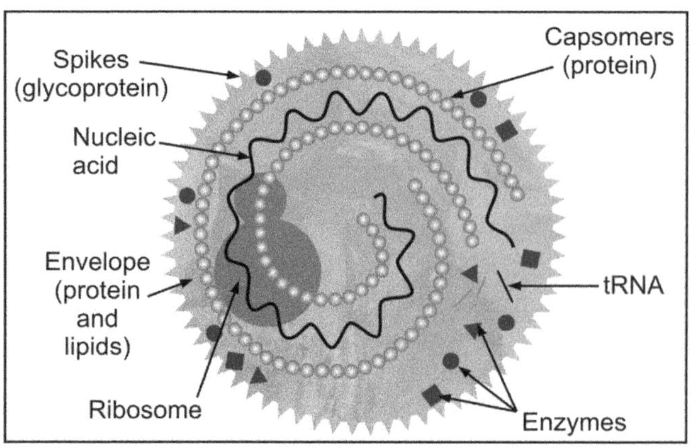

Fig. 2.33 Envelope of virus

2.9.2 Classification

I. ICTV Classification

Since 1971, the International Committee on Taxonomy of Viruses (ICTV) operating on behalf of the world community of virologists has taken on the task of developing a single, universal taxonomic scheme for all viruses infecting animals (vertebrate, invertebrates, and protozoa), plants (higher plants and algae), fungi, bacteria, and archaea. International committee on Taxonomy of viruses, the agency responsible for standardizing the classification of all viruses.

Virus Taxonomy: 2014 Release

I.	**Order Candovirales**	**(3 Families)**
II.	**Order Herpesvirales**	**(3 Families)**
III.	**Order: *Ligamenvirales***	**(2 Families)**
IV.	**Order: *Mononegavirales***	**(5 Families)**
V.	**Order: *Nidovirales***	**(4 Families)**
VI.	**Order: *Picornavirales***	**(5 Families)**
VII.	**Order: *Tymovirales***	**(4 Families)**
	Virus families not assigned to an order	**(77 Families)**

I. The **Caudovirales** are an order of viruses also known as the *Tailed bacteriophages*. Under the Baltimore classification scheme, the *Caudovirales* are group I viruses as they have double stranded DNA (dsDNA) genomes, which can be anywhere from 18,000 base pairs to 500,000 base pairs in length. The virus particles have a distinct shape; each virion has an icosohedral head that contains the viral genome, and is attached to a flexible tail by a connector protein. The order encompasses a wide range of viruses, many of which containing genes of similar nucleotide sequence and function. Some tailed bacteriophage genomes can vary quite significantly in nucleotide sequence, however, even among the same genus. Due to their characteristic structure and possession of potentially homologous genes, it is believed these bacteriophages possess a common origin.

II. **Herpesvirales** The taxonomy of herpesviruses has been updated by the International Committee on Taxonomy of Viruses (ICTV). The former family *Herpesviridae* has been split into three families, which have been incorporated into the new order Herpesvirales. The revised family Herpesviridae retains the mammal, bird and reptile viruses, the new family. *Alloherpesviridae* incorporates the fish and frog viruses, and the new family *Malacoherpesviridae* contains a bivalve virus. Three new genera have been created in the family Herpesviridae, namely *Proboscivirus* in the subfamily Betaherpesvirinae and Macavirus and *Percavirus* in the subfamily *Gammaherpesvirinae*. These genera have been formed by the transfer of species from established genera and the erection of new species, and other new species have been added to some of the established genera. In addition, the names of some nonhuman primate virus species have been changed. The family Alloherpesviridae has been populated by transfer of the genus Ictalurivirus and addition of the new species Cyprinid herpesvirus 3. The family Malacoherpesviridae incorporates the new genus Ostreavirus containing the new species Ostreid herpesvirus.

III. **Ligamenvirales** is an order of linear viruses that infect Archaea of the kingdom Crenarchaeota and have double-stranded DNA genomes. The order was established by D. Prangishvili and M. Krupovic in 2012.

The name is derived from the Latin **ligamen**, meaning *string* or *thread.*

There are two families in this order – *Lipothrixviridae* and *Rudiviridae.*

The virons are filamentous with a helical nucleocapsid. At either end are attached either fibers or more complex structures involved in host adhesion.

The major coat proteins of both lipothrixviruses and rudiviruses have an unusual four-helix bundle topology. Viruses from the two families share up to ten genes.

The genome is non segmented linear double stranded DNA

IV. The order **Mononegavirales** is the taxonomic home of numerous related viruses. Members of the order that are commonly known are, for instance, Ebola virus, human respiratory syncytial virus, measles virus, mumps virus, *Nipah virus*, and *Rabies virus*. All of these viruses cause significant disease in humans. Many very important pathogens of nonhuman animals and plants are also members of this order

V. **Nidovirales** is an order of viruses with animal hosts. It includes the families *Coronaviridae*, *Arterivirus Roniviridae* and *Mesoniviridae.*

The order Nidovirales is named for the Latin *nidus*, meaning nest, as all viruses in this order produce a 3' co-terminal nested set of subgenomic mRNA's during infection

VI. The **Picornavirales** are an order of viruses with vertebrate, insects and plant hosts. This group consists of viruses which have (+) sense single stranded RNA genomes.

Five families within this group - Caliciviridae, Dicistroviridae, Picornaviridae, Potyviridae and Sequiviridae share a number of common features:

It has been suggested that the evolution of these viruses may have preceded the separation of eukaryotes into the extant crown groups

VII. The **Tymovirales** are a newly established order of viruses in the 2009 classification with four genera. This group consists of viruses which have (+) sense single stranded RNA genomes without DNA intermediates. Their genetic material is protected by a special coat protein

Group IV (+)ssRNA; Families

Alphaflexi viridae,Gammaflexi viridae,Betaflexi viridae,Gammaflexi viridae,Tymo viridae.

Table 2.9 Properties used for Classification of Viruses

Primary characteristics	Secondary characteristics
Chemical nature of nucleic acid: RNA or DNA; single or double stranded; (+) or (–) strand; molecular weight • Structure of virion • Site of replication	**Host range:** Mode of transmission specific surface structures

II. Classification of viruses on the basis of differences in their transcription processes

The **Baltimore classification**, developed by David Baltimore, is a virus classification system that groups viruses into families, depending on their type of genome (DNA, RNA, single-stranded (ss), double-stranded (ds), etc.) and their method of replication.

Group I: dsDNA viruses (e.g. Adeno viruses, Herpes viruses, Pox viruses)

Group II: ssDNA viruses (+ strand or "sense") DNA (e.g. Parvo viruses)

Group III: dsRNA viruses (e.g. Reoviruses)

Group IV: (+) ssRNA viruses (+ strand or sense) RNA (e.g. Picornaviruses, Polioviruses,Togaviruses)

Group V: (–) ssRNA viruses (– strand or antisense) RNA (e.g. Orthomyxoviruses, Rhabdoviruses)

Group VI: ssRNA-RT (Reverse Transcribing) viruses (+ strand or sense) RNA with DNA intermediate for replication in life-cycle (e.g. Retroviruses)

Group VII: dsDNA-RT (Reverse Transcribing) viruses (e.g. Hepadnaviruses)

III. Classification of Eukaryotic Viruses on the basis of Nucleic Acid

Major groups of viruses are distinguished on the basis of their nucleic acid content as:

- **DNA Viruses**
- **RNA Viruses**

Subsequent subdivisions are based largely on other properties of nucleic acids. The RNA viruses can be ssRNA or dsRNA, although most are ssRNA.

(A) DNA Viruses

Important Characteristics:

- DNA as its genetic material
- Replicationoccurs in the nucleus using a DNA-dependent DNA polymerase
- DNA can be ssDNA or dsDNA and may be linear or circular

Important groups of DNA viruses are: Adenoviridae, Herpesviridae, Poxviridae, Papovaviridae, Hepadnaviridae, and /Parvoviridae.

The dsDNA viruses are further separated in families on the basis of the shape of their DNA (linear or circular), their capsid shape and the presence or absence of an envelope. Only one family of viruses has ssDNA (as shown in Table 2.3)

Table 2.10 Different Groups of Viruses, Characteristics and their Clinical Significance

Group	Virus	Characteristics	Clinical importance
Double Stranded DNA viruses			
Poxviruses (fam:poxviridae)	Variola	Large particles; 200-250 nm: complex symmetry	Smallpox virus
Adenoviruses (fam:Adenoviridae) Linear DNA;Naked	Adenovirus	Icosahedra particles 80 nm in diameter	Causes upper respiratory infections
Herpesviruses (fam:Herpesviridae) Linear DNA	Herpes simplex virus (HSV1 and HSV2)	Enveloped, icosahedral particles; 150 nm in diameter	HSV1 infections in children HSV2 for recurrent genital herpes
	Varicella zoster virus	Enveloped, icosahedral particles; 150 nm in diameter	Chickenpoxin children
Cytomegalovirus (CMV) (fam:Herpesviridae) Linear DNA		Enveloped, icosahedral particles; 150 nm in diameter	Pneumonia, hepatitis, encephalitis in immunocomprimised patients.
Epstein-Barr virus (EBV) (fam:Herpesviridae)		Enveloped, icosahedral particles;150nm in diameter	Glandular fever, sever EBV infection & facial tumors in tropical Africa
Hepatitis viruses (Fam:Hepadnaviridae) Circular DNA	Hepatitis B virus (HBV)	Spherical enveloped particle 42 nm in diameter enclosing an inner icosahedral 27 nm nucleocapsid	Children are infected by prenatal transmission; infection spread by blood transfusion and sexual intercourse; chronic infection with HBV can progress to liver cancer.
Papova viruses (Fam: Papova viridae) (Single stranded DNA) Circular DNA RNA viruses	Papilloma virus	Naked icosahedral; 50 nm in diameter	Cause warts; some associated with cervical carcinoma

Table 2.10 *Contd...*

Group	Virus	Characteristics	Clinical importance
Myxoviruses (fam: Myxoviridae)	Influenza virus	Enveloped particles;100 nm diameter with helically symmetric capsid	Produce new antigenic variation cause pandemics of influenza
Paramyxoviruses (Fam: Paramyxo viridae) ssRNA with mRNA complementary in base sequence to virion RNA (-) sense	Mumps virus	Enveloped particles size range 110-170 nm in diameter, helical capsid	Mumps infection to parotid and submallillary salivary glandsin children& neurological complication in adults.s
	Measles virus	Enveloped particles size range 120-250 nm in diameter, helical capsid	Childhood fever, immunity is life long.
Rhabdoviruses (Fam:Rhabdoviridae) (-) sense	Rabies virus	Bullet shaped particles, 75-180 nm, enveloped, helical capsids	Infecting all mammals;dogs,cats and cattle ; Rabies a deadly infection
Reoviruses (Fam:Reoviridae) (double stranded RNA virus)	Rotavirus	Icosahedral shell of 70 nm diameter particles	Gastroenteritis in infants
Picornaviruses (Fam:Picornaviridae) ssRNA with mRNA identical in base sequence to virion RNA (+) sense	poliovirus	Naked icosahedral particles 28 nm in diameter	polio
Rhinoviruses (Fam:Picornaviridae)		Naked icosahedral 30 nm in diameter	Common cold, there are 100 antigenically distinct types
	Hepatitis a virus	Naked icosahedral 27 nm in diameter	Infectious hepatitis
Togaviruses (Fam: Togaviridae) (+) sense	rubella	Spherical particles; 70 nm in diameter; envelop surrounding icosahedral capsid	German measles in children
Flaviviruses (Fam:Flaviviridae) (+) sense	Yellow fever virus	Spherical particles 40 nm in diameter with lipid envelope	Jaundice and fever
	Hepatitis C virus (HCV)	Spherical particles 40 nm in diameter with lipid envelop	Infection Milder than HBV.

Table 2.10 *Contd...*

Group	Virus	Characteristics	Clinical importance
Filoviruses (Fam: Filoviridae) ssRNA with mRNA complementary in base sequence to virion RNA	Ebola virus	Long filamentous rods with lipid envelop; helical nucleocapsid;1000 nm long,80 nm diameter	Wide spread among monkeys,spread to humans contact with body fluids of primates;haemorrhagic fever;90%fatality rate.
Retroviruses (Fam: Retroviridae) ssRNA with DNA intermediate in their growth (+) sense	Human T-cell leukaemia virus (HTLV-1)	Spherical enveloped virus 100 nm in diameter;icosahedral core	Human T-cell leukaemia in adults
	HIV	The core is cone-shaped rather than icosahedral	HIV;principal target for the virus is the CD4+ T-lymphocyte cells. Depletion of these cells induce immunodeficiency.
Hepatitis viruse (Fam: Unassigned)	Hepatitis D virus (HDV)	Can replicate in cells co-infected with HBV. The spherical coat of HDV is composed of HBV capsid protein	Severe hepatitis HBV

(B) RNA viruses

Important Characteristics:

- RNA as their genetic material
- Genome may be ssRNA or dsRNA
- ssRNA viruses may be of **positive (+) sense** or **negative (-) sense**
- Replicationoccurs in the cytoplasm using a RNA-dependent RNA polymerase
- RNA dependent RNA polymerases are not having proofreading activity and hence replicate their templates with a higher error rate.

Positive (+) sense viral RNA is similar to mRNA and thus can be immediately translated by the host cell. *Flaviviruses, Togaviruses, Poliovirus* are some examples of (+) sense RNA viruses.

Negative (-) sense viral RNA is complementary to mRNA and thus must be converted to positive (+) sense RNA by an RNA dependent RNA polymerase before translation. Influenza virus, Measles virus, Rabies virus are some examples of negative (-) sense RNA viruses.

Double-stranded RNA viruses need to package an RNA dependent RNA polymerase to make their mRNA after infection of the host cell. Examples of dsRNA viruses are *Rotaviruses* which belong to family *Reoviruses.*

Important groups of RNA viruses are:

- *Picornaviridae, Togaviridae, Flaviviridae, Retroviridae, Paramyxoviridae, Orthomyxoviridae, Bunyaviridae, Reoviridae.*

The different families of RNA viruses are distinguished from one another by their nucleic acid content, their capsid shape and presence or absence of an envelope.

2.9.3 Virus Cultivation

Viruses are obligate intracellular parasites so they depend on host for their survival. They cannot be grown in non-living culture media or on agar plates alone, they must require living cells to support their replication.

The primary purpose of virus cultivation is:

1. To isolate and identify viruses in clinical samples.
2. To do research on viral structure, replication, genetics and effects on host cell.
3. To prepare viruses for vaccine production.

Cultivation of viruses

1. Animal inoculation
2. Inoculation into embryonated egg
3. Cell cultures

1. **Animal inoculation:** Viruses which are not cultivated in embryonated egg and tissue culture are cultivated in laboratory animals such as mice, guinea pig, hamster, rabbits and primates are used.

   The selected animals should be healthy and free from any communicable diseases.

   Suckling mice (less than 48 hours old) are most commonly used,because they are susceptible to *Togavirus* and *Coxsackie* virus. The inoculation is done by intracerebral and intranasal route.

   Viruses can also be inoculated by intraperitoneal and subcutaneous route.

   After inoculation, virus multiply in host and develops disease. The animals are observed for symptoms of disease and death.

   Then the viruses are isolated and purified from the tissue of these animals.

   Advantages of animal inoculation:

   1. Diagnosis, pathogenesis and clinical symptoms are determined.
   2. Production of antibodies can be identified.
   3. Primary isolation of certain viruses

4. Mice provide a reliable model for studying viral replication.
5. Used for the study of immune responses, epidemiology and oncogenesis.

Disadvantages of animal inoculation:

1. Expensive and difficulties in maintenance of animals.
2. Difficulty in choosing of animals for particular virus
3. Some human viruses cannot be grown in animals, or can be grown but can not cause disease.
4. Mice do not provide models for vaccine development
5. It will lead to generation of escape mutants
6. Issues related to animal welfare systems.

2. **Inoculation in embryonated egg:** Pasteur in 1931 first used the embryonated hen's egg for the cultivation of virus.

It depends on the type of egg used, and chick embryo of 7-12 days old.

Eggs are first prepared for cultivation; the shells surface is first disinfected with iodine and penetrated with a small sterile drill for inoculation.

After inoculation, the opening is sealed with gelatin or paraffin and incubated at 36 ° C for 2-3 days.

After incubation the egg is broken and virus is isolated from tissue of egg.

Viral growth and multiplication in the egg embryo is indicated by the death of the embryo, by embryo cell damage, or by the formation of typical pocks or lesions on the egg membranes.

Viruses can be cultivated in various parts of egg like chorioallantoic membrane, allantoic cavity, amniotic sac and yolk sac.

Advantages of inoculation into embryonated egg:

1. Widely used method for the isolation of virus and growth
2. Ideal substrate for the viral growth and replication.
3. Isolation and cultivation of many avian and few mammalian viruses
4. Cost effective and maintenance is much easier
5. Less labor is needed.
6. The embryonated eggs are readily available.
7. Sterile and wide range of tissues and fluids.
8. They are free from contaminating bacteria and many latent viruses.
9. Specific and non specific factors of defense are not involved in embryonated eggs.
10. Widely used method to grow virus for some vaccine production.

***Disadvantages of inoculation into embryonated egg*:**

1. The site of inoculation varies with type of virus.

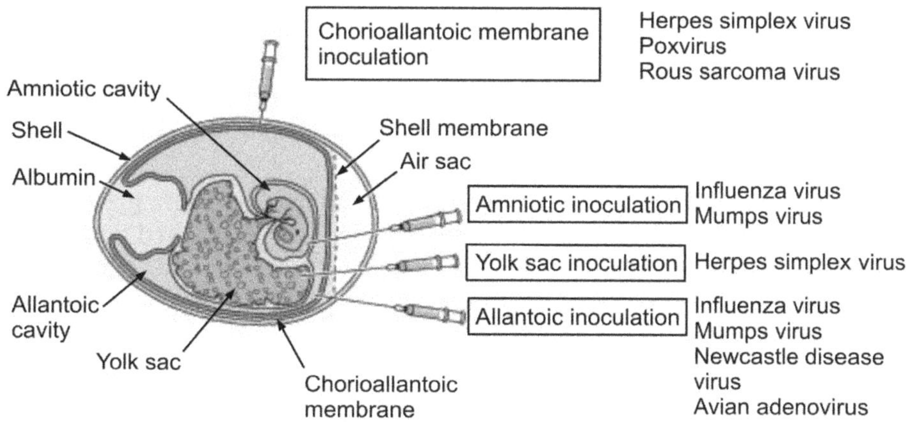

Table 2.11 Showing the details of virus cultivation in different membranes of chick embryo and their properties

S.No.	Type of Membrane of Chick embryo	Properties of virus cultivation
1	Chorioallantoic Membrane (CAM)	1. For growing pox virus, herpes simples virus. 2. Visible lesions (pocks) are observed on grey white are in transparent CAM. 3. Single virus gives single pocks 4. Suitable for plaque studies
2	Allantoic cavity	1. For production of vaccine of influenza virus, yellow fever, rabies. 2. Most avian viruses can be isolated.
3	Amniotic sac	1. For isolation of influenza virus and mumps virus. 2. Detection of virus is done by haemagglutination assay.
4	Yolk sac	1. Simplest method for growth and multiplication of virus. 2. For cultivation some viruses,and bacteria (Chlamydia & Rickettsiae) 3. Immune interference mechanism can be detected in most of avian viruses.

3. **Cell cultures (Tissue Culture):** There are three types of tissue culture; Organ culture, Explant culture and Cell culture

   Organ cultures are mainly done for highly specialized parasites of certain organs e.g. tracheal ring culture is done for isolation of corona virus.

   Explant culture is rarely done.

   Cell culture is mostly used for identification and cultivation of viruses.

   Cell culture is the process by which cells are grown under controlled conditions.

   Cells are grown in vitro on glass or a treated plastic surface in a suitable growth medium.

   At first growth medium, usually balanced salt solution containing 13 amino acids, sugar, proteins, salts, calf serum, buffer antibiotics and phenol red are taken and the host tissue or cell is inoculated.

   On incubation the cell divide and spread out on the glass surface to form a confluent monolayer.

Table 2.12 Type of cell culture

S.No.	Type of cell culture	Properties
1	Primary cell culture	1. These are normal cells derived from animal or human cells. 2. They are able to grow only for limited time and cannot be maintained in serial culture. 3. They are used for primary isolation of viruses and production of viral vaccines. Examples are Monkey kidney cell culture, Human amnion cell culture
2	Diploid cell culture (semi-continuous cell lines)	1. They are diploid and contain the same number of chromosomes as the parent cells. 2. They can be sub-cultured upto 50 times by serial transfer following senescence and the cell strain is lost. 3. They are used for the isolation of some fastidious viruses and production of viral vaccines. Examples are Monkey embryonic lung strain, Rhesus embryo cell strain.
3	Heteroploid cultures (continuous cell lines)	1. They are derived from cancer cells. 2. They can be serially cultured idenfinitely so named as continuous cell lines. 3. They can be maintained either by serial subculture or by storing in deep freeze at -70°C. 4. They are not useful for vaccine preparation. 5. Examples HeLa(Human carcinoma of cervix cell), HEP-2(Human Epithelioma of larynx cell line, Vero (Vervet monkey) kidney cell lines, BHK-21 (Baby Hamster Kidney cell line).

***Advantages of cell culture*:** Relative ease, broad spectrum, cheaper and sensitivity

Disadvantage of cell culture:

1. The process requires trained technicians with experience in working on a full time basis.
2. State health laboratories and hospital laboratories do not isolate and identify viruses in clinical work.
3. Tissue or serum for analysis is sent to central laboratories to identify viruses.

Cultivation of plant viruses and bacteriophages

Cultivation of plant viruses: There are some methods of cultivation of plant viruses such as plant tissue cultures, cultures 9 of separated cells, or cultures of protoplasts, etc. viruses can be grown in whole plants.

Leaves are mechanically inoculated by rubbing with a mixture of viruses and an abrasive. When the cell wall is broken by the abrasive, the viruses directly contact the plasma membrane and infect the exposed host cells. A localized necrotic lesion often develops due to the rapid death of cells in the infected area. Some plant viruses can be transmitted only if a diseased part is grafted onto a healthy plant.

Cultivation of bacteriophages: Bacteriophages are cultivated in either broth or agar cultures of young, actively growing bacterial cells.

2.9.4 Viruses Replication

Introduction to Life Cycle of Viruses

(A) Lytic Cycle: These are also known as virulent cycle because phages multiply inside the host and lyse the cell at the end of its life cycle.After attachment of tail fibre to host, genetic materials are injected inside the host. The time period between the entry of genetic material inside the host and release of mature phage after end of life cycle is termed as eclipse period. Synthesis of phage components and its packaging into mature phages takes place in this period. After infection, the genetic material of phages uses host biosynthetic machinery for replication, transcription and translation. Structural proteins of phages (capsid, tail etc.) are also synthesized inside the host using host biosynthetic machinery. After synthesis, genetic materials are packed inside the capsid and tail is attached on it. This process is called as maturation of phages. In lytic phage, phages also synthesized lysis protein. Bacterial cells are lysed due to accumulation of phage lysis protein and mature phages are released into the medium. Around 10-1000 phages are released from the bacterial cell. The average yield of phages per infected bacterial cell is known as burst size.

(B) Lysogenic cycle: These are also known as temperate phage because phages multiply via the lytic cycle or may enter a dormant state inside the cell. After entry of genetic material into the host cell, the phage DNA integrates into the host chromosome and starts replication along with it and passed to the daughter cells of host. Integration of phage DNA to host chromosome is termed as prophage and bacteria is termed as lysogenic bacteria. Due to integration of phage DNA to host chromosome, extra genes carried by phage get expressed in the host cell and it may change the properties of bacterial cell. This process is termed as lysogenisc or phage conversion.

Due to exposure to UV rays, ionizing radiations, mutagenic chemicals etc, DNA of phage is released from host chromosome and separated phage DNA initiates lytic cycle resulting in the lysis of cell and release of phages into the medium.

Steps in Virus Replication

1. **Adsorption:** It occurs after a chance collision between phage particles and bacteria i.e. an attachment site on the virus attaches to a complimentary receptor cite on the bacteria cell. The Adsorption process occurs in two steps: The first step involves preliminary attachment by ionic bonds or charges and is easily reversed by a shift in pH or salt concentration. The second step appears more specific and it is irreversible. Molecular entities on the surface of cells act as receptor for viruses.
2. **Penetration:** The penetrations of animal viruses into attached cells occur by one of two mechanisms.
   - One mechanism consists of engulfment of whole virions by the cells in a phagocytic process called viropexis followed by uncoating or removal of the capsid. This takes place due to the action of enzymes called lysosomal proteus.
   - The second mechanism occurs in the enveloped viruses; the viral lipoprotein envelope fuses with the host cell's surface membrane. This fusion results in the release of viral nucleocapsid material into the cytoplasm of the host cell. Uncoating again occurs within the host cell.

   In the T – phages, penetration is achieved when:

   (ii) The tail fibres of the virus attach to the cell and hold the tail firmly against the cell wall.

   (iii) The sheath contracts, driving the tail core into the cell through the cell wall and membrane and

   (iv) The virus injects its DNA.

3. **Replication and bio synthesis of virus-specific molecules:** Shortly after penetration, there follows an interval of time called the latent period. During the latent period uncoating of the virion takes place.
   - The uncoating process varies from one virus to another. Some viruses are uncoated in the cytoplasm, while others are uncoated in the nucleus.
   - Transcription of the viral nucleic acid into mRNA is the next step for all viruses except those RNA viruses (eg: picornaviruses) whose viral RNA acts directly as mRNA.
   - Transcription is catalyzed by a viral RNA polymerase released during uncoating.
   - The biosynthetic processes of viral specific molecule can be divided into early and late events. Thus in most viruses, only part of the nucleic acid of the infecting virion is initially transcribed into mRNA.
   - Generally, early mRNA codes for early enzymes required for nucleic acid replication and for proteins that inhibit synthesis of cellular macromolecules and break down cellular polyribasomes, making them available for the transcription of the viral genes.
   - Replication process may take place in the cell nucleus or cytoplasm.
   - Nucleic acid replication serves as demarcation line between early and late events in the viral replication process. Since late mRNA is not synthesized until after viral DNA replication has begun, it is transcribed from progeny genomes.
   - Late protein synthesis is defined as the process taking place after nucleic acid replication.
   - Late mRNA usually specifies structural proteins of the virion.
   - Translation of mRNA into proteins takes place in the host cell cytoplasm and uses ribosomes, transfer RNAs, and enzymes in the cytoplasm.
4. **Assembly and release:**
   - Only after the synthesis of various viral components, then the phage components begin to assemble into mature phages.
   - The DNA viruses, with the exception of the poxviruses, are assembled in the nucleus
   - The RNA viruses are generally assembled in the cytoplasm.
   - Release of the completed virions from the host cell is the final step in virus multiplication.
   - In some animal virus infections, the host cell lyse, releasing the virions.
   - Naked virions are released in a burst like fashion from the cells as they lyse.
   - Enveloped animal viruses are released by budding.
   - The yield of virus particles per cell varies with the virus, the type of cell, and the growth conditions.

2.9.5 Bacteriophages

Bacteriophage: A virus that lives within a bacterium, replicating itself and eventually destroying the bacterial cell. Bacteriophages have been very helpful in the study of bacterial and molecular genetics. They are sometimes simply called phages.

2.9.5.1 Morphology and Classification

Morphologically phages vary from exceedingly simple such as the small, single standard DNA phage, Φx 174, to phages with a complex tadpole – like shape, the T – even phage shown in Fig. 2.34 and 2.35.

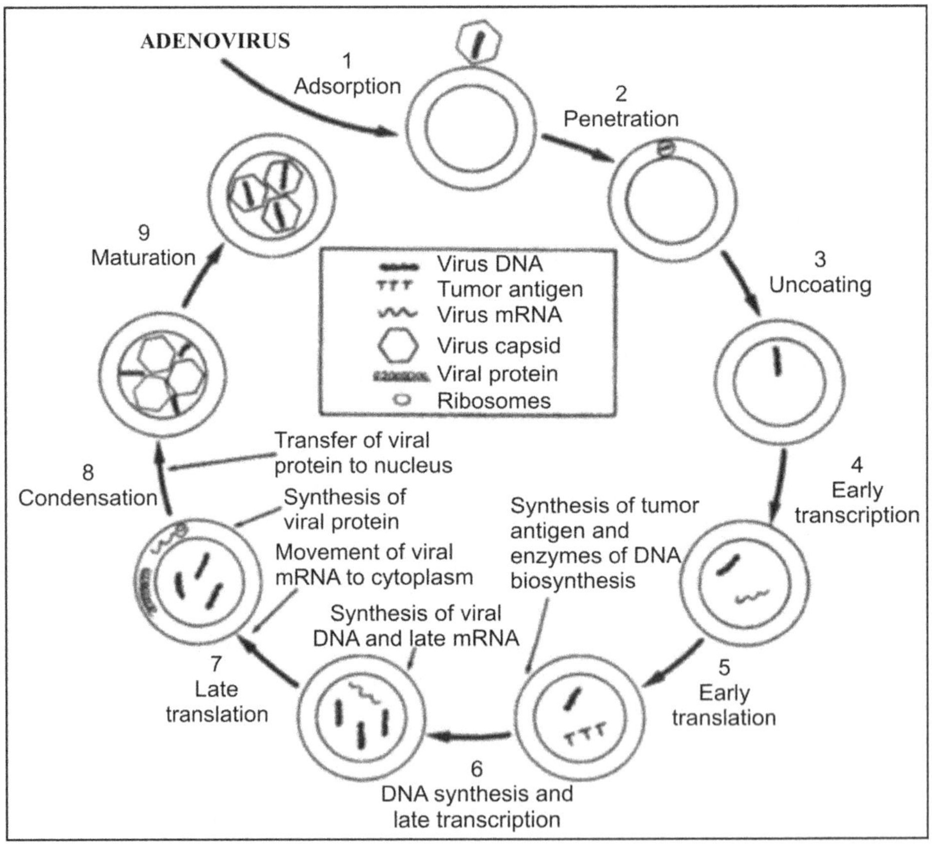

Fig. 2.34 Characterization, classification and identification of bacteriophage

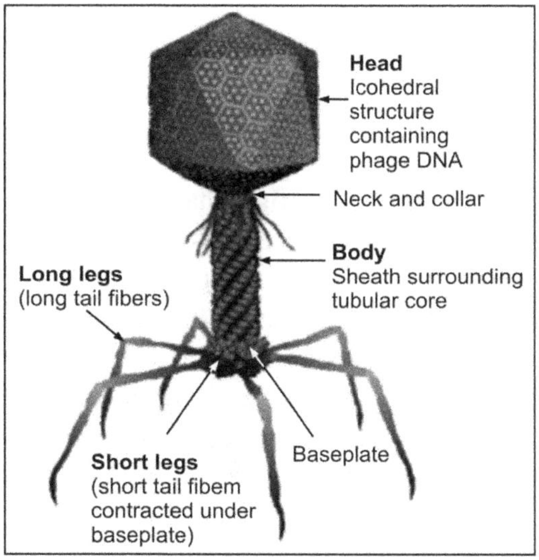

Fig. 2.35 Bacteriophage structure

A number of phages known to attack Escherichia coli described by Bradly are listed in below.

Table 2.13 Types of Bacteriophages

Bradly Type	Examples (colliphages)	Description	Nucleic Acid Type
A	T – even	Angular head, contractile tail	2 – DNA
B	T_1, T_5	Angular head, long– Non – contractile tail	2 – DNA
C	$T_3 - T_7$	Angular head, short – Non – contractile tail	2 – DNA
D	Φ x 174	Angular virion, no tail	1 – DNA
E	f_2, R_{17}, f_r	Angular head, contractile tail	1 – DNA
F	F_d, m_{13}, f_1	Flexible filament	1 – DNA

Phages can be classified as virulent or temperate on the basis of the response they produce in their host cells. Infection of a sensitive bacterium with a virulent phage results in the replication of the virus, lysis of the cell and release of new infectious progeny phage particles. Temperate phages can produce this lytic cycle response, but they are also capable of a symbiotic response in which the invading viral genome does not take over the direction of cellular activity, the cell survives the infection and the viral nucleic acid becomes incorporated into the bacterial chromosome, where it is termed prophage. Cells carrying viral genes in this way are referred to as lysogenic virus.

Applications of Bacteriophages

1. ***Phage therapy:*** Many phage biologists believe it is possible to use phage or phage products (such as phage-encoded enzymes) as disease therapy or in other ways to solve our bacterial problems. With a few exceptions, these techniques are in research stages rather than in actual use. In fact, bacterial infections can be treated with bacteriophages: viruses that have the ability to infect and fight harmful bacteria, culminating in their destruction. Bacteriophage or phage therapy is therefore very useful in various fields like medicine, veterinary science, dentistry, and even agriculture. Eli Lilly began the commercialization of phage therapy in the US during the 1940s. During the Second World War, phages were used to treat bacterial diseases among soldiers of the Soviet Union, particularly gangrene and dysentery. The development of antibiotics in the 1950s led to a temporary setback on phage therapy as the use of antibiotics became more favourable. However, there has been a renewed interest in the development and employment of phage therapy in more applications.

   It may be less difficult for phages to overcome bacterial or viral resistance compared to antibiotics. Because phages are target specific, meaning only a one or very few bacterial strains are targeted upon, it is easier to develop new phages than new antibiotics. A time period of only a few days or weeks are needed to acquire new phages for resistant strains of bacteria, whereas it can take years to obtain new antibiotics. When resisting bacteria evolve, the assigned phages also evolve, so when super bacterium appears, an equivalent super phage fights it as long as the phage is derived from the same environment. Phages are and have for decades been widely used as tools in recombinant DNA technology: important in applications and developing applications ranging from medical diagnostics and forensics to basic research.

   Compared to antibiotics, phages go deeper into the infected area.

   Secondary resistance does not happen among phages. Certain infections in people and experimentally infected animals have been proven to be more effectively treated with phage therapy than using antibiotics.

   It can be the key to fighting the NDM-1, a gene that can be included in the DNA of bacteria, enabling them to resist antibiotics. Waste water from sewage systems are not really considered waste because it is a rich source of phage strains for various kinds of bacteria that lead to the most up-to-date medicines. Skin grafting for extensive wounds, trauma, burns, and skin cancer can also be improved by using phage therapy to lessen the *Psuedomonas aeruginosa* infection. Some experiments for cells in tissue culture have also discovered antitumor agents in phages. Bacteria cause food to spoil faster, and phages have been studied for their potential to increase the freshness of food and decrease the incidents of food spoilage.

2. ***Phage display:*** Phage Display is a method wherein a library of phage particles that express very diverse peptides is generated. The objective is to choose those that will bind a desired target; the target can be a protein, a peptide, or a piece of DNA.

   The fast isolation of particular ligands through phage display has a wide variety of applications like epitope mapping, analyzing different protein interactions, vaccine development, drug design, and therapeutic target validation. Phage display is also used to pick inhibitors for the active and allosteric sites of G-protein binding modulatory peptides, enzymes, and receptor antagonists and agonists.

   Determining the proper protein partners can be useful to identify the functions of various proteins. For drug discovery and design, Phage Display is employed in protein engineering or *in vitro* protein evolution. Therapeutic targeting with phage display is also primarily used to diagnose and determine tumour antigens, which is useful for cancer research.

   Antibody Phage Display significantly improved the discovery and development of antibody drugs. Phage display for antibody libraries paved the way for rapid vaccine design and therapy. These libraries are used to learn more about the human immune system and to create human antibodies *in vitro* with the use of diverse synthetic substances.

   Phage Display can be used in conjunction with other techniques, and with enough support and studies, more applications for it can be discovered.

   The challenges before us are how the phage-based therapeutic agent is to be delivered to the patient, and how to protect the phage-based agent from immune attack by the patient's body, and how to handle the expected development of phage-resistant pathogens.

3. ***Miscellaneous applications***: New characteristics are acquired using lysogenic conversion.

   Insertional mutation can be induced in bacterial chromosome by random insertion of genes or nucleotides.

   Latent infection in mammalian cells by retroviruses can be studied using Lambda phage as model system.

   In genetic engineering, phages are used extensively where they serve as cloning vectors.

   Phages are used to maintain libraries of genes and monoclonal antibodies

   Natural removal of bacteria from water bodies can be done using bacteriophages.

2.9.6 Plant Viruses

The beginnings of plant virology dates back to the late 19th century, when Dutch microbiologist Martinus Beijerinck and Russian researcher Dmitrii Iwanowski were investigating the cause of a mysterious disease of tobacco (Scholthof 2001). These researchers independently described an unusual agent that caused mosaic disease in tobacco (Zaitlin 1998). What distinguished this agent from other disease-causing agents was its much smaller size compared to that of other microbes. This agent, later named *Tobacco mosaic virus* (TMV), was the first virus to be described. Since then, a large number of diverse viruses have been found in plants, animals, fungi, and bacteria. The current estimate of recognized viruses is approaching 4,000, of which about 1,000 are plant viruses. The main reason that we study plant viruses is the negative impact that viral diseases have on crop production. For instance, plant viruses are being used to produce large quantities of proteins of interest in plants (Pogue et al. 2002) and to develop safe and inexpensive vaccines against human and animal viruses (Walmsley and Arntzen 2000).

Major Plant Viruses

Tobacco Mosaic Virus

Cucumber Mosaic Virus

Barley Yellow Dwarf

Bud Blight,

Sugarcane Mosaic Virus,

Cauliflower Mosaic Virus

Lettuce Mosaic Virus

Maize Mosaic Virus,

Peanut Stunt Virus

2.9.7 Viroids

Genomes of non-defective viruses range in size from 2,400,000 bp of dsDNA (*Pandoravirus salinus*) to 1,759 bp of ssDNA (porcine circovirus). Whereas even smaller viral genomes possible are available in the subviral agents called viroids. *provide.*

Viroids, the smallest known pathogens, are naked, circular, single-stranded RNA molecules that do not encode protein yet replicate autonomously when introduced into host plants. Potato spindle tuber viroid, discovered in 1971, is the prototype; 29 other viroids have since been discovered ranging in length from 120 to 475 nucleotides. Viroids only infect plants; some cause economically important diseases of crop plants, while others appear to be benign. Two examples of economically important viroids are coconut cadang-cadang viroid (which causes a lethal infection of coconut palms) and apple scar skin viroid (which causes an infection that results in visually unappealing apples).

The 30 known viroids have been classified in two families. Members of the *Pospiviroidae*, named for *po*tato *spi*ndle tuber viroid, have a rod-like secondary structure with small single stranded regions, a central conserved region, and replicate in the nucleus. The *Avsunviroidae*, named for *av*ocado *sun*blotch viroid, have both rod-like and branched regions, but lack a central conserved region and replicate in chloroplasts. In contrast to the *Pospiviroidae*, the latter RNA molecules are functional ribozymes, and this activity is essential for replication.

There is no evidence that viroids encode proteins or mRNA. Unlike viruses, which are parasites of host translation machinery, viroids are parasites of cellular transcription proteins: they depend on cellular RNA polymerase for replication. Such polymerases normally recognize DNA templates, but can copy viroid RNAs.

In plants infected with members of the *Pospiviroidae*, viroid RNA is imported into the nucleus, and copied by plant DNA-dependent RNA polymerase II. The viroid is copied by a rolling circle mechanism that produces complementary linear, concatameric, RNAs. These are copied again to produce concatameric, linear molecules, which are cleaved by the host enzyme RNAse III. Their ends are joined by a host enzyme to form circles.

In plants infected with members of the *Avsunviroidae*, viroid RNA is imported into the chloroplast, and complementary concatameric RNAs are produced by chloroplast DNA-dependent RNA polymerase. Cleavage of these molecules is carried out by a ribozyme, an enzyme encoded in the viroid RNA.

After replication, viroid progeny exit the nucleus or chloroplast and move to adjacent cells through plasmodesmata, and can travel systemically via the phloem to infect other cells. Viroids enter the pollen and ovule, from where they are transmitted to the seed. When the seed germinates, the new plant becomes infected. Viroids can also be transmitted among plants by contaminated farm machinery and insects.

Symptoms of viroid infection in plants include stunting of growth, deformation of leaves and fruit, stem necrosis, and death. So far there are no known human pathogens in this category, although human hepatitis D virus shares some features in commons with viroids, and may have originated from them. Because viroids do not produce mRNAs, it was first proposed that disease must be a consequence of viroid RNA binding to host proteins or nucleic acids. The discovery of RNA silencing in plants lead to the hypothesis that small interfering RNAs derived from viroid RNAs guide silencing of host genes, leading to induction of disease. In support of this hypothesis, peach latent mosaic viroid small RNAs have been identified that silence chloroplast heat shock protein 90, which correlates with disease symptoms. The different disease patterns caused by viroids in their hosts might all have in common an origin in RNA silencing.

Our current understanding is that the disease-causing viroids were transferred from wild plants used for breeding modern crops. The widespread prevalence of these agents can be traced to the use of genetically identical plants (monoculture), worldwide distribution of breeding lines, and mechanical transmission by contaminated farm machinery. As a consequence, these unusual pathogens now occupy niches around the planet that never before were available to them.

The origin of viroids remains an enigma, but it has been proposed that they are relics from the RNA world, which is thought to have been populated only by non-coding RNA molecules that catalysed their own synthesis. Viroids have properties that make them candidates for survivors of the RNA world: small genome size (to avoid error catastrophe caused by error-prone replication), high G+C content (for greater thermodynamic stability), circular genomes (to avoid the need for mechanisms to prevent loss of information at the ends of linear genomes), no protein content, and the presence of a ribozyme, a fingerprint of the RNA world. Today's viroids can no longer self-replicate, possibly having lost that function when they became parasites of plants. What began as a search for virus-like agents that cause disease in plants has lead to new insights into the evolution of life.

2.9.8 Prions

A **prion** is a protein that can fold in multiple, structurally distinct ways, at least one of which is transmissible to other **prion** proteins. It is this form of replication that leads to disease that is similar to viral infection.

Prion disease represents a group of conditions that affect the nervous system in humans and animals. In people, these conditions impair brain function, causing changes in memory, personality, and behavior; a decline in intellectual function (dementia); and abnormal movements, particularly difficulty with coordinating movements (ataxia). The signs and symptoms of prion disease typically begin in adulthood and worsen with time, leading to death within a few months to several years.

These disorders are very rare. Although the exact prevalence of prion disease is unknown, studies suggest that this group of conditions affects about one person per million worldwide each year. Approximately 350 new cases are reported annually in the United States.

Between 10 and 15 percent of all cases of prion disease are caused by mutations in the *PRNP* gene. Because they can run in families, these forms of prion disease are classified as familial. Familial prion diseases, which have overlapping signs and symptoms, include familial Creutzfeldt-Jakob disease (CJD), Gerstmann-Sträussler-Scheinker syndrome (GSS), and fatal familial insomnia (FFI).

The *PRNP* gene provides instructions for making a protein called prion protein (PrP). Although the precise function of this protein is unknown, researchers have proposed roles in several important processes. These include the transport of copper into cells, protection of brain cells (neurons) from injury (neuroprotection), and communication between neurons. In familial forms of prion disease, *PRNP* gene mutations result in the production of an abnormally shaped protein, known as PrP^{Sc}, from one copy of the gene. In a process that is not fully understood, PrP^{Sc} can attach (bind) to the normal protein (PrP^{C}) and promote its transformation into PrP^{Sc}. The abnormal protein builds up in the brain, forming clumps that damage or destroy neurons. The loss of these cells creates microscopic sponge-like holes (vacuoles) in the brain, which leads to the signs and symptoms of prion disease.

The other 85 to 90 percent of cases of prion disease are classified as either sporadic or acquired. People with sporadic prion disease have no family history of the disease and no identified mutation in the *PRNP* gene. Sporadic disease occurs when PrP^{C} spontaneously, and for unknown reasons, is transformed into PrP^{Sc}. Sporadic forms of prion disease include sporadic Creutzfeldt-Jakob disease (sCJD), sporadic fatal insomnia (sFI), and variably protease-sensitive prionopathy (VPSPr).

Acquired prion disease results from exposure to PrP^{Sc} from an outside source. For example, variant Creutzfeldt-Jakob disease (vCJD) is a type of acquired prion disease in humans that results from eating beef products containing PrP^{Sc} from cattle with prion disease. In cows, this form of the disease is known as bovine spongiform encephalopathy (BSE) or, more commonly, "mad cow disease." Another example of an acquired human prion disease is kuru, which was identified in the South Fore population in Papua New Guinea. The disorder was transmitted when individuals ate affected human tissue during cannibalistic funeral rituals.

Rarely, prion disease can be transmitted by accidental exposure to PrP^{Sc}-contaminated tissues during a medical procedure. This type of prion disease, which accounts for 1 to 2 percent of all cases, is classified as iatrogenic.

Familial forms of prion disease are inherited in an autosomal dominant pattern, which means one copy of the altered *PRNP* gene in each cell is sufficient to cause the disorder. In most cases, an affected person inherits the altered gene from one affected parent. In some people, familial forms of prion disease are caused by a new mutation in the gene that occurs during the formation of a parent's reproductive cells (eggs or sperm) or in early embryonic development. Although such people do not have an affected parent, they can pass the genetic change to their children.

The sporadic, acquired, and iatrogenic forms of prion disease, including kuru and variant Creutzfeldt-Jakob disease, are not inherited.

2.10 Identification of Micro-organisms

1. **Staining:** A stain is a dye or colouring substance that adheres to a cell giving the cell colour. The presence of colour gives the cell significant contrast so are much more visible. Staining techniques are most frequently used for identification, observation or the morphological characteristics of bacteria. Staining is an auxillary technique used in microscopy to enhance contrast in the microscopic image and highlight structures.

The advantages of staining are:

1. Bacteria have nearly the same refractive index as water therefore when they are observed under a microscope they are opaque or nearly invisible to the naked eye. Different types of staining methods are used to make the cells and their internal structures more clearly visible under the light microscope after they are coloured.
2. Differences between cells of different species and within the same species can be demonstrated by use of appropriate staining solutions.

The essential steps in preparing a fixed, stained smear are:

1. Preparation of the film or smear of the microbial culture on a clean glass slide with incoculating loop.
2. Fixation of the smear without heat is aimed to preserve the shape of the cell. Fixing with heat is to kill, adhere and alter the specimen so it will accept the stain.
3. Application of one or more staining solutions on the smear.

2. **Microbiological Stains:** A large number of coloured organic compounds are available for staining micro-organisms.

   These compounds are generally complex in terms of molecular structure and can be classified into groups such as triphenyl methane dyes, oxazine dyes and thiazine dyes.

   A more practical classification is based on the chemical behaviour of the dye namely acid, basic and neutral.

   An Acidic (Anionic) Dye is one in which the charge on the dye ion is negative and they stain basic cell components.Acidic dye bind to positively charged cell structure like some proteins used to provide background staining like capsule staining. Examples Nigrosine, Picric acid, Eosin, Acid Fuschin, India Ink.

   A **Basic Dye** is one in which the charge on the dye ion is positive and they stain acidic cell components like Nucleic acids, Carboxylic group and Alcohol group. Basic dyes are most commonly used in Bacteriology. Examples are Crystal violet, Mythelene blue, Saffranin, and Basic Fuschin.

   A **Neutral Dye** is a complex salt of an acidic dye with a basic dye.Neutral dye stains nucleic acid and cytoplasm E.g., Eosinate of methylene blue and Geimsa stain.

   Bacteria are slightly negatively charged at pH 7.0, so basic dye stains bacteria and acidic dye stains background.

   The process of staining may involve ion-exchange reactions between the stain and active sites at the surface or within the cell.

   E.g., Coloured ions of dye may replace other ions on cellular components.

2.10.1 Simple Staining

The colouration of bacteria by applying a single solution of a stain to a fixed smear is termed as simple staining. The fixed smear is flooded with a dye solution for a specified period of time, after which the solution is washed off with water and the slide blotted dry.

When methylene blue is used, some granules of the interior cell may appear more deeply stained than the rest indicating a different type of chemical substance.

2.10.2 Differential Staining

Staining procedures use two or more stains and allow the cells to be categorized into various groups or types. It is the technique that makes visible the differences between bacterial cells or parts of a bacterial cell.

(a) Gram's staining: Gram's staining is one of the most important and widely used differential staining techniques in microbiology.

It is invented by Hans Christian Gram in 1884.

In this process the bacterial smear is subjected to staining reagents such as crystal violet Gram's Iodine solution, Alcohol and Safranin.

Procedure (shown in Table 2.4)

1. Prepare and heat-fix smears.
2. Prepare the smears of *S. epidermidis* and *N. sicca* on a second slide.
3. Heat-fix.
4. Stain the slides as follows:
5. Flood the **crystal violet** for one minute (primary stain).
6. Pour off excess dye and wash gently in tap water and drain the slide against a paper towel.
7. Expose the smears to **Gram's iodine** for one minute by washing with iodine, then adding more iodine and leaving it on the smear until the minute is over (mordant).
8. Wash with tap water and drain carefully. (Do not blot.)
9. Wash with **95% alcohol** for 30 seconds (decolorization agent).
10. Wash with tap water at the end of the 30 seconds to stop the decolorization. Drain.
11. Counterstain with **0.25% safranin** for 30 seconds.
12. Wash, drain, blot, and examine under oil.

Draw the cells showing morphology, grouping, and relative sizes. Color a few of the cells of each bacterial species to show the Gram reaction.

Bacteria stained by gram method fall in two groups:

(i) Gram positive bacteria (ii) Gram negative bacteria

Table 2.14 Steps in gram's staining procedure

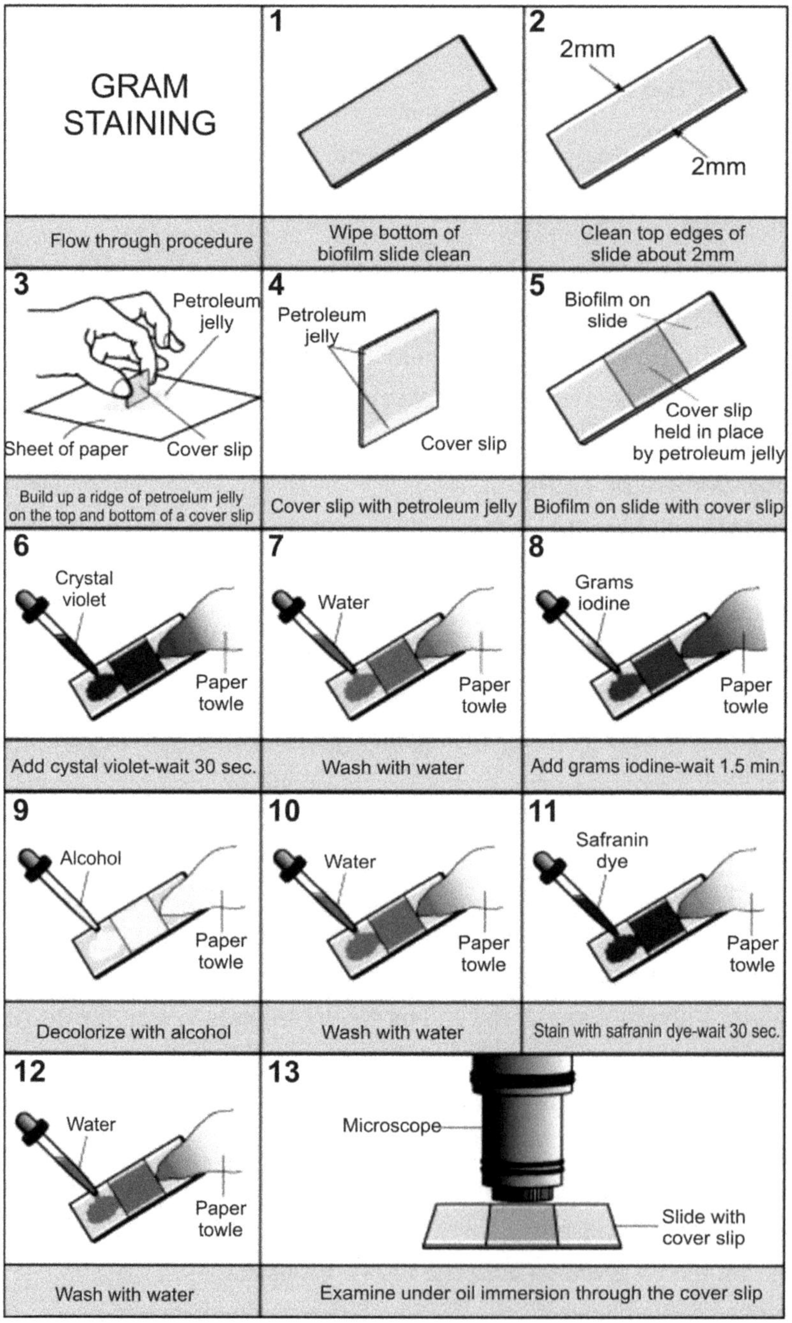

Gram +ve bacteria retain the crystal violet and appear deep blue in colour.

Gram –ve bacteria lose crystal violet, are counter stained by safranin and appear red in colour.

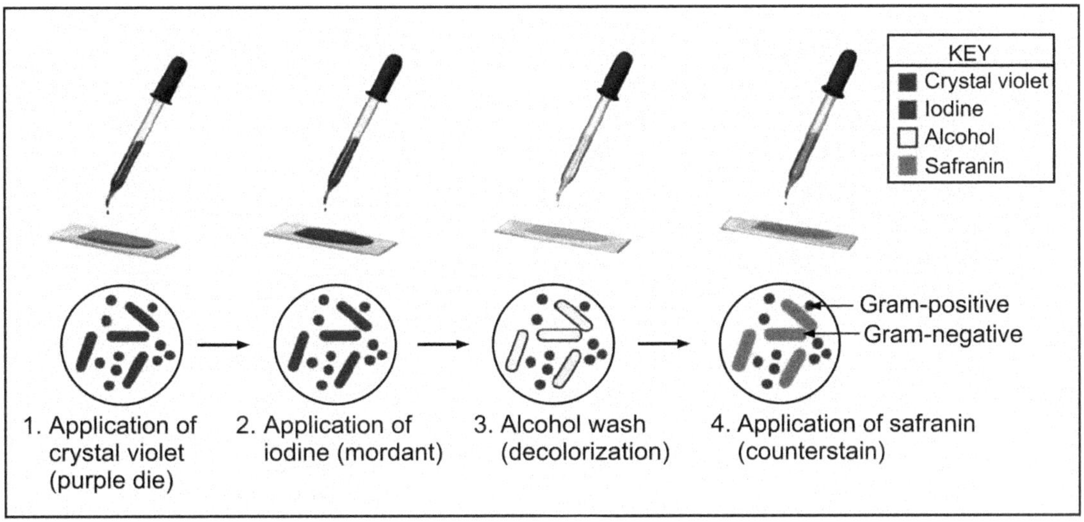

Fig. 2.36 (Colour Plate 2.1) Gram's staining method and results

Mechanism of Gram's Staining

Gram Positive Bacteria: When applied to both Gram-positive and Gram-negative cells, Crystal Violet (CV) and then Iodine (I) readily enter the cells. Inside the cells, the crystal violet and iodine combine to form the crystal violet-iodine (CVI) complex. The purple dye (Crystal Violet, CV) and the Iodine (I) combine in the cytoplasm of each bacterium and color it dark violet or purple. Bacteria that retain this color even after the alcohol (decolorizing agent) has attempted in vain to decolorize the CVI complex which is trapped in the wall following ethanol treatment,: which causes a diminution in the diameter of the cell wall peptidoglycon. They appear dark violet or purple color, so they are classified as Gram-positive.

Gram Negative Bacteria: When applied to both Gram-positive and Gram-negative cells, Crystal Violet (CV) and then Iodine (I) readily enter the cells. Inside the cells, the crystal violet and iodine combine to form the crystal violet-iodine (CVI) complex. In gram-negative cells, however, the alcohol wash disrupts the outer lipopolysaccharide layer and the CVI complex is washed out through the thin layer of peptidoglycon. As walls of Gram-negative bacteria have a very much small amount of peptidoglycon, which is less extensively cross-linked and pores in the peptidoglycon remain sufficiently large after ethanol treatment and allow CVI complex to be extracted. As a result, Gram negative cells are colorless until counterstained with safranin, after which they are stained in pink color.

Table 2.15 Differences between Gram +ve and Gram –ve

Gram +ve	Gram -ve
1. They contain magnesium ribonucleate	1. Not sensitive to triphenyl methane dyes.
2. They are very sensitive to triphenyl methane dyes.	2. Less sensitive to triphenyl methane dyes.
3. Sensitive to penicillin	3. Sensitive to streptomycin
4. They are resistant to alkalies; not dissolved by 1% KOH Isoelectric range pH – 2.5–4	4. Sensitive to alkalies dissolved by 1% KOH. Isoelectric range pH – 4.5–5.5
5. They may be acid fast	5. Never acid-fast
6. Gram + ve contain a lower content of lipids ranging from 4.8% in s citreus to 8.9% in S. aureus	6. Gram -ve contain higher content of lipids, ranging from 13.2% in E. coli to 27.7% in R. Pneumoniae.
7. Gram +ve can be rendered gram –ve by increasing acidity.	7. Grarn-ve organisms can be rendered gram +ve by increasing alkalinity.
8. Cell wall is thicker	8. Cell wall is thinner
9. Lower percentage of lipids	9. Higher percentage of lipids
10. Higher percentage of Peptidoglycan	10. Lower percentage of peptidoglycan

Examples of Gram-positive Bacteria

Cocci-*Staphylococcus, Streptococcus, Enterococcus*

Bacilli- *Listeria, Corynecaterium, Nocardia, Actinomyces, Clostridium.*

Examples of Gram-negative Bacteria

Cocci: *Neisseria, Moraxella*

Bacilli: *Escherichia, Klebsiella, salmonella, Shigella, Enterobacter, Citrobacter, Proteus, Yersinia, Pseudomonas, Acinetobacter,*

Curved Bacilli: *Campylobacter, Helicobacter and Vibrio*

2.10.3 Acid Fast Staining

2.10.3.1 Mycobacteria

Gram-resistant (waxycell walls), non-motile, pleomorphic rod, related to actinomyces. Most mycobacteria are found in habitats such as water or soil. However, a few are intracellular pathogens of animals and humans. *Mycobacterium tuberculosis*, along with *M.bovis*, *M.africanum*, and *M.microti* all cause the diseas known as tuberculosis (TB) and are members of the pathogenic for humans while *M.bovis* is usually pathogenic for animals. Mycolic acids are long fatty acids found in the cell walls of the *mycolata taxon*, a group of bacteria that includes *Mycobacterium tuberculosis*, the causative agent of the disease tuberculosis. They form the major component of the cell wall of *mycolata species*.

Mycolic Acid: Mycolic acids are composed of a longer beta-hydroxy chain with a shorter alpha-alkyl side chain. Each molecule contains between 60 and 90 carbon atoms. The exact number of carbons varies by species and can be used as an identification aid. Most mycolic acids also contain various functional groups. *M. tuberculosis* produces three main types of mycolic acids: alpha-, methoxy-, and keto-. Alpha-mycolic acids comprise at least 70% of the mycolic acids present in the organism and contain several cyclopropane rings.

Acid–Fast cells contain large amount of lipids and waxes in their cell walls primarily mycolic acid. Acid fast bacteria usually are members of the genus *Mycobacterium* or *Nocardia*.

This staining technique is used to diagnose *Mycobacterium tuberculosis*, *Mycobacterium leprae* which causes tuberculosis and leprosy respectively. Zeil Neelsen's –hot stain /Kinyoun's –cold stain and some modifications are the staining techniques used. The Basic fuchsin is a mixture of P – Rosaniline, Rosaniline and Magenta – II.

New fuchsin (Magenta – III) in pure form is employed in the acid fast staining method.

New fuchsin with three methyl groups is the deepest in shade and p-rosaniline with no methyl groups is lightest in shade.

Deeper the shade of stain used in the acid fast stain, the better will be the degree of differentiation.

Steps (Fig. 2.37)

1. Make a smear, airdry and heat fix.
2. Flood smear with carbolfuchsin stain (a lipid soluble, phenolic compound, which can penetrate the cell wall)
3. Cover flooded smear with filter paper
4. Steam for 10 minutes. Add more carbolfuchsin stain as needed.
5. Cool slide
6. Rinse with deionized water
7. Flood slide with acid alcohol (leave 15 seconds). The acid alcohol contains 3% HCl and 95% ethanol, or 20% H_2SO_4 can be used instead of acid alcohol.
8. Tilt slide 45° over the sink and add acid alcohol dropwise until the red colour stops streaming from the smear

9. Rinse with deionized water
10. Add Loeffler's methylene blue stain (counter stain). This stain adds blue colour to non-acid fast cells. Leave methylene blue stain on smear for 1 minute.
11. Rinse slide, blotdry.
12. Use oil immersion objective to view.

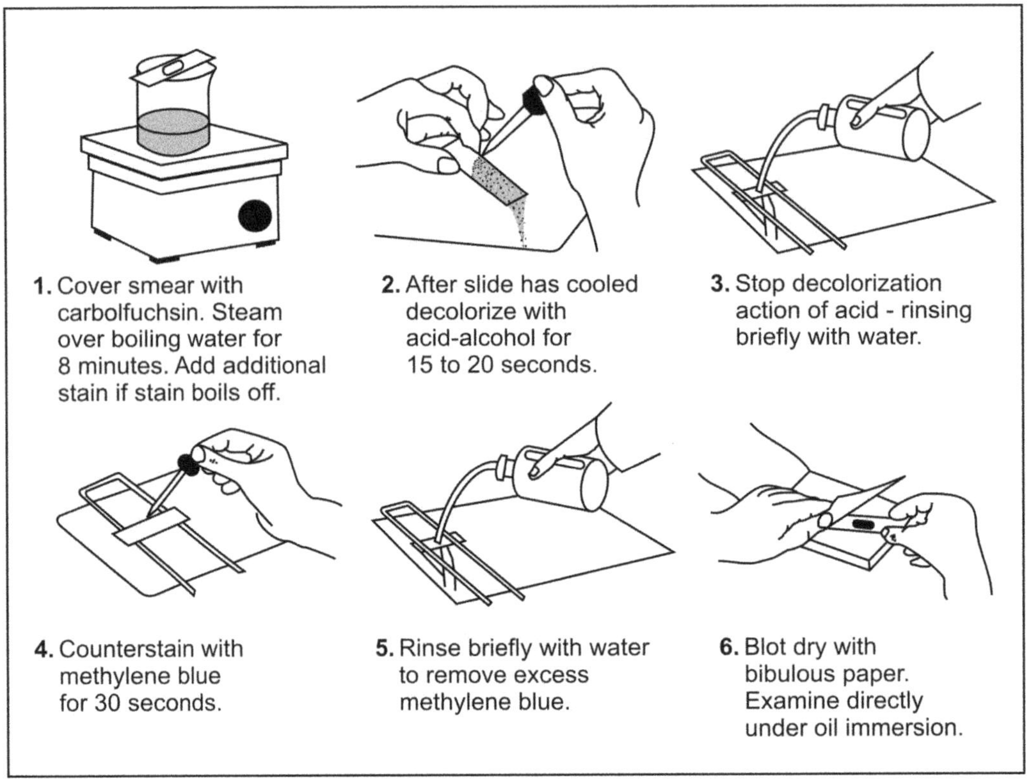

Fig. 2.37 Acid fast staining method

Result: Acid fast bacilli stains red and the other background remains blue shown in (Fig. 2.38 (Colour Plate 2.2).

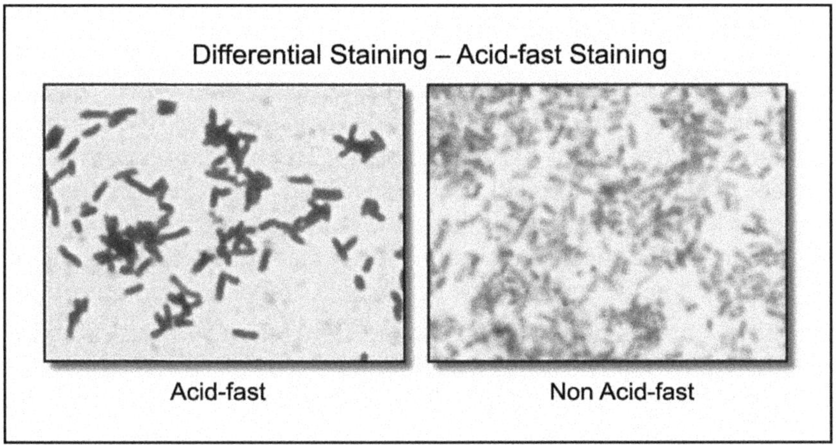

Fig. 2.38 (Colour Plate 2.2) Slides showing acid-fast and non-acid fast results

2.10.4 Kinyoun's Stain

It is the method of staining acid-fast micro-organisms which do not involve heating the slides being stained. The Kinyoun staining method uses carbol fuchsin as a primary stain, followed by decolorization with an acid-alcohol solution and methylene blue as a counterstain. Kinyoun carbol fuchsin has a greater concentration of phenol and basic fuchsin and does not require heating in order to stain properly.

Advantage: As heating is not needed, it facilitates examination in large numbers of epidemiological studies.

Auramine O stain is the Fluorescent stain used to stain *Mycobacterium tuberculosis.*

Mechanism of Acid Fast Staining

Acid-fast organisms are characterized by wax-like, nearly impermeable cell walls; they contain mycolic acid and large amounts of fatty acids, waxes, and complex lipids. Acid-fast organisms are highly resistant to disinfectants and dry conditions.

The primary stain used in acid-fast staining, carbolfuchsin, is lipid-soluble and contains phenol, which helps the stain penetrate the cell wall. This is further assisted by the addition of heat. The smear is then rinsed with a very strong decolorizer, which strips the stain from all non-acid-fast cells but does not permeate the cell wall of acid-fast organisms. The decolorized non-acid-fast cells then take up the counterstain methylene blue.

2.10.5 Feulgen Staining Protocol

The Feulgen technique selectively stains DNA, and under controlled conditions, can be used for the photometric determination of DNA content. The reaction consits of two steps. Fixed material is treated for 8-10 min with 1N HCl in a water bath or oven at 60°C. Afterwards, the material is immediately transferred into Schiff's reagent at room temperature (for at least 30 min or until the tissue stains deep purple). The material is then squashed in acetocarmine or aceto-orcein. It is recommended that the material be analyzed the same day, however, it can be kept at **4 °C for a several days if necessary.**

Acid hydrolysis removes purin bases from the DNA, thereby unmasking free aldehyde groups. The aldehyde groups then react with Schiff's reagent, which results in the purple staining. RNA is not hydrolyzed by the HCl treatment and, thus, the reaction is DNA-specific.

Schiff's Reagent

Schiff's reagent is prepared by pouring 200 mL of boiling distilled water over 1-g basic fuchsin. Shake thoroughly, cool to 50 °C, filter, and add 30 mL 1N HCl to the filtrate. Cool to room temperature and add 1 g potassium metabisulfite ($K_2S_2O_5$). Allow the solution to stand overnight in the dark or until a light straw or faint pink color develops. If not completely decolorized, add 0.5 g charcoal powder, shake, filter through a coarse filter, and refrigerate in a tightly-stoppered bottle in the dark. Commercially prepared Schiff's reagent can be obtained from several companies.

2.10.6 Staining of Corynebacterium Diptheriae

It is the identification test for diphtheria, Stain one of the smears with gram staining. If the smear shows morphology of *Corynebacterium diptheriae* proceed to do Albert staining which demonstrates the presence or absence of metachromatic granules.

Albert-I composition: Toluidine blue 0.15 gm, Malachite green 0.20 gm, Glacial acetic acid 1-00 mL, alcohol 95% 2.00 ml and distilled water 100 mL.

Albert-II composition: Iodine 2.0 gm, Potassium iodide 3.0 gm and distillled water 300 mL.

Procedure

1. Cover the heat fixed smear with Albert-I and let it stand for 2 minutes.
2. Wash with water.
3. Cover the heat fixed smear with Albert-II and let it stand for 2 minutes.
4. Wash with water.
5. Blot dry.
6. Examine for metachromatic granules of *Corynebacterium diptheriae.*

Metachromatic granules appear **Bluish black**

Corynebacterium diptheriae body appear **Green or bluish green.**

Apart from the above mentioned Albert stain, Ponder stain, Neisser stain and Christian Pugh's stain are also used to stain metachromatic granules of *Corynebacterium diphtheria.*

2.10.7 Miscellaneous Staining Methods

The other numerous differential staining techniques designed to identify some particular features of cell structure or compositions include the following staining methods which are shown in Table 2.16.

Table 2.16 Miscellaneous staining methods and their applications

Name of staining technique	Application
(a) Endospore staining	Demonstrates spore structure in bacteria as well as free spores. E.g. genera of bacillus & clostridium which causes Anthrax, Tetanus and gangrene.
(b) Capsule staining/Negative staining	Indian Ink stain or Negrosin are used to demonstrate the presence of capsules surrounding cells. E.g. *Cryptococcus neoformans & Streptococcus pneumoniae*
(c) Flagella staining	Demonstrates presence and arrangement of flagella
(d) Silver impregnation method Leifson stain	Laptospira and Flagella
(e) Cytoplasmic inclusion stains	Identifies intracellular deposits of starch, glycogen, polyphosphates, hydroply butyrate and other substances
(f) Giemsa stain	Applicable for staining Rickettsia, Chlamydia and some protozoa.
(g) Macchia vello stain	Stains Rickettsia
(h) Warthin-Starry stain; Dieferle stain	Spirochetes are stained
(i) Levaditi stain	Treponemas in tissue sections

2.11 Bio Chemical Tests for Identifying unknown Micro-organisms

1. **Carbohydrate Utilization:** Bacteria produce acidic products when they ferment certain carbohydrates.

The carbohydrate utilization tests are designed to detect the change in pH which would occur if fermentation of the given carbohydrate occurred.

- Acids lower the pH of the medium, which will cause the pH indicator (phenol red) to turn yellow.
- If the bacteria do not ferment the carbohydrate then the media remains red.
- If gas is produced as a by product of fermentation, then the Durham tube will have a bubble in it.

The carbohydrate tests that we perform are:

(a) Glucose (Dextrose) test

(b) Lactose test

(c) Sucrose test

During the fermentation process, an organic substrate serves as the final electron acceptor. The end-product of carbohydrate fermentation is an acid or acid with gas production. Various end-products of carbohydrate fermentation can be produced. The end-product depends on the organisms involved in the fermentation reaction, the substrate being fermented, the enzymes involved, and environmental factors such as pH and temperature. Common end-products of bacterial fermentation include lactic acid, formic acid, acetic acid, butyric acid, butyl alcohol, acetone, ethyl alcohol, carbon dioxide, and hydrogen.

Fermentation reactions are detected by the color change of a pH indicator when acid products are formed.

Phenol red is commonly used as a pH indicator in carbohydrate fermentation tests because most of the end-products of carbohydrate utilization are organic acids.

Phenol red carbohydrate broth

Trypticase or proteose peptone no. 3 10 g

Sodium chloride (NaCl) 5 g

Beef extract (optional) 1 g

Phenol red 0.018 g

(7.2 ml of 0.25% phenol red solution)

Distilled and deionized water 1,000 ml

Carbohydrate 10 g

Prepare broth medium by mixing all ingredients in 1,000 ml of distilled and deionized water; heat gently to dissolve. Use a single carbohydrate for each batch of medium prepared. Fill test tubes with 4 to 5 ml of phenol red carbohydrate broth. Insert an inverted fermentation tube or Durham tube to detect gas production. Sterilize media by autoclaving for 15 minutes at 116 to 118°C. The sterilization process will also drive the broth into the inverted fermentation tube or Durham tube. When using arabinose, lactose, maltose, salicin, sucrose, trehalose, or xylose, autoclave at 121°C for only 3 minutes as these carbohydrates are subject to breakdown by autoclaving. Broth medium will be a light red color. The final pH should be 7.4 ± 0.2.

Alternatively, mix all ingredients except carbohydrate in 800 ml of distilled and deionized water to prepare the base broth. Heat while mixing. Fill test tubes with 4.5 ml of base broth. Insert an inverted fermentation tube or Durham tube to detect gas production. Sterilize base broth by autoclaving for 15 minutes at 121°C. Cool sterilized base broth in a 42 to 50°C water bath before adding carbohydrates. Prepare carbohydrate solution by dissolving 10 grams of desired carbohydrate in 200 ml of distilled and deionized water and sterilize by filtering the solution through a bacteria-retaining membrane filter with a 0.45-μm pore size.

Aseptically add 0.5 ml of filtrate to each tube of sterilized and cooled broth. Shake gently to mix. Broth medium will be a light red color. The final pH should be 7.4 ± 0.2.

Cool all media before use. Store prepared media at 4 to 10°C. Refrigerated media has a shelf life of approximately 6 to 8 weeks. Run controls to check for possible breakdown of carbohydrates.

Protocol

A. ***Inoculation of media:*** Aseptically inoculate each test tube containing medium with the test micro-organism using an inoculating needle or loop. Make sure to avoid the Durham tube, if present. Swirl the tube gently to mix contents. Avoid contact of liquid with tube cap. Alternatively, inoculate each test tube with 1 to 2 drops of an 18- to 24-hour broth culture of the desired organism. Examples of broth media that could be used include brain heart infusion, nutrient agar, and tryptic soy agar.

B. ***Incubation:*** Incubate tubes at 35 to 37 °C for 18 to 24 hours. Longer incubation periods may be required to confirm a negative result.

C. ***Interpretation of results:***

1. *Fermentation results*: When using phenol red as the pH indicator, a yellow color indicates that enough acid products have been produced by fermentation of the sugar to lower the pH to 6.8 or less. A delayed fermentation reaction may produce an orange color. In such cases, it is best to reincubate the tube.
2. *Gas production results*: Bubbles trapped within the Durham tube indicate the production of gas. Even a single bubble is significant and denotes evidence of gas production. No bubbles within the Durham tube indicate a non-gas-producing or anaerogenic organism.
3. *Negative results*: Reddish or pink color indicates a negative reaction. In negative tubes, the presence of turbidity serves as control for growth. A reddish or pink color in a clear tube could indicate a false negative (Fig. 2.39 (Colour Plate 2.3).

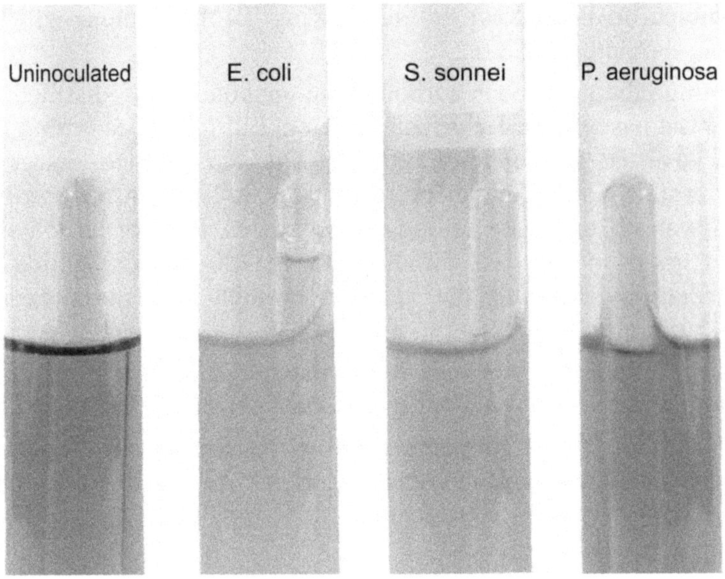

Fig. 2.39 (Colour Plate 2.3) Peptone media with bromocresol purple indicator. From left to right: uninoculated tube; *E. coli*, glucose fermenter with gas production (visible air bubble in the inverted Durham tube); *S. sonnei*, glucose fermenter without gas production (no visible air bubble in the inverted Durham tube); *P. aeruginosa*, nonfermenter.

2. **Citrate Utilization:** Koser's citrate medium has citrate as the sole source of carbon. The ability to use this substance is indicated by the production of turbidity in the medium

   Tests for the ability of bacteria to convert citrate (an intermediate of the Kreb's cycle) into oxaloacetate (another intermediate of the kreb's cycle)

   In this media, citrate is the only carbon source available to the bacteria.

   - If the bacteria cannot use the citrate, then it will not grow.
   - If it can use the citrate, then the bacteria will grow and the media will turn to bright blue as a result of an increase in the pH of the media.
   - This test is useful in the identification and classification of enteric gram negative bacteria.

Procedure for Citrate Utilization Test

1. Inoculate Simmons Citrate Agar (Simmons Citrate Agar is a modification of Koser's medium) lightly on the slant by touching the tip of a needle to a colony that is 18 to 24 hours old.
2. Incubate at 35°C to 37°C for 18 to 24 hours. Some organisms may require up to 7 days of incubation due to their limited rate of growth on citrate medium.
3. Observe the development of blue color; denoting alkalinization shown in (Fig. 2.40 (Colour Plate 2.4)).

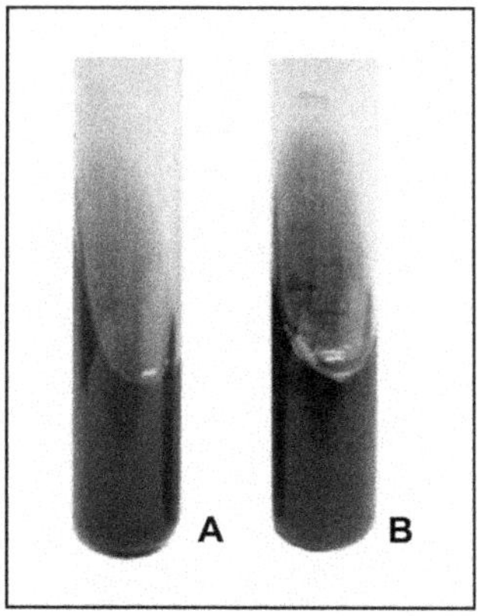

Fig. 2.40 (Colour Plate 2.4)
A-negative B- Positive citrate utilization test

Simmons Citrate Agar Medium

Ingradient	gm/litre
Magnesium sulphate	0.200
Ammonium dihydrogen phosphate	1.000
Dipotassium phosphate	1.000
Sodium citrate	2.000
Sodium chloride	5.000
Bromothymol blue	0.080
Agar	15.000
Final pH at 25°C	6.8± 0.2

Quality Control strains used in citrate utilization test

- Positive: *Klebsiella pneumoniae*
- Negative: *Escherichia coli*

List of Bacteria which give positive citrate utilization test

1. *Citrobacter* spp
2. *Klebsiella pneumoniae*
3. *Enterobacter aerogenes*

Uninoculated Negative, Positive

3. **Gelatin Utilization:** This media is used to test if bacteria can digest the protein gelatin, To digest, the bacteria must make an enzyme called gelatinase.

The procedure for this method is as follows:

1. To inoculate this media, use a transfer needle to stab the gelatin.

2. After incubating the inoculated media for at least 48 hr, transfer the tube into a refrigerator.
3. The tube should be completely chilled prior to observation

The observations that are made are:

(a) If the media is solid after refrigeration then the test is concluded as negative because the bacteria did not digest the gelatin.

Nutrient gelatin composition:

Peptone	5.0	g/liter
Beef extract	3.0	g/liter
Gelatin	120.0	g/liter
Final pH:	6.8 ± 0.2 at 25°C.	

Prepare medium by mixing all ingredients in 1,000 ml of distilled or deionized water and heating gently to dissolve. Dispense 2 to 3 ml of medium into 13- by 100 -mm culture tubes. Autoclave medium at 121 °C (15 psi) for 15 minutes. Allow the tubed medium to cool in an upright position before use. Store the prepared medium at 2 to 8 °C. Tubed medium stored at 2 to 8 °C may be used until its expiration date. Do not use tubed medium if it shows signs of microbial contamination, discoloration, drying, or other signs of deterioration.

Protocol

Nutrient gelatin stab method: There are several methods for determining gelatinase production, all of which make use of gelatin as the substrate. The standard and most commonly employed method is the nutrient gelatin stab method (Fig. 2.41). This method offers an easy and accurate interpretation of results (medium liquefaction) and eliminates the use of reagents or chemicals that may be hazardous to health.

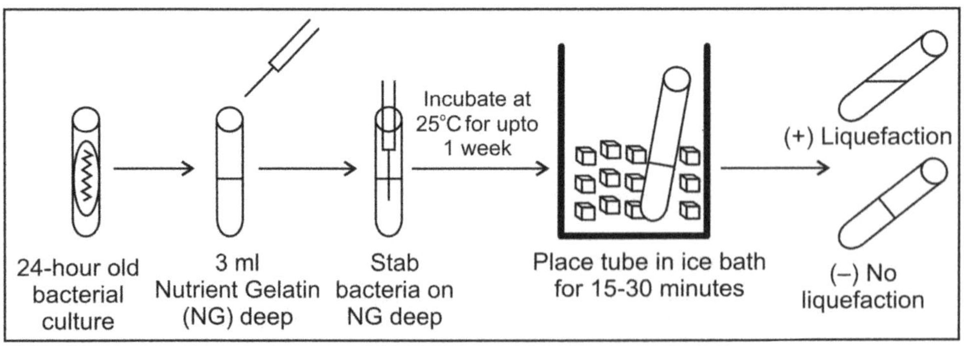

Fig. 2.41 A schematic diagram of the gelatin hydrolysis test using the nutrient gelatin stab method. The use of screw-capped test tubes is recommended.

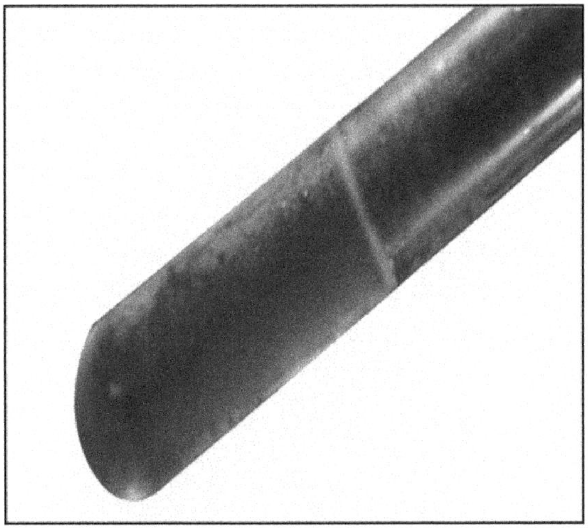

Fig. 2.42 (Colour Plate 2.5) Gelatin hydrolysis test result A-Gelatin hydrolysis Test Control (Uninoculated)

In this method, a heavy inoculum of 18- to 24-hour-old test bacteria is stab-inoculated into tubes containing nutrient gelatin. The inoculated tubes and an uninoculated control tube are incubated at 25 °C, or at the test bacterium's optimal growth temperature, for up to 1 week, and checked everyday for gelatin liquefaction. Gelatin normally liquefies at 28 °C and above, so to confirm that liquefaction shown in Fig. 2.42 (Colour Plate 2.5) and 2.43 (Colour Plate 2.6) was due to gelatinase activity, the tubes are immersed in an ice bath for 15 to 30 minutes. Afterwards, tubes are tilted to observe if gelatin has been hydrolyzed. Hydrolyzed gelatin will result in a liquid medium even after exposure to cold temperature (ice bath), while the uninoculated control medium will remain solid. For weak positive results, incubate the inoculated nutrient gelatin tube longer until complete liquefaction is observed. The hydrolysis of gelatin indicates the secretion of gelatinase by the test organism into the medium. Note that some bacterial species, e.g., *Proteus vulgaris*, may require up to 14 days of incubation to yield a positive result. Aseptic techniques and appropriate biosafety protocols should always be strictly observed and practiced in the microbiology laboratory.

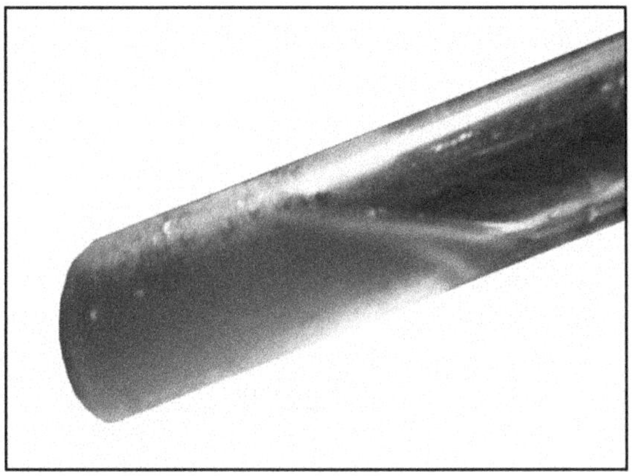

Fig. 2.43 (Colour Plate 2.6) Gelatin hydrolysis test. After 30 minutes in an ice bath, a nutrient gelatin tube inoculated with Bacillus subtilis exhibited positive gelatin hydrolysis as shown by medium liquefaction (A) while the uninoculated control remained solid
(B) Gelatin hydrolysis was observed after 3 days of incubation.

Nutrient Gelatin Plate Method: A suggested alternate test to detect gelatin hydrolysis is the nutrient gelatin plate method. In this method, a heavy inoculum of 18- to 24-hour-old test bacteria is stab-inoculated onto culture plates prefilled with nutrient gelatin (23 g/liter nutrient agar, 8 g/liter gelatin). Inoculated nutrient gelatin plates are incubated at 35°C for 24 hours. Gelatin hydrolysis is indicated by clear zones around gelatinase-positive colonies (Fig. 2.44). In some cases, plates are flooded with saturated ammonium sulfate to precipitate unhydrolyzed gelatin, making the clear zones easier to see. Results are often observed within 5 to 10 minutes after flooding with saturated ammonium sulfate

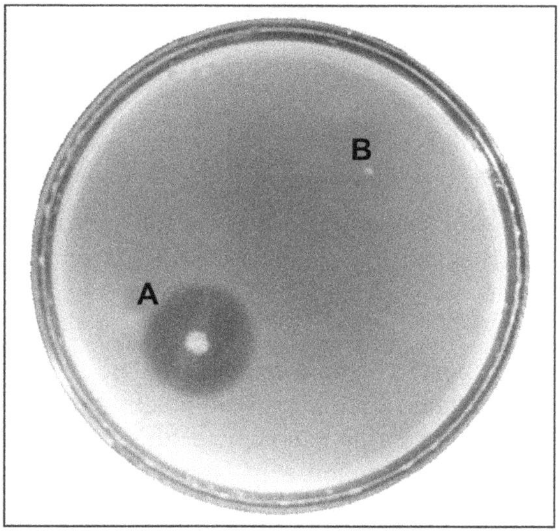

Fig 2.44 Gelatin hydrolysis test using nutrient gelatin plate method. (A) Positive gelatin hydrolysis exhibited by *Bacillus subtilis* indicated by the clear zone around the colony after the addition of saturated ammonium sulfate. (B) Negative gelatin hydrolysis exhibited by *Escherichia coli* indicated by the absence of a clear zone around the colony. Inoculated culture plates were incubated for 24 hours.

Another suggested medium for the nutrient gelatin plate method contains 4 g/liter of peptone, 1 g/liter of yeast extract, 12 g/liter of gelatin, and 15 g/liter of agar. In most cases, this medium gives a visible zone without treatment by saturated ammonium sulfate.

4. **Starch Hydrolysis:** This test is used to detect the enzyme amylase, which breaks down starch

***The Procedure is as follows*:**

1. For this a starch plate is used and the media is placed 48 hr for incubation.
2. After incubation the plate is treated with Gram's iodine.

Starch agar is a differential medium that tests the ability of an organism to produce certain exoenzymes, including α-amylase and oligo-1,6-glucosidase, that hydrolyze starch. Starch molecules are too large to enter the bacterial cell, so some bacteria secrete exoenzymes to degrade starch into subunits that can then be utilized by the organism.

Starch Agar Medium composition:

Meat extract	3.0	g/liter
Peptic digest of animal tissue	5.0	g/liter
Starch soluble	2.0	g/liter
Agar	15.0	g/liter
Final pH:	7.2 ± 0.1 at 25°C.	

Starch agar is a simple nutritive medium with starch added. Since no color change occurs in the medium when organisms hydrolyze starch, we add iodine to the plate after incubation. Iodine turns blue, purple, or black (depending on the concentration of iodine) in the presence of starch. A clearing around the bacterial growth indicates that the organism has hydrolyzed starch Fig. 2.45 (Colour Plate 2.7).

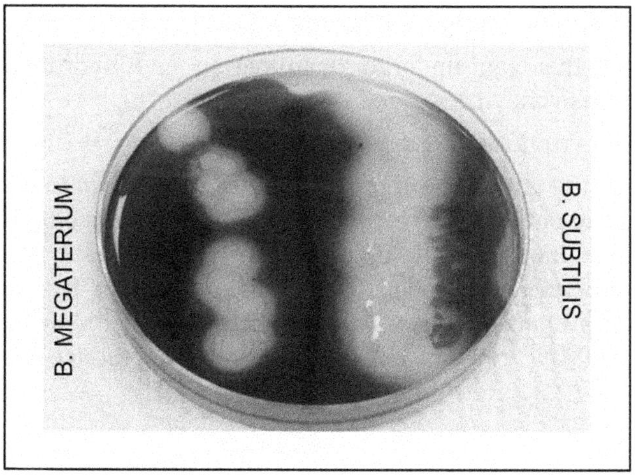

Fig. 2.45 (Colour Plate 2.7) Starch hydrolysis test positive result

Positive Result: Iodine has been added to this starch agar plate. The zone of clearing surrounding *Bacillus megaterium* and *Bacillus subtilis* indicate that both were able to hydrolyze starch.

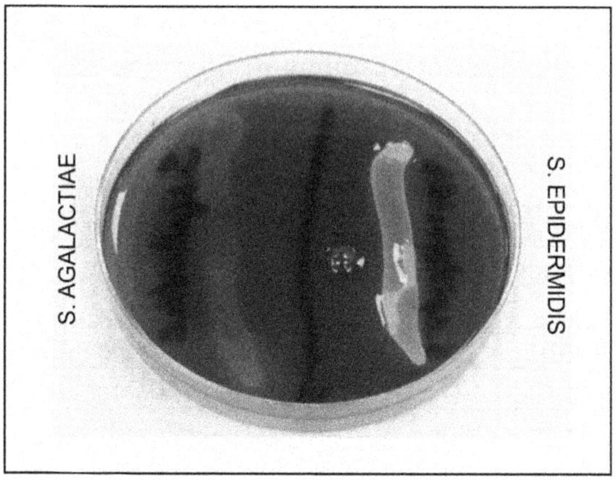

Fig. 2.46 (Colour Plate 2.8) Starch hydrolysis negative result

Negative Result: Iodine has been added to this starch agar plate. The absence of any clearing indicates that neither *Streptococcus agalactiae* nor *Staphylococcus epidermidis* were able to hydrolyze starch Fig. 2.46 (Colour Plate 2.8).

5. **Indole Production:** As far back as 1889, the indole test was used as a means to distinguish between *Escherichia coli* and *Enterobacter aerogenes*. This test plays the central role in the characterization of coliforms (gram-negative nonsporulating bacilli that ferment lactose, producing acid and gas). The indole test is still used as a classic test to distinguish indole-positive *E. coli* from indole-negative *Enterobacter* and *Klebsiella*.

Purpose

The indole test screens for the ability of an organism to degrade the amino acid tryptophan and produce indole. It is used as part of the IMViC procedures, a battery of tests designed to distinguish among members of the family Enterobacteriaceae.

Tryptophan is an amino acid that can undergo deamination and hydrolysis by bacteria that express tryptophanase enzyme.

Tryptophan + water = indole + pyruvic acid + ammonia

The chief requirement for culturing an organism prior to performing the indole test is that the medium contains a sufficient quantity of tryptophan. The presence of indole when a microbe is grown in a medium rich in tryptophan demonstrates that an organism has the capacity to degrade tryptophan. Detection of indole, a by-product of tryptophan metabolism, relies upon the chemical reaction between indole and p-dimethylaminobenzaldehyde (DMAB) under acidic conditions to produce the red dye rosindole.

Tryptone broth (2)

Ingredient	Amount
Tryptone	10.0 g
Sodium chloride	5.0 g

Dissolve the ingredients in 1 liter of sterile water. Dispense 4 ml per tube. Cap tube and autoclave at 121°C under 15 psi pressure for 15 minutes. Store the tubes in the refrigerator at 4 to 10 °C.

Kovács reagent

Ingredient	Amount
Amyl or isoamyl alcohol, reagent grade (butyl alcohol may be substituted)	150.0 ml
p-Dimethylaminobenzaldehyde (DMAB)	10.0 g
HCl (concentrated)	50.0 ml

Dissolve DMAB in the alcohol. Gentle heating might be required to get the aldehyde into solution.

Slowly add the acid to the aldehyde-alcohol mixture. The solution should be a pale yellow color and is only stable for a short time. Store the mixture in a brown glass bottle in the refrigerator. Kovács reagent also is commercially available.

Protocol

Inoculate the tube of tryptone broth with a small amount of a pure culture. Incubate at 35 °C ± 2°C for 24 to 48 hours.

To test for indole production, add 5 drops of Kovács reagent directly to the tube.

A positive indole test is indicated by the formation of a pink to red color ("cherry-red ring") in the reagent layer on top of the medium within seconds of adding the reagent (Fig. 2.47b (Colour Plate 2.8).

If a culture is indole negative, the reagent layer will remain yellow or be slightly cloudy (Fig. 2.47c (Colour Plate 2.9)).

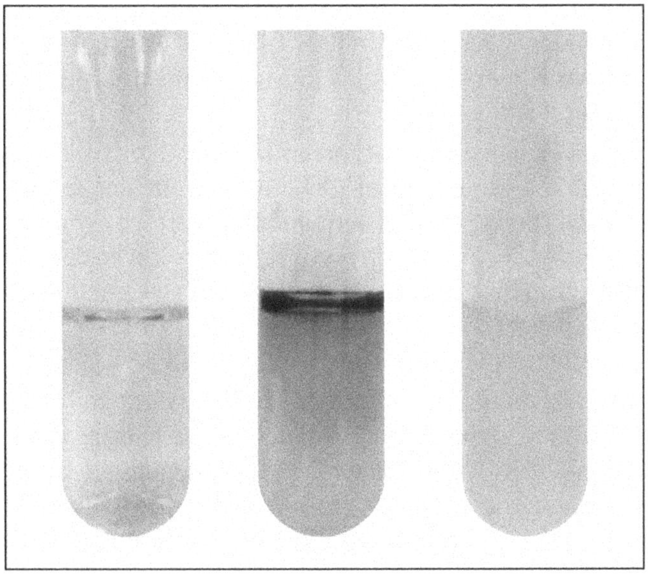

(a) (b) (c)

Fig. 2.47 (Colour Plate 2.9) The indole test. **(a)** An uninoculated tube of tryptone broth. **(b)** A positive indole test. The 48-hour *Escherichia coli* culture grown at 37°C tests positive for the presence of indole as indicated by the red reagent layer after the addition of Kovács reagent. **(c)** A negative indole test. The 48-hour *Enterobacter aerogenes* culture incubated at 37°C has not broken down the tryptophan in the medium and thus no color change occurs upon addition of the Kovács reagent. The reagent appears as a thin yellow layer on top of the culture medium.

6. **MRVP (Methyl red – Voges Proskauer):** The methyl red and Voges-Proskauer tests are part of a battery of biochemical tests known as IMViC used in the clinical lab.

The acronym IMViC stands for indole, methyl red, Voges-Proskauer and citrate). The "i" in the acronym is added for pronunciation purposes.
Originally the paired MR-VP tests were used to distinguish between members of the family *Enterobacteriaceae*, but now they are used to characterize other groups of bacteria including *Actinobacteria* .

Both the Methyl Red and Voges-Proskauer tests are commonly used in conjunction with the indole and citrate tests, to form a group of tests known as IMViC which aid in the differentiation of *Enterobacteria.*

Methyl red

Principle: *Escherichia coli* and other members of the low-ratio organisms described by Clark and Lubs ferment sugars by the mixed acid pathway resulting in a low ratio of CO_2 to H_2 gas produced by fermentation. The mixed acid pathway gives 4 mol of acidic products (mainly lactic and acetic acid), 1 mol of neutral fermentation product (ethanol), 1 mol of CO_2, and 1 mol of H_2 per mol of glucose fermented. The large quantity of acids produced causes a significant decrease in the pH of the culture medium.

In contrast, *Enterobacter aerogenes* and other members of the high-ratio organisms (those that produce a high ratio of CO_2 to H_2 from the fermentation of glucose) ferment sugars via the butanediol fermentation pathway, producing only 1 mol of acid per mol of glucose. This pathway results in a lower degree of acidification of the culture medium. The pH indicator methyl red (p-dimethylaminoaeobenzene-O-carboxylic acid) has been found to be suitable to measure the concentration of hydrogen ions between pH 4.4 (red) and 6.0 (yellow).

When the culture medium turns red after addition of methyl red, because of a pH at or below 4.4 from the fermentation of glucose, the culture has a positive result for the MR test (Fig.2.48A (Colour Plate 2.10)). A negative MR test is indicated by a yellow color in the culture medium (Fig. 2.48B (Colour Plate 2.10)), which occurs when less acid is produced (pH is higher) from the fermentation of glucose.

Voges-Proskauer

Principle: Bacteria fermenting sugars via the butanediol pathway produce acetoin (i.e., acetyl methyl carbinol or 3-hydroxybutanone) as an intermediate which can be further reduced to 2,3-butanediol.

2 pyruvate = acetoin + $2CO_2$ acetoin + NADH + H^+ = 2,3-butanediol + NAD^+ In the presence of KOH the intermediate acetoin is oxidized to diacetyl, a reaction which is catalyzed by α-Naphthol. Diacetyl reacts with the guanidine group associated with molecules contributed by peptone in the medium, to form a

pinkish-red-colored product. The α-Naphthol in the Barritt's modification of the VP test serves as a color intensifier.

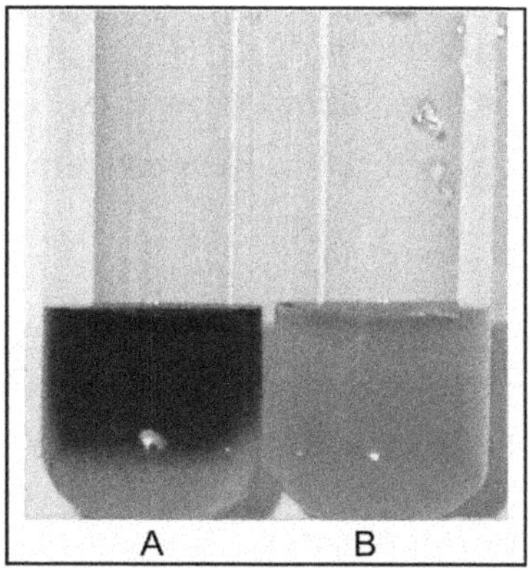

Fig. 2.48 (Colour Plate 2.10) Methyl red reaction. *E. coli* (A) and *E. aerogenes* (B) were grown for 48 hours at 35°C in MR-VP medium. After incubation, 5 drops of a 0.05% methyl red solution (per 2.5 ml) were added to each culture. The MR-positive *E. coli* (A) shows a red coloration as a result of high acid production and a decrease in the pH of the culture medium to 4.4. The MR-negative *E. aerogenes* culture (B) has a yellow color indicating a less acidic medium.

Medium: Buffered peptone-glucose broth
(commercially available as MR-VP broth)

Buffered peptone 7.0 g (can be replaced by 3.5 g of peptic digest of animal tissue and 3.5 g of pancreatic digest of casein)

Completely dissolve Dipotassium phosphate 5.0 g

Dextrose 5.0 g

Procedure: Add 1 liter of deionized water for a final pH of 6.9 (± 0.2) at 25°C. Gently heat to completely dissolve the ingredients and distribute 5 ml aliquots into culture tubes. Sterilize via autoclaving at 121°C and 15 psi for 15 minutes. After the medium cools down it can be store in a refrigerator until use.

This medium is a modification of the original Clark and Lubs medium using the decreased concentration of glucose (0.5%) as well as peptone. It was shown that this amount of glucose allowed for an identification of MR-positive organisms. The reduced amount of peptone results in a less-colored medium, making the interpretation of the color reaction easier.

Methyl red solution 0.1 g of methyl red in 300 ml of ethanol (95%). Add 200 ml of deionized water to make 500 ml of a 0.05% (wt/vol) solution in 60% (vol/vol) ethanol. Store the prepared methyl red solution at 4°C.

Voges-Proskauer reagents

Barritt's reagent A: 5% (wt/vol) a-naphthol in absolute ethanol shown in Fig. 2.49A.

Barritt's reagent B: 40% (wt/vol) KOH in deionized water (this might be replaced by a 40% (wt/vol) NaOH solution) shown in (Fig. 2.49B (Colour Plate 2.11)).

Reagents must be prepared fresh. Reagents are also referred to as VP-1 and VP-2 or VP-A and VP-B.

Other materials

Sterile culture tubes containing 5 ml of MR-VP broth; sterile culture tubes; test and control bacterial strains (commonly used controls are *Escherichia coli* and *Enterobacter aerogenes*) from trypticase soy agar or broth; inoculation loop (disposable or have additional equipment available for sterilization of the inoculation loop); transfer pipettes

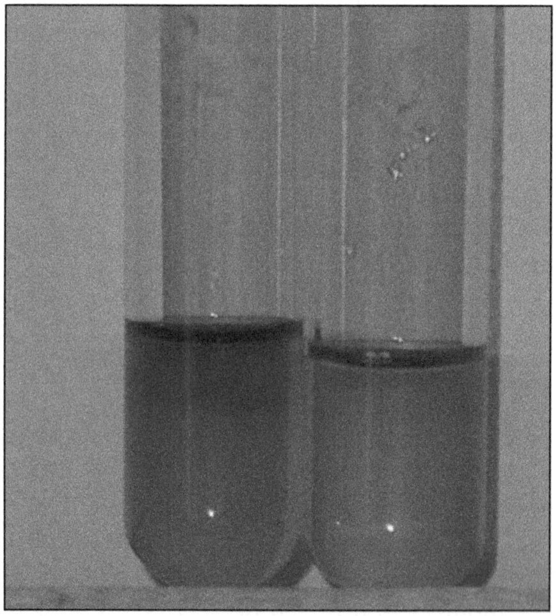

A B

Fig. 2.49 (Colour Plate 2.11) Voges-Proskauer reaction. *E. aerogenes* (A) and *E. coli* (B) were grown in MR-VP-broth for 48 hours at 37°C and Barritt's reagents A and B were added. VP-positive *E. areogenes* (A) shows red coloration on top of the culture, whereas VP-negative *E. coli* (B) has a yellowish color.

Protocol

A. Inoculation of medium: Prepare MR-VP broth as described above or as directed by the manufacturer. Prior to use, allow the medium to come to room temperature.

Inoculate one tube of MR-VP broth from a fresh (18 to 24 hours) pure culture (e.g., grown on trypticase soy agar) of the test culture. Transfer a light inoculum from an isolated colony and resuspend it in the 5 ml MR-VP broth tube. Note that the use of a heavy inoculum may result in aberrant results. For comparision it is suggested that *Escherichia coli* (MR+, VP-) and *Enterobacter aerogenes* (MR-, VP+) be used as control cultures.

B. Incubation: Incubate test and control cultures at 35°C (±- 2°C) for 48 hours.

C. Methyl red test and interpretation of results

1. Transfer 2.5 ml of culture into a new sterile culture tube.
2. Add 5 drops of the methyl red reagent.
3. Compare the test organism to the control cultures to immediately interpret the result, MR positive (e.g., *E. coli*) (Fig. 1A) or MR negative (e.g., *E.aerogenes*).

False-negative results or an inconclusive orange color may occur due to insufficient length of incubation. In this case, it is recommended that the test be repeated with a culture that was incubated an additional 24 to 48 hours.

An increase in glucose concentration in the medium might lead to false-positive results in the MR test. Clark and Lubs showed that increased glucose concentration also led to high hydrogen ion concentration in high-ratio cultures which, under standard test conditions, are MR negative.

D. Voges-Proskauer test and interpretation of results

1. Use the remaining 2.5 ml of culture grown in MR-VP broth.
2. Add 0.6 ml (or 12 drops) of Barritt's reagent A.
3. Add 0.2 ml (or 4 drops) of Barritt's reagent B.
4. Carefully shake the tube for 30 seconds to 1 minute to expose the medium to atmospheric oxygen (necessary for oxidation of acetoin to obtain a color reaction).
5. Allow the tube to stand for at least 30 minutes.
6. Within 1 hour, compare the test result to control cultures to determine if the culture is VP positive like *E. aerogenes* or VP negative like *E. coli*. Delayed reading of the result may lead to an erroneous reading; over time α-naphthol and KOH may react to give a copper-like color.

Incubation times shorter or longer than 48 hours may result in false-negative results since either the amount of acetoin accumulated is too low to be detected or acetoin will be further reduced to 2,3-butanediol.

7. **Triple Sugar Iron (TSI) – A Hydrogen Sulfide Production (H_2S):** Triple sugar iron (TSI) agar is a tubed differential medium used in determining Carbohydrate fermentation and H_2S production. TSI is most frequently used in the identification of the *Enterobacteriaceae*, although it is useful for other gram-negative bacteria.

Medium: TSI contains three carbohydrates: glucose (0.1%), sucrose (1%), and lactose (1%). TSI is similar to Kligler's iron agar, Phenol red is the pH indicator, and agar is used to solidify the medium. During preparation, tubes containing molten agar are angled. The slant of the medium is aerobic, while the deep (or butt) is anaerobic.

Principle: When any of the carbohydrates are fermented, the drop in pH will cause the medium to change from reddish-orange (the original color) to yellow. A deep red color indicates alkalization of the peptones. Sodium thiosulfate in the medium is reduced by some bacteria to hydrogen sulfide (H_2S), a colorless gas. The Hydrogen sulfide will react with ferric ions in the medium to produce iron sulfide, a black insoluble precipitate.

Procedure: Inoculate the TSI slant by first stabbing the butt down to the bottom, withdraw the needle, and then streak the surface of the slant. Use a loosely fitting closure to permit access of air shown in Fig. 2.50 (Colour Plate 2.12).

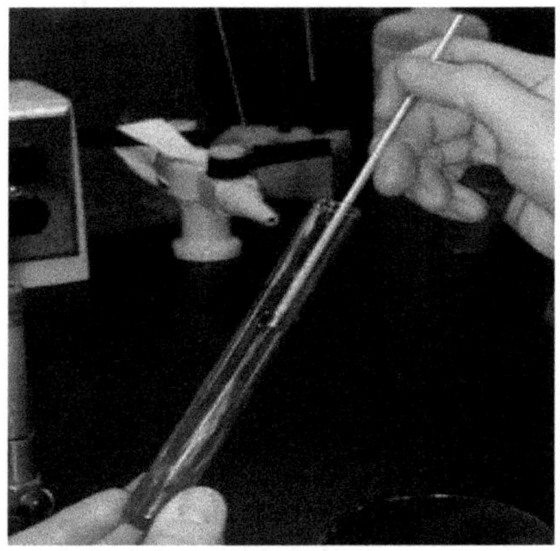

Fig. 2.50 (Colour Plate 2.12)
Triple sugar iron test

Read results after incubation at 37 °C for 18 to 24 h. Three kinds of data may be obtained from the reactions. If we look at the fermentation of glucose, lactose, and sucrose and checks if hydrogen sulfide is produced in the process.

Inference: Basically a pH indicator will change the color of the media in response to fermentation.Where that color change occurs in the tube will indicate what sugar or sugars were fermented.

The presence of a black color indicates that H_2S was produced.

In this media H_2S reacts with the ferrous sulfate in the media to make ferrous sulfide, which is black. In addition to TSI media, SIM media can be used to determine if H_2S is produced. A black color in the SIM medium following inoculation and incubation indicates that H_2S is made by the bacteria shown in Table 2.17.

Table 2.17

Slant color	Interpretation
Red	Does not ferment either lactose or sucrose
Yellow	Ferments lactose and or sucrose

Butt Color / condition	Interpretation
Red	No fermentation of glucose
yellow	Some fermentation of glucose has occurred, acid has been produced
Gas formed	Seen as cracks in the agar, bubbles, or the entire slant may be pushed out of the tube. (caution: these gassy fermenters may have bacteria close to the opening)
Black	H_2S has been produced

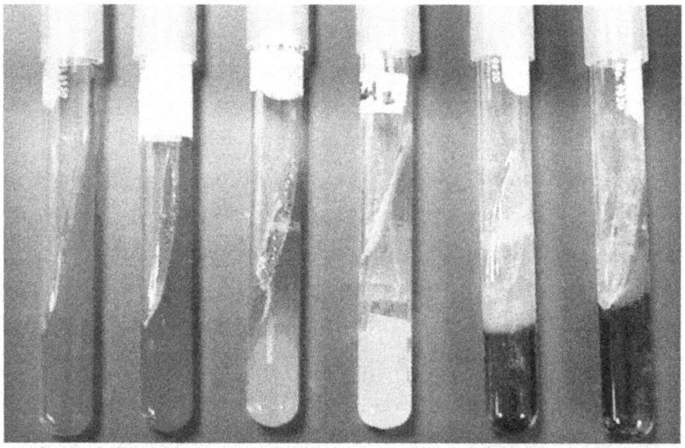

Fig. 2.51 (Colour Plate 2.13) Hydrogen sulphide production test results

From Left to right

(a) Uninoculated control

(b) Red slant and red butt, no black color = no fermentation of glucose, sucrose, or lactose

No hydrogen sulfide produced

(c) Red slant and black butt = no lactose or sucrose fermentation, H_2S has been produced

(d) Red slant with yellow butt = no lactose or sucrose fermentation, Lactose is fermented, no H_2S has been produced.

(e) Yellow slant and yellow butt and black coloration = lactose, sucrose and glucose fermented, and H_2S has been produced

(f) Yellow slant, yellow butt and lifting / or cracking of media, no black coloration = lactose, sucrose and glucose fermented, H_2S has not been produced but gas has been produced.

(g) Yellow slant, yellow butt and no lifting and or cracking of media, no black coloration = lactose, sucrose and glucose fermented H_2S has not been produced nor has gas been produced

8. Urea Test: The urease test identifies those organisms that are capable of hydrolyzing urea to produce ammonia and carbon dioxide. It is primarily used to distinguish urease-positive *Proteus* from other *Enterobacteriaceae.* Urease is a constitutively expressed enzyme that hydrolyzes urea to carbon dioxide and ammonia.

$$(NH_2)_2CO + H_2O \rightarrow CO_2 + 2NH_3$$

Urease test media contain 2% urea and phenol red as a pH indicator. An increase in pH due to the production of ammonia which is a base that increases pH i.e., a color change from yellow (pH 6.8) to bright pink (pH 8.2).

Urea broth (Stuart's urea broth) is a highly buffered medium requiring large quantities of ammonia to raise the pH above 8.0 resulting in a color change. This medium provides all essential nutrients for *Proteus*, for which it is differential. Urea agar (Christensen's urea agar) has reduced buffer content and contains peptones and glucose. This medium supports the growth of many *enterobacteria* allowing for the observation of urease activity.

Two media types are commonly used to detect urease activity. Christensen's urea agar is used to detect urease activity in a variety of micro-organisms. Stuart's urea broth is used primarily for the differentiation of *Proteus* species. Both media types are available commercially as prepared tubes or as a powder.

Christensen's Urea Agar

Ingredient	Amount
Peptone	1 g
Dextrose	1 g
Sodium chloride	5 g
Potassium phosphate, monobasic	2 g
Urea	20 g
Phenol red	0.012 g
Agar	15 to 20 g

- To prepare the urea base, dissolve the first six ingredients in 100 ml of distilled water and filter sterilize (0.45-mm pore size). Suspend the agar in 900 ml of distilled water, boil to dissolve completely, and autoclave at 121 °C and 15 psi for 15 minutes. Cool the agar to 50 to 55 °C. Aseptically add 100 ml of filter-sterilized urea base to the cooled agar solution and mix thoroughly. Distribute 4 to 5 ml per sterile tube (13 x 100 mm) and slant the tubes during cooling until solidified. It is desirable to have a long slant and short butt. Prepared media will have a yellow-orange color. Store the prepared media in the refrigerator at 4 to 8 °C until needed. Once prepared, do not reheat the medium as the urea will decompose.

Protocol

Christensen's Urea Agar

Use a heavy inoculum from an 18- to 24-hour pure culture to streak the entire slant surface. Do not stab the butt as it will serve as a color control Fig.2.42C. Incubate tubes with loosened caps at 35 °C. Observe the slant for a color change at 6 hours, 24 hours, and every day for up to 6 days. Urease production is indicated by a bright pink (fuchsia) color on the slant that may extend into the butt. Note that any degree of pink is considered a positive reaction. Prolonged incubation may result in a false-positive test due to hydrolysis of proteins in the medium. To eliminate protein hydrolysis as the cause of a positive test, a control medium lacking urea should be used shown in Fig. 2.52 (Colour Plate 2.14).

Rapidly urease-positive *Proteeae* (*Proteous* spp., *Morganella morganii*, and some *Providencia stuartii* strains) will produce a strong positive reaction within 1 to 6 hours of incubation. Delayed-positive organisms (e.g., *Klebsiella* or *Enterobacter*) will typically produce a weak positive reaction on the slant after 6 hours, but the reaction will intensify and spread to the butt on prolonged incubation (up to 6 days). The culture medium will remain a yellowish color if the organism is urease negative).

9. **<u>Catalase Test</u> (Fig. 2.53 (Colour Plate 2.15)):** Catalase is an enzyme, which is produced by micro-organisms that live in oxygenated environments to neutralize toxic forms of oxygen metabolites; H_2O_2. The catalase enzyme neutralizes the bactericidal effects of hydrogen peroxide and protects them. Anaerobes generally lack the catalase enzyme.

   Catalase mediates the breakdown of hydrogen peroxide H_2O_2 into oxygen and water. To find out if a particular bacterial isolate is able to produce catalase enzyme, small inoculums of bacterial isolate is mixed into hydrogen peroxide solution (3%) and the rapid elaboration of oxygen bubbles occurs. The lack of catalase is evident by a lack of or weak bubble production.

   Catalase-positive bacteria include strict aerobes as well as facultative anaerobes. They all have the ability to respire using oxygen as a terminal electron acceptor.

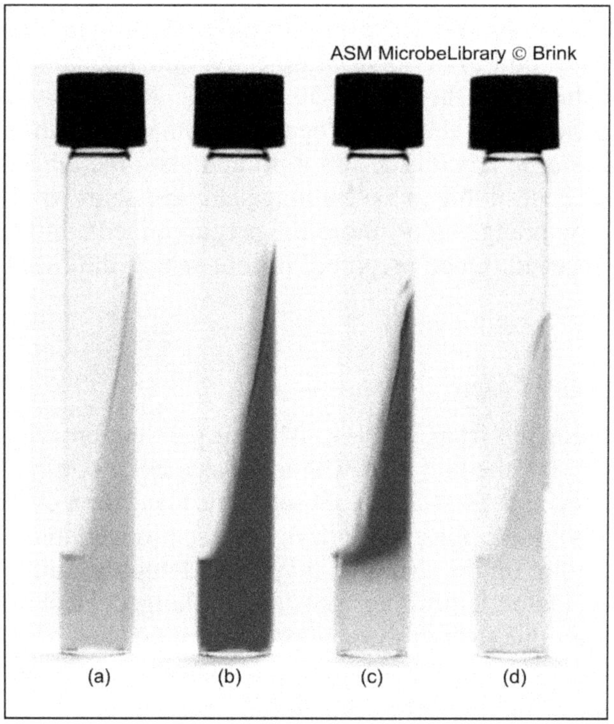

Fig. 2.52 (Colour Plate 2.14) Urea agar test results. Urea agar slants were inoculated as follows: **(a)** uninoculated, **(b)** *Proteous mirabilis* (rapidly urease positive), **(c)** *Klebsiella pneumoniae* (delayed urease positive), **(d)** *Escherichia coli* (urease negative). All samples were incubated at 37 °C for 16 hours.

Uses of Catalase Test

1. The catalase test is primarily used to distinguish among Gram-positive cocci: Member of the genus *Staphylococcus* are catalase-positive, and members of the genera *Streptococcus* and *Enterococcus* are catalase-negative.
2. Catalase test is used to differentiate aerotolerant strains of *Clostridium*, which are catalase negative, from *Bacillus* species, which are positive.
3. Semiquantitative catalase test is used for the identification of *Mycobacterium tuberculosis*
4. Catalase test can be used as an aid to the identification of *Enterobacteriaceae*. Members of *Enterobacteriaceae* family are Catalase positive.

Procedure of Catalase Test (Fig. 2.53 (Colour Plate 2.13))

1. Transfer a small amount of bacterial colony to a surface of clean, dry glass slide using a loop or sterile wooden stick
2. Place a drop of 3% H_2O_2 on to the slide and mix.

3. A positive result is the rapid evolution of oxygen (within 5-10 sec.) as evidenced by bubbling.
4. A negative result is no bubbles or only a few scattered bubbles.
5. Dispose of your slide in the biohazard glass disposal container.

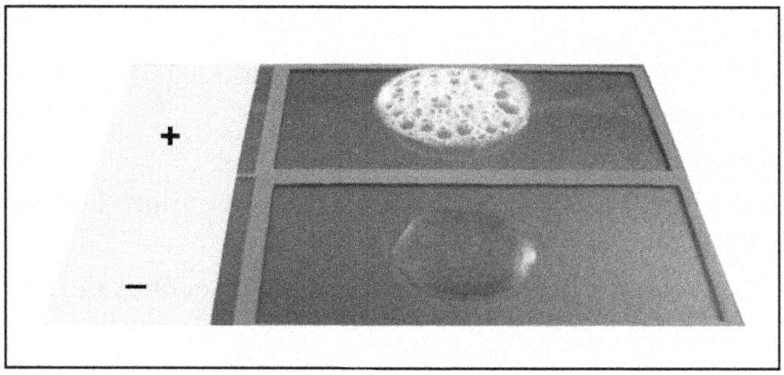

Fig. 2.53 (Colour Plate 2.15) Catalase test

10. **<u>Oxidase Test</u> (Fig. 2.54 (Colour Plate 2.16)):** This test depends on the presence of cytochrome oxidase in gram-negative bacteria that will catalyze the transport of electrons between electron donors and redox dye. Tetramethyl-p-phenylene diamine dihydrochloride in the reagent is reduced to deep purple color. This test is used for the screening of *Pseudomonas, Vibrio, Neisseria, Brucella* and *Pasteurella*, which give positive test. *Enterobacteriaceae* are oxidase negative.

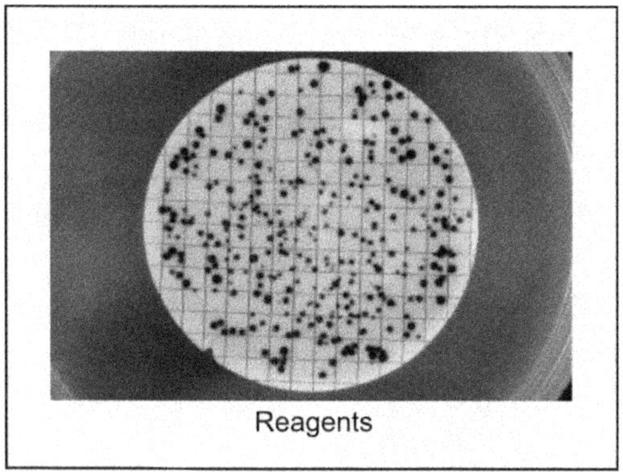

Fig. 2.54 (Colour Plate 2.16) Oxidase test

Oxidase reagent is specially prepared as 10 g/l or 1% solution of tetramethyl-p-phenylene diamine dihydrochloride.

Procedure

Filter Paper Method

Place a piece of filter paper in petri dish and add 3 drops of freshly prepared oxidase reagent. Using a sterile glass rod, remove a colony of test organisms from a culture plate and smear it on the filter paper.

Interpretation

Oxidase positive organisms give blue color within 5-10 seconds, and in oxidase negative organisms, color does not change.

Dry slide method

To perform this test simply swab some of the test culture into one of the boxes on an oxidase dry slide.

If a color change to purple or blue is evident at 30 seconds (1 min) then the result is positive.

Note: It is very important that the test is read by one minute to ensure accurate results (avoid false negative and false positives)

11. <u>Litmus Milk Test</u> (Fig. 2.55 (Colour Plate 2.17))

Applications of Litmus milk test: It is a milk-based medium used to distinguish between different species of bacteria.

The lactose (milk sugar), litmus (pH indicator), and casein (milk protein) contained within the medium can all be metabolized by different types of bacteria.

Since milk is usually the first substrate used to maintain bacteria, this test allows for accurate depiction of bacterial types.

The addition of litmus, other than explaining the pH type, acts as an oxidation-reduction indicator.

The test itself tells whether the bacterium can ferment lactose, reduce litmus, form clots, form gas, or start peptonization.

Materials required: 24-48 hours cultures of organisms grown in Tryptic Soy Broth

Litmus milk broth (pH-6.8) composition:

Skim milk powder	100 g
Litmus	0.075 g
Distilled water	1,000.0 ml

Autoclave at 12lb pressure for 15 minutes

Procedure

1. Using sterile technique, inoculate each experimental organism into its appropriately labeled tube by means of a loop inoculation. The last tube will serve as a control.
2. Incubate all cultures for 24 to 48 hours at 37 °C.

Expected Results

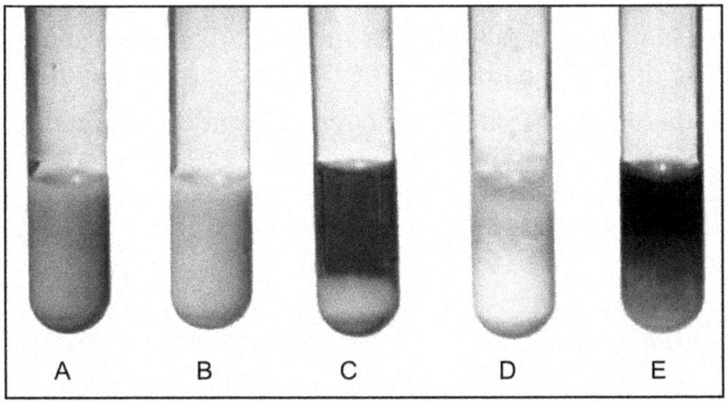

Fig. 2.55 (Colour Plate 2.17) Litmus milk reactions: (A) Alkaline. (B) Acid. (C) Upper transparent portion is peptonization; solid white portion in bottom is coagulation and litmus reduction; overall redness is interpreted as acid. (D) Coagulation and litmus reduction in lower half; some peptonization (transparency) and acid in top portion. (E) Litmus indicator is masked by production of soluble pigment.

S.No.	Organism	Litmus Reaction
1.	*Escherichia E.coli*	Acid production (Pink) with or without reduction, curd formation and gas.
2.	*Bacillus cereus*	Peptonization with an alkaline reaction and rennet curd.
3.	*Proteus vulgaris*	Alkaline reaction
4.	*Streptococcus lactis*	Reduction with red band of acid on top, curd formation.
5.	*Lactobacillus acidophilus*	Acid clot (Pink)
6.	*Enterococcus foecalis*	Acid and reduction (white to colorless)
7.	*Clostridium sporogenes*	Acid clot and peptonization.
8.	*Morasella osloenals*	No change
9.	*Alcallegenes foecalis*	Alkaline reaction
10.	*Pseudomonas aeruginosa*	Peptonization (clearing)

Limitations

1. Litmus milk is a complex medium that can produce a diversity of results. Because of this, litmus milk can give quite unreliable results (i.e., the results often give negative results when something positive should happen). Thus, you would be advised to use litmus milk as a confirmatory test but not a definitive test (except as a last resort).

2. A clot formation is simply recorded as "clot" and cannot clearly differentiate between a clot and curd formation in this medium.

In this test there may be no change in the medium, or acid or alkali may be produced; or sometimes clotting of milk, peptonization or saponification may occur.

The clot may be disrupted by the gas produced (stormy fermentation)

Essay Questions

1. Explain the different types of Reproduction in bacteria
2. Explain the Replication of virus
3. Write a note on special groups of bacteria along with distinguishing features
4. Explain the Taxonomy and classification of microbes
5. Explain the different techniques of staining
6. Write a note on fungal growth and metabolism

Multiple Choice Questions

1. The amino acid sequence of proteins directly reflect
   (a) RNAs
   (b) t RNA
   (c) m RNA
   (d) DNA
2. 5 Kingdom classification was given by
   (a) Robert Whittaker
   (b) Zuckerkandi
   (c) Pauling
   (d) Bergy
3. Bacterial flagella are
   (a) Cylindrical appendages
   (b) Helical appendages
   (c) Linear appendages
   (d) Circular appendages
4. Assemblage of unrelated fungi existing in their anamorphic state are now placed in the special class of
   (a) Zygomycetes
   (b) Deuteromyctes
   (c) Ascomycetes
   (d) basidiomyctes
5. Survival of adverse environmental conditions such as desiccation, low nutrient supply anaerobiosis is provided by
   (a) Pellicle
   (b) Plasma lemma
   (c) Cysts
   (d) Shells
6. The most common and most important type of cell division in bacterial growth is
   (a) Fragmentation
   (b) Budding
   (c) Spores formation
   (d) Binary fission
7. Virus infecting bacteria are called
   (a) Bacteriophage
   (b) Heliophage
   (c) Microphage
   (d) plasmophage

Answers

1. (c)	2. (a)	3. (b)
4. (b)	5. (c)	6. (d)
7. (a)		

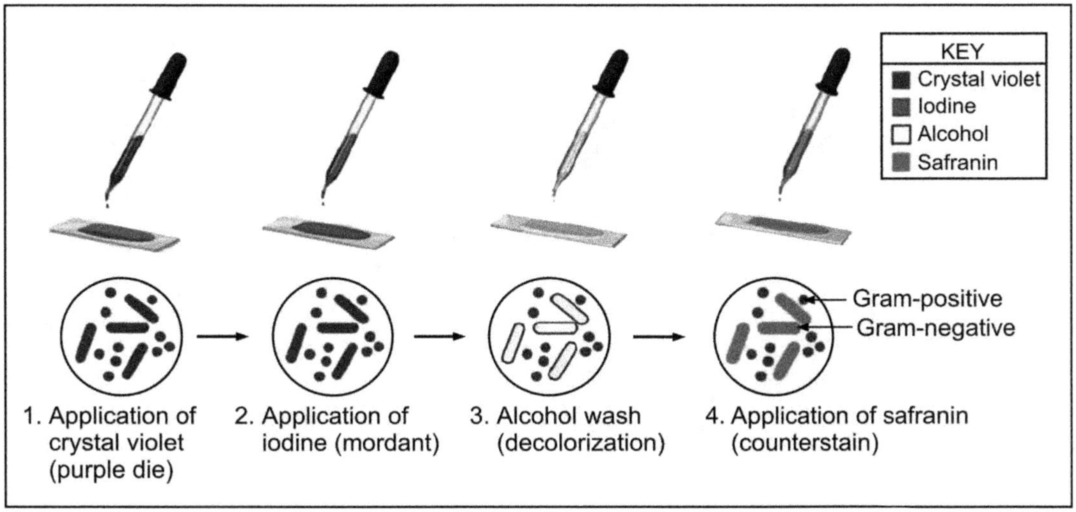

Colour Plate 2.1 (Fig. 2.36; Pg. 147) Gram staining method and results

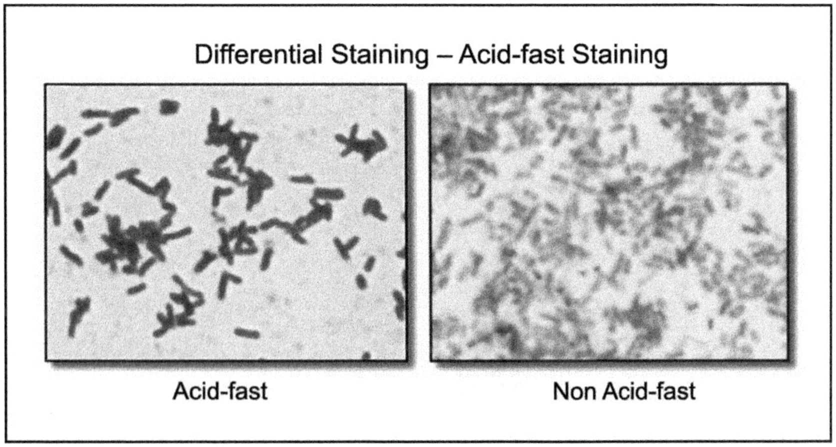

Colour Plate 2.2 (Fig. 2.38; Pg. 151) Slides showing acid-fast and non-acid fast results

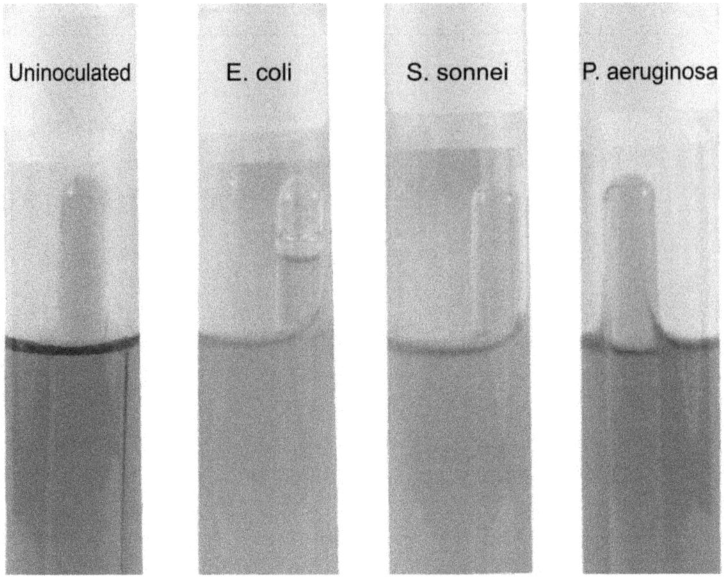

Carbohydrate Utilization Test

Colour Plate 2.3 (Fig. 2.39; Pg. 156) Peptone media with bromocresol purple indicator. From left to right: uninoculated tube; *E. coli*, glucose fermenter with gas production (visible air bubble in the inverted Durham tube); *S. sonnei*, glucose fermenter without gas production (no visible air bubble in the inverted Durham tube); *P. aeruginosa*, nonfermenter.

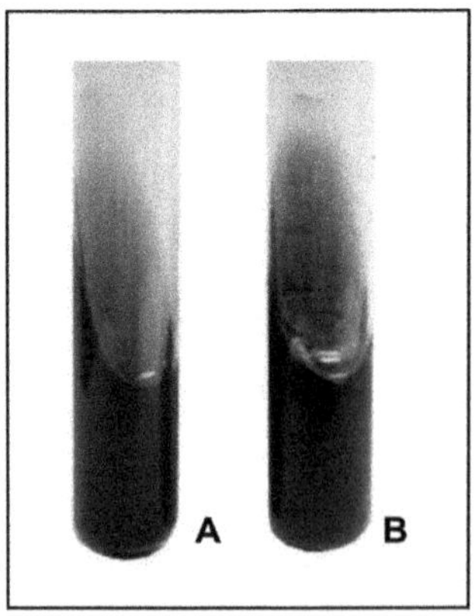

Colour Plate 2.4 (Fig. 2.40; Pg. 157) A-negative B- Positive citrate utilization test

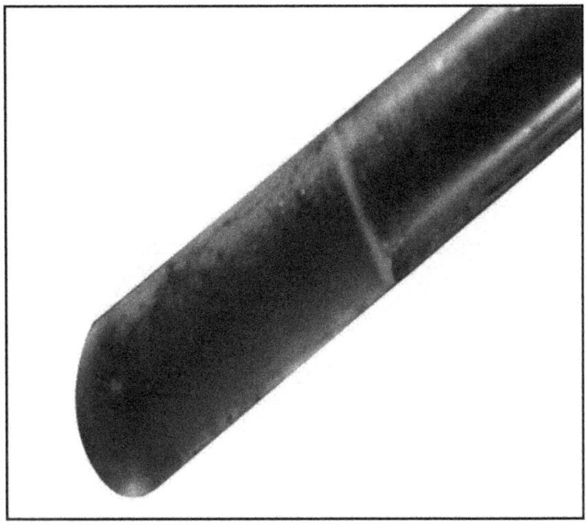

Colour Plate 2.5 (Fig. 2.42; Pg. 159) Gelatin hydrolysis test result
A-Gelatin hydrolysis Test Control (Uninoculated)

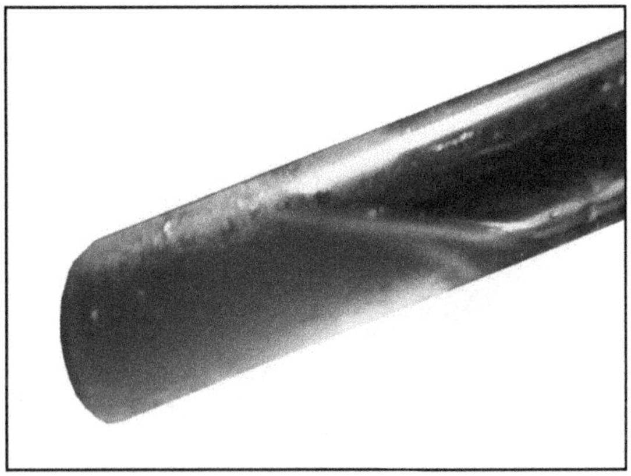

Colour Plate 2.6 (Fig. 2.43; Pg. 159) Gelatin hydrolysis test. After 30 minutes in an ice bath, a nutrient gelatin tube inoculated with Bacillus subtilis exhibited positive gelatin hydrolysis as shown by medium liquefaction (A) while the uninoculated control remained solid (B) Gelatin hydrolysis was observed after 3 days of incubation.

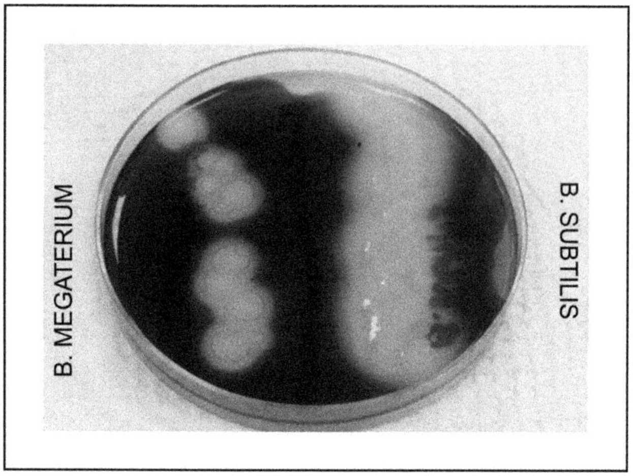

Colour Plate 2.7 (Fig. 2.45; Pg. 161) Starch hydrolysis test positive result

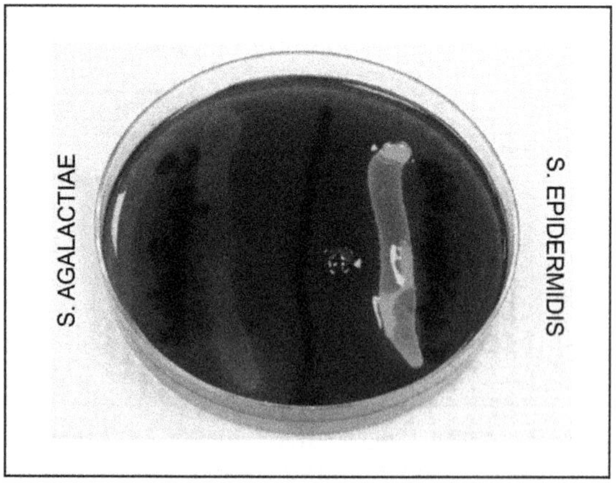

Colour Plate 2.8 (Fig. 2.46; Pg. 161) Starch hydrolysis negative result

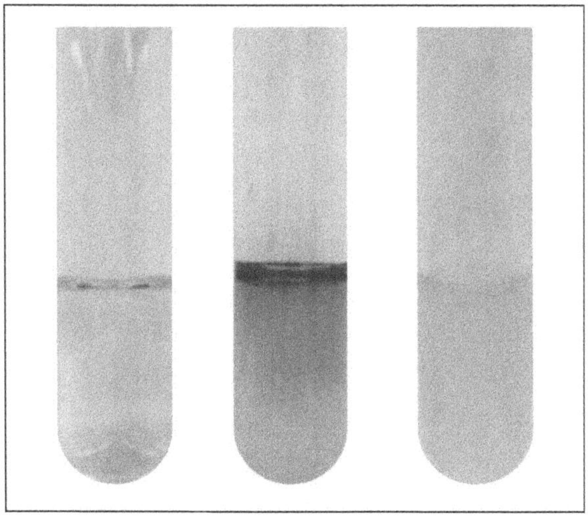

(a) (b) (c)

Colour Plate 2.9 (Fig. 2.47; Pg. 163) The indole test. **(a)** An uninoculated tube of tryptone broth. **(b)** A positive indole test. The 48-hour *Escherichia coli* culture grown at 37°C tests positive for the presence of indole as indicated by the red reagent layer after the addition of Kovács reagent. **(c)** A negative indole test. The 48-hour *Enterobacter aerogenes* culture incubated at 37°C has not broken down the tryptophan in the medium and thus no color change occurs upon addition of the Kovács reagent. The reagent appears as a thin yellow layer on top of the culture medium.

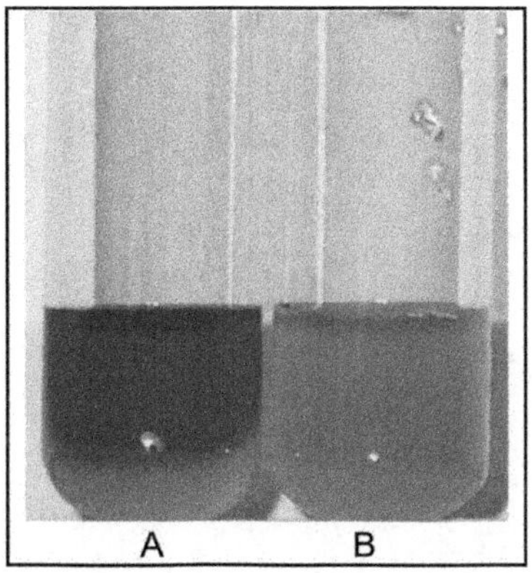

Colour Plate 2.10 (Fig. 2.48; Pg. 165) Methyl red reaction. *E. coli* **(A)** and *E. aerogenes* **(B)** were grown for 48 hours at 35°C in MR-VP medium. After incubation, 5 drops of a 0.05% methyl red solution (per 2.5 ml) were added to each culture. The MR-positive *E. coli* **(A)** shows a red coloration as a result of high acid production and a decrease in the pH of the culture medium to 4.4. The MR-negative *E. aerogenes* culture **(B)** has a yellow color indicating a less acidic medium.

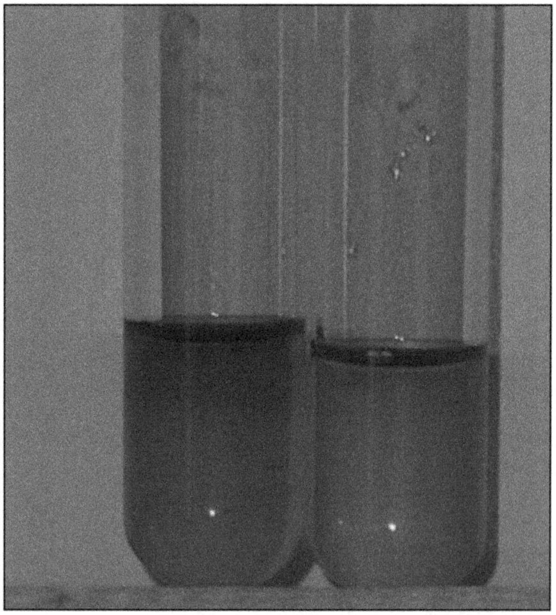

A B

Colour Plate 2.11 (Fig. 2.49; Pg. 166) Voges-Proskauer reaction. *E. aerogenes* (**A**) and *E. coli* (**B**) were grown in MR-VP-broth for 48 hours at 37°C and Barritt's reagents A and B were added. VP-positive *E. areogenes* (**A**) shows red coloration on top of the culture, whereas VP-negative *E. coli* (**B**) has a yellowish color.

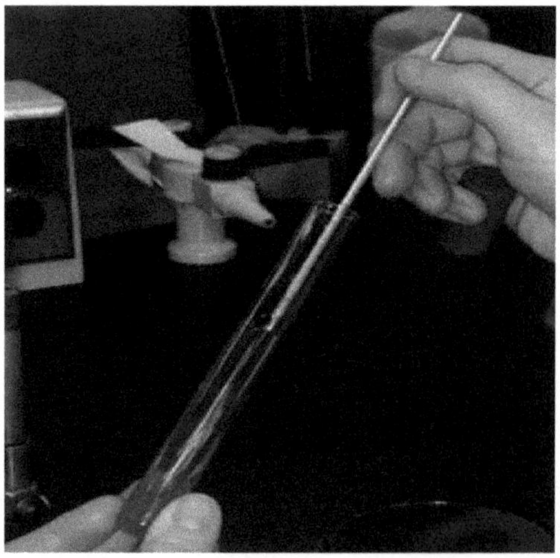

Colour Plate 2.12 (Fig. 2.50; Pg. 168) Triple sugar iron test

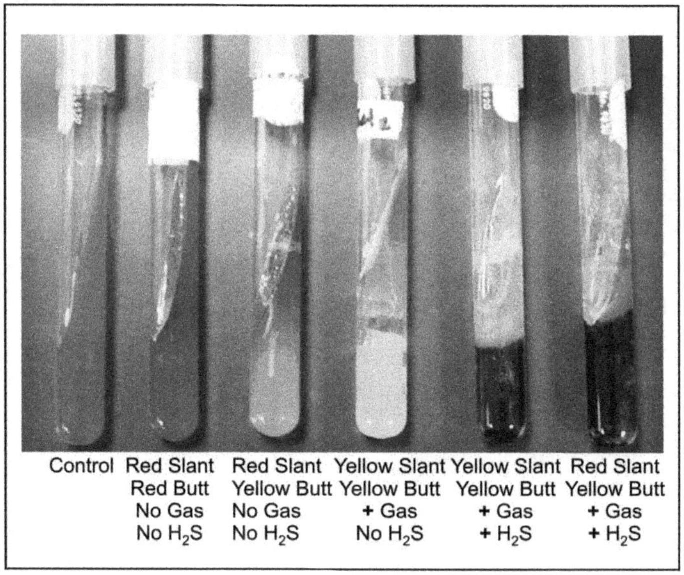

Colour Plate 2.13 (Fig. 2.51; Pg. 169) Hydrogen sulphide production test results

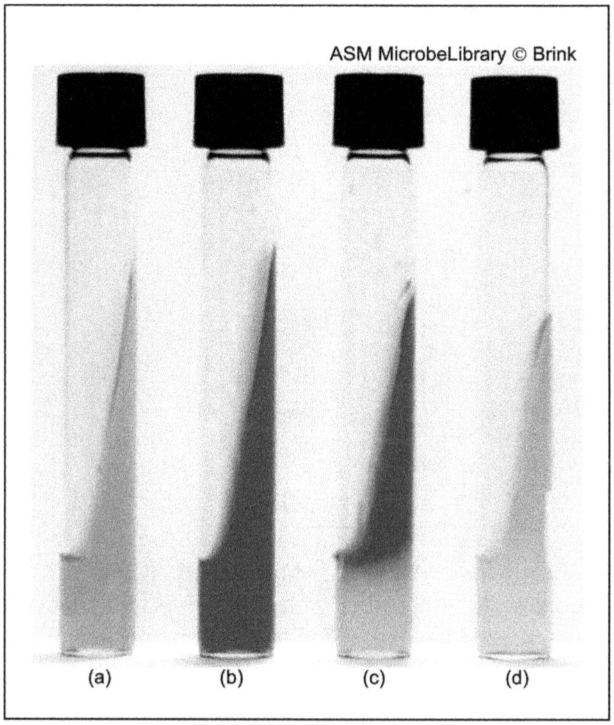

Colour Plate 2.14 (Fig. 2.52; Pg. 172) Urea agar test results. Urea agar slants were inoculated as follows: (a) uninoculated, (b) *Proteous mirabilis* (rapidly urease positive), (c) *Klebsiella pneumoniae* (delayed urease positive), (d) *Escherichia coli* (urease negative). All samples were incubated at 37 °C for 16 hours.

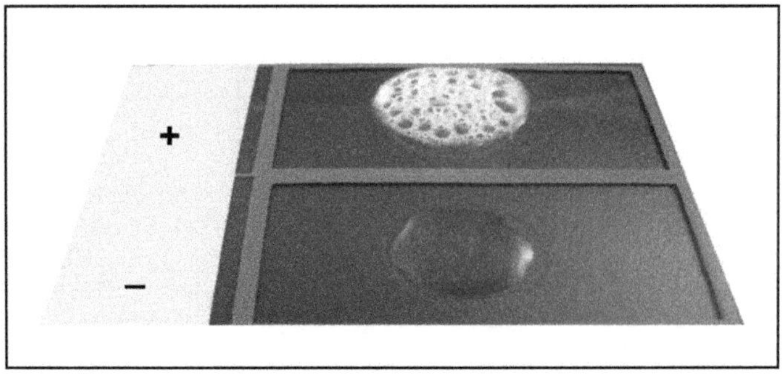

Colour Plate 2.15 (Fig. 2.53; Pg. 173) Catalase test

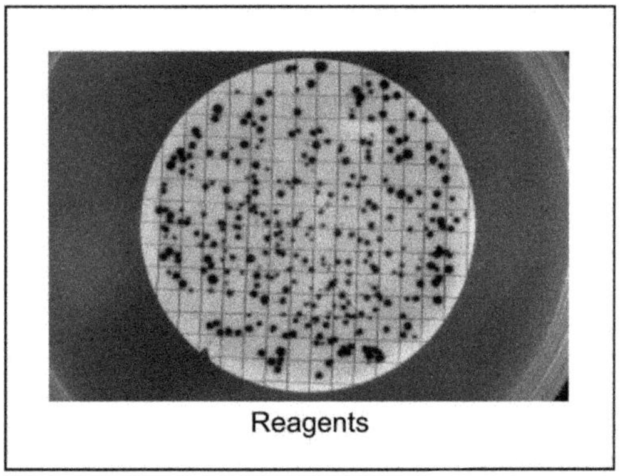

Colour Plate 2.16 (Fig. 2.54; Pg. 173) Oxidase test

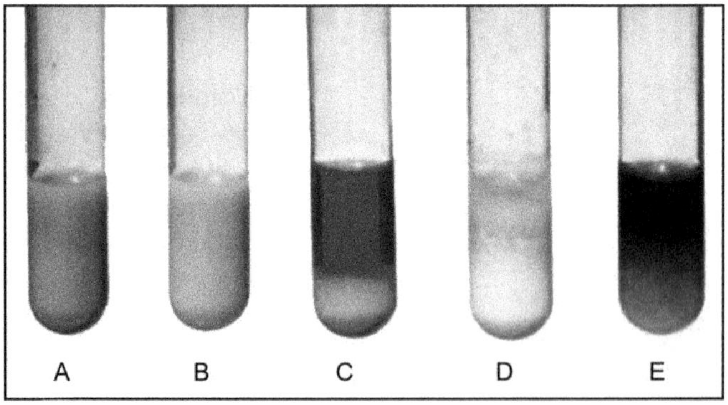

Colour Plate 2.17 (Fig. 2.55; Pg. 175) Litmus milk reactions: **(A)** Alkaline. **(B)** Acid. **(C)** Upper transparent portion is peptonization; solid white portion in bottom is coagulation and litmus reduction; overall redness is interpreted as acid. **(D)** Coagulation and litmus reduction in lower half; some peptonization (transparency) and acid in top portion. **(E)** Litmus indicator is masked by production of soluble pigment.

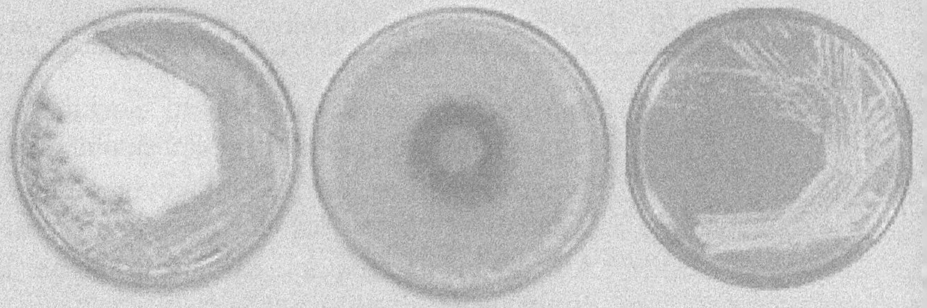

3 NUTRITION AND GROWTH

LEARNING OBJECTIVES

After studying the chapter, the students familiarize themselves with concepts in:

Understanding the nutritional types of bacteria

Understanding techniques involved in cultivation of bacteria

Understanding the various methods of isolating pure cultures

Develop an understanding on growth of bacteria

Understanding various methods involved for bacterial count

Introduction

Except for certain ecological studies where bacterial populations are examined in their natural habitats, bacteria are usually cultivated and studied under laboratory conditions. Numerous media (single medium) have been developed for bacterial cultivation. Nutritional requirements of bacteria vary widely. Chemical compositions of media also vary. Bacteria exhibit wide differences with respect to the physical conditions favoring their growth.

Examples of physical conditions are temperature, pH and gaseous environment.

3.1 Nutritional Requirements

(i) All organisms require a source of energy. Some rely on chemical compounds for their energy and are designated as chemotrophs. Others can utilize radiant energy (light) and are phototrophs.

(ii) All organisms require a source of electrons for the metabolism.

Some organisms can use reduced inorganic compounds as electron donors and are termed lithotrophs (some may be chemolithotrophs, others photolithotrophs).

Other organisms use organic compounds as electron donors and are called organotrophs (some are chemo organotrophs, others photo organotrophs).

(iii) All organisms require carbon in some form for use in synthesizing cell components.

All organisms require at least small amounts of CO_2. However, some can use CO_2 as their major, or even sole source of carbon; such organisms are termed autotrophs. Others require organic compounds as their carbon source and are termed heterotrophs.

(iv) All organisms require nitrogen in some form for cell components. Bacteria are extremely versatile in this respect.

Some bacteria can use atmospheric nitrogen. Others grow on inorganic nitrogen compounds such as nitrates, nitrites, or ammonium salts.

Other derives nitrogen from organic compounds such as amino acids.

(v) All organisms require oxygen, sulfur and phosphorus for cell components.

Oxygen is provided in various forms, such as water, component atoms of various nutrients; or molecular oxygen.

Sulfur is needed for synthesis of certain amino acids (cysteine, cystine, and methionine).

Some bacteria require organic sulfur compounds, some are capable of utilizing inorganic sulfur compounds, and some can even use elemental sulfur.

Phosphorous is supplied in the form of phosphate, is an essential component of nucleotides, nucleic acids, phospholipids, teichoic acids, and other compounds.

(vi) All organisms require metal ions, such as K^+, Ca^{+2}, Mg^{+2} and Fe^{+2} for normal growth.

Other metal ions needed at very low concentrations, such as Zn^{2+}, Cu^{2+}, Mn^{2+}, MO^{6+}, $Ni2^+$, B_3^+ and CO_2^+. These are often termed trace elements.

Certain marine bacteria, cyanobacteria, and photosynthetic bacteria members of archaeobacteria (red extreme halophiles) require more than 12 to 15 percent NaCl for their growth.

This high level requirement of NaCl is for maintenance of the integrity of their cell walls and for the stability and activity of certain of their enzymes.

(vii) All living organisms contain vitamins and vitamin like compounds.

These function either as coenzymes for several enzymes or as the building blocks for coenzymes.

Some bacteria are capable of synthesizing their entire requirement of vitamins from other compounds in the culture medium.

Others grow only if the required vitamins are supplied in the medium.

(viii) All living organisms require water. All nutrients must be aqueous solution before they can enter the cells of bacteria.

Water is highly polar, it dissolves or disperses cellular components and provides a suitable milieu for various metabolic reactions of cell.

High specific heat of water provides resistance to sudden transient temperature changes in the environment.

Water is a chemical reactant, being required for the many hydrolytic reactions carried by cell.

3.2 Nutritional Types of Bacteria

On the basis of nutritional requirements bacteria can be divided into many groups. The major separation is into two groups, phototrophs and chemotrophs.

Phototrophs

Among the phototrophic bacteria are species that use inorganic compounds as their source of electrons (i.e., photolithotrophs).

For example, *Chromatium okenii* uses H_2S as its electron donor, oxidizing it to elemental sulfur.

Some phototrophic bacteria use organic compounds such as fatty acids and alcohol as electron donors and are therefore photoorganotrophs.

E.g., *Rhodospirillum rubrum* can use succinate as an electron donor.

Under some circumstances a phototrophic bacterium can grow as a chemotrophic.

E.g., In the absence of oxygen R.*rubrum* is dependent on light as its source of energy and lives as a photo organotroph; however, in the presence of oxygen it can grow in the dark as chemoorganotroph.

Chemotrophs

Among the chemotrophic bacteria are species that use inorganic compounds as their source of electrons (i.e., chemolithotrophs).

E.g., *Nitrosomonas* use ammonia as their electron source, obtaining energy by oxidizing ammonia to nitrite.

Many other chemotrophic bacteria use organic compounds such as sugars and amino acids, as electron donors and are therefore chemoorganotrophs.

E.g., *Pseudomonas pseudoflava* can use either the organic compound glucose or the inorganic compound H_2 as its source of electrons.

Autotrophs and Heterotrophs

Autotrophs: Organisms that can use CO_2 as their sole source of carbon for assimilation are termed autotrophs. Most of chemolithotrophs obtain energy by utilizing inorganic electron donors.

Some autotrophs are facultative autotrophs; i.e., they can either live as autotrophs, deriving their carbon from CO_2, other can live as heterotrophs. Examples of autotrophsa are cyanobacteria, green and purple sulfur bacteria and red algae.

Heterotrophs: Organisms that can use organic compounds as their carbon source are termed Heterotrophs. Heterotrophic bacteria have been studied more extensively than the autotroph, because heterotrophic species cause diseases to human beings and other animals and plants.

Comparison chart of Autotrophs and Heterotrophs

Autotrophs	Heterotrophs
1. An organism that is able to form nutritional organic substances from simple inorganic substances such as carbon dioxide.	1. Heterotrophs cannot produce organic compounds from inorganic sources and therefore rely on consuming other organisms in the food chain.
2. Types are Photoautotroph, Chemoautotroph	2. Types are Photoheterotroph, Chemoheterotroph
3. Examples are Plants, algae, and some bacteria	3. Examples are Herbivores, omnivores, and carnivores
4. Produce own food	4. Do not Produce own food
5. Produce their own food for energy.	5. They eat other organisms to get proteins and energy
6. Food chain level is Primary	6. Food chain level is Secondary and tertiary

3.3 Types of Nutrient Media

To meet these needs the microbiologist has available numerous media which on the basis of their application or function, may be classified as follows.

1. **Selective media:** These media favor the growth of a particular bacterium by inhibiting the growth of undesired bacteria and allowing growth of desirable bacteria. *Examples*: MacConkey agar, Lowenstein-Jensen media, Tellurite media (Tellurite inhibits the growth of most of the throat organisms except *Diphtheria bacilli*). Antibiotic may be added to a medium for inhibition.

- For instance one wants to isolate only cellulose utilizing organisms present in the soil sample which may be containing other kinds of bacteria, in the medium cellulose only must be added as carbon source.
- The isolation of the *gonorrhoea* causing organism, *Neisseria Gonorrhoea* from a clinical specimen is facilitated by the use of media containing certain antibiotics; these antibiotics do not affect *N.gonorrhoea* but do inhibit the growth of contaminating bacteria.

2. **Differential (indicator) media:** Certain reagents or supplements, when incorporated into culture media, may allow differentiation of various kinds of bacteria.
   - One can distinguish between hemolytic and nonhemolytic bacteria by inoculating mixture of bacteria onto a blood containing agar medium.
   - Hemolytic bacteria present in the mixed culture may hemolyze (destroy) the red blood cells; others do not.
   - An indicator is included in the medium. A particular organism causes change in the indicator, *e.g.*, Blood, Neutral red, Tellurite. Examples: Blood agar and MacConkey agar, Cystein lactose electrolyte deficient agar (CLED), Thiosulphate citrate bile salts-sucrose agar (TCBS), Xylose lysine deoxycolate agar (XLD) are indicator media. Many special purpose media are needed to facilitate recognition, enumeration and isolation of certain types of bacteria.
3. **Assay media:** For the assay of vitamins, amino acids and antibiotics, media of prescribed compositions are used. Example: Antibiotic assay medium No.19 of Sigma Aldrich, Antibiotic Agar No.1 (Penassay seed agar, Grove and Randall Antibiotic Agar No.1)

   Media of special composition are also available for testing disinfectants.
4. **Media for enumeration of bacteria:** Special kinds of media are used for determining the bacterial content of such materials as milk and water.

   Their composition must adhere to prescribed specifications. Example RCPB agar; M-MRS agar
5. **Media for characterization of bacteria:** A wide variety of media are conventionally used to determine the type of growth produced by bacteria, as well as to determine their ability to produce certain chemical changes. Depending on the growth requirements of the bacteria and the information that the microbial scientist wants to gain, various types of growth media are available for cultivating bacteria, in a microbiology laboratory environment. Culture media contain the nutrients and other substances required to cultivate bacteria. There are several characteristics that any culture media must have:
6. **Maintanance media:** Satisfactory maintanance of the viability and physiological characteristics of a culture over time may require a medium different form that which is optimum for growth.

Prolific, rapid growth may also be associated with rapid death of the cells at end of the growth phase.

Glucose in a medium frequently enhances growth, but may produce acid which is harmful to the cells.

Omission of glucose is preferable in maintanance medium.

7. **Enriched media:** The media are enriched usually by adding blood, serum or egg. Examples: Enriched media are blood agar and Lowenstein-Jensen media, Chocolate agar and Loffler's serum slope *Streptococci* grow in blood agar media.
8. **Transport media:** These media are used when specimen cannot be cultured soon after collection. Examples: Cary-Blair medium, Amies medium, Stuart medium and Sach's buffered glycerol saline.
9. **Storage media:** Media used for storing the bacteria for a long period of time. Examples: Egg saline medium, chalk cooked meat broth.
10. **Synthetic media:** These are chemically defined media prepared from pure chemical substances. It is used in research work. The constituents of a chemically defined media include: a basal media (such as DMEM, F12, or RPMI 1640 containing amino acids, vitamins, inorganic salts, buffers, antioxidants and energy sources), which is supplemented with recombinant albumin, chemically defined lipids, recombinant insulin and/or zinc, recombinant transferrin or iron, selenium and an antioxidant thiol such as 2-mercaptoethanol or 1-thioglycerol.
11. **Chemically defined media** also allows researchers who are studying in the field of cell physiology (especially extracellular) and or molecule–cell interactions to eliminate any variables that may arise due to the effects of unknown components in the medium. It is composed of exact amounts of chemically pure, specifically indentified organic or inorganic components. Examples Glucose salt broth or Inorganic synthetic broth.
12. **Basal media:** Basal media are those that may be used for growth (culture) of bacteria that do not need enrichment of the media. Examples: Nutrient broth, Nutrient agar and Peptone water. *Staphylococcus* and *Enterobacteriaceae* grow in these media.
13. **Anaerobic media:** Anaerobic bacteria need special media for growth because they need low oxygen content, reduced oxidation-reduction potential and extra nutrients. Example Robertson Cooked Meat Broth (RCMB).

3.4 Bacteriological Media

Chemically defined media are used for the cultivation of autotrophs. For routine cultivation of heterotrophs, certain complex raw materials such as peptone, meat extract and yeast extract are used, and the resulting media support the growth of a wide variety of heterotrophic bacteria.

Solidifying agent is usually agar (concentration of 1.5 to 2.0%) forms firm, transparent gels that are not degraded by most bacteria. Agar melts at 95 °C and solidifies at 45 °C, it does not contribute or has any nutritive property. It is usually free from growth-promoting or growth-retarding substances.

Examples of relatively simple liquid and solid media that support the growth of many common heterotrophs are **Nutrient broth** and **Nutrient agar**.

Yeast extract contains several of the B vitamins and other growth promoting substances, it improves the nutrient quality.

For the cultivation of certain fastidious heterotrophs, supplements like bovine rumen fluid, animal blood, blood serum, or extracts of plant and animal tissues may be required.

3.4.1 Fungal Media

1. Potato Dextrose Agar Medium (PDA)
2. Corn Meal Agar Medium (CMA)
3. Czapek Dox Agar Medium(CzDA) pH 6-6.5
4. Malt peptone agar
5. Sugar assimilation agar
6. Sabouraud agar
7. Christensen urea agar containing glucose
8. Sugar fermentation medium

Sabouraud's agar composition:

Dextrose	40.0 g
Mycological Peptone	10.0 g
Agar	15.0 g
Distilled water	1000.0 ml
pH	5.6 ± 2

3.4.2 Classification of Media Basing on the Consistency

(a) Solid media: Solid and semisolid media are widely used for cultivation of bacteria.

Solid media are useful for isolating bacteria or for determining the characteristics of colonies.

Agar is included as non-nutritive solidifying agent when a solid medium is desired.

Silica gel is sometimes used as an inorganic solidifying agent for autotrophic bacteria.

Bacteria growing on the surface of agar reveal their colony morphology - their characteristic appearance when growing in a group of bacteria that arose from one parent cell. Being able to view species colony morphology can provide helpful, albeit general, information on the identity of unknown bacteria. Mixed bacteria can be separated easily on solid media.

(b) **Semisolid media** prepared with agar at the conc. of 0.5% or less have soft, custard like consistency. This medium is useful for the cultivation of microaerophilic bacteria, and for determination of bacterial motility.

(c) **Liquid media (nutrient broth):** Nutrient broth is a liquid bacterial growth medium made of powdered beef extract and short chains of amino acids that have been dissolved in water. Liquid medium is convenient to use for growing bacteria in test tubes, and can reveal information about the oxygen requirements of bacteria growing within. Bacteria that require oxygen will grow close to the water's surface, and bacteria that cannot tolerate the presence of oxygen will grow at the bottom of the test tube.

(d) **Biphasic media:** A biphasic medium consisting of a solid and a liquid phase in the same blood culture bottle that was developed by Castaneda and others. Castaneda system for blood culture is used for suspected brucellosis.

3.4.3 Preparation of Media

Naturally occurring substances like milk (skimmed milk), sterilized before use is used to cultivate bacteria.

Media are prepared by compounding the required individual ingredients. Or by adding water to a dehydrated product which contains all ingredients.

Steps for preparation of bacteriological media

1. Each ingredient, or the complete dehydrated medium, is dissolved in the appropriate volume of distilled water.
2. The pH of the fluid medium is determined and adjusted if necessary.
3. For solid medium, agar is added and boiled to dissolve agar.
4. The medium is dispensed into tubes or flasks. Ingredients that are heat labile are sterilized by filtration.

3.4.4 Physical Conditions required for Growth

It is necessary to know the physical environment in which the organisms will grow best. Bacteria show diverse responses to physical conditions such as temperature, gaseous conditions, and pH.

3.4.4.1 Temperature

Since all processes of growth are dependent on chemical reactions and since the rate of these reactions are influenced by temperature, the pattern of bacterial growth can be profoundly influenced by this condition.

Bacterial species may not manifest the same characteristics in every detail when grown at different temperatures.

E.g., *Serrati marcescens* forms a blood-red to orange pigment when cultured at 25 °C but produces little or no pigment when cultured at 37-26 °C.

Lactobacillus plantarum does not require the amino acid phenylalanine for growth when cultured at 25 °C but does require it at 37-23 °C.

Optimum growth temperature: The temperature that allows for most rapid growth during a short period of time (12 to 24 hr) is known as the optimum growth temperature.

Optimum growth temperature may not necessarily be optimum for other cellular activities.

The maximum temperature at which growth occurs is usually quite close to the optimum temperature, whereas the minimum temperature for growth is usually much lower than the optimum.

On the basis of their temperature relationships, bacteria are divided into three main groups:

(a) ***Psychrophiles*****:** These are able to grow at 0 °C or lower, though they grow best at higher temperatures. They can grow at 0 °C but have optimum temperature of 15 °C or lower and a maximum of about 20 °C.

Psychrotrophs or facultative psychrophiles those grow at 0 °C but which grow best between 20 to 30 °C. Samples for isolation should be maintained at cold temperatures.

Strict psychrophiles die if they are temporarily exposed to room temperature.

Even at optimum temperature it takes two or three weeks for colonies of psychrophiles to develop.

Heat instability of ribosomes and various enzymes, increased leakage of cell components, and impaired transport of nutrients above the maximum temperature are the root causes for psychrophiles restricted growth temperature. Examples are *Arthrobacter* sp., *Psychrobacter* sp. and members of the genera *Halomonas*, *Pseudomonas*, *Hyphomonas*, and *Sphingomonas*.

(b) ***Mesophiles*****:** Grow best within a temperature range of approximately 25 to 40 °C. Bacteria pathogenic to human and warm blooded animals are mesophiles, most grow best at about body temperature 37-30 °C. Thermophiles grow best at temperatures above 45 °C. The growth range of many thermophiles extends into the mesophilic region; these species are designated facultative thermophiles. Bacterial infections in humans are mostly caused by mesophilic bacteria that find their optimum growth temperature around 37 °C (98.6 °F), the normal human body temperature. Examples of common mesophilic bacteria are *Listeria monocytogenes, Pesudomonas maltophilia, Thiobacillus novellus, Staphylococcus aureus, Streptococcus pyrogenes, Streptococcus pneumoniae, Escherichia coli, and Clostridium kluyveri.*

(c) ***Thermophiles*****:** Those cannot grow in the mesophilic range; these are termed true thermophiles, obligate thermophiles, or stearothermophiles. Increased thermal stability of ribosomes, membranes, and various enzymes are the factors that have been implicated in the ability to grow at high temperature.

Examples of thermophilic eubacteria are *Thermus aquaticus, Thermotoga maritima*, and thermophilic archaeobacteria are *Sulfolobus solfataricus, Pyrococcus furiosus and Thermus thermophilus*

(i) The ***True thermophiles*** show no growth, or only very feeble growth, below 40 to 45 °**C**. Their development requires temperatures above 50 °**C**., and some are able to develop at a temperature of 80 °**C**., though most abundant growth is shown at 60 to 70 °**C.**

(ii) ***Stearothermophiles*** will grow within a temperature range of 30-75 °**C** degrees Celsius.

(iii) ***Obligate thermophiles*** (Extreme thermophiles) Thermophiles, meaning heat-loving organisms, are organisms with an optimum growth temperature of 50 °C or more, a maximum of up to 70 °C or more, and a minimum of about 40 °C, but these are only approximate. Some extreme thermophiles (hyper thermophiles) require a very high temperature (80 °C to 105 °C) for growth. Their membranes and proteins are unusually stable at these extremely high temperatures.

Loss of fluidity (lipid bilayer) of the cytoplasmic membrane may be a factor governing the minimum temperature.

3.4.4.2 Gaseous Requirements

The principal gases that affect bacterial growth are oxygen and carbon dioxide.

Bacteria display a wide variety of responses to free oxygen, based on this bacteria are divided into four groups.

1. **Aerobic bacteria** require oxygen for growth and can grow when incubated in air atmosphere (i.e., 21% oxygen).

Examples of Aerobic bacteria: *Staphylococcus species, Streptococcus species, Enterobacteriacae species, Mycobacterium tuberculosis, Bacillus, Nocardia and Pseudomonas aeruginosa.*

2. **Anaerobic bacteria** do not use oxygen to obtain energy; moreover oxygen is toxic for them and they can not grow when incubated in an air atmosphere.

   Some can tolerate low levels of oxygen (non stringent or tolerant anaerobes), but others (stringent or strict anaerobes) cannot tolerate even low levels and may die upon brief exposure to air.

   Examples of Anaerobic bacteria are
   Clostridium tetani which causes tetanus,
   Clostridium botulinum which causes food poisoning,
   Escherichia coli, Klebsiella , Actinomyces.

3. ***Facultative anaerobic bacteria*** do not require oxygen for growth, although they may use it for energy production if it is available. They are not inhibited by oxygen and usually grow as well under an air atmosphere as they do in the absence of oxygen.

   Some examples of facultative anaerobic bacteria are *Staphylococcus* spp., *Streptococcus* spp., *Escherichia coli*, *Listeria* spp. and *Shewanella oneidensis.* Certain eukaryotes are also facultative anaerobes, including fungi such as *Saccharomyces cerevisiae* and many aquatic invertebrates such as Nereis polychaetes (worm).

4. ***Microaerophilic bacteria*** require low levels of oxygen for growth but cannot tolerate the level of oxygen present in an air atmosphere.

   Examples of microaerophilic bacteria: *Borrellia burgdorferi* causing Lyme disease in cattle and humans, *Helicobacter pylori* causing gastritis and *Campylobacter* causing food poisoning.

3.4.4.3 Oxygen Toxicity

Oxygen is both beneficial and poisonous to living organisms.

Oxygen's beneficial effect: Its strong oxidizing ability makes it an excellent terminal electron acceptor for the energy yielding process known as respiration.

Oxygen's toxic effect: Oxygen is quite a reactive molecule which likes to be reduced (*i.e.,* oxidise something else). It may be toxic to obligate anaerobes for several reasons.

(i) A common reason is that oxygen is easily partially reduced to highly reactive species such as hydrogen peroxide (H_2O_2) or superoxide radicals (O_2). These can react with proteins and cell membrane lipids and kill the cell. Hydrogen peroxide (powerful oxidizing agent) is highly toxic to many kinds of cells.

   Aerobic organisms possess enzymes to remove reactive oxygen species, such as catalases, peroxidases and superoxide dismutases, but these are often absent or present in low concentration in obligate anaerobes *Bacteroides fragilis Gram-negative*, rod-shaped bacterium.

(ii) Another reason for oxygen toxicity in anaerobes is that many of their enzymes are oxygen-sensitive. This is especially so for the metalloenzymes that makes up the alternative respiratory chains. These proteins often have metals such as iron, molybdenum or tungsten at the active site, which are reactive towards oxygen and make the protein unstable if oxygen is present.

(iii) Oxygen inactivation of enzymes. Molecular oxygen O_2 can directly oxidize certain essential reduced groups, such as thiol (–SH) groups, or enzymes, resulting in enzyme inactivation.

For instance, the enzyme complex known as nitrogenase, responsible for nitrogen fixation, is irreversibly destroyed by even small amounts of oxygen.

(iv) According to recent studies production of even more toxic substance such as hydroxyl radical (oH) by means of the following reactions. Hydroxyl radical (most reactive free radical) can damage almost every kind of molecule found in living cells.

(v) Another toxic derivate of oxygen is an energized form known as singlet oxygen, $(^1\Delta_g)O_2$, which is produced in biological systems by certain photochemical reactions.

Aerobic and facultative organisms have developed various protective mechanisms against the toxic forms of oxygen Fig. (3.1).

$$O_2 + \bar{e} \rightarrow \bar{O}_2 .$$

$$2\bar{O}_2 + 2H^+ \rightarrow O_2 + H_2O_2$$

$$\bar{O}_2 . + H_2O_2 \rightarrow O_2 + OH^- + OH$$

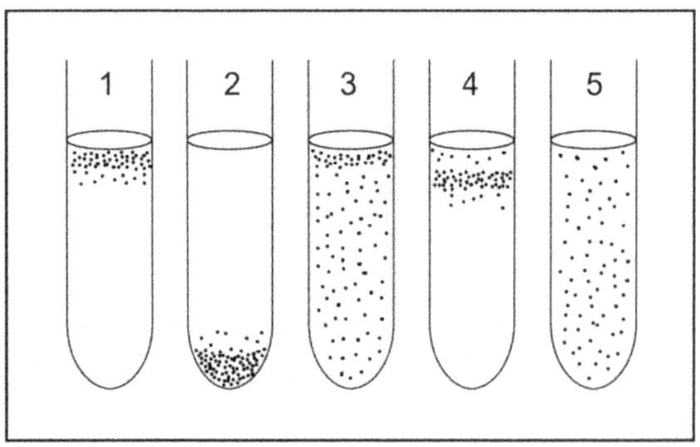

1. Obligate aerobes
2. Obligate anaerobes
3. Facultative anaerobes
4. Microaerophiles
5. Aerotolerant organisms

Fig. 3.1 Growth patterns of bacteria with different oxygen requirements in liquid medium

3.4.4.4 Cultivation of Aerobic Bacteria

1. Incubating in tubes or small flasks containing medium, under normal atmospheric conditions is generally satisfactory.
2. To grow in large quantities, medium should be exposed to the atmosphere, by dispensing the medium in shallow layers (in special containers), and constant shaking of inoculated liquid cultures.

3.4.4.5 Cultivation of Anaerobic Bacteria

Stringent anaerobes can be grown only by taking special precautions to exclude all atmospheric oxygen from the medium.

1. ***Prereduced media*:** During preparation, the culture medium is boiled for several minutes to drive off most of the dissolved oxygen. A reducing agent e.g., cysteine, is added to further lower the oxygen content. Oxygen-free N_2 is bubbled through the medium to keep it anaerobic. The medium is then dispensed into tubes which are being flushed with oxygen free N_2, stoppered tightly, and sterilized by autoclaving. During inoculation, the tubes are continuously flushed with oxygen-free CO_2 by means of a cannula, restoppered, and incubated.

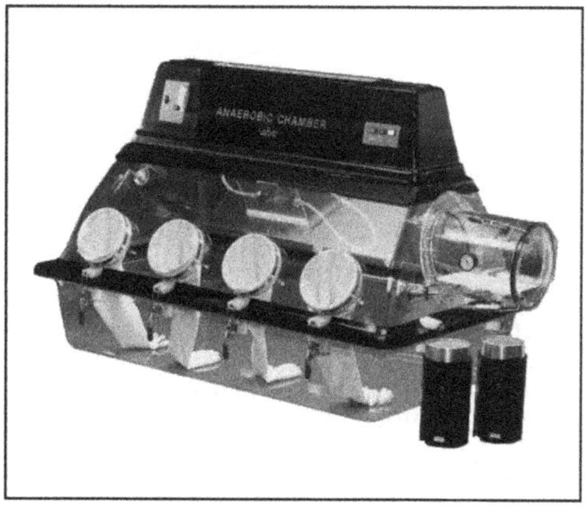

Fig. 3.2 Anaerobic chamber

2. ***Anaerobic chamber (Fig. 3.2)*:** This refers to a plastic anaerobic glove box that contains an atmosphere of H_2, CO_2, and N_2. Culture media are placed within the chamber by means of an air lock which can be evacuated and refilled with N_2. From the air lock the media are placed within the main chamber.

   Any O_2 in the media is slowly removed by reaction with the H_2, forming water; this reaction is aided by a palladium catalyst. After being rendered oxygen-free, the media are inoculated within the chamber (by means of the glove ports) and incubated (also within the chamber).
3. ***Anaerobic Jar (Fig. 3.3)*:** Non-stringent anaerobes can be cultured within an anaerobic jar. Inoculated media are placed in the jar along with an H_2 + CO_2 generating system. After the jar is sealed, the oxygen present in the atmosphere within the jar, as well as that dissolved in the culture medium, is gradually used up through reaction with the hydrogen in the presence of a catalyst.

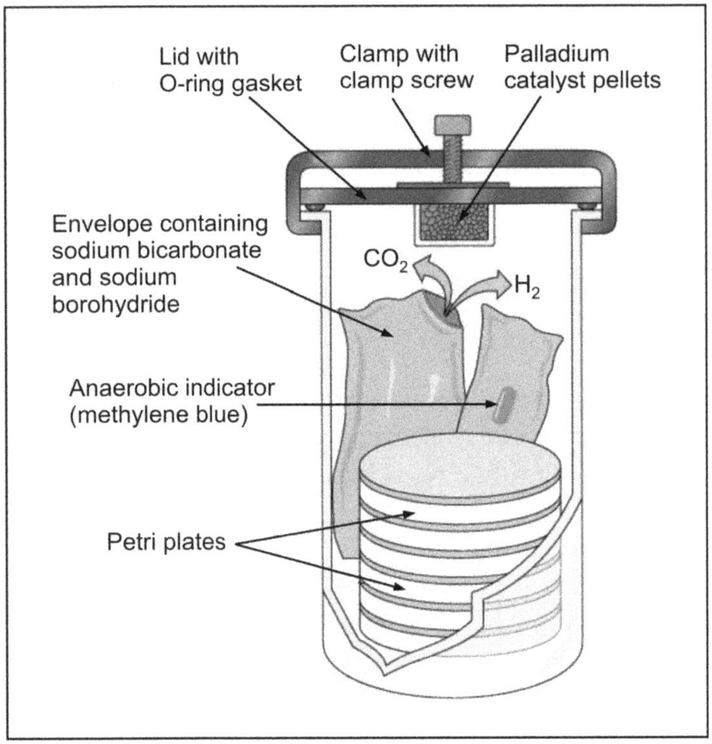

Fig. 3.3 Anaerobic jar

3.4.4.6 Acidity or Alkalinity (pH)

For most bacteria the optimum pH for growth lies between 6.5 and 7.5, and the limits generally li0065 somewhere between 5 and 9. Few bacteria such as *Thiobacillus thiooxidans* has an optimum pH of 2.0 to 3.5 and can grow in a range of pH 0.5 and 6.0.

An unclassified bacterium isolated from an alkaline spring in California was found to grow best at a pH of 9.0 and 9.5 and could grow within range from 8.0 to 11.4.

Bacteria are cultivated in a medium originally adjusted to a given pH, if a carbohydrate is present in the medium, that carbohydrate may be fermented or oxidized to organic acids, thus that acid decreases the pH of the medium.

If the salt of an organic acid is supplied, as a carbon source (*e.g.*, sodium malate), oxidation of the salt, by bacteria will cause an increase in pH.

Such shifts in pH may be so great that further growth of the organism is eventually inhibited.

Radical shifts in pH can be prevented by incorporating a buffer (substance that resists change in pH) into the medium. A buffer is a mixture of a weak acid and its conjugate base (*e.g.*, acetic acid (CH_3COOH) and acetate (CH_3COO). Some of the nutritional ingredients of the medium, such as peptones, also possess some buffering capacity because the component amino acids provide weak acid/conjugate base systems.

Some large fermentation apparatuses are equipped with automatic controls that maintain a constant pH.

Miscellaneous Physical Requirements

Some bacteria have additional requirements. For example, phototrophic bacteria must be exposed to a source of illumination, since light is their source of energy. Bacterial growth may also be influenced by hydrostatic pressure which is measured in tons per square inch. Bacteria isolated from the deepest ocean trenches will not grow in the laboratory unless the medium is subjected to a similar pressure.

Choice of Media and Conditions of Incubation

To grow bacteria successfully the microbiologist must provide the proper kind of medium and an appropriate set of physical conditions. A great deal of information with respect to choice of media, preparation of media, and the physical and nutritional conditions required for the cultivation.

3.5 Pure Culture

If the bacterial species being sought comprises a suitably high proportion of the mixed population, it can be isolated in pure culture. The descendents of a single isolation in pure culture comprise strain.

A strain is usually made up of a succession of cultures and is often derived from a single colony (however, the number of bacteria which gave rise to the original colony) is usually unknown.

If a strain is derived from a single parent cell, it is termed as clone. Each strain is designated by an identifying number and it's history recorded.

A variety of techniques have been developed whereby isolation into pure culture can be accomplished. Each technique has certain advantages and limitations, and there is no one method that can be used for all bacteria.

3.5.1 Methods of Isolating Pure Cultures

(i) **The streak-plate technique:** By means of a transfer loop, a portion of the mixed culture is placed on the surface of an agar medium and streaked across the surface. This manipulation thins out the bacteria on the agar surface so that some individual bacteria are separated from each other. When streaking is properly performed, the bacterial cells will be sufficiently far apart in some areas of the plate to ensure that the colony developing from one cell will not merge with that growing from another (Fig. 3.4).

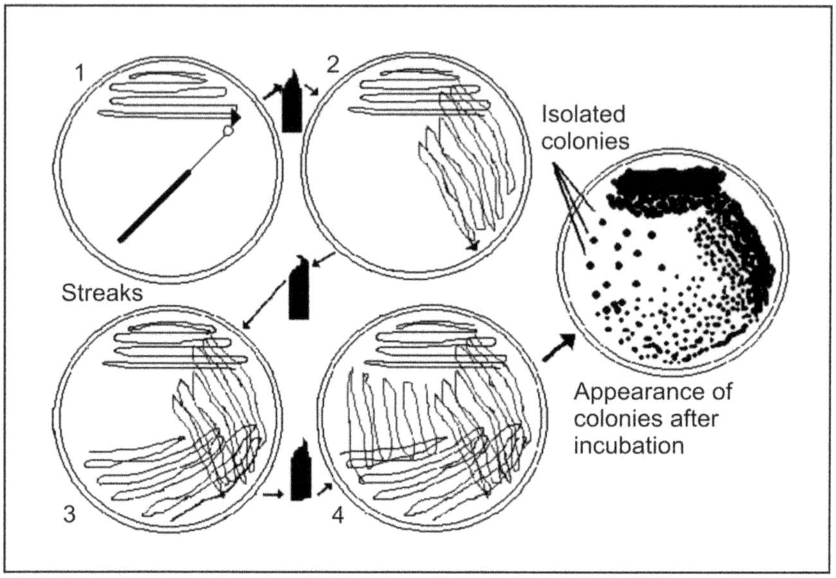

Fig. 3.4 Isolation by streak plate method

(ii) Roll-Tube Technique: It is a modification of streak-plate technique. This technique is used for the isolation of stringent anaerobes. One should recognize that sub culturing a colony from a single streak plate does not automatically assure purity. The colony may have been derived from two or more different kinds of bacteria. So it is advisable to streak a culture several times in succession, preferably on nonselective media, in order to ensure purity.

(iii) The Pour Plate Technique: Mixed culture is first diluted to provide only a few cells per milliliter before being used to inoculate media. Since the number of bacteria in the specimen is not known beforehand, a series of dilutions is made so that at least one of the dilutions will contain a suitably sparse concentration of cells (Fig. 3.5).

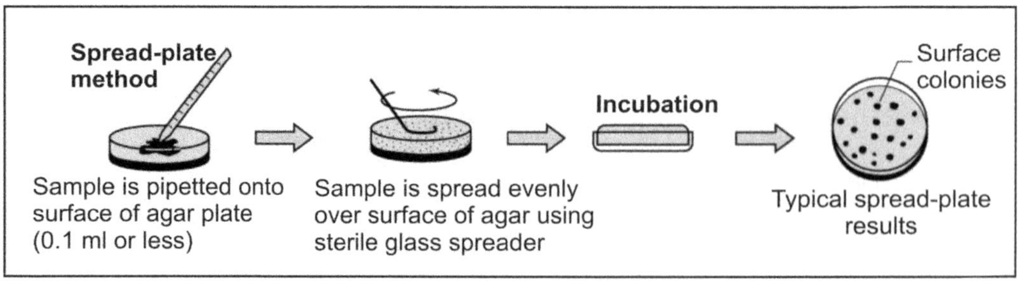

Fig. 3.5 Isolation by pour plate method

The mixed culture is diluted directly in tubes of liquid (cooled) agar medium. The medium is maintained in liquid state at a temperature of 45 °C to allow through distribution of the inoculums. The inoculated medium is dispensed into Petri dishes, allowed to solidify, and then incubated. A series of agar plates show decreasing numbers of colonies resulting from the dilution procedure can be obtained. Some of the organisms are trapped beneath the surface of the medium when it gels, and therefore both surface and subsurface colonies develop. The subsurface colonies can be transferred to fresh media.

The organisms being isolated must be able to withstand temporary exposure to the 45 °C temperature of the liquid agar medium.

This method is unsuitable for isolating psychrophilic bacteria.

(iv) **Spread-plate method:** The mixed culture is not diluted in the culture medium; instead it is diluted in a series of tubes containing a sterile liquid usually water or physiological saline. A sample is removed from each tube, placed onto the surface of an agar plate, and spread evenly over the surface by means of a sterile, bent glass rod. On at least one plate of the series the bacteria will be in numbers sufficiently low as to allow the development of well-separated colonies. Only surface colonies develop; moreover, the organisms are not required to withstand the temperature of liquid agar.

The pour-plate and spread-plate techniques may be performed in a quantitative manner to determine the number of bacteria present in a specimen (Fig. 3.6).

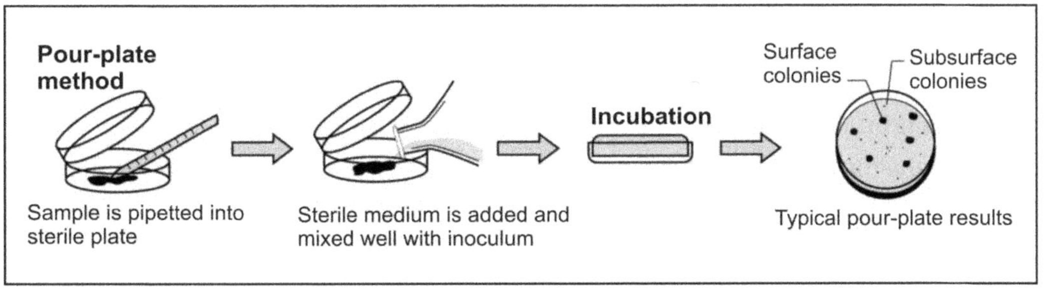

Fig. 3.6 Isolation by spread plate method

(v) **Micromanipulator techniques:** A device called the micromanipulator can be used in conjunction with a microscope to pick a single bacterial cell from a mixed culture. The micromanipulator permits the operator to control the movements of a micropipette or a microprobe (a fine needle) so that a single cell can be isolated. This technique requires a skilled operator and is reversed for studies in which a clone must be obtained unequivocally (Fig. 3.7).

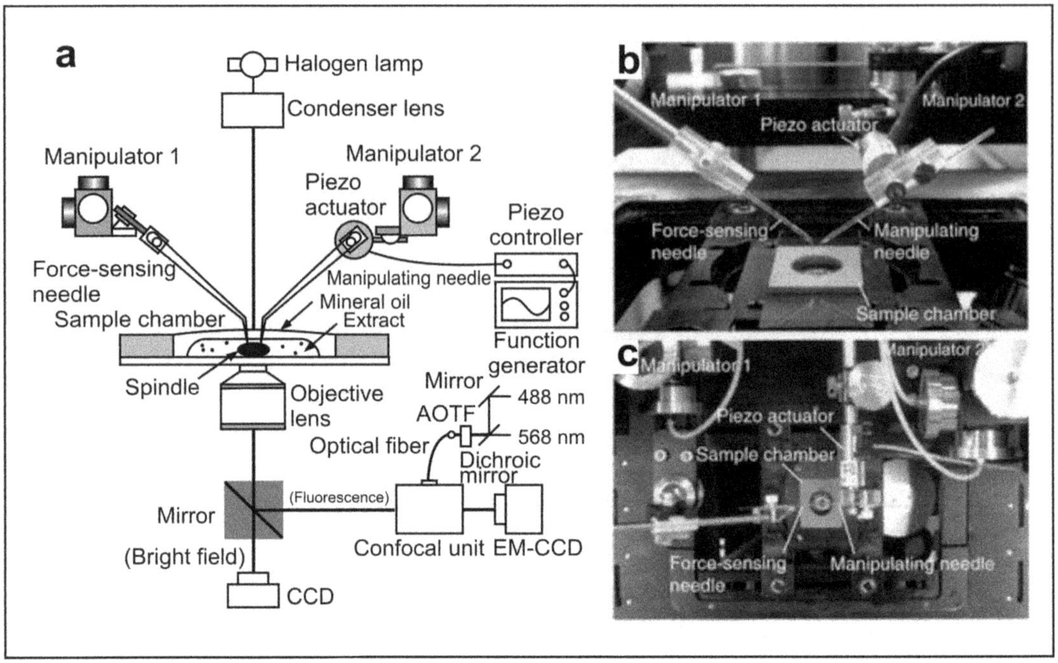

Fig. 3.7 Micromanipulator flow chart

3.5.2 Maintenance and Preservation of Pure Cultures

Most microbiology laboratories maintain a large collection of strains, frequently referred to as a stock-culture collection.

Need for maintaining Stock Cultures

These organisms are needed for laboratory classes and research work, as test agents for particular procedures, or as reference strains for taxonomic studies. The strains are used for screening of new, potentially effective chemotherapeutic agents; as assay tools for vitamins and amino acids; as agents for the production of vaccines, antisera, antitumor agents, enzymes, and organic chemicals; and as reference cultures that are cited in company patents.

For several reasons it is extremely important to have properly identified and cataloged strains of bacteria available.

Several different methods have been developed to preserve and store bacteria until they are needed. The objective is to maintain strains alive and uncontaminated and to prevent any change in their characteristics.

3.5.3 Methods of Maintenance and Preservation

Strains can be maintained by periodically preparing a fresh stock culture from the previous stock culture. The culture medium, the storage temperature and the time interval at which the transfers are made vary with the species and must be ascertained beforehand. Preservation of microbial cultures was critical for all individuals and firms engaged in the search for patentable products from and patentable processes by micro-organisms.

1. **Periodic Transfer to Fresh Media:** The temperature and the type of medium chosen should support a slow rather than a rapid rate of growth so that the time interval between transfers can be as long as possible. Many common heterotrophs remain viable for several weeks or months on NA.

   Disadvantage: It fails to prevent changes in the characteristics of a strain due to the development of variants and mutants.

2. **Preservation by overlaying Culture with Mineral Oil:** Many bacteria be successfully preserved by covering the growth on an agar slant with sterile mineral oil. The oil must cover the slant completely; to ensure this, the oil should be about 1/2 inch above the tip of the slanted surface.

3. **Serial Transfer:** Based upon its ease of use, serial transfer is often the first "preservation" technique used by microbiologists.

   The disadvantages of relying upon this method for culture maintenance include contamination, loss of genetic and phenotypic characteristics, high labor costs, and loss of productivity.

4. **Preservation in Distilled Water:** This method (Castellani method, 50 years ago) was extensively tested on 594 fungal strains: 62% of the strains growing and maintaining their original morphology.

   In another study, 76% of yeasts, filamentous fungi and *Actinomycetes* survived storage in distilled water for 10 years.

   The pathogenic fungus *Sporothrix schencki* which can infect humans as well as animals and is the causative agent of "sporotrichosis", commonly known as "rose handler's disease concluded that even though long-term survival was good when this procedure was used, there was a noted loss in virulence.

   Castellani technique should be considered as one of the options for practical storage of fungal isolates.

5. **Preservation under Oil:** One of the earlier preservation methods was the use of mineral oil to prolong the utility of stock cultures. The oil must cover the slant completely; to ensure this, the oil should be about ½ inch above the tip of the slanted surface.

   Sterile mineral oil has been found to prevent evaporation from the culture and Decrease the metabolic rate of the culture by limiting the supply of oxygen.

This method is more suitable than lyophilization for the preservation of non-sporulating strains.

6. **Lyophilization:** One of the best methods for long-term culture preservation of many micro-organisms is freeze-drying (lyophilization). In Lyophilization, or freeze drying, there is a water is frozen, followed by its removal from the sample, initially by sublimation (primary drying) and then by desorption (secondary drying). In this process, the moisture content of the product is reduced to such a low level that does not support biological growth or chemical reactions, which gives the stability to the formulation (Fig. 3.8).

   The commonly used cryoprotective agents are skim milk (15% [w/v] for cultures grown on agar slants and 20% for pelleted broth cultures) or sucrose (12% [w/v] final concentration).

   It should be noted that some plasmid--containing bacteria are successfully preserved by this method (Fig. 3.9).

7. **Storage over Silica Gel:** Neurospora a genus of **Ascomycete** fungi has successfully been preserved over silica gel.

8. **Preservation on Paper:** Drying the spores on some inert substrates can preserve spore-forming fungi, Actinomycetes, and unicellular bacteria.

   Fruiting bodies of the myxobacteria, containing *myxospores*, may be preserved on pieces of sterile filter paper and stored at room temperature or at 6 °C for 5 to 15 years.

9. **Preservation on Beads:** The method involving preservation on beads (glass, porcelain), developed by Lederberg, is successful for many bacteria.

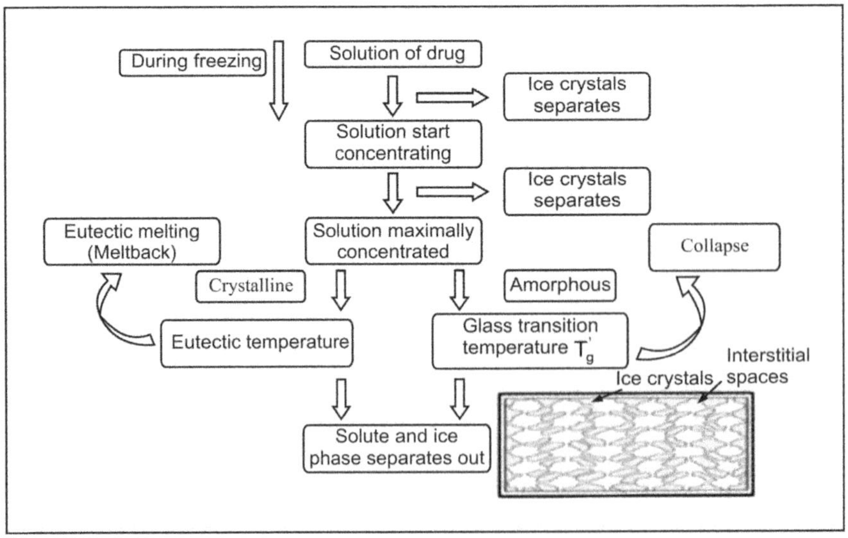

Fig. 3.8 Flowchart of primary drying steps in lyophilization

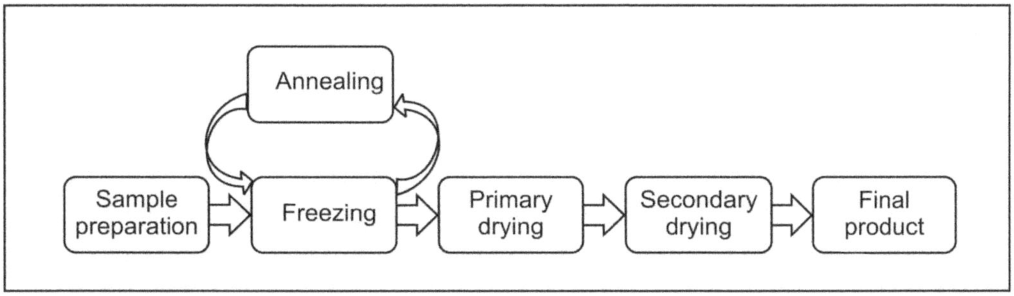

Fig. 3.9 Lyophilization cycle

10. **Liquid Drying:** To avoid the damage that freezing can cause a liquid drying preservation process is applied.

    It has effectively preserved organisms such as anaerobes that are damaged by or fail to survive freezing.

    This procedure was preferred over lyophilization for the maintenance of the biodegradation capacity of six gram--negative bacteria capable of degrading toluene.

    Malik's liquid-drying method was also found to be markedly superior to lyophilization for the preservation of unicellular algae.

11. **Cryopreservation:** Micro-organisms may be preserved at –5 to –20 °C for 1 to 2 years by freezing broth cultures or cell suspensions in suitable vials.

    Deep freezing of micro-organisms requires a cryoprotectant such as glycerol or dimethyl sulfoxide (DMSO) when stored at -70 °C or in the liquid nitrogen at –156 to –196 °C.

    Broth cultures taken in the mid--logarithmic to late logarithmic growth phase are mixed with an equal volume of 10 to 20% (vol/vol) glycerol or 5 to 10% (vol/vol) DMSO.

    Alternatively, a 10% glycerol-sterile broth suspension of growth from agar slants may be prepared.

12. **Preservation in Liquid Nitrogen:** Storage in liquid nitrogen is clearly the preferred method for preservation of culture viability.

    Protocol for Cryopreservation with Cryoprotectants by a Two-stage Freezing Process, and Revival of Culture:

    After centrifugation the supernatant is removed and the pellet, consisting of microbial cells, is dissolved in an ice-cold solution containing polyvinyl ethanol (10% [wt/vol]) and glycerol (10% [wt/vol]) in a 1:1 ratio.

    Due to the presence of polyvinyl ethanol, a viscous thick cell suspension is obtained, which is kept for about 30 minutes in an ice bath for equilibration.

    During equilibration, an aliquot of 0.5 to 1.0 mL of the cell suspension is dispensed into each plastic cryovial or glass ampoule.

They are tightly closed, clamped onto labeled aluminum canes, and placed at –30 °C for about 1 h or for a few minutes in the gas phase of liquid nitrogen to achieve a freezing rate of about 1°C/min.

The canes are then placed into canisters, racks, or drawers and frozen rapidly at 80 °C or in liquid nitrogen.

For revival of cultures, the frozen ampoules are removed from the liquid nitrogen.

For thawing, they are immediately immersed to the neck in a water bath at 37 °C for a few seconds.

The thawed cell contents of the ampoule or vial are immediately transferred to membranes to form a thick layer.

The resulting bacterial membranes with immobilized cells are used as a biological component of a biosensor for activity measurements.

3.6 Physiology of Growth

When bacteria are inoculated into a suitable medium and incubated under appropriate conditions, a tremendous increase in the number of cells occurs within a relatively short time.

The term growth is commonly applied to bacteria and other micro-organisms usually refers to changes in the total population rather than an increase in the size or mass of an individual organism.

Growth denotes the increase in number beyond that present in the original inoculums.

Growth determination requires quantitative measurement of the total population of cells or cell crops at the time of inoculation and again after incubation.

3.6.1 Growth

The most common means of bacterial reproduction is binary fission, one cell divides producing two cells.

If we start with a single bacterium, the increase in population is by geometric progression i.e., $1 - 2^2 - 2^3 - 2^4 - 2^5 - \ldots\ldots\ldots 2^n$ where n = no. of generations.

Each succeeding generation, assuming no cell death, doubles the population. The total population 'N' at the end of a given time period is expressed as

$$N = 1 \times 2^n$$

Under practical conditions, the number of bacteria N_0 inoculated at time zero is not 1 but several thousand, so the formula becomes

$N = N_0 \times 2^n$

$\text{Log}_{10} N = \log_{10} N_0 + n \log 10^2$

$$n = \frac{\log_{10} N - \log_{10} N_0}{\log_{10}{}^{2}}$$

But $\log_{10} 2 = 0.301$

$$n = \frac{\log_{10} N - \log_{10} N_0}{0.301}$$

$$n = 3.3 (\log_{10}N - \log_{10} N_0)$$

Thus, by above equation, no. of generations can be calculated if we know initial population and the population after growth has occurred.

Normal Growth Cycle (Growth curve) of Bacteria

Assume that a single bacterium has been inoculated into a flask of liquid culture medium which is subsequently incubated. Eventually the bacterium will undergo binary fission and a period of rapid growth will ensure in which cells multiply at an exponential rate.

During this period of rapid growth, if we use the theoretical number of bacteria which should be present at various intervals of time then plotted the data in two ways. (Logarithmic number of bacteria and arithmetic number of bacteria versus time).

We would obtain the curve shown in (Fig. 3.10).

The Lag Phase: The addition of inoculums to a new medium is not followed immediately by a doubling of the population.

The population remains temporarily unchanged. But this does not mean that the cells are quiescent or dormant; on the contrary, during this stage the individual cells increase in size beyond their normal dimensions. Physiologically they are very active and are synthesizing new protoplasm. Bacteria may be deficient in enzymes or coenzymes required for chemical machinery of the cell.

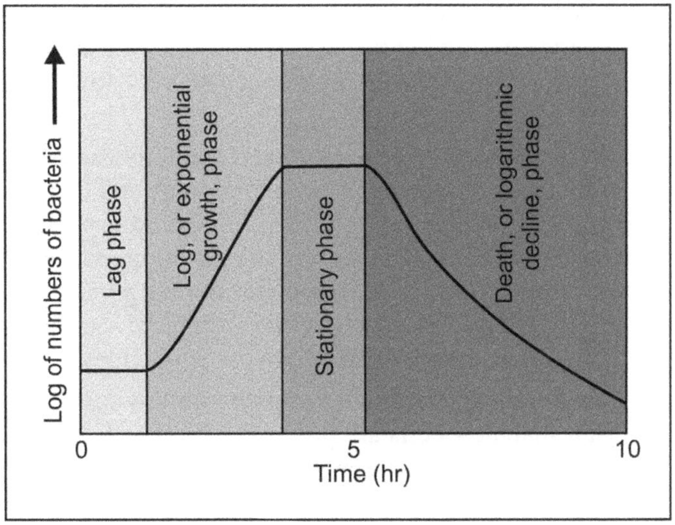

Fig. 3.10 Typical bacterial growth curve

Time for adjustments in the physical environment around each cell may be required. Organisms are metabolizing but there is a lag in cell division.

At the end of the lag phase each organism divides. However, since not all organisms complete the lag period simultaneously, there is a gradual increase in the population until the end of this period, when all cells are capable of dividing at regular intervals.

The Logarithmic or Exponential Phase: During this period the cells divide steadily at a constant rate, and the log of the number of cells plotted against time results in a straight line. The population is most nearly uniform in terms of chemical composition of cells metabolic activity, and other physiological characteristics. Since bacteria are commonly "overfed" in laboratory culture, they can multiply at a constant exponential rate for many generations before the substrate level becomes low enough to affect this rate. In general, cells in the logarithmic phase of growth are the most uniform and are in a more clearly defined condition than in any other phase, log-phase cultures are commonly used for studies of microbial metabolism.

The generation time g (the time required for the population to double) can be determined from the number of generations n that occur in a particular time interval t using eq. for n, the generation time can be calculated by the following formula:

$$G = t/n = t/3.3\ (\log_{10}N - \log_{10} N_0)$$

During exponential growth, the growth rate (i.e., the number of generations per hour), termed R, is the reciprocal of the generation time g. It is also the slope of the straight line obtained when the log number of cells is plotted against time:

$$R = 3.3\ (\log_{10}N - \log_{10} N_0)/t$$

How this growth rate remain constant during the logarithmic phase of growth even though the concentration of substrate is continually decreasing through utilization by the organisms. If you study the effect of nutrient (substrate) concentration upon the growth rate of bacterial culture, you can understand this. The level of substrate provided in a bacterial culture is sufficiently high so that, even though the bacteria use up some substrate during log phase of the growth, the growth rate does not decrease appreciably. It is only when substrate levels become very low that the growth rate begins to be severely affected.

***The Stationary Phase*:** The logarithmic phase of growth begins to taper off after several hours, again in a gradual fashion represented by the transition from a straight line through a curve to another straight line. This trend toward cessation of growth can be attributed to a variety of circumstances, particularly the exhaustation of some nutrients and less often, the production of toxic products during growth. The population remains constant for a time, perhaps as a result of complete cessation division or perhaps because the reproduction rate is balanced by an equivalent death rate.

***The Phase of Decline or Death*:** Following the stationary phase the bacteria may die faster than new cells are produced, if indeed some cells are still new cells are produced, if indeed some cells are still reproducing. A variety of conditions contribute to bacterial death, but the most important are the depletion of essential nutrients and the accumulation of inhibitory products, such as acids, the number of viable cells decrease exponentially, essentially the inverse of growth during the log phase.

Bacteria die at different rates, just as they grow at different rates. Some species of Gram-negative cocci die very rapidly, i.e., after 72 hr or less. Other species die so slowly that viable cells may persist for months or even years.

Transitional Periods between Bacterial Growth Phases

Note that a culture proceeds gradually from one phase of growth to the next. This means that not all the cells are in an identical physiological condition toward the end of a given phase of growth. Time is required for some to catch up with others.

Synchronous Growth (Fig. 3.11)

Various aspects of bacterial growth, organization, and differentiation to a particular stage of the cell divisions are related in the aspects of microbiological research. Since it is not feasible to analyze a single bacterium, if all cells in a culture were to be in the same stage of the division cycle, the result from analysis of the cell crop could be interpreted as that for a single cell.

When the growth of cultures is manipulated so that all the cells will be in the same stage of their growth cycle such conditions is termed as synchronous growth.

The synchrony generally lasts only a few generations, since even the daughters of a single cell soon get out of phase with one another.

A Population can be Synchronized by

1. Manipulating the physical environment
2. The chemical composition of the medium.

The cells may be inoculated into a medium at a suboptimal temperature; if they are kept in these conditions for some time, they will metabolize slowly but will not divide, when the temperature is subsequently raised, the cells will undergo a synchronized division. The smallest cells in a log-phage culture are those which have just divided and separated out by filtration or by differential centrifugation. They are reasonably well synchronized with each other.

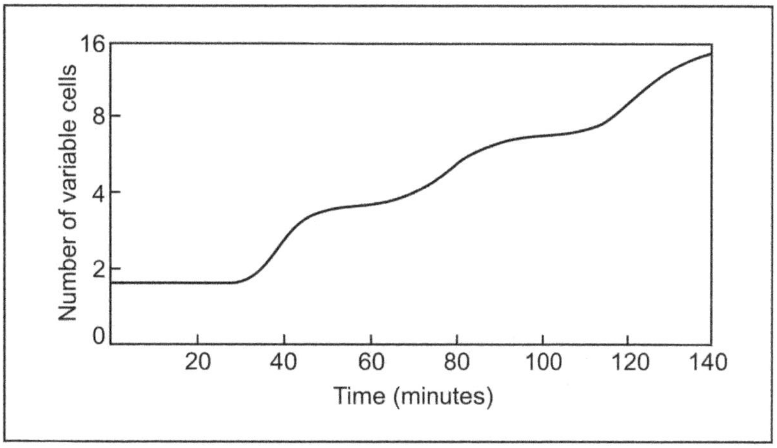

Fig. 3.11 Synchronous growth curve of bacteria

3.7 Reproduction

The most common mode of cell division in the usual growth cycle of bacterial populations is transverse binary fission, in which a single cell divides after developing a transverse septum (cross wall). Transverse binary fission is an asexual reproductive process.

New Cell Formation (Macromolecular Synthesis)

A bacterial cell inoculated into a fresh medium selectively takes up nutrients from its environment. Many biochemical syntheses then take place. The nutrients are converted into cell substance – RNA, DNA, proteins, enzymes, and other macromolecules. Cell mass and cell size increases, and new cell wall building blocks are synthesized. Subsequently, the process of binary fission is initiated, ultimately resulting in the formation of two new cells.

Septum Formation

In transverse binary fission, septum formation does not begin until the chromosome content of the cell has been doubled; i.e., cell division is triggered by completion of DNA replication. Material continually being destroyed and new, inner material continually being added as the cell elongates.

Particularly in gram positive cells, it may have a role in the synthesis of new membrane material.

The next step is the inward growth of the cell wall to form a septum that splits to allow separation of the two daughter cells.

E.g., During growth of gram positive coccus *Streptococcus faecalis*, all of the new wall material formed by dividing cell is made during synthesis of septum. Septum formation begins beneath an equatorial ridge in the cell-wall. New cell-wall material is synthesized in this region and the septum forms; this material becomes one half of the wall of each daughter cell. In order for the new wall to achieve its final hemisphere shape, some plasticity must be present.

This is due to two factors:

1. The turgor pressure of the protoplast against the newly synthesized wall.
2. Certain amount of reorganization of the peptidoglycon due to breakage of some of the chemical bonds by hydrolytic enzymes and subsequent formation of new bonds at different locations.

In gram positive rods such as *Bacillus subtilis* the transverse septum is formed, but not ridge is present at the middle of the cell.

Only about 15% of the new wall of the daughter cell is derived from the formation of septum.

The remainder is synthesized along the cylindrical part of the cell, since bacillus grows mainly by elongation rather by septum formation.

Budding

Some bacteria, such as *Rhodopseudomonas acidophila*, reproduce by budding, a process in which a small protuberance bud develops at one end of the cell; this enlarges and eventually develops into a new cell which separates from the parent. In some budding bacteria, such a *Hyphomicrobium* species, the bud may develop at the end of a prostheca.

Fragmentation

Bacteria that produce extensive filamentous growth, such as *Nocardia* species, reproduce by fragmentation of the filaments into small bacillary or coccoid cells, each of which gives rise to new growth.

Formation of Conidiospore or Sporangiospores

Species of the genus streptomyces and related bacteria produce many spores per organism by developing cross walls (septation) at the hyphal tips; each spore gives rise to a new organism.

3.8 Continuous Culture

To maintain a bacterial population growing at a particular rate in the exponential or log phase is known as steady-stage growth. Steady-stage growth is desirable in both experimental research and in industrial processes.

In the process the culture volume and the cell concentration are both kept constant by allowing fresh sterile medium to enter the culture vessel at the same rate that 'spent' medium, containing cells, is removed from the growing culture. Under these conditions, the rate at which new cells are produced in the culture vessels is exactly balanced by the rate at which cells are being lost through the overflow from the culture vessel.

The Chemostat

Widely employed system for continuous cultivation is the chemostat shown in Fig.3.12. The principle involved is the concentration of an essential nutrient (substrate) within the culture vessel is in turn controlled by the dilution rate. That means the rate at which fresh medium is being added to the culture (flow rate) divided by the volume of the culture vessel. Therefore by adjusting the dilution rate we can control the growth rate.

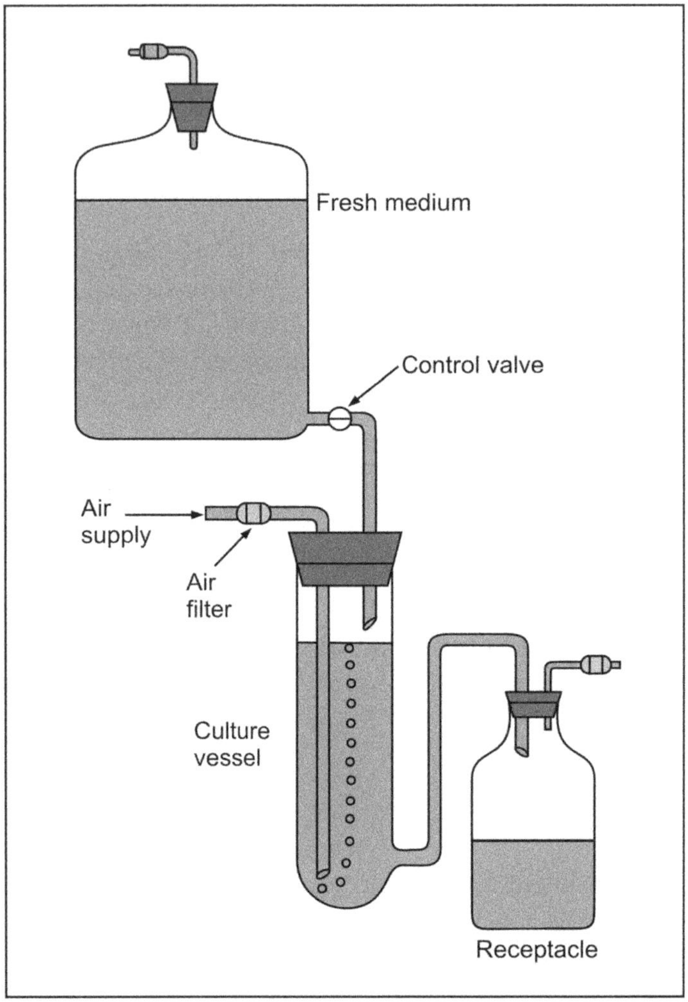

Fig. 3.12 Apparatus for continuous cultivation of bacteria. The system can be regulated for continuous addition of fresh sterile medium to and removal of spent medium (and cells) from the culture vessel

Chemostats are continuous cultures grown in fermentors with control systems, which are widely used for research in microbial physiology. Parameters, like temperature, pH, and concentration of dissolved gases in the growth medium, can be monitored and controlled. Fresh medium is supplied to the culture at a constant flow rate (F), and removed from the fermentor at the same rate, thus maintaining a constant culture volume (V). At steady state, the growth rate of the culture equals to the dilution rate, D = F/V, and the biomass concentration and other free parameters stabilize at levels depending on the dynamics of the fermentation. Hence, chemostats allow continuous exponential growth to occur for many generations under constant physicochemical conditions. Crucially, chemostat culture allows the experimenter to control the growth rate (flux) at any value below a maximum value termed the maximum specific growth rate (μ_{max}). This contrasts with batch cultures, where biomass concentration and the environmental conditions (in terms of pH, nutrient concentration etc.) change significantly during the (limited) time course of the fermentation, and the experimenter has no control over growth rate (flux).

The factor that determines the growth rate of a cell population in a chemostat is dilution rate, i.e., the rate of supply of the limiting nutrient. In a chemostat operating at a low dilution rate, the limiting nutrient is present at very low concentrations at the steady state. Therefore, most of the nutrient is converted into cells and the biomass concentration is high (close to the cell concentration of an equivalent batch culture at late exponential phase). As the dilution rate is increased, the availability of the limiting nutrient increases; however, the rate of removal of cells from the growth vessel is also higher and so the biomass concentration falls. At values of $D–\mu_{max}$, nutrient limitation entirely disappears as there are too few cells in the culture to utilize the available nutrients. Those cells remaining in the culture vessel grow at their maximum growth rate since even the limiting nutrient is present in excess. Finally, at $D> \mu_{max}$, a steady state can no longer be maintained and the number of cells in the fomenters starts to fall since the rate at which new cells are produced is insufficient to overcome dilution by the addition of fresh medium, which leads to the washout of the cells from the growth vessel.

A second type of Continuous Culture Apparatus is the Turbidostat

In this a photoelectric device continuously monitors the cell density within the culture vessel and controls the dilution rate to maintain the cell density at a constant value.

If the density becomes too high the dilution rate is increased; if the density becomes too low, the dilution rate is decreased.

The turbidostat differs from the chemostat in many ways. The dilution rate in a turbidostat varies rather than remaining constant and its culture medium lacks a limiting nutrient. The turbidostat operates best at high dilution rates; the chemostat is most stable and effective at low dilution rates.

Turbidostat

In a turbidostat the system includes an optical sensing device (photoelectric device) which controls the culture density in the growth vessel and controls the dilution rate to maintain the culture under rate.

Turbidostats are continuous cultures (Fig. 3.13) in which the cells, rather than the experimenter, control the growth rate. A turbidostat employs a positive feedback control system that senses, and responds to, the biomass concentration in the fermenter. If the culture is growing faster than the rate imposed by the current dilution rate, then the biomass concentration will rise as a result of the positive difference between the biomass production rate and the rate of removal of cells from the culture vessel. In such circumstances, a control loop is activated that increases the dilution rate by increasing the speed at which a pump introduces fresh medium into the culture. This continues until the biomass concentration is decreased to some set point (which, in our experiments, represents the biomass concentration of a mid-exponential phase batch culture growing in the same medium under the same conditions). Contrariwise, if the culture is growing slower than the current dilution rate, the biomass concentration will fall jto below the set point, and the control loop acts to decrease the rate at which fresh medium is pumped into the growth vessel. Hence the turbidostat equilibrates at a dilution rate equal to the actual growth rate of the culture and the cell concentration stays constant. As our set point is equivalent to the biomass concentration of a mid-exponential phase batch culture, the turbidostat equilibrates at a maximum specific growth rate of the yeast strain used.

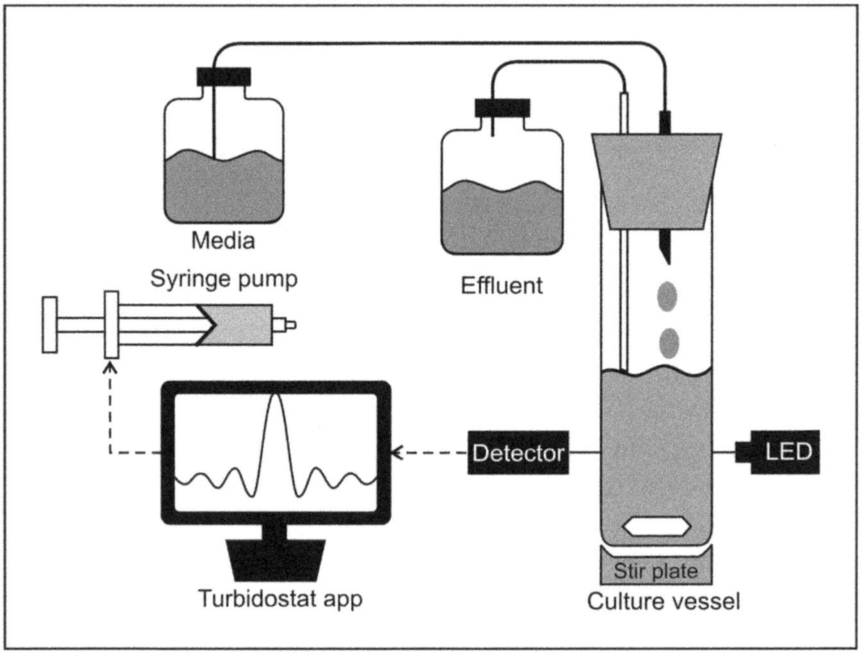

Fig. 3.13 Continuous culture system

The problem of growth or other materials fouling the optical surfaces of whatever method is used to measure turbidity has not been solved. While a turbidostat may operate well for a brief time, the control signal for turbidity soon becomes unreliable.

3.9 Bacterial Counts

Growth can be determined by numerous techniques based on one or more of the following types of measurement.

1. **Cell count:** Directly by microscopy or by using an electronic particle counter, or indirectly by a colony count.
2. **Cell mass:** Directly by weighing or by a measurement of cell nitrogen, or indirectly by turbidity
3. **Cell activity:** Indirectly by relating the degree of biochemical activity to the size of the population.

3.9.1 Methods for Bacterial Count

1. **Direct microscopic count:** Bacteria can be counted easily and accurately with the Petroff – Hausser counting chamber. This is a special slide accurately ruled into squares that are 1/400 mm^2 in area; a glass cover slip rests 1/50 mm above the slide, so that the volume over a square is 1/20,000 mm^3 (1/20,000,000 cm^3). A suspension of unstained bacteria can be counted in the chamber, using a phase – contrast microscope.
   If for example an average of five bacteria is present in each ruled square, there are 5 × 20,000,000, or 10^8, bacteria per milliter.

   Advantages: Direct microscopic counts can be made rapidly and simply with a minimum of equipment.

   The morphology of bacteria can be observed as they are counted.

   Very dense suspensions can be counted if they are diluted appropriately.

   Disadvantage: Suspensions having low numbers of bacteria, e.g., at the beginning of growth curve cannot be counted.
2. **Electronic enumeration of cell numbers:** In this method, the bacteria suspension is placed inside the electronic particle counter, within which the bacteria are passed through a tiny orifice 10 to 30 micrometers in diameter. This orifice connects the two compartments of the counter which contains an electrically conductive solution. As each bacterium passes through the orifice, the electrical resistance between the two compartments increases momentarily. This generates an electrical signal which is automatically counted.

   Drawbacks: Although this method is rapid, it requires sophisticated electronic equipment

   The orifice tends to become clogged.

   There is no way to determine whether the cells being counted are *viable.*
3. **The plate-count method:** A measured amount of the bacterial suspension is introduced into a Petri dish, after which the agar medium (maintained in liquid form at 45 °C) is added and the two were thoroughly mixed by rotating the plate. When the medium solidifies, the organisms are trapped in

the gel. Each organism grows; reproducing itself until a visible mass of organism–a colony–develops. One organism gives rise to one colony.

Hence, a colony count performed on the plate reveals the viable microbial population of the inoculums. The original sample is usually diluted so that the number of colonies developing on the plate will fall in the range of 30 to 300. The possibility of interference of the growth of one organism with that of another is minimized and the count can be accurate. Counting of colonies is done by dark-field illumination from below so that they are easily visible. Various electronic techniques have been developed for the counting of colonies.

Limitations: The bacteria that can utilize provided medium, and provided incubation conditions only can grow but not other bacteria. This can be an important consideration if a mixture of bacteria is to be counted.

4. **Membrane filter count:** It is a very useful variation on the plate-count technique and is based on the use of molecular or membrane filters. These filters have a known uniform porosity of predetermined size sufficiently small to trap micro-organisms. The membrane with its trapped bacteria is then placed in a special plate containing a pad saturated with the appropriate medium. Special medium and dyes can be used to make it easier to detect certain types of organisms than with the conventional plate count. During this incubation the organisms grow into colonies which appear on the membrane surface.

   This technique is particularly valuable in determining the number of bacteria in a large sample that has a very small number of viable cells.

5. **Turbidimetric methods:** Bacteria in a suspension absorb and scatter the light passing through them, so that a culture of more than 107 to 108 cells per milliliter appears turbid to the naked eye. A spectrophotometer or colorimeter can be used for turbidimetric measurements of cell mass.

   Simple, rapid method for measuring growth

   Culture grown is deeply colored media or cultures that contain suspended material other than bacteria counts cannot be measured.

   Dead and living cells contribute to turbidity.

   The relation of turbidity measurement of direct expressions of growth: It is frequently desirable to relate measurements of growth made by an indirect method, e.g., turbidity, to a direct measurement, *e.g.*, dry weight of the cell crop. By measuring the bacterial suspension simultaneously by the two methods and establishing a relationship between the values obtained.

6. **Determination of nitrogen content:** The major constituent of cell material is protein, and since nitrogen is a characteristic part of proteins, one can measure a bacterial population or cell crop in terms of bacterial nitrogen.

Bacteria average approximately 14 percent nitrogen on a dry-weight basis. To measure growth one must first harvest the cells and wash them free of medium and then perform a quantitative chemical analysis for nitrogen.

- Method is somewhat laborious
- It can be performed only on specimens free of all other sources of nitrogen.
- The method is applicable only for concentrated population.
- The procedure is used primarily in research.

7. **Determination of the Dry Weight of Cells:** The most direct approach for quantitative measurement of a mass of cells.

   It can be used only with very dense suspensions.

   Cells must be washed free of all extraneous matter.

   Dry weight may not always be indicative of the amount of living material in cells.

   The intracellular reserve material poly-β-hydroxy butyrate can accumulate and finally can comprise of 74 percent of the dry weight of the cells thus the dry weight may continue to increase without corresponding cell growth.

8. **Measurement of Specific Chemical Change Produced on a Constituent of the Medium:** We may take a species that produces an organic acid from glucose fermentation. The assumption is that the amount of acid produced, under specified conditions and during a fixed period of time, is proportional to the magnitude of the bacterial population.

   It is indirect method, and is applicable only in special circumstances.

The selection of Procedure to Measure Growth

Each method has its particular advantages and limitations, and no one method can be recommended universally.

The colony count (Fig. 3.14) is the most widely used procedure for general microbiological work.

It reflects the viable count. Discrepancies may occur in results of growth of bacterial population when measured by two different methods.

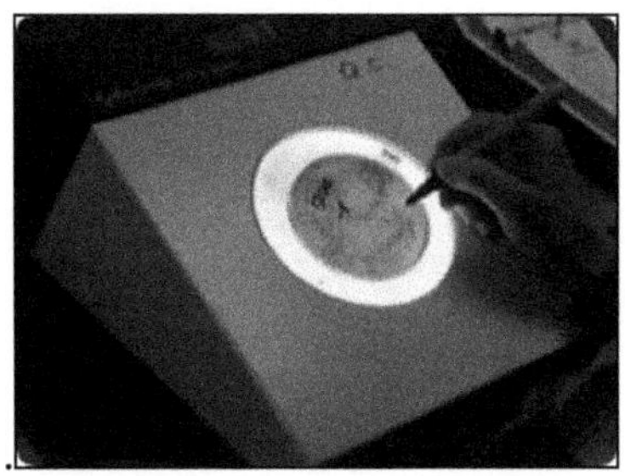

Fig. 3.14 Colony counter

Essay Questions

1. Explain the different nutritional types of bacteria
2. Write a note on techniques involved in cultivation of bacteria
3. Explain the different methods involved for bacterial count

Multiple Choice Questions

1. Spontaneous generation theory is also known as
   (a) Biogenesis (b) Abiogenesis
   (c) Neobiogenesis (d) Microbiogenesis
2. Chemotrophs that use ammonia as their electron source, obtaining energy by oxidizing ammonia to nitrite
   (a) Psuedomonas
   (b) Nitrosomonas
   (c) lithotrophs
   (d) chemolithotrophs
3. Yeast extract contain several of
   (a) A vitamins (b) B vitamins
   (c) C vitamins (d) D vitamins
4. Mesophiles grow best with the temperature of
   (a) 15 to 20 °C
   (b) 20-25 °C
   (c) 30-35 °C
   (d) 35-40 °C
5. The main disadvantage of direct microscopic count is
   (a) Lag phase cannot be estimated
   (b) stationary phase cannot be estimated
   (c) Growth curve cannot be counted
   (d) Decline phase cannot be counted
6. The most direct approach for quantitative measurement of mass cells is
   (a) Determination of Nitrogen content
   (b) Determination of dry weight of cells
   (c) Plate count method
   (d) Membrane filter count

Answers

1. (b)	2. (b)	3. (b)
4. (d)	5. (b)	6. (b)

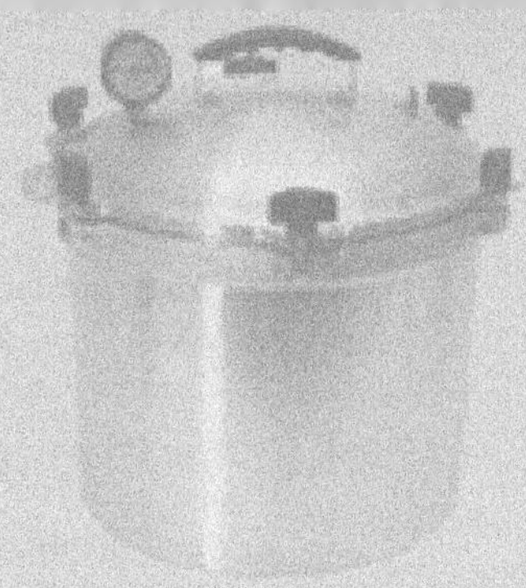

4 DISINFECTANTS, ANTISEPTICS AND CONTROL OF MICRO-ORGANISMS

LEARNING OBJECTIVES

After studying the chapter the students familiarize themselves with concepts in:

- *Analyzing different disinfectant compounds along with their structure and modes of action*
- *Understanding the chemotherapeutic properties of the agents*
- *Understanding different tests for the effectiveness of disinfectants*
- *Develop an understanding on Antimicrobial action of drugs*

4.1 Introduction

Antiseptics and disinfectants are extensively used in hospitals and other health care settings for a variety of topical and hard-surface applications. A wide variety of active chemical agents (biocides) are found in these products, many of which have been used for hundreds of years, including alcohols, phenols, iodine, and chlorine etc. Most of these active agents demonstrate broad-spectrum antimicrobial activity; In particular, they are an essential part of infection control practices and aid in the prevention of nosocomial infections. Mounting concerns over the potential for microbial contamination and infection risks in the food and general consumer markets have also led to increased use of antiseptics and disinfectants by the general public.

The ability to kill or deactivate etiologic agents is required for worker safety, to prevent contamination of experiments and proper disposal of biohazardous waste. Typically, these are physical controls (e.g., heat) and chemical controls (e.g., bleach). The ability to kill or deactivate organisms by any means is related to the construction of the organism, the method used, and the amount of time the method is applied.

4.2 Some Important Definitions

Biocide: The term biocide is increasingly being used to describe compounds with antiseptic, disinfectant or, sometimes, preservative activity. A compound might be used in only one such capacity or possess two or even all of these properties.

Antiseptic: Acting against or opposing sepsis, putrefaction, or decay by either preventing or arresting the growth of micro-organisms. Examples are chlorhexidine(CHX), Alcohols, and Iodophors etc.

Sepsis: Poisoning by the products of putrefaction; a severe toxic state resulting from an infection with pyogenic micro-organisms.

Aseptic: Free of pathogenic micro-organisms: *aseptic surgical instruments*.

Disinfection: The act of disinfecting, using specialized cleansing techniques that destroy or prevent growth of organisms capable of infection. Examples are phenol, methyl phenol, hydrogen peroxode, sulfur dioxide, & Dettol (chloroxylenol + trepenol).

Terminal disinfection: Disinfection of a sick room and its contents at the termination of a disease.

Disinfectant: An agent that frees from infection by killing the vegetative cells of microorganism.

Bactericide: An agent that destroys bacteria. Examples are Anicarthiazole, Bismerthiazole, chloramphenicol, cresol, formaldehyde etc.

Bacteriostatic: Inhibiting the growth of bacteria without killing them.

Fungicide: An agent that kills or destroys fungi. Examples are Benzimidazoles, Dicarosimide, Piperazine and Triazole etc.

Fungistat: A substance that inhibits the growth of fungi.

Virucide: An agent that kills viruses. A **virucide** is an agent (physical or chemical) that deactivates or destroys viruses. This differs from an antiviral drug which inhibits the development of the virus. Examples are Cyanovirin-N, Griffithsin, Scytoririn, and Lysol.

Virustatic: Pertaining to the inhibition of the growth and development of viruses, as distinguished from their destruction.

Sterilization: The process of making sterile; the killing of all forms of life.

Sterilization (or sterilisation) is a term referring to any process that eliminates (removes) or kills all forms of microbial life, including transmissible agents (such as fungi, bacteria, viruses, spore forms, etc.) present on a surface, contained in a fluid, in medication, or in a compound such as biological culture media.[1][2] Sterilization can be achieved by applying heat, chemicals, irradiation, high pressure, and filtration or combinations thereof.

Sanitizer: An agent that reduces to levels judged safe by public health authorities the microbial flora in minerals or on such articles as eating utensils. Examples are Hypochlorites, Chlorine Dioxide, Peroxyacetic Acid (PAA) and Iodophors.

4.2.1 Desirable Properties of Disinfectant

1. It should be able to kill all kinds of microbes, in a very much diluted form, in a relatively short time.
2. Its efficacy should not be reduced in presence of blood, face or other organic matter.
3. It should be chemically inert and non caustic.
4. It should have good wetting and penetrating properties.
5. It should be soluble in water and have reasonable shelf life.
6. It should be non toxic to humans or animals and non-offensive
7. It should not separate in standing, should penetrate well and should not corrode instruments.
8. It should be cheap and easily available.

4.2.2 Factors Affecting Disinfectants

(i) Concentration: It is expected that a concentrated disinfectant should act rapidly while a diluted one should take more time.

- However the effectiveness is generally related to concentration exponentially, not linearly.
- There is an optimum concentration of phenol at about 1%. Beyond this concentration the disinfecting effectiveness becomes increasingly less.

(ii) Time of Contact: Sufficient time of contact must be allowed for the disinfectant to exert its action. This depends on the nature of disinfectant, concentration, p^H, temperature, nature of the organism and variability of susceptibility of the bacterial cell population.

(iii) Temperature:

- Disinfection can be treated as a first order reaction and the effect of temperature on bactericidal activity may be expressed quantitatively by means of a temperature coefficient.
- The temperature coefficient per degree rise in temperature is denoted by θ whereas per 10° rise in temperature is expressed by Q_{10} values, which can be calculated as follows.

$$\theta(T_2 - T_1) = \frac{t_1}{t_2}$$

t_1 = extinction time at T_1 °C

t_2 = extinction time at T_1 + 1 °C = T_2 °C

If the value θ for a disinfectant is 2 then the increase in activity for a 5 °C rise in temperature is 2^5 or 32 – fold.

$$Q_{10} = \frac{\text{Time to kill at } T^o}{\text{Time to kill at } (T_1 + 10)^o}$$

The value for Q_{10} for phenol is 4, which means that over the 10 °C range used to determine Q_{10} (actually 20 °C – 30 °C) the activity will be increased by a factor of 4.

(iv) Type, Number and Condition of the Organism Present:

- In general, disinfectants and antiseptics may have a greater effect on Gram + positive bacteria.
- The endospores of bacteria and cysts of protozoa are also highly resistant to disinfectants and antiseptics, as are some viruses.
- Larger the population of bacteria, higher may be concentration of disinfectant and/or longer contact time.

(v) Presence of Organic Matter and Other Inactivators:

- The presence of organic matter may reduce the effect of a disinfectant by adsorbing or inactivating it.
- Extraneous matter may form a protective coat around the cell and prevent the penetration of the disinfectant to its site of action.

(vi) pH: The bacterial growth is optimal in the pH range 6-8 and the growth declines outside this range.

- A change of pH during the disinfection process can affect
  - (i) The rate of growth of inoculum
  - (ii) The potency of the disinfectant
  - (iii) The ability of the disinfectant to combine with site on the cell surface.

(vii) Surface Tension:

- The contact between aqueous solutions of disinfectants is facilitated if they have surfactant properties also. This helps in adsorption of surfactant disinfectants on the surface of cells as well as in wetting and spreading properties of the solutions.

- Phenol and related compounds lower surface tension. Thus a combination of soap with crude phenol (carbolic acid) has excellent disinfecting properties; Lysol (cresol with soap) is such a marketed product.

Besides these factors, the chemical structures influence the disinfection action.

4.2.3 Major Groups of Disinfectants and Antiseptics

Chemicals used for biologic decontamination are called sterilizers, disinfectants, sanitizers, antiseptics and germicides. Based on strength, length of exposure and susceptibility of the organism, these are considered high, intermediate and low level disinfectants, in that order.

Chemical agents most commonly used as disinfectants and antiseptics are

(i) Phenol and phenolic compounds
(ii) Alcohols
(iii) Halogens
(iv) Heavy metals and their compounds
(v) Dyes
(vi) Synthetic Detergents
(vii) Quaternary ammonium compounds
(viii) Aldehydes
(ix) Gaseous agents

4.3 Phenol and Phenolic Compounds

Phenolic compounds: Contact time: 10 minutes. At a concentration of 1-5%, phenolic compounds are effective against vegetative bacteria, fungi and lipid-containing viruses. They have an unpleasant odor, can easily be absorbed through the skin and are irritants to the mucous membrane and respiratory tract. *Examples*: Amphyl, Lysol I.C.

Phenolic compounds can cause rapid and permanent eye damage-always wear safety glasses, Nitrile gloves and Labcoat, and prepare in chemical fume hood, when using or preparing phenolic solutions.

- Phenol was being used in the 1880's by Joseph Lister, a surgeon to reduce infection,
- 5% aqueous solution of phenol rapidly kills vegetative cells but spores are much more resistant.

- Antimicrobial activity is enhanced by the addition of chemical substitutions in the phenol ring structure.

(a) Hexyl Resorcinol: A derivative of phenol is marketed in a solution surface of glycerin and water. Hexyl Resorcinol 37 indicates the value of surface tension.

- Hexyl Resorcinol preparations employed as general antiseptics
- It is more active against Gram negative and Gram positive bacteria

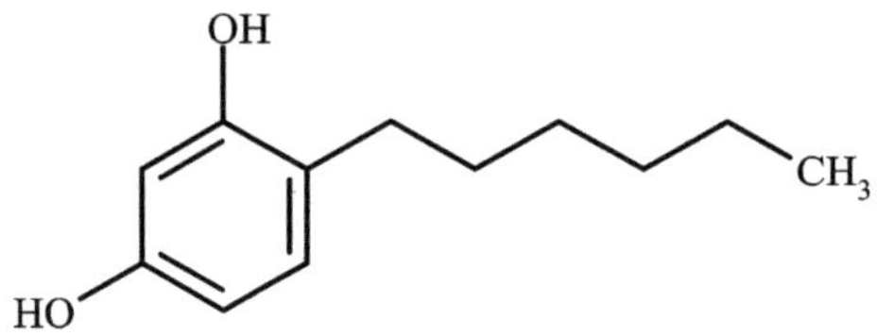

(b) Chlorhexidine (CHX): It is another biphenol which is commercially available as 4% solution for disinfecting and 0.2% solution is most effective antiplague and antigingivites agent.

Cresols, xylenols and chloroxylenols are other phenolic compounds.

- Chloroxylenol is more effective against Gram positive bacteria.
- Cresol is a mixture of ortho, meta and para methyl xylenols.
- It is effective for disinfecting faeces, bedpours, lavatories, floors and laboratory equipment.
- One of the widely used phenolic derivatives O – phenylphenol.

Mode of Action: Antiseptic like Chlorhexidine (CHX) contains a positively charged hydrophobic and lipophilic molecule which can combine with the molecules of phospholipids and lipo-polysaccharides on the cell membrane of microorganism.

Due to this interaction, CHX enters in the cell through active or passive transport mechanism. This interaction affects the osmotic equilibrium of cell, hence increase the permeability of membrane which further allowing the reactant molecule in cell and cause damage of cell. The presence of antiseptic inside the microbe cell directly affects the intracellular constituents like nucleic acid and collapse the bacterial cell. This antiseptic shows its activity in acidic medium at pH 5.5 - 0.7.

A specific mode of action is that the lethal effect is associated with physical damage to the membrane in the cell surfaces, which initiates further deterioration.

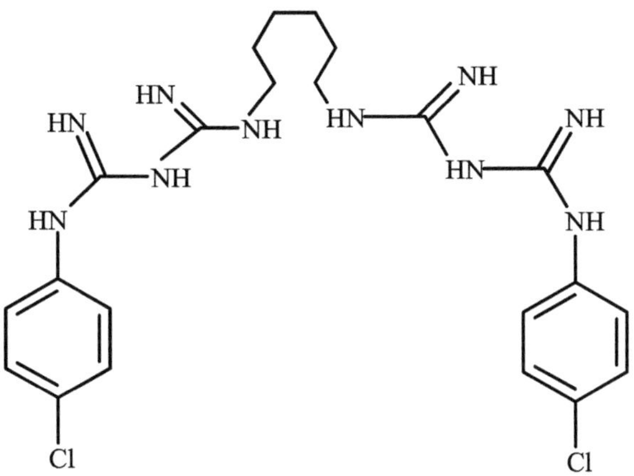

4.3.1 Alcohols

Alcohols: Contact time: immediate to 10 minutes. A 70% ethanol or isopropyl solution is made by adding three parts water to seven parts 95% ethanol. Always keep ethanol and isopropyl solutions away from potential sources of ignition. These solutions should be labeled and dated, with an expiration date of 180 days.

Ethyl alcohol, in concentrations between 50% and 90% is effective against vegetative or non spore forming cells.

- For practical application of 70% concentration of alcohol is generally used.
- **Methyl alcohol** is less bactericidal than ethyl alcohol.
- Methyl alcohol is highly poisonous because even the fumes of this compound may produce permanent injury to the eyes, and is not generally employed for the destruction of micro-organisms.
- There is a progressive increase in germicidal power as the molecular weight of alcohol increases.
- **Propyl** and **Isopropyl alcohols** in concentration ranging from 40% to 80% are bactericidal for vegetative cells.

Mode of Action: Alcohols are protein denaturants, and this property is responsible for antimicrobial activity.

- Alcohols are also solvents for lipids, and hence they may damage lipid complexes in the cell membrane. They are also dehydrating agents.
- Very high concentration of alcohol may remove much water from the cell and the alcohol is unable to penetrate.

Practical Applications

- Alcohol is effective in reducing the microbial flora of skin and for the disinfection of clinical oral thermometers.
- Alcohol concentrations above 60% are effectively influenced considerably by the amount of extraneous protein material in the mixture.

4.3.2 Halogens

Iodine: Iodine is one of the oldest and the most effective germicidal agent, used in the form of 'tincture of iodine'.

- It is soluble in alcohol and aqueous solution of sodium and potassium iodine.
- Iodine is also used in the form of substances known as Iodophores.
- Iodophores are mixture of iodine and surface active agent which act as carriers and solubilizers for the iodine. *Ex*: Poly vinil pyrrolidone
- Iodine is released slowly from this complex expressed as pup – I.
- **Iodophor Disinfectant (Wescodyne):** Contact time: 10 minutes. Prepare this solution according to the instructions on the label. Final concentration should be 0.47%. These solutions should be labeled and dated, with an expiration date of 365 days (one year).
- Iodophores have germicidal characteristics in addition they have non staining and low irritant properties.

Iodine preparations include 2% I_2 + 2% NaI diluted in alcohol

7% I_2 + 5% KI in 83% alcohol

5% I_2 + 10% KI in aqueous solution

Mode of Action: Iodine is an oxidizing agent. Oxidizing agents irreversibly oxidize and inactivate essential metabolic compounds such as proteins with sulfhydryl groups. The action also involves the halogenating of tyrosine units and other cellular proteins requiring tyrosine for activity.

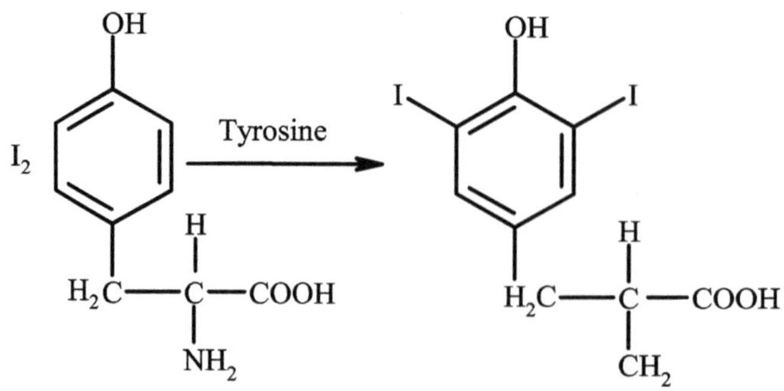

Practical Applications

1. Iodine is highly effective bactericidal agents and also possesses sporicidal activity, fungicidal and to some extent possesses virucidal activity.
2. Iodine solutions are chiefly used for disinfection of skin, water, air and sanitization of food utensils.

Chlorine Dioxide: Contact time: 10 minutes. Chlorine dioxide (ClO_2) is a strong and fast-acting germicide, disinfecting agent, and oxidizer, often reported to be active at concentrations lower than those needed by chlorine as bleach. However, it has a shelf-life of only one day for activated solutions, so if it is used a fresh solution must be made each day. Chlorine dioxide is unstable as a gas; however, chlorine dioxide is soluble in water and stable in an aqueous solution. Chlorine dioxide can be obtained by ordering its stabilized form, which is then activated on-site when required.

Of the oxidizing biocides, chlorine dioxide is the most selective oxidant. Ozone and chlorine are much more reactive than chlorine dioxide, and they will be consumed by most organic compounds

Chlorine and Chlorine Compounds

- Chlorine can be used in the form of gas or in the form of chemical combinations.
- Chlorine and its compounds are more conveniently handled than free chlorine.
- Chlorine in the form of compressed gas popularly used for purification of municipal water supplies.

Chlorine Compounds include: hypochlorites

Calcium hypochlorite Ca $(OCl)_2$ (also known as chlorinated lime sodium hypochlorite (NaOCl)

Chloramines

Class of chlorine compounds used as disinfectants, sanitizing agents or antiseptics.

Chemically they have one or more hydrogen atoms in an amino group of a compound replaced with chlorine.

E.g., monochloramine, chloramines – T, azochloramide

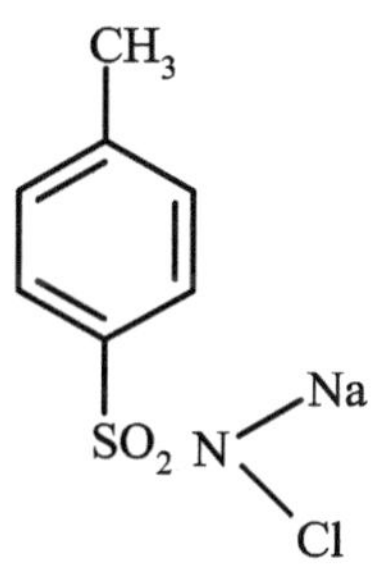

Chloramine - T

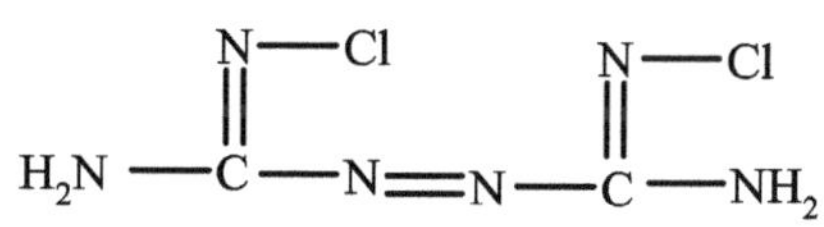

Azochloramide

- Advantage of chloramines is that they have greater stability.

Mode of action: The antimicrobial action of chlorine comes from the hypochloric acid formed when chlorine is added to water.

$$Cl_2 + H_2O \rightarrow HCl + HClO$$

Hypochlorites and chloramines undergo hydrolysis, with the formation of *hypochloric acid*. The *hypochloric acid* formed is further decomposed to

$$HClO \rightarrow HCl + O$$

The oxygen release in this reaction (nascent oxygen) is a strong oxidizing agent, and through its action on cellular constituents, micro-organisms are destroyed.

Practical Applications

- Chlorine compounds are widely used in water treatment, domestic used, food industry and in medicine.
- Calcium hypochlorite used for sanitizing dairy equipment and eating utensils.
- Sodium hypochlorite 1% concentration used as personal hygiene and a household disinfectant; at higher concentrations household bleaches and disinfectants.
- Chlorine compounds have been used to treat athletes' foot, to disinfect open wounds.

Hypochlorite (Bleach): Contact time: 10 minutes. A 10:1 bleach solution/Sodium Hypochlorite (also called 10% bleach solution) is made by adding nine parts water to one part laboratory bleach (sodium hypochlorite). Bleach solution is corrosive to stainless steel; therefore, thorough rinsing must follow its use in the biosafety cabinet.

Hypochlorite solutions are classified as irritant and corrosive. Appropriate precautions should be taken when using hypochlorite products to prepare disinfectant bleach solutions:

Using 12.5% hypochlorite (Top-Chlor) in a 1:10 dilution (one part Top-Chlor and nine parts water) yields 12,500 ppm or a 1.25% hypochlorite solution, for use within 30 days. Likewise 1:20.1:5.1:10 dilutions are used.

4.3.3 Heavy Metals and Compounds

Heavy metals and their compounds exert detrimental effect on micro-organisms.

E.g., mercury, silver and copper

Mode of Action: Heavy metals and their compounds act antimicrobially by combining with cellular proteins and inactivating them.

Mercuric chloride show effect on the sulfhydryl groups of enzyme and inhibits them.

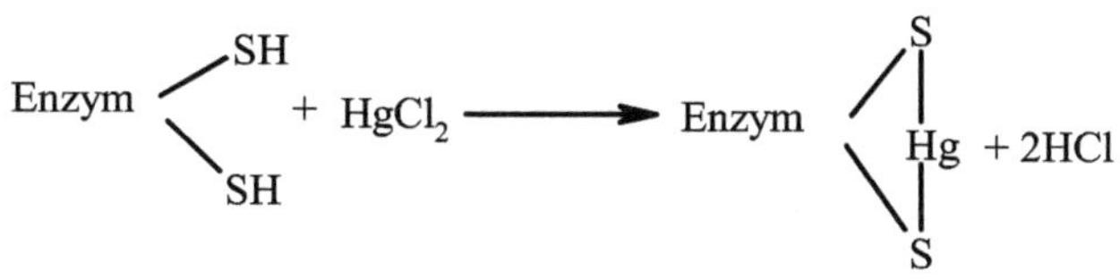

High concentrations of salts of heavy metals coagulate cytoplasmic proteins and cause damage or death to the cell.

Mercury

Inorganic Mercury Compounds

These are bactericidal, highly toxic to animals. Their effectiveness is reduced in the presence of organic matter. Limited use because of corrosive action.

E.g., Mercuric chloride

Organic Mercury Compounds

They are less irritating and less toxic than inorganic compounds. They are employed as antiseptics. They may be bactericidal or bacteriostatic. Example Phenyl mercuric borate, Thiomersal

Mechanism of Action

Mercury compounds are bacteriostatic. This is based on the inhibition of bacterial sulfhydryl containing enzymes by the metal ions, leading to an accompanying inhibition in metabolic function and growth. This appears to be the case with all bacteria, susceptible viruses, and bacterial spores. It is recently reported that they inhibit penicillinase (β-lactamase) producing strains of *Neisseria gonorrhoeae* (PPNG) and non-PPNG strains.

Silver

They are employed in the form of colloidal silver compounds and consists of proteins in combination with metallic silver or silver oxide. They show bacteriostatic or bactericidal function. Silver nitrate ($AgNO_3$) is most widely used.

Mechanism of Action

The antimicrobial properties of silver are due to its ionized form, Ag^+, and its ability to cause damage to cells by interacting with thiol-containing proteins and DNA, i.e., fragmentation of DNA, formation of shrunken cells and apoptosis are induced by high concentrations of silver nitrate. Silver compounds are more preferred because of their low toxicity to humans and there is ever increasing number of antibiotic-resistant strains of bacteria.

Copper

It is used in the form of $CuSO_4$. It is much more effective against algae and moulds than bacteria. It is mostly used in the form of Bordeaux mixture. i.e., fungicidal used to treat plant diseases.

Mechanism of Action

Science suggests that copper surfaces affect bacteria in two sequential steps: the first step is a direct interaction between the surface and the bacterial outer membrane, causing the membrane to rupture. The second is related to the holes in the outer membrane, through which the cell loses vital nutrients and water, causing a general weakening of the cell.

- Causing leakage of potassium or glutamate through the outer membrane of bacteria.
- Disturbing osmotic balance.
- Binding to proteins that do not require copper.
- Causing oxidative stress by generating hydrogen peroxide.

4.3.4 Dyes

Triphenyl/Methane Dyes

These include malachite green, brilliant green and crystal violet.

- Gram-Positive organisms are more susceptible to lower concentrations of these compounds than Gram-negative.
- Crystal violet 1: 200000 to 1: 300000 about 10 times this concentration is required to inhibit *E.Coil* which is gram-negative.

Applications

- Certain media can be made selective by incorporation of low concentration of these dyes.
- Susceptibility to various dyes is useful for identification of bacteria.
- Crystal violet also used as fungicide.

Mode of Action*:* They exert inhibitory effect by interfering with cellular oxidation process.

Acridine Dyes

The two examples of dyes derived from acridine are acroflavin and tryptoflavin.

Applications

- Antifungal activity.
- Treatment of burns and wounds and for ophthalmic application and bladder irrigation.

4.3.5 Synthetic Detergents

Surface tension depressants or wetting agents employed for cleansing surface are called detergents.

Soap is an example for detergent. But soap is poor detergent in hard water. Hence synthetic detergents developed, called surfactants.

Advantages

1. Surfactants do not form precipitants in alkaline or acid water.
2. They do not produce deposits, with minerals found in hard water.
3. They are extensively used in laundry, dish washing powders, shampoos.

***Chemically Detergents Classified as*:**

Anionic Detergents

Anionic detergents are those which ionize with the detergent property and resident in the anion.

E.g., Sodium lauryl Sulphate

↓

$[C_{12}H_{25}\,OSO_3]^- \; Na^+ [C_{19}\,H_{19}\,COO^-]\; Na^+$

Soap

Cationic Detergents

Cationic detergents are those which ionize with the detergent property and resident in the cation.

E.g., Cetylpyridinium Chloride

Non Ionic Detergents

This category of detergents are nonionic, do not ionize and do not possess antimicrobial activity.

Mode of Action*:* Soaps reduce the surface tension and increase the wetting power of water in which they are dissolved. Soapy water has the ability to emulsify and disperse the oil and dirt. Micro-organisms get enmeshed within the soap lather.

4.3.6 Quaternary Ammonium Compounds

Quaternary Ammonium Compounds (Quats): Contact time: 10 minutes. Quats are used to disinfect at concentrations of 0.1-2% for vegetative bacteria and non-lipid-containing viruses. Quaternary ammonium compounds are not effective against spores and may be neutralized by anionic detergents. *Example:* Lysol I.C.

Most compounds of germicidal cationic detergent class are 4° ammonium compounds.

- The bactericidal power of quaternaries is more for Gram-positive.
- The action of these compounds demonstrates to distinguish between static and lethal activity in test procedure.
- Quaternaries are fungicidal and destructive to pathogenic protozoa.
- Viruses are much more resistant than bacteria and fungi.

Applications

- Detergent action, low toxicity, high solubility, stability, non corrosiveness, germicidal activity which resulted in its application as disinfectants and sanitizing agents.
- Skin disinfectants, preservation in ophthalmic solution, cosmetic preparation.
- Dairy, egg, fishing industry.
- Sanitize food and beverage utensils.

Mode of Action: The action includes denaturation of protein, interfering with glycolysis and membrane damage.

4.3.7 Aldehydes

Formalin: Contact time: 10 minutes. At an aqueous concentration of 0.2-0.8%, formaldehyde (formalin) has good disinfectant properties against vegetative bacteria, spores and viruses. It has an irritating odor and is a suspected human carcinogen. Formaldehyde is not recommended for daily disinfection. Use only with proper ventilation control (*e.g.*, chemical fume hood). *Example: Sterac.*

***Formaldehyde*:** Formaldehyde gas has been used for fumigation of rooms and hospital blankets.

- It is the gas that is stable only in high concentrations and at elevated temperature.
- At room temperature it polymerizes to solid substance.
- Formaldehyde also marketed in aqueous solution as formalin which contains 37-40% formaldehyde
- The important polymer is paraformaldehyde, formaldehyde upon heating.

Mode of Action: It combines with vital organic nitrogen compounds such as proteins and nucleic acids. Interaction of formaldehyde with these cellular substance accounts for its antimicrobial action.

Applications

- Formaldehyde gas has been used for fumigation of rooms and hospital blankets.
- Formaldehyde in solution is useful for sterilization of certain instruments.

Advantages

- It kills all bacteria including spores, fairly and rapidly.
- It is also effective virucide in gaseous as well as in solution form.

Disadvantages

- It is bactericidal agent with poor penetrating power.
- It is irritant and pungent.
- The fumes are noxious.

Glutaraldehyde: (also called a "Cold Disinfectant"): Contact time: 15 minutes. Two-percent solutions exhibit good activity against vegetative bacteria, spores and viruses. Glutaraldehyde is toxic, a sensitizer and is generally not used for laboratory surface disinfectant, and is capable of eye damage. Use only with proper ventilation control, such as a chemical fume hood or specially designed slot hood. *Example*: Cidex.

- A 2% solution of glutaraldehyde is an effective disinfector. It is less irritating than formaldehyde and is used to disinfect hospital and laboratory equipment.
- It is used in sterilizing urological instruments, lensed instruments and respiratory therapy equipment.

Mode of action: Glutaraldehyde polymerizes and then interacts with amino acids in proteins. As a result, the proteins are alkylated and cross linked to other proteins, which inactivates them.

The amino groups in peptidoglycan are also alkylated and cross linked which prevents them from participating in other chemical reactions such as those involved in peptidoglycan synthesis.

4.3.8 Gaseous Agents

E.g., Ethyleneoxide, β – propiolactone, formaldehyde. Certain kinds of medical devices that need to be available in sterile condition are made of materials that are damaged by heat.

E.g., Plastic syringes, blood transfusion apparatus, plastic pipettes, petridishes and other equipment, i.e., packaged and sterilized to use.

Sterilization by means of gaseous agents is effective and practical for such situations.

Ethylene Oxide

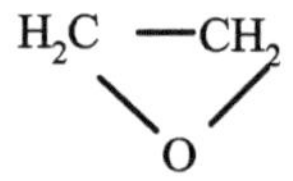

- It is a liquid at temperature below 10.8°C (51.4°F). Above this temperature it vaporizes rapidly.
- Vapors of this compound in air are highly flammable even in low concentrations, so, this can be overcome by preparing mixtures of ethylene oxide in CO_2 or Freon.
- The CO_2–ethylene oxide or Freon–ethylene oxide mixtures are non flammable, and there is no alteration of the microbicidal activity of the ethylene oxide.

Mode of Action*:* The mode of action is by alkylation reaction with organic compounds such as enzymes and other proteins. Alkylation consists of the replacement of active H_2 atom in an organic compound.

E.g., The hydrogen atom in a free carboxyl, amino or sulphydryl group, with an alkyl group.

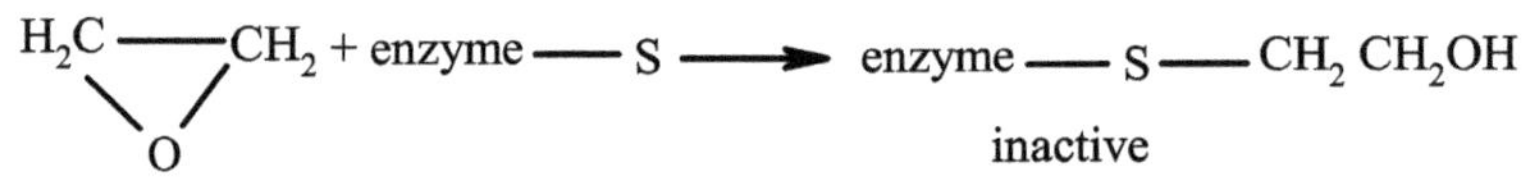

Applications

- It is an effective sterilizing agent for heat and moisture sensitive materials.
- It has been used in the space programs by both Americans and the Russians for decontaminating space craft components.
- It is effective at relatively low temperature include spices, biological preparations, soil, plastics, certain medical preparations and contaminated laboratory equipment.

Advantages

- Final shipping containers can also be sterilized by this gas.
- It will pass through and sterilize large packages of materials, bundles of cloth and even certain plastics.

Disadvantages

- Its ability to penetrate and diffuse in liquids is limited.

β-Propiolactone

This compound is a color less liquid at room temperature with a high boiling point (155 °C)

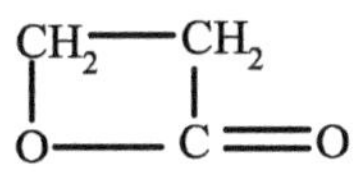

β-Propiolactone

- It is not flammable like ethylene oxide but is vesicant and lachrymator and must be handled with care.
- A concentration of 2-5 mg of β-Propiolactone is required for sterilization purposes.
- It is very effective in destroying micro-organisms on surfaces.

Uses

- It is sporicidal, fungicidal and virucidal.
- It is highly bactericidal and used in concentration of 5 mg/Litre or less.
- It has been used to sterilize blood plasma, vaccines, tissue grafts, surgical instruments and enzymes.

Advantages

- It is more active against micro-organisms.
- It is very effective in destroying micro-organisms on surface.

Disadvantages

- The penetrating power of β-Propiolactone is low.
- It is irritant and carcinogenic to animals and needs careful handling.
- The use of - Propiolactone is limited to decontaminating rooms, chambers and buildings.

4.3.9 Hydrogen Peroxide and Peracetic Acid

Contact time: 10 minutes. Like chlorine, hydrogen peroxide (H_2O_2) and peracetic acid are strong oxidants and can be potent broad-spectrum germicides. They are also safer than chlorine to humans and the environment. However, they have a short shelf-life of just five days for dilute solutions, so fresh solution must be made frequently if used.

Hydrogen peroxide can be used for the decontamination of work surfaces of laboratory benches and biosafety cabinets, and stronger solutions may be suitable for disinfecting heat-sensitive medical/dental devices. The use of vaporized hydrogen peroxide or peracetic acid (CH_3COOOH) for the decontamination of heat-sensitive medical/dental devices requires specialized equipment.

Hydrogen peroxide and peracetic acid can be corrosive to metals such as aluminum, copper, brass, and zinc, and can also decolorize fabrics, hair, skin, and mucous membranes. Articles treated with them must be thoroughly rinsed before contact with eyes and mucous membranes. They should always be stored away from heat and protected from light.

4.4 Evaluation of Disinfectants

- A disinfectant does not necessarily sterilize an object because viable spores and a few micro-organisms may remain.
- Optimicrobial agent often begins with an initial screening test to see if they are effective and at what concentrations. This may be followed by more realistic in- use testing.

The different types of tests are:

(i) Rideal-Walker (RW) test (phenol coefficient test)

(ii) Use-Dilution test

(iii) Chick VU Martin test

(iv) Kelsey-Sykes (KS) test

Rideal-Walker test is the best known method.

4.4.1 Rideal-Walker (RW) Test

Phenol Coefficient Test Principle: Bacterial potency is assessed by measuring the rate of killing a selected range of bacteria under specified conditions. Bactericidal power of a particular disinfectant as compared with that of pure Phenol, minimum time of 10 minutes. Usually employed cultures are *S. typhi*. Phenol coefficient is considered to be 1.

- RW coefficient is a measure of effectiveness of an antiseptic or disinfectant as compared to phenol.
- Higher than 1 RW coefficient value indicates that the chemical is more effective than phenol. While lower than 1 RW coefficient value indicates poorer disinfecting power of the test disinfectant than phenol.
- The method prescribed under Drugs and cosmetic rules (Rule 126, schedule 0) is briefly explained below.

Preparation of Broth

- Broth is prepared by dissolving

  20 g – Meat extract

  20 g – Peptone

  10 g – NaCl

  1000 mL – H_2O

  p^H is adjusted to 7.6 and it is sterilized by autoclaving
- The filtered broth is placed in 5 mL quantities in sterilized broth tubes and the tubes are autoclaved.

- The test organism *Salmonella typhi* is sub cultured on a nutrient agar slope and incubated for 24 hr at 37 °C.
- A little of the growth from the recent subculture in nutrient slope is placed in the broth and incubated for 23 hours at 38 °C.
- A standard loopful is then transferred to a second tube and incubated as above. This is done for at least 3 times before a test is carried out.

Preparation of Standard

- A 5% w/v solution of pure phenol is prepared in sterile distilled water.
- Test dilutions are prepared from this stock solution containing 1 gm of phenol in each 95, 100, 105, 110, 115 mL of the solution made.

Preparation of Unknown Dilutions

- Test dilutions of unknown disinfectant are prepared by dissolving 5 mL portion into sufficient sterilized water to make 500 mL, with thorough mixing in a sterile measuring cylinder and further dilutions are made in sterile distilled water from this stock solution.
- 5 mL of 4 chosen dilutions of the disinfectants are taken in 4 tubes, placed in a rack provided with a water bath maintained at a temperature between 17 °C and 19 °C, with the strongest dilution at the left.
- The 5th tube containing 5 mL of the particular phenol dilution is placed on the right.
- After temperature equilibration of the tubes and broth cultures of the test organism, starting at zero time, 0.2 mL of the culture is added to the left tube and shaken gently.
- After 30 seconds the next tube is inoculated similarly and the process is repeated with each successive tube at intervals of 30 seconds until the phenol control has been inoculated.
- 30 seconds after this last addition (i.e., 2.5 min from 0) a loopful of the well – shaken content of the tube at the extreme left is withdrawn and placed in the tube containing 5 mL of the broth culture.
- The procedure is repeated at an interval of 30 seconds with each of the 5 tubes until 4 sets of cultures have been made i.e., 2.5, 5, 7.5 and 10 minutes respectively after exposure.
- The inoculated broth tubes are incubated for 48 to 72 hrs at 37 °C. When the tubes showing the growth of the test organism will be recognized by turbidity of the broth. The sample calculation is made and RW coefficient calculated as:

Determination of the RW Coefficient

+ = indicates growth

– = indicates no growth

Table 4.1

Disinfectant	Dilution	Time of exposure (min)			
		2.5	5	7.5	10
Phenol (control)	1: 100	+	+	–	–
	1: 1000	–	–	–	–
	1: 1100	+	–	–	–
	1: 1200	+	+	–	–
	1: 1300	+	+	–	–

$$\text{Rw coefficient} = \frac{\text{Dilution of Unknown which kills in 7.5 but not in 5min}}{\text{Dilution of phenol which kills in 7.5 but not in 5min}}$$

Hence, from the above table

$$\text{RW coefficient} = \frac{1200}{100} = 12$$

Drawbacks

(i) The test is performed in a laboratory rather than in a real-life situation.

(ii) Factors such as tissue toxicity, activity in the presence of organic matter, or variations in temperature; are not taken into account.

(iii) This is also known as phenol coefficient test because the test disinfectant is tested against phenol as standard.

Table 4.2 Phenol Coefficient of some Common Disinfectant and Antiseptics

Disinfectant/Antiseptic	S . typhi	S . aureus
H_2O_2	0.01	–
formalin	0.7	0.3
phenol	1.0	1.0
lysol	3.2	5.0
Tincture iodine	5.8	6.3
C_2H_5OH	6.3	6.3
Chloramine	100.0	133.0
Mercury chloride	143.0	100.0

4.4.2 Use-Dilution Test

- The disinfectants are actually used in diluted form and the dilution in which disinfectant must be used can be determined by the use dilution test.
- The current standard is prescribed by the American official analytical chemists which employs 3 strains of bacteria: *Staphylococcus aureus, Salmonella choleraesuis* and *Pseudomonas aeruginosa.*

- Standardized cultures of the test organisms are grown in liquid media, standardized metal carrier rings are dipped into and removed, and dried at 37 °C for a short time.
- The dried cultures are then placed into a solution of the disinfectant at the concentration recommended by the manufacturer and left there for 10 min at 20 °C.
- Following this exposure, the carrier rings are transferred to a culture medium that will allow the growth of any surviving organism.
- The effectiveness of the disinfectant is then determined by the number of organisms in resulting cultures.

4.4.3 Chick-Martin Test

- The phenol coefficient test is conducted in the laboratory and its drawbacks are explained. Those disinfectants were required to act in the presence of organic matter, was pointed by Chick and Martin in 1908 who recommended that dried human feces should be added to the test system.
- Later, Garrod suggested the use of dried yeast as a substitute.
- The test is conducted by inoculating *Salmonella typhi* (test organism) into solution containing graded concentrations of the test substance, or phenol as standard: all solutions containing dried yeast.
- The contact period is 30 min at 20 °C and at the end of this period subcultures are made in duplicate into nutrient broth.
- The subculture tubes are incubated for 48 hours at 37 °C and the presence or absence of growth is noted.
- The concentration of phenol, which prevents growth in broth, is determined and the mean value calculated, a similar value is obtained for the unknown.
- The coefficient is calculated by dividing that value found for phenol by the value found for the unknown.
- A test such as the RW or Chick Martin may be performed with any test organism and at any temperature; the test is then described as a phenol coefficient test, never as a modified RW or chick martin, and the conditions i.e., organisms and temperature used, should be clearly stated.

Table 4.3 Comparison of Rideal Walker Test and Chick Martin Test

Parameter in the test	Rideal Walker test	Chick Martin Test
Volume Medium	5.0ml	10 ml
Diluent for test disinfectant	water	Yeast suspension
Reaction temperature	17.5± 0.5°C	30°C
Organism	Salmonella typhi	Salmonella typhi & Staphylococcus aureus
Sampling Times	2.5,5.0,7.5,10.0 minutes	30 minutes
Calculation of coefficient	Dilution test killing in 7.5 min.devided by same for phenol	Mean concentration of phenol showing no growth after 30 minutes. devided by same for test.

4.4.4 Kelsey-Sykes Test

- It is a capacity use-dilution test introduced in 1960's where the capacity of the disinfectant to destroy successive dilutions of a bacterial culture is tested.
- The test is performed using four test organisms and *Proteus vulgaris.*
- The organisms are cultivated on a synthetic medium and survival is tested in a broth containing tween 80 (a nonionic surfactant).
- The disinfectant solution is carried at 20 °C and recovery of organisms at 32 °C.
- The test is carried out under clean and dirty conditions, the later being simulated by dried yeast as in the chick martin test.
- Calibrated and dropping pipettes rather than loops are used for inoculation and other liquid manipulations, and disinfectants diluted at approximately the dilutions recommended for use are made in hard water.
- The disinfectant is assessed on its ability to kill micro-organisms and not by comparison with phenol.
- The KS suspension test is not a capacity test it reports the data as pass or fail and not as a coefficient, and it uses a range of micro-organisms.

4.5 Dynamics of Disinfection

The disinfection process does not take place at once but is a gradual operation in which the number of organisms killed in unit time is greater at the beginning and becomes less as the exposure period is increased.

- If the number of survivors in unit volume are plotted against time, the points fall on smooth curves.

- If the logarithms of the numbers of bacteria surviving in unit volume are plotted against time, a straight line is obtained.

  E.g., Results of anthrax spores treated with 5% phenol and incubated at 33 minutes/3 °C are plotted. The curved line represents the numbers of anthrax spores surviving in unit volume, and the straight line the corresponding logarithms of the numbers of surviving bacteria.

- The disinfection process appears to follow the law of mass – action and to proceed in accordance with the monomolecular equation, or a reaction of first order, provided the disinfectant is present in large excess

$$\frac{-dN}{dt} = KN \quad \text{or} \quad \frac{1}{t_2 - t_1} \log \frac{N_1}{N_2} = K$$

  N_1 and N_2 represent the number of surviving bacteria in unit volume after times t_1 and t_2.

Importance of Logarithmic Survivor Curves (Fig. 4.1)

- In the destruction of bacteria by various agents, the greater the number of cells present, the longer will be the time necessary for complete sterilization.

E.g., A suspension contains 200,000 organisms per milliliter. If the bacteria are destroyed at the rate of 90% per minute, the number of survivors at the end of 7 min will be

200,000 → 20,000 → 2000 → 200 → 20→ 2 → 0.2→ 0.02

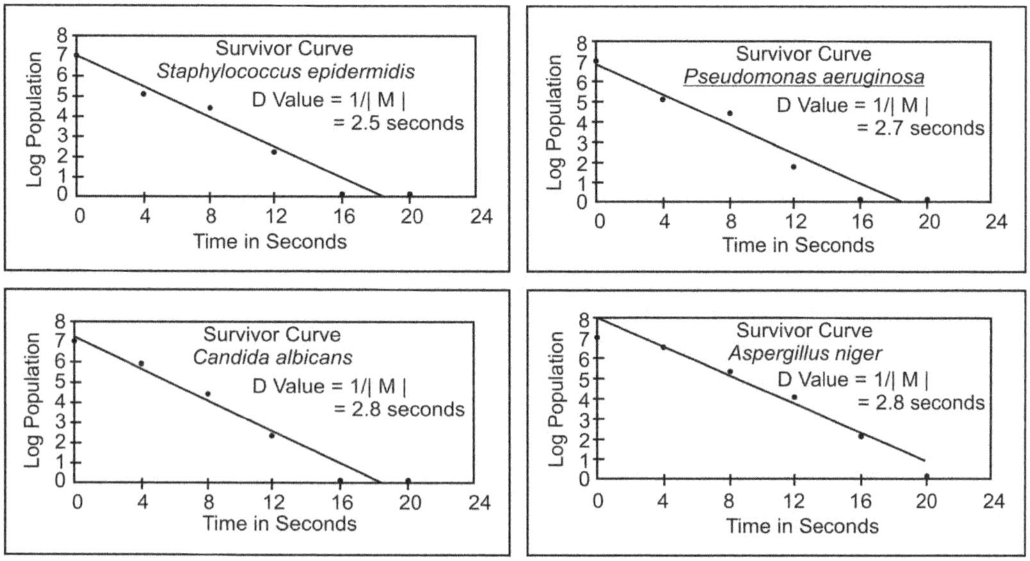

Fig. 4.1 Logarithmic survivor curves

If instead of 200,000 the suspension contains only 200 organisms per milliliter, the time required to reduce the count to 2 bacteria per 100 ml will be only 4 min

$$200 \rightarrow 20 \rightarrow 2 \rightarrow 0.2 \rightarrow 0.02$$

The relationship between bacterial numbers and the time required to produce complete sterilization are important

Uses

1. In canning and dairying industries
2. In bacteriology
3. In surgery

4.6 Sterilization

Sterilization is derived from Latin word ***Sterilis*** which means unable to produce offspring. Sterilization may be defined as a process by which an article, surface or medium is free of all micro-organisms either in vegetative or spore state. Sterility is the condition of freedom from living organisms. It is an absolute term.

The physical means most frequently used in sterilization are dry heat, moist heat, and incineration. Autoclaves may provide dry or moist heat, with moist heat being the most effective. Heat is effective against most viruses and bacteria encountered, and may be effective against spores and fungi. Prions, spores, and temperature-resistant organisms may require additional time and adjunct chemical means to be completely deactivated. The amount of time the material is heated and the sustained temperature can be modified to achieve higher levels of decontamination.

The following is a comparison of the different types of sterilization and efficacy in different circumstances.

Steam Heat (Autoclave) requires approximately 15 psi pressure with a chamber temperature of at least 250 °F (121 °C). The cycle time begins when the materials being sterilized reach the predetermined temperature. The duration required is dependent upon the volume of the load (usually 30-60 minutes).

Each autoclave that uses steam sterilization must be biologically challenged using a biological indicator (*Bacillus stearothermophilus*) at least monthly. Upon failure, the unit must pass two consecutive tests prior to use.

Dry Heat is less effective than steam and requires more time (two to four hours) and a higher temperature (320-338 °F or 160-170 °C). Monitor effectiveness with a biological indicator.

Each unit that uses dry heat must be biologically challenged using a biological indicator (*Bacillus subtilis*) at least weekly. Upon failure, the unit must pass two consecutive tests prior to use.

4.6.1 Methods and Equipment Used for Sterilization Purposes

I Application of high temperature for destruction of micro-organisms include.
  (a) Moist-Heat Sterilization
  (b) Dry-Heat Sterilization
II Low temperature methods
III Desiccation
IV Osmotic pressure
V Radiation
  (i) UV-light
  (ii) X-rays
  (iii) γ-rays
  (iv) Cathode rays
VI Surface and Interfacial tension
VII Filtration
  1. Bacteriological filters
  2. HEPA filters

4.6.1.1 High Temperature Methods

4.6.1.1.1 Moist Heat Sterilization

Steam under Pressure: Heat in the form of saturated steam under pressure is the most practical and dependable agent for sterilization. Steam under pressure provides temperature above those obtainable by boiling.

Advantages

- Rapid heating
- Penetration
- Moisture in abundance which facilitates the coagulation of proteins.

The laboratory apparatus designed to use steam under regulated pressure is called an autoclave is shown in Fig. 4.2.

Autoclave is essentially a double-jacketed steam chamber equipped with devices which permit the chamber to be filled with saturated steam and maintained at a designated temperature and pressure for any period of time.

The mode of operation may depend upon the material to be sterilized. The sterilization cycle consists of the following stages.

(i) Loading and packaging the autoclave

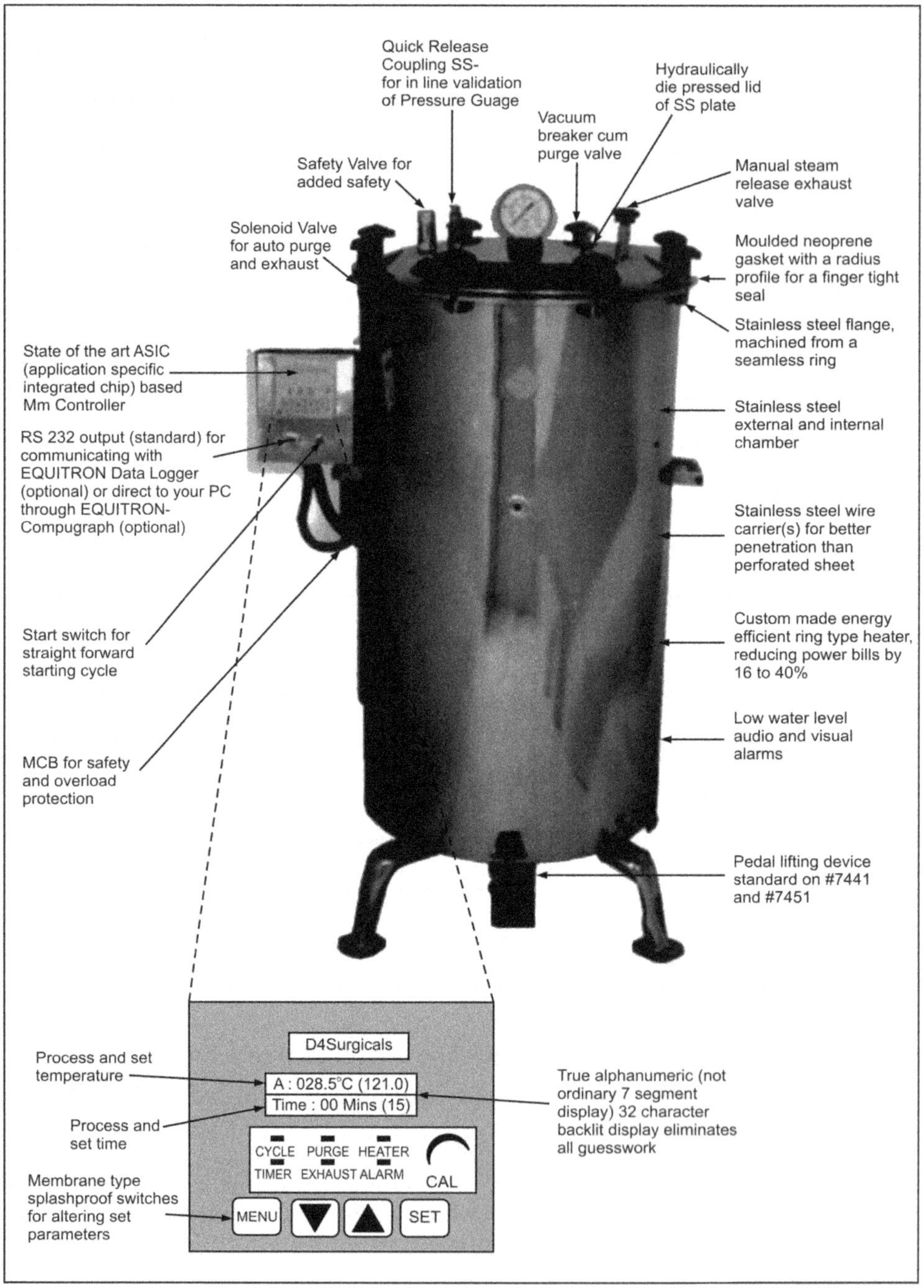

Fig. 4.2 Autoclave

(ii) Raising the temperature and pressure
(iii) Holding the load at this level for a specified time
(iv) Cooling and unloading

- In the operation of an autoclave it is absolutely essential that the air in the chamber be completely replaced by saturated steam.
- If air is present, it will reduce the temperature obtained within the chamber.
- Many media, solutions, discarded cultures and contaminated materials are routinely sterilized with autoclave.
- Auto clave is operated at a pressure of approximately 15 *l*b/in^2.

E.g., 1000 test tubes containing 10 mL each of a liquid medium can be sterilized in 10-15 minutes at 121 °C; 10 litres of the same medium contained in a single container would require 1 hour or more at the same temperature.

The Stages of Operation

1. **Air Removed and Steam Admission:** In the operation of an autoclave it is absolutely essential that the air in the chamber replaced by saturated steam. If air is present, it will reduce the temperature steam were under the same pressure. It is not the pressure that kills the organisms but the temperature of the steam.

   Air can be removed from steam sterilizers either by downward displacement with steam, evacuation or a combination of the two.

   In the downward displacement sterilizer, the heavier cool air is forced out of the discharge, channel by incoming hot steam.

   This has the benefit of warming the load during air removal, which aids the heating-up process. It finds widest application in the sterilization of bottled fluids where bottle breakage may occur under combined stress of evacuation and high temperature.

   For more air retentive loads (dressings) mechanical evacuation of air is essential before administration of steam.

   Small packages entrain air and this must be removed with near-to-steam thermostatic valve incorporated in the discharge channel.

   It is common practice to package sterile fluids in flexible plastic containers; these can develop a considerable pressure in the air space above the fluids and it is necessary to maintain proportion of air within the chamber to produce sufficient overpressure to prevent these containers from bursting (air ballasting). Air removal is therefore unnecessary, but air layering must be controlled.
2. **Heating-up and Exposure:** When the sterilizer reaches its operating temperature and pressure the sterilization stage begins. The duration of exposure may include a heating-up time in addition to the holding time and this will normally be established using thermocouples in dummy articles.
3. **Drying or Cooling:** Dressings, packs and other porous loads may become dampened during the sterilization process and must be dried before removal from the chamber.

This is achieved by steam exhaust and application of vacuum, often assisted by heat from the steam-filled jacket if fitted. After drying, atmospheric pressure within the chamber is restored by admission of sterile filtered air.

For bottled fluids the final stage of sterilization process is cooling, and this needs to be achieved as rapidly as possible to minimize thermal degradation of the product and to reduce processing time. This is achieved by circulating water in the jacket that surrounds the chamber or spray-cooling with retained condensate.

Mechanism of Action of Moist Heat Sterilization: Moist heat kills viruses, bacteria, and fungi by degrading nucleic acids, denaturing enzymes and other essential proteins. Saturated steam may also disrupt cell membranes, destroy vegetative cells and endospores.

Condensate can be removed. Temperature is monitored within an opening of the discharge channel and by thermocouples in dummy packages; jacket and chamber pressures are followed using pressure gauges. In hospitals and industry, it is common practice to operate sterilizers on an automatic cycle, each stage of operation being controlled by a timer responding to temperature or pressure sensing devices.

Advantages of Autoclaving

(i) Because of greater penetrating power of the steam under pressure micro-organisms are destroyed more efficiently than the dry heat and therefore shorter exposure at a lower temperature.

(ii) The method is suitable for large load.

(iii) For sterilizing porous materials, dry saturated steam can be supplied.

Disadvantages

(i) Unsuitable for anhydrous materials such as powder and oils and also for materials, which cannot withstand heating at 115 °C and above.

(ii) Auto claves should be frequently checked for their performance and all the sterilized materials should invariably be subjected to tests for sterility.

4.6.1.1.2 Fractional Sterilization (Tyndallization)

The sterilization of materials by heating to 100 °C on 3 successive days with incubation period in between, called fractional sterilization. This method was developed by John Tyndall.

- Some microbiological media, solutions of chemicals, biological materials cannot be heated above 100 °C without being damaged.
- Resistant spores germinate during the incubation period on subsequent exposure to heat; the vegetative cells will be destroyed.
- If spore are present and do not germinate during the incubation periods, the material will not be sterilized.

- Steam Arnold apparatus is used for this technique and an autoclave with free flowing steam can also be used.

4.6.1.1.3 Boiling Water

Contaminated materials or objects exposed to boiling water cannot be sterilized with certainity, but all the vegetative cells will be destroyed within minutes by exposure to boiling water, but some bacterial spores can withstand this condition for many hours.

- The practice of exposing instruments for short periods of time in boiling water is more likely to bring about disinfection rather than sterilization.
- Boiling water cannot be used in the laboratory as a method of sterilization.

4.6.1.1.4 Pasteurization

Milk, cream and certain alcoholic beverages are subjected to a controlled heat treatment called pasteurization.

- This method kills micro-organisms of certain types but does not destroy all organisms.
- The temperature for pasteurization is 62.8 °C for 30 minutes.
- Methods of pasteurization of milk used commercially include a low temperature holding method and a high temperature short time method 55 (HTST methods).
- The holding method or vat pasteurization, expose milk to 145 °F for 30 minutes in appropriately designed equipment.
- The HTST process employs equipment capable of exposing milk to a temperature of 161 °F for 15 seconds.
- Ultra high temperature –138 °C for 1-2 sec is used for preparing milk powders.
- Precautions should be taken to prevent recontamination after pasteurization.
- The finished product should be stored at a low temperature to retard growth of micro-organisms which survive pasteurization.

4.6.1.2 Dry-Heat Sterilization

4.6.1.2.1 Hot Air Sterilization

Dry–heat or hot air sterilization is recommended when steam under pressure makes direct and complete contact with the materials to be sterilized.

- Destruction of micro-organisms by dry heat is primarily on oxidation process.
- This method is used for the sterilization of oils, talcum powder, glass and metallic apparatus.

(a) **Flaming:** It is the simplest method for applying dry heat and is used for the sterilization of forceps, needles, scalpels, and metal spatulas, the mouths of culture tubes, bottles and platinum loops.

- The method consists of applying the hot part of a Bunsen flame to the surface for approximately 5 seconds.

(b) **Hot Air Oven:** The modern hot air oven consists of a double walled chamber of aluminum or stainless steel separated from the outer case by a thick layer of insulation made of fibre glass.

- Insulation is also filled in the hollow flanged door, which carries an asbestos jacket that provides a tight seal.
- Heating is affected by electrical heating elements and thermostats automatically control temperature.
- This equipment has a vent at the outside of the aluminum case. A fan is fixed at the inner side of the case.
- A regulator is provided at the outside which is used to adjust the temperature changes and to set the desired temperatures.

Principle: Heat transfer from the source to the material takes place by conduction, convection and radiation.

Conditions

- Substances that are hot heat – liable and can tolerate temperatures of 140 °C to 260 °C may be rendered sterile by means of dry heat in a hot air oven.
- For laboratory glass ware, a 2 hour exposure to a temperature of 160 °C is sufficient for sterilization.

4.6.1.2.2 Incineration

Destruction of micro-organisms by burning is practiced routinely in the laboratory, where the transfer needle is introduced into the flame of the Bunsen burner.

- When the transfer needle is sterilized, care should be exercised to prevent spattering.
- The danger of spattering can be greatly reduced or eliminated by using a Bunsen burner or an electric heat coil equipped with a tube into which the transfer needle can be inserted.
- Incineration is used for the destruction of carcasses, to be disposed off.

4.6.1.3 Low Temperature

- Low temperatures are useful for preservation of cultures, since micro-organisms have a unique capacity for surviving extreme cold.
- Agar – slant cultures of some bacteria, yeasts and molds are stored for long periods of time at refrigeration temperatures of about 4 to 7 °C.
- Many bacteria and viruses can be maintained in a deep – freeze unit at temperatures from –20 to –70 °C.

- Liquid nitrogen, at a temperature of – 196 °C, is used for preserving cultures of many viruses and micro-organisms, as well as stocks of mammalian tissue cells used in animal virology and many other types of research.

4.6.1.4 Desiccation

Desiccation causes a cessation of metabolic activity, followed by a decline in the total viable population.

- The time of survival of micro-organisms after desiccation varies, depending on the following factors
  1. The kind of microorganism.
  2. The material in or on which the organisms are dried.
  3. The completeness of the drying process.
  4. The physical conditions to which the dried organisms exposed. *E.g.*, light, temperature and humidity.
- Species of Gram negative Cocci such as *Gonocooci* and *Meningococci* are very sensitive to desiccation; they die in a matter of hours.
- *Streptococci* are much more resistant.
- The tuberclei bacillus dried in sputum remains viable for even longer periods of time. Dried spores of micro-organisms are known to remain viable indefinitely.

In the process of lyophilization, organisms are subjected to extreme dehydration in the frozen state and then sealed in a vacuum. In this condition, desiccated (lyophilized) cultures of micro-organisms remain viable for many years.

4.6.1.5 Osmotic Pressure

- When two solutions with differing concentration of solute are separated by a semi permeable membrane, there will occur a passage of water, through the membrane in the direction of higher concentration. The trend is toward equalizing the concentration of solute on both sides of a membrane.
- If cells are exposed to solutions with higher solute concentration, water will be drawn out of the cell. The process is called plasmolysis.
- The reverse process i.e., passage of water from a low solute concentration into the cell, is termed plasmoptysis. The pressure built up within the cell as a result of this water intake is termed as osmotic pressure.
- Plasmolysis results in dehydration of the cell, and as a consequence metabolic processes are retarded partially or completely. The antimicrobial effect is similar to that caused by desiccation.

- Because of the great rigidity of microbial cell walls, the cell wall structure does not exhibit distortions as a result of plasmolysis or plasmoptysis.
- Shrinkage of the protoplast from the cell wall can be observed during plasmolysis.

4.6.1.6 Radiation

- The influence of sunlight in preventing the spread of infection has been known for centuries but it was realized only towards the end of the 19th century that the radiations primarily responsible lie in the UV range of wave lengths.
- Radiation is commonly classified as electromagnetic and particulate. Electromagnetic radiation comprises of photons of energy including UV, gamma, X-rays and cosmic radiation.
- Beta particles or electrons are the particulate form of radiations.

Radiation sterilization is also known as cold sterilization as it is non thermal method.

4.6.1.6.1 Ultraviolet Radiation

- It is commonly employed in the reduction of airborne contamination in the maintenance of aseptic areas and rooms within the processing environment in a pharmaceutical industry.
- The most common source of artificial UV radiation is the UV lamps.
- Ultraviolet radiation in the region of 253.7A^{o} has been shown to possess the greatest activity in destroying micro-organisms.
- The bactericidal effectiveness is primarily a function of the intensity of radiation and duration of exposure and varies with the susceptibility of the organism.

Mode of Action: UV light is absorbed by the Nucleic acids of the cell where it does the greatest damage. The absorption and subsequent reactions are predominantly in the pyrimidines of nucleic acids causing the formation of pyrimidine dimer in which two adjacent pyrimidines become bonded in DNA molecule. The effect of UV radiation on DNA are shown in Fig. 4.3.

The method has been used to destroy the viruses by homologous serum jaundice in blood serum and to inactivate viruses and bacteria in vaccine production.

Ionizing Radiations: It is an excellent sterilizing agent and penetrate deep into objects. It will destroy bacterial endospores and vegetative cells, both prokaryotic and eukaryotic.

- Ionizing radiations destroy micro-organisms by stopping reproduction as a result of lethal mutations.

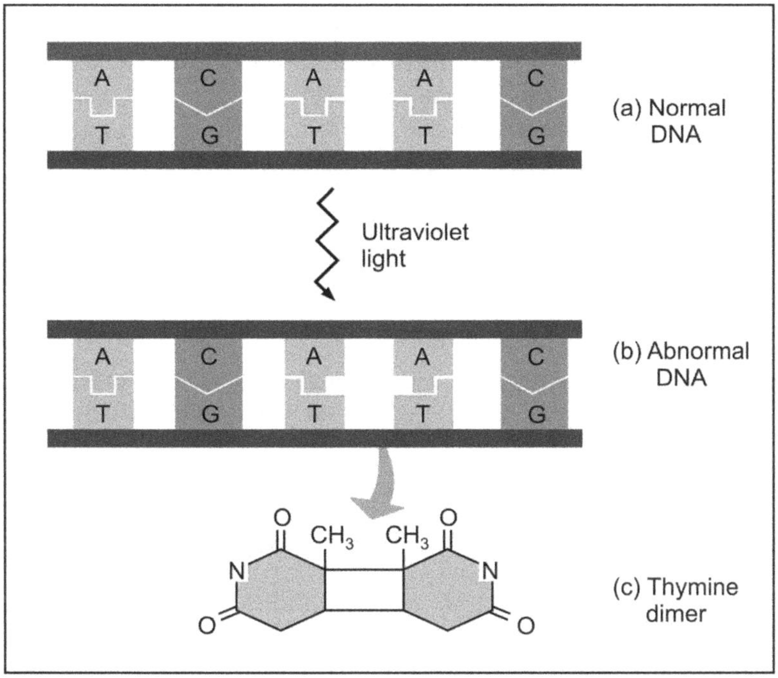

Fig. 4.3 Effect of UV radiation on DNA

4.6.1.6.2 X–rays (Roentgen Rays)

X-Rays are lethal to micro-organisms and higher forms of life. They have better penetrating power than UV radiations. However their use for controlling microbial population is impracticable because

(i) They are very expensive to produce in quantity

(ii) They are difficult to utilize efficiency, since radiations are given off in all directions from their point of origin

But X-rays have been widely used to produce microbial mutants.

4.6.1.6.3 Gamma Radiations

Gamma radiations are high energy radiations emitted from certain radioactive isotopes such as ^{60}C Isotopes which have become available as by product of atomic fission are potential sources of gamma radiations.

- Gamma rays are similar to X-rays but are of shorter wavelength and higher energy.
- They are capable of great penetration into matter, and they are lethal to all life, including micro-organisms
- Gamma radiation has also been used to sterilize and pasteurize meat and other food.

4.6.1.6.4 Cathode Rays (Electron Beam Radiation)

When a high voltage potential is established between a cathode and an anode in an evacuated tube, the cathode emits beams of electrons called cathode rays (or) electron beams. These intense beams of accelerated electrons are microbicidal as well as having other effects on biological and non biological materials.

- One of the unique feature of the process is that the material can be sterilized after it has been packaged.
- Electron beam radiation has limited power of penetration.

4.6.1.7 Surface and Interfacial Tension

- The interface or boundary between a liquid and a gas is characterized by unbalanced forces of attraction between the molecules in the surface of the liquid and in the interior.
- Molecules in the surface of the liquid-air interface is pulled strongly towards the interior of the liquid beneath it.
- Molecules in the interior of the liquid are attracted uniformly in all directions.
- This behaviour of molecular forces at the liquid air interface imparts a distinctive characteristic to the surface of a liquid, known as surface tension.
- Surface forces also exist between two immiscible liquids and at the interface between a solid and a liquid; they are referred to as interfacial tension.
- Changes in surface tension may alter the permeability characteristics of the cytoplasmic membrane, causing leakage of cellular substances, which results in damage to the cell.

4.6.1.8 Filtration

Filtration is a mechanical method of controlling the growth of micro-organisms.

- For many years varieties of filters have been available to the microbiologist, which can remove micro-organisms from liquids (or) gases.
- These filters are made up of different materials like
  - (i) An asbestos pad in the Seitz filter (Fig. 4.4)
  - (ii) Diatomaceous earth in the Berkefeld filter (Fig. 4.5)
  - (iii) Porcelain in Chamberland-Pasteur filters (Fig. 4.5)
  - (iv) Sintered glass disks in other filters
- The mean diameter in these bacteriological filters ranges from one to several micrometers.
- Factors such as electric charge of the filter, electric charge carried by the organisms, the nature of fluid being filtered and porosity prevent the passage of organisms.

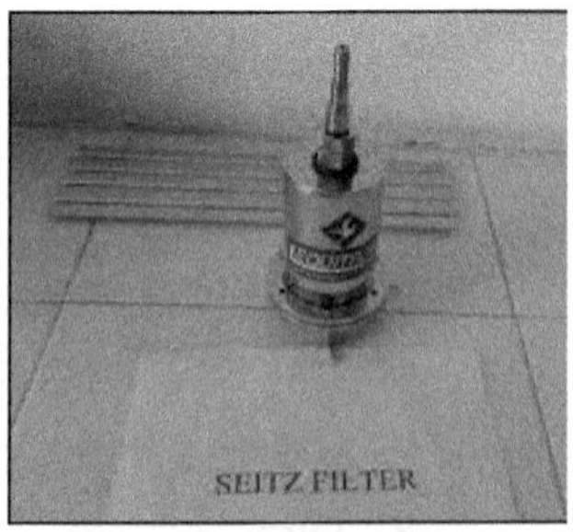

Fig. 4.4 Seitz filter

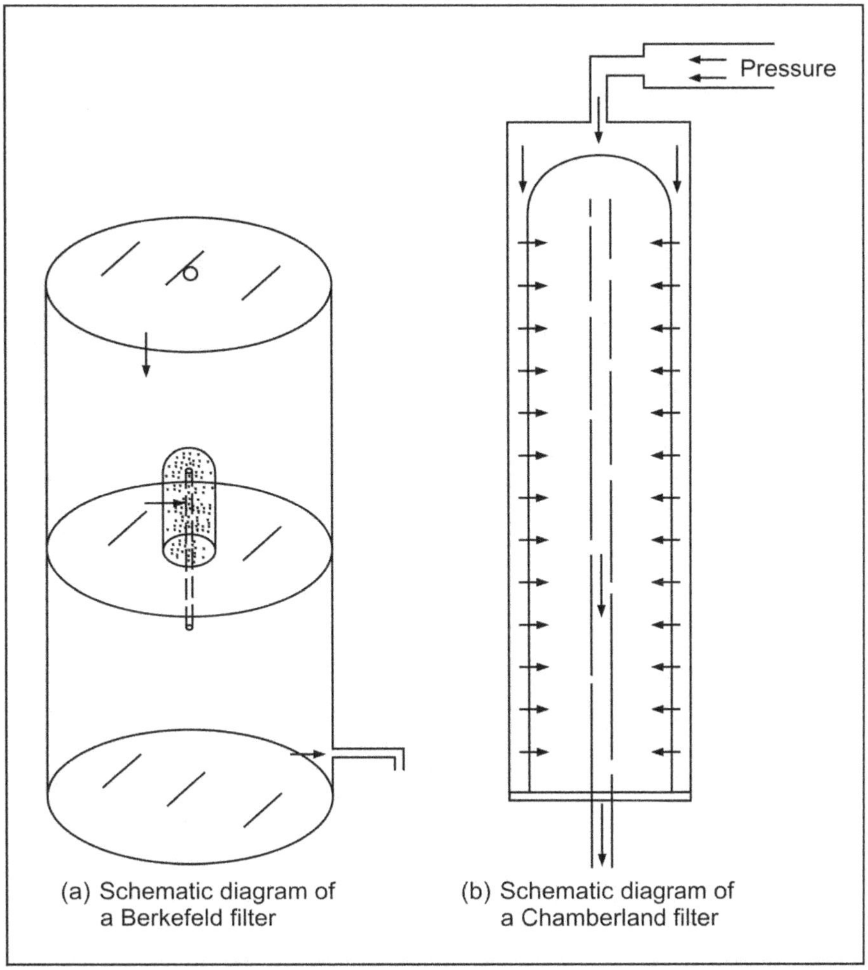

Fig. 4.5 Schematic diagram of **(a)** Berkefeld filter **(b)** Chamberland filter

4.6.1.8.1 Membrane or Molecular Filters

The pores are of uniform and specific predetermined size.

- They are composed of biologically inert cellulose esters.
- They are prepared as circular membrane of about 150 μm thickness and contain millions of microscopic pores of very uniform diameter.
- Two types of pressure can be applied in filtration process
- Negative pressure can be applied on the fluid in the filter flask by the use of vacuum.
- Positive pressure can be imposed above the fluid.

- Molecular or membrane filters are used extensively in laboratory and in industry to sterilize fluid materials
- Filters of this type can be produced with known porosities ranging approximately 0.01 to 10 μm.
- After completion of filtration, precautions must be taken to prevent contamination of the filtered material when it is transferred to other containers.

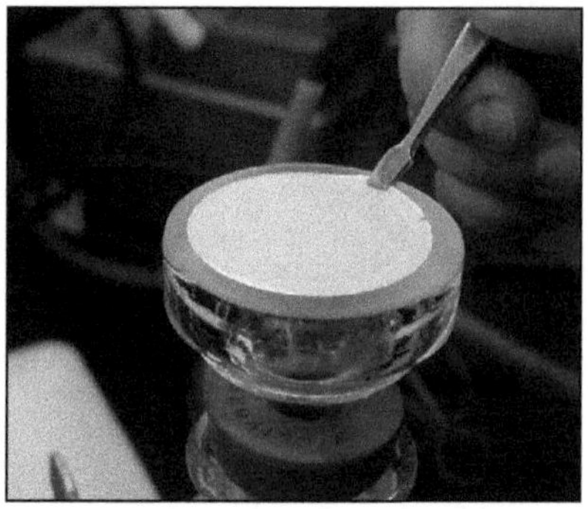

Fig. 4.6 Membrane filter

Membrane filters covering pore sizes from 0.015 to 12 μm is shown in Fig 4.6. membrane materials (PTFE, regenerated cellulose, nylon, cellulose nitrate, polycarbonate, aluminum oxide, etc.) provides the user with an array of solvent compatibility options, porosities, and pore sizes according to individual specific needs. Some membrane materials are also available in sterile format.

Membrane filters are typically used in both liquid and air filtration. They offer accurately controlled pore size distribution with high strength and flexibility and are a suitable choice for a wide range of applications such as basic research, environmental testing, and pharmaceutical as well as food and beverage industries. Products in the pharmaceutical industry must be tested for micro-organisms at specific critical points during the production process.

Sterile Membrane Filters for Microbiology

Two types of materials for microbiology membrane filters:

- Cellulose mixed ester membranes: ME Standard type and ME 25 Select with improved recovery rate
- Cellulose nitrate membranes: Micro Plus type

Sterilization of Parenterals by Filtration

Filtration is a preferred method of sterilizing drug product solutions. A sterilizing grade filter should be validated to reproducibly remove viable micro-organisms from the process steam. Whatever filter or combination of filters is used, validation should include microbiological challenges to simulate worse case production conditions for the material to be filtered and integrity test results of the filters used for the study. The microorganism *Brevundimonas* - ATCC 19146 - when properly grown, harvested and used, is a common challenge microorganism for 0.2 m rated filters because of its small size - 0.3 m mean diameter.

Membrane Filtration

Membrane filters are thin, uniform porous sheets that trap all particles larger in size than the pores in the membrane or larger than their interstices. Particle entrapment by sieving alone is an excessively simplistic interpretation of what happens to particles during membrane filtration.

In reality, by spatial sequestration, membrane filters are also capable of retaining particles that are dimensionally smaller than their pores. These mechanisms are:

(a) Spatial entrapment applies equally to liquid and gas filtration; they include inertial impaction to the walls or surfaces of the pores and lodgment in crevices and dead-end.

(b) Physicochemical interactions with the filter medium can be very complex and differ according to the types of particles, the fluid in which they are suspended, and the dynamics of the filtration system.

(c) Electrostatic forces are of more importance in gas filtration than in liquid filtration.

(d) Adsorption of surfactants from liquid suspensions to both particles and pore surfaces may result in mutually repulsive ionic forces that encourage the passage of particles.

(e) Liquid suspensions through covalent bonding, and through attraction by Van der Walls forces when zeta potentials of both particles and pore surfaces are low - usually less than 30 mV.

Microbial Particle Passage

Pore size is clearly not the only factor influencing the retention of micro-organisms on or in membrane filters. The FDA's microbiological particle passage standard, that a sterilizing filter should be capable of retaining a challenge of at least 107 micro-organisms of a particular type per cm2, is an end-result criterion.

Applications of Sterilizing Filtration

There are two main occasions for the use of filtration in the sterilization of fluids. The first is when fluids are damaged or destroyed by exposure to other sterilization processes; the second is when the scale of sterilization is too large to be addressed through other sterilization processes.

Aseptic processing of liquid pharmaceutical formulation implies the use of sterile filtration. Filtration should not be the method of choice ahead of thermal sterilization, but it is not out of the question; some heat-stable pharmaceutical liquid products are currently being filter-sterilized and aseptically processed. Sterilizing membranes for this purpose should have a pore size rating no greater than 0.22 m.

4.6.1.8.2 High Efficiency Particulate Air Filters (HEPA)

The development of HEPA filters has made it possible to deliver clean air to an enclosure such as cubicle or a room. This type of air filtrations together with a system of laminar flow is now used extensively to produce dust and bacteria free environment.

HEPA filters are employed to remove 99.97% of 0.3 μm particles.

Working with dangerous agents such as *mycobacterium tuberculosis* and tumor viruses needs laminar air flow cabinets.

4.7 Large Scale Sterilization Equipments

Pharmaceutical Sterilizers

Sterilizers are special large scale sterilization equipments used to make a product free from live bacteria or other microorganisms. The industries such as pharmaceuticals and health care have become more concerned about safety issues and thus sterilizers become an essential component for controlling microbial contamination. Sterilization can be achieved through application of heat, chemicals, irradiation, or filtration.

There are several kinds of sterilization equipment using different technology and processes, according to the application.

- Moist steam Sterilizer
- Dry Heat Sterilizer
- ETO Sterilizer
- Sterilizing Tunnel
- CIP System
- SIP System

4.7.1 Moist Steam Sterilizer

Principle and working: Moist heat sterilization technology is the most widely used given its versatility and effectiveness for heat resistant products. Depending on the type of product to be sterilized, different techniques are used:

- Steam sterilization
- Steam-air mixture sterilization
- Steam-water mixture sterilization

Steam sterilization technique is basically used to sterilize different types of solid materials: clothing, stainless steel equipment, filters, component parts of other equipment, etc., and also for liquids in sealed or ventilated containers, etc.

Steam-air mixture and steam-water mixture sterilization autoclaves have been specially designed for the terminal sterilization of liquid solutions in sealed glass or plastic containers and the process controls the differential pressure existing between the inside of the container and the chamber.

In moist steam sterilizers, steam destroys microorganisms by the irreversible denaturation of enzymes and structural proteins. The temperature at which denaturation occurs varies inversely with the amount of water present. Sterilization in saturated steam thus requires precise control of time, temperature, and pressure.

Pressure serves as a means to obtain the high temperatures necessary to quickly kill microorganisms. Specific temperatures must be obtained to ensure the microbicidal activity. Minimum sterilization time should be measured from the moment when all the materials to be sterilized have reached the required temperature throughout.

The most widely used steam sterilizer for steam sterilization technique is autoclave. The name comes from Greek 'auto'-, ultimately meaning 'self' and Latin 'clavis' meaning 'key' a self-locking device. This is medical equipment that was initially created by a French microbiologist Charles Chamberlain in 1879.

Industrial autoclaves are industrial devices that are used to treat various components and materials at extremely high pressures and temperatures. Autoclaves are extremely useful in applications where chemical reactions need to be carried out under controlled conditions.

Design and Construction

In essence, autoclaves are another type of pressure vessel. As they apply extreme amounts of heat and pressure, the body of the vessel needs to be capable of withstanding the extreme conditions within the interior chamber. For this reason, high grade steel is the general material of choice when it comes to designing and constructing the autoclave. The vessel can be constructed with varying levels of thickness depending on the industry it will be used in, and the kind of components that will be placed within it.

One solution driven design factor is the fast opening door. When the heating process is at full pressure, the force upon the door is more than 1,000 tons. Thus, it protects engineers from the heat and pressure inside the chamber. It is also designed in a manner that an engineer can quickly and easily open it to remove the components without compromising on his safety. Various sources can be used to heat the autoclave. The most popular source is gas; however, there are electrically powered autoclaves as well.

Applications

As one can imagine, autoclaves can be used in variety of applications to heat numerous components. A few typical application examples are given below.

- Heat treating metal
- Vulcanizing rubber

- Composites manufacturing
- Sterilization of medical instruments
- Aerospace components manufacturing

4.8 Industrial Large Scale Autoclave

Advantage: Steam sterilizers provide a cost-effective solution to sterilize medical waste, infectious waste and other material. Manufacturers can design customized sterilizers to suit the needs of individual clients and the waste treating capacity varies depending on the size of the plant.

- Some of the other types of steam sterilizers used in pharmaceutical and biotech industries is the following:

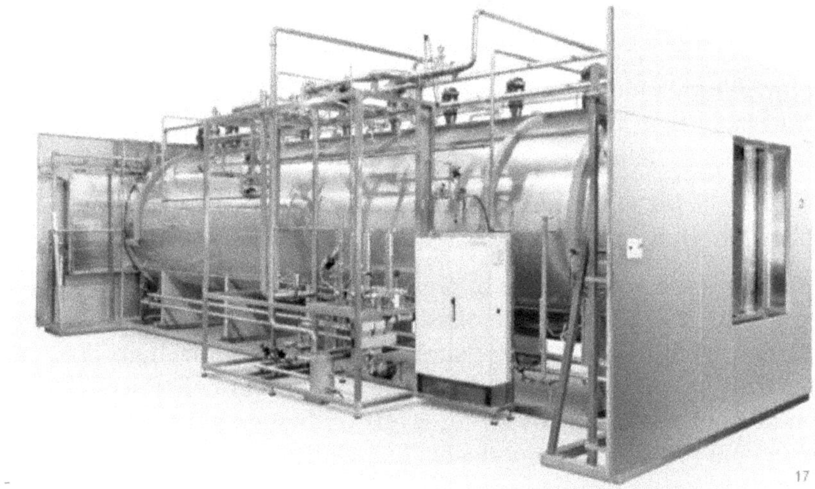

Fig. 4.7 Industrial large scale autoclave

4.8.1 Fully Automatic Horizontal Cylindrical High Pressure Steam Sterilizer (Class-B Autoclave)

***Salient features*:**

- Fully automatic PLC based control system
- Numeric keyboard 4 line display +18 keys

- Shortcut keys for fixed sterilization programs, appliance, dressing, packing instrument, liquid
- Sterilization pressure, temperature and drying time can be adjusted
- Automatic sterilization by pre-programming the cycle
- Triple walled unit, the sterilizer consist of a chamber with steam jacket and outer insulation cover - all are made of heavy gauge
- SS304/316 grade stainless steel
- Working pressure: 1.2 kgf/cm & 2.1 kgf/cm; Temperature: 121°C & 134°C

Sterilizer Control System

- Automatic free steaming
- A venting period during heating, which greatly improves temperature distribution by encouraging air removal
- Media warming: At end of the cycle the autoclave is kept warm to keep media at a ready to sterilize temperature.

GT View: The PLC can be connected with system to view all functions

WORKING

Pre – cycle vacuum

- A powerful vacuum pump draws a series of evacuations to ensure removal of stale air from difficult loads. This is combined with pulsed free steaming to achieve excellent steam penetration
- Post – cycle vacuum
- Vacuum cooling after a cycle to accelerate the cooling of waste loads to safe opening temperature
- Vacuum drying after a cycle for fabric and wrapped loads using water chamber hot air to reduce condensation onto the load

Process Printer: Temperature and time are printed at key stages of the cycle. Pressure and load temperature printing and data logging options are also available. USB connectivity & SD card support facility to store and preview data.

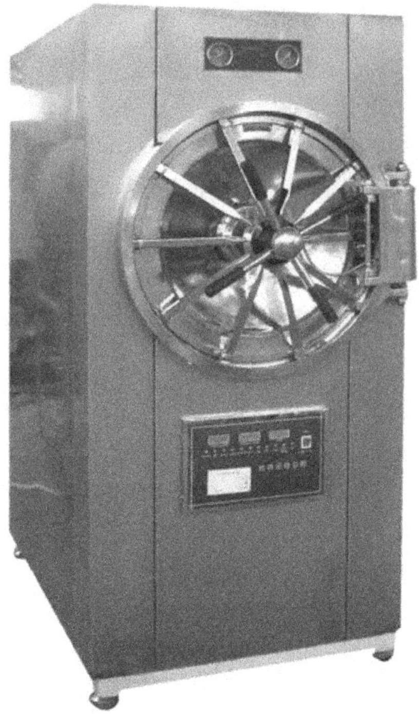

Fig. 4.8 Highpressure steam sterilizer (Class-B Autoclave)

4.8.2 Fully Automatic Steam Storage Vertical High Pressure Steam Sterilizer with Drying System - Triple Walled

Sailent features

- Fully automatic PLC based control system
- Automatic sterilization by pre-programming the cycle
- Triple walled unit, the sterilizer consists of a chamber with steam jacket and outer insulation cover - all are made of heavy gauge SS304/316 grade stainless steel
- Steam storage - Subsequent sterilization can be in quick succession as steam generated is retained even when the load chamber is opened
- Drying system - Mechanical ejector system for drying the working chamber
- Standard features: Chamber condensate line with Solenoid valve, steam release valve, pressure gauge, compound gauge, thermometer, sight glass, silicone gasket
- Working Pressure: 1.2 kgf/cm & 2.1kgf/cm; Temperature: 121°C & 134°C

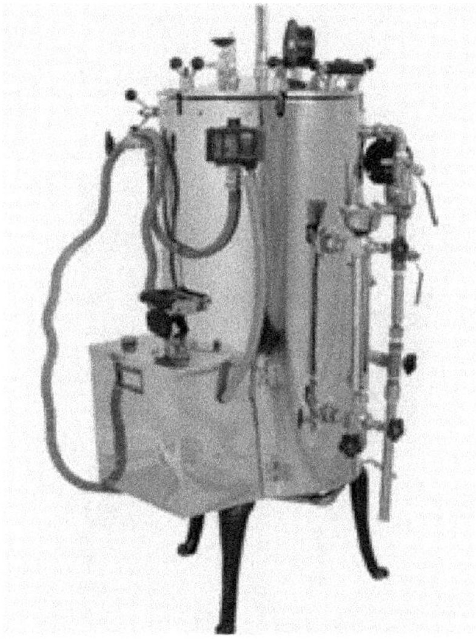

Fig. 4.9 Fully automatic steam storage vertical high pressure steam sterilizer with drying system – Triple walled

4.8.3 Fully Automatic Vertical High Pressure Steam Sterilizer – Triple Walled

Sailent features:

- Fully automatic PLC based control system
- Shortcut keys for fixed sterilization programmes, appliance, dressing, packing instrument, liquid
- Automatic sterilization by pre-programming the cycle
- Triple walled unit has steam jacket, working chamber, outer insulation cover - all made of 304 grade stainless steel
- Safety devices: Pressure switch, safety valves, vacuum breaker, low water level cut-off
- Standard features: Solenoid valve, steam release valves, pressure gauge, condensate valve, sight glass, silicone gasket
- Working Pressure: 1.2 kgf/cm & 2.1kgf/cm; Temperature: 121°C & 134°C

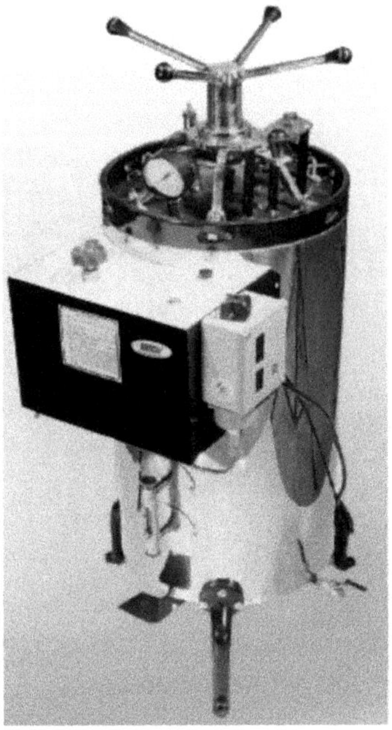

Fig. 4.10 Fully automatic vertical high pressure steam sterilizer (Triple walled)

4.8.4 Dry Heat Sterilizer

Mainly three types of dry-heat sterilization systems are utilized in the pharmaceutical industry today. I. Batch Sterilizer Ovens II. Tunnel Sterilizers

I. Batch Sterilizer/oven Sterilizer

Batch sterilizer is consists of a conical shaped vessel fully closed jacketed in which material need to be sterilized is loaded. The vessel is then subjected to vacuum and the material is subjected to steam **sterilization**. At the same time the material is tumbling inside the vessel. This methos provides the proper mixing cum perfect **sterilization** of the required product.

Principle and Working

This is the type of dry heat unit widely used in the pharmaceutical industry. There are four stages involved in oven sterilization. 1) Drying 2) heat-up 3) exposure 4) Cool down. It uses the principle of convective heat transfer to heat the load.

The two types of convection heating include:

- Natural: as a result of the buoyancy forces generated by differences in density

- Forced convection heating: (HEPA)-filtered air is heated by passage over the electric heating elements of the oven and then this heat is transferred from the air to the product by forced convection.

1. Air - Circulation fan
2. Water cooled battery (for the cooling phase)
3. Circulation HEPA filters
4. Launch/recovery bulkheads
5. Trolley and load
6. Discharge duct
7. HEPA filter on the discharge duct to prevent back-flow contamination
8. Variable-speed fan for chamber pressurization (proportionally controlled)
9. Prefilter and HEPA filter on the chamber pressurization loop
10. Electric heater (proportionally controlled)
11. Four flexible pt100 4-wire RTDs
12. Main control Pt100 4-wire RTD
13. Pressure transducer

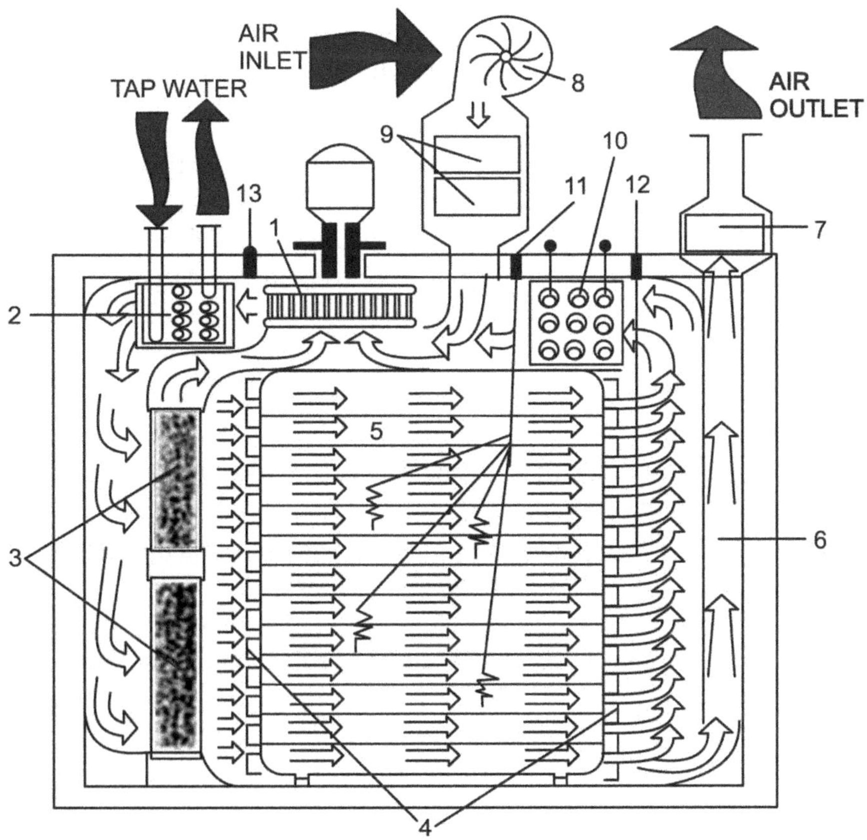

Fig. 4.11 Forced convection batch sterilizer

Applications

- **Batch sterilizer**; is one of the appropriate technique for the dry **sterilization** as it enables proper mixing cum perfect **sterilization** of the product
- The Vacuum inside the chamber ensures that the microbiological and organoleptic properties of the product are preserved
- It does not destroy the microbiological properties of the products that can be proteins denaturation.

Sterilizing Tunnels

Sterilizer is a fully automated system which utilizes dry heat by means of forced convection of filtered air, through high efficiency particulate air filter to achieve sterilization and depyrogenation of washed empty pharmaceutical glassware used of parentral product packing. Continuous dry heat sterilizer ensures the glassware to expose for depyrogenation temperature. The Sterilization Depyrogenation cycle is based on selection of cycle times and exposure of temperature that will sterilize or depyrogenate the glassware to an acceptable low probability level of contamination, without adversely affecting the critical parameters of the product.

Principle and Working

The destruction process of microorganisms is a function of time and temperature. The rate of destruction is linear logarithmic, means in a given time interval and at a given temperature, the same percentage of the bacterial population will be destroyed.

The Forced Conventional Dry Sterilizer consists of Drying Zone to raise the temperature of the glassware and evaporate the wash water from the glassware. The Sterilizing Zone sterilizes the glassware at higher temperature and the third section consists of cooling & sterilizing zone to restore the glassware temperature to ambient.

Applications

- Dry-heat tunnel sterilization is a continuous conduction process in contrast to the batch processes in ovens.
- This is only found in large-scale processes, and the main application of this process is in the sterilization and depyrogenation of glass.
- When a product is sterilized in a tunnel, it is dried, heat- treated by radiant heat or hot air, and then cooled. A typical tunnel sterilization exposure time is 3 or 4 min at 300 ^{0}C or more.

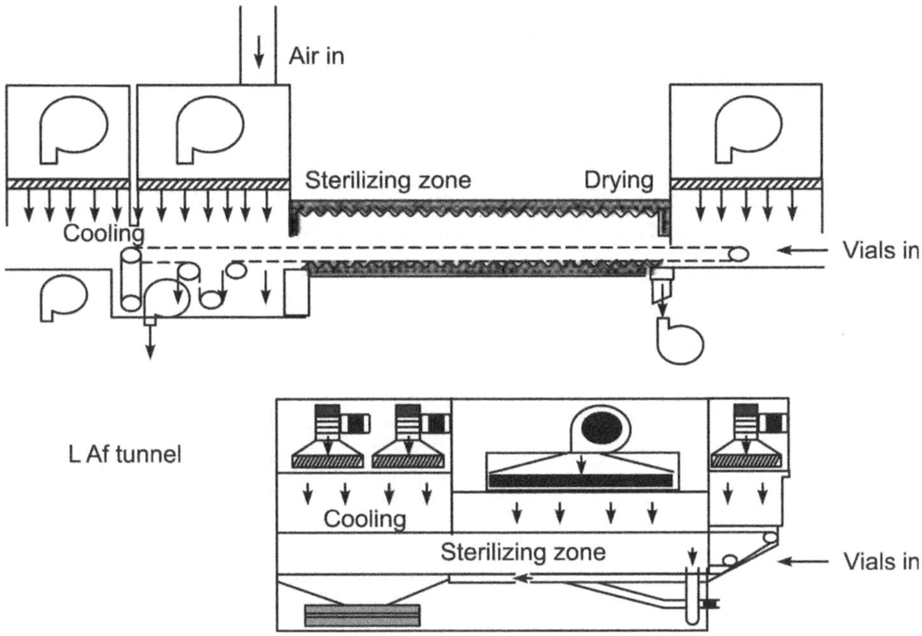

Fig. 4.12 Sterilizing tunnels

Chemical Sterilization Equipment: ETO Sterilizer

Sailent features:

- Ethylene oxide, ETO sterilizers are potent in killing pathogens and consist of electrical heating jackets and provide excellent steam and temperature distribution in the heating chamber.
- The heating chamber is generally made of stainless steel and enclosed with aluminum or stainless steel panels.
- The machines are also equipped with automatic temperature control mechanism. In ETO sterilization bacteria die from the coagulation or denaturation of the protein constituents.

Principle and Working

An effective ETO process can be properly designed for almost every type of medical device and permeable packaging configuration, provided that all variables are assessed through thorough process design and development. Typically, the ETO process can be broken down into four basic phases, each of which needs careful planning to ensure a safe and efficacious process. The four phases are: (1) air removal, (2) steam injection and conditioning dwell, (3) ETO injection and gas dwell, and (4) gas purge and air in-bleed

Benefits of ETO Sterilizer

- E.T.O Gas Sterilizer types of gear are extremely powerful and dependable in annihilating the obsessive miniaturized scale life forms alongside their spores.
- They are ideal for gadgets and substances that can't endure excessive temperature.
- This procedure is perfect for stickiness delicate devices as well.
- They are material perfect. They are able to perform the sterilization procedure on almost any type of material.

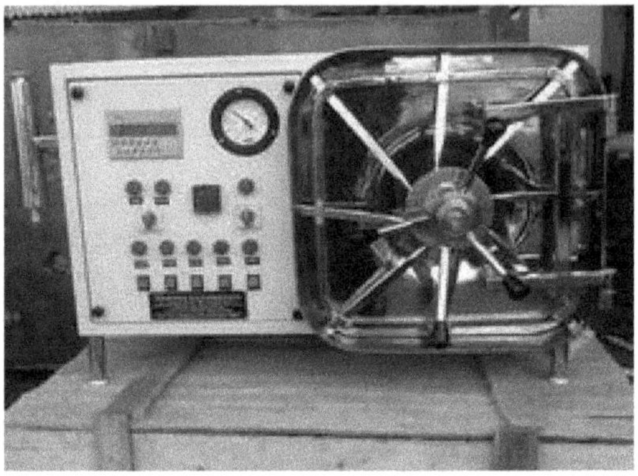

Fig. 4.13 ETO Sterilizer

CIP System

***Salient features*:**

Cleaning in Place or CIP systems are widely used in the pharmaceutical and biotechnology industry to clean and decontaminate tanks, reactors, decanting pumps, and transfer lines etc.

CIP integration starts with the proper selection of the CIP System to deliver the required cleaning parameters to the intended targets. The variables of temperature, velocity/pressure, chemical concentration, and exposure time are precisely controlled by the CIP System, which can be configured with many options not only to deliver the specified CIP parameters in a reliable, repeatable and verifiable manner. CIP system ensures improved hygiene and sanitize more effectively than manual cleaning.

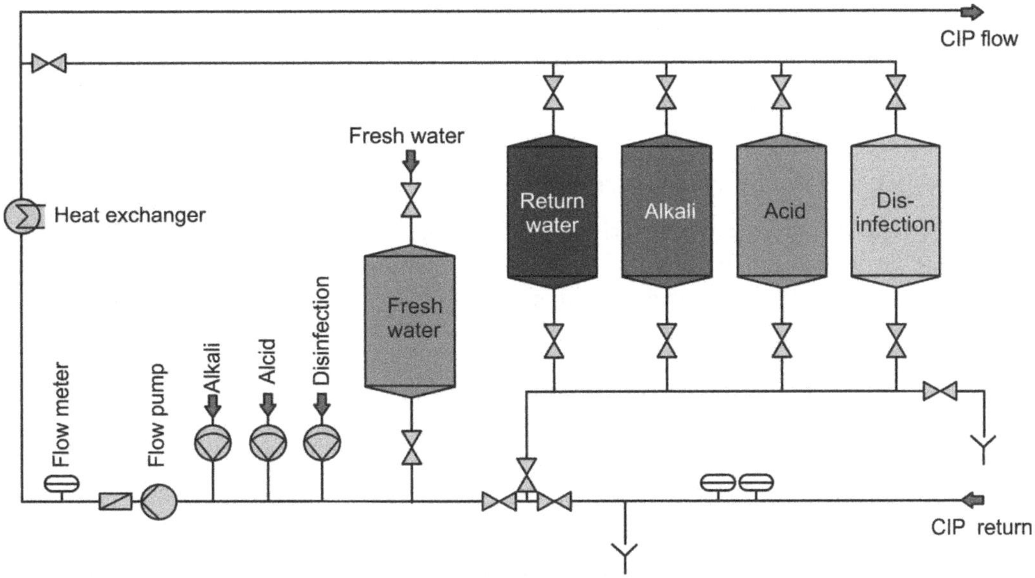

Fig. 4.14 Clean in place (CIP) systems

SIP System

***Salient features*:**

Pharmaceutical Sterilization-in-Place (SIP) systems are designed to sterilize a collection of process equipment after a batch of product is completed.

- Equipment such as bioreactors, fermentors and the accompanying tubing must be cleaned and/or sterilized before a new production cycle.
- The steam pressures seen are typically in the 20-30 psi range with corresponding temperatures ranging from 121°C to 135°C.
- The relationship between pressure and temperature is a given, however sterilization times will range depending on the temperature and the nature of the item being sterilized.
- In general, the lower the temperature, the longer it takes to sterilize.
- The sterilization time/temperature relationship in a typical SIP process will occur at about 121°C for 30-40 minutes.
- For systems with hard to reach components, times can increase.

SIP Advantages

- It is the only technique for large equipment obviates the need for large autoclaves
- Reduces clean room operation activity

- Enhanced system integrity or reduction of aseptic connections or reduction of flexible hoses

Water for Injection Systems (WFI)

Water for Injection (WFI) System comprises of multicolumn Distillation Plant, WFI Storage System and Pure Steam Generator.

The pre-treatment system comprises of: Pressure Filters, Activated Carbon Filters, D.M. Plant or Reverse Osmosis system (with Softner), Ultra-Filtration system, UV Sterilizer, Storage and Distribution loop system

Multicolumn Distillation Plant

To industries where 100% pure Pyrogen - free water-for injection plays role, Multicolumn Distillation Plant is the perfect solution. Available in capacities ranging from 80 - 5000 LPH, the Multicolumn Distilled plant is used for its economy, low maintenance and low operation costs.

Distilled Water Storage Tank

Vertical / Horizontal Distilled Water Storage Tank is available in both jacketed and non jacketed design. The tank is designed to withstand pressure as well as vacuum. Therefore it can be steam sterilized.

Pure Steam Generator

Pure Steam Generator for the Pharmaceutical and Biotech Industries is the most reliable technology for producing pure, Pyrogen free sterile Steam. Pure Steam is defined as uncondensed Water for Injection and meets the Indian, British and the United States Pharmacopoeia.

Advantages

- Pure Pyrogen free sterile steam is available for Sterilization.
- Pure Steam when condensed will give WFI quality water. This is very advantageous, as steam which gets condensed after sterilization will not be a source of contamination.
- It is ideal in sterilization of Pipelines, Tanks, Fermentors etc.

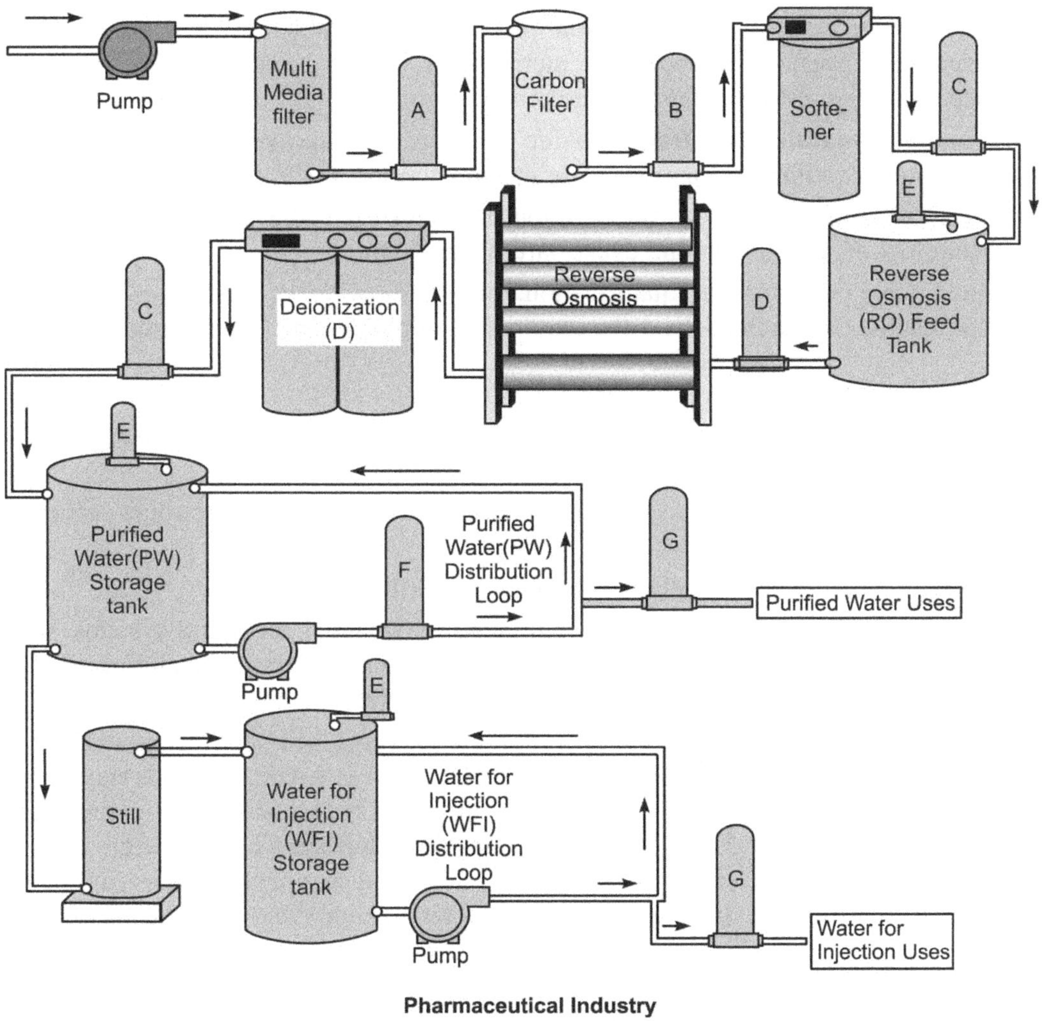

Fig. 4.15 Water for injection systems

4.9 Sterilization Indicators

4.9.1 Validation of Sterilization Process

Validation is defined as the documented procedure for obtaining; recording process will consistently comply with predetermined specifications.

- The efficiency of any sterilization process can only be assured, it cannot be guaranteed because a process of sterilization cannot be verified by subsequent inspection and testing of the finished product.

Performance Qualification Data provide evidence that the process equipment will produce a product with an acceptable assurance of sterility.

- Physical performance of qualification provides that the specified sterilization conditions are attained within every part of the product.
- Biological performance qualification provides evidence that the specialized sterilization conditions deliver the required microbial lethality to the product.

Physical Methods

Heat distribution within the sterilizer chamber or load is usually measured using thermocouples.

- Pressure gauges or pressure transducers connected to electronic recording instruments.
- Physical measurement of relative humidity in sterilizers is difficult
- Microprocessor controlled sterilizers utilize multichannel recording systems, which are able to handle large amounts of data from physical instruments and give a more detailed control and monitoring of sterilization cycle.

Mechanical monitoring: sterilizer operation must be watched carefully to observe the machine's dials and gauges and listen as it functions to make sure it sounds normal. For example, a steam sterilizer that makes a hissing noise or has difficulty getting up to pressure may need a new door gasket. Although some sterilizers have recording devices that document these physical parameters of time and temperature for each cycle, handwritten records of the date, run number, time, temperature, and pressure will suffice.

Chemical Methods

Chemical monitoring is based on the ability of the sterilization process to produce sufficient change in the physical and or chemical characteristics of chemical substances which are detected visually or by physically instrumentation.

(i) CI types and uses: One type of chemical monitoring involves the use of CIs that change color or physical form when exposed to certain temperatures. Examples would be autoclave tape and special markings on sterilization pouches and bags. This type of indicator is commonly used as an external indicator on the outside of every pack, pouch, or cassette to indicate that the item has at least been processed through a heat sterilizer. This distinguishes the items that have been heat-processed from those that have not; otherwise, the two types may appear identical. In turn, this helps prevent the accidental clinical use of unprocessed items.

(ii) A second type of CI, an integrated indicator, changes color or form more slowly, and responds to a combination of time and temperature or to a process involving time, temperature, and the presence of steam. Integrated indicators commonly are used on the inside of every pack, pouch, or cassette to ensure that the instruments inside the packaging material all have been exposed to sterilizing conditions. If these CIs placed inside paper/plastic peel pouches are visible from the outside, there is no need to use an external CI.

When it comes to instrument processing and sterilization, better to use all three methods of monitoring mechanical, chemical, and biologic to help ensure sterility. Mechanically monitor each sterilizer load and chemically monitor each package in each load. Biologically monitor every sterilizer at least once a week. Accurate records on all monitoring should be kept. Of the three methods, biologic monitoring is regarded as the most valid for monitoring the sterilization process, for it uses live, highly resistant bacterial spores. Chemical monitoring uses, heat-sensitive or heat-time-steam-sensitive chemicals that change color. It may also help to immediately detect certain sterilizer malfunctions and help to earmark procedural problems. In addition, use of mechanical monitoring by observing the time, temperature and pressure of sterilizer cycles may provide early detection of a mechanical problem.

4.10 Biological Indicators

A biological indicator is a preparation of micro-organisms usually bacterial spores that is carried either directly by some of the items to be sterilized or by adventitious carriers such as filter papers, threads and porcelain cylinders and that serves as a challenge to the effectiveness of a given sterilization process (or) cycle.

Types of BIs: BIs contain the bacterial spores used for monitoring. The spores used are *Geobacillus stearothermophilus* (for testing steam or chemical vapor sterilization) or *Bacillus subtilis* (for testing dry-heat or ethylene oxide gas sterilization).

(i) Spore strips. BIs are packaged in different varieties. Spore strips are one-inch paper strips that contain one or both types of monitoring spores. The spore strip is enclosed in a protective glassine envelope. After processing through the sterilizer, the strip is aseptically removed from the envelope and placed in a tube of appropriate Tryptic-soy broth medium that in turn is incubated for two to seven days at 55 °C/131°F (for *G. stearothermophilus*) or at 37 °C/98.6 °F (for *B. subtilis*). If live bacterial spores still are present, they will grow and produce cloudiness and/or change the color of the growth medium, indicating sterilization failure. Spore strip BIs can be used to monitor all forms of heat sterilization.

(ii) Self-contained vial. Another type of BI is a self-contained vial. This comprises both a spore strip or disk and an ampoule filled with growth medium, contained in a plastic vial with a vented cap to permit entrance of the sterilizing agent into the vial. After processing through the sterilizer, either the vial is squeezed or the cap is pushed down to break the internal ampule, which mixes the growth medium with the spores. The vial is then incubated at 55 °C/131 °F, and if live bacterial spores still are present, they will grow and change the color of the growth medium, indicating sterilization failure. Moist heat sterilization (autoclaving) – spores of *Bacillus Stearothermophilus*

I.P 1996 Recommends the following Biological Indicators

(i) *Clostridium sporogens*

Dry heat sterilization

Ethylene oxide sterilization

Spores of *Bacillus subtilis var. niger.*

Radiation Sterilization

(ii) *Spores* of *Bacillus pumilis*

- Biological indicator should be used only for the sterilization process for which they are intended and strictly in accordance with the manufacturer's directions

D-Value: Decimal reduction time, it has gained wide acceptance. The decimal reduction time is the time required to kill 90% of the micro-organisms or spores in a sample at a specified temperature. D values are used to estimate the relative resistance of micro-organisms to different temperature through the calculation of the Z value.

Z-Value: Z-value is the increase in the temperature required to reduce D-value to $1/10^{th}$ of its value (or) to reduce it by one log cycle. When D is plotted against temperature Z-value is used in the calculation of time-temperature relationships for survival of a test microorganism based on D-value responses at various temperatures. The Z-value is the increase in temperature needed to reduce the decimal reduction time (D) to 10% of its original value.

F-Value: F–value is the time in minutes at a specified temperature (usually 250°F or 121.1 °C) needed to kill a population of cells or spores.

4.11 Quality Control of Microorganism: Sterility Testing

Introduction

Sterility testing is a crucial step in quality control that must be taken to ensure the safety of products in the cosmetic, pharmaceutical, medical device and diagnostic equipment industries.

The principle is that the testing looks for both aerobic & anaerobic contamination of the product undergoing the sterility test.

According to Indian pharmacopoeia (1996) the STERILITY TESTS are intended for detecting the presence of viable forms of micro-organisms in or on the pharmacopoeial preparations.

4.11.1 Definitions

(a) **Colony Forming Unit (CFU):** Visible outcome of growth of micro-organisms arising from a single or multiple cells.

(b) **Growth Promotion Test:** Also referred to as fertility or nutritive properties test, which is performed on the media used during the sterility test to demonstrate that it is capable of supporting the growth of micro-organisms

(c) **Negative Controls:** Refers to the sterility test controls that may be used to identify a "false positive" test result'. Growth in the media sterility test, or environmental monitoring, or negative product controls may contribute to the verification of a "false positive" test finding and an invalid test result.

(d) **Negative Product Controls:** Product or simulated product of known or undoubted sterility that is tested during the same test session as the product test samples. Negative product controls should be exposed to a terminal sterilization process, such as exposure to steam sterilization, gamma – irradiation etc., and be packaged in terms of manipulations required of the test operator.

(e) **Positive Controls:** Refers to the sterility test controls that may be used to define a "false negative" test result. An absence of growth of test challenge micro-organisms in the growth promotion, validation or "stasis" tests would result in a "false negative" test finding & an invalid test result.

(f) **Stasis Test:** Also referred to as an inhibition test, which is performed to ensure that there are no inhibitory substances remaining in the product and that the media is still capable of supporting the growth of micro-organisms at the end of the sterility test incubation period. This test is not mandatory but it may be useful to confirm the inactivation of antimicrobial substances in products. Where a marginal test methodology is employed routinely, after an initial successful test validation.

In practice, the sterility of a product is defined by the absence of viable & actively multiplying micro-organisms. When tested in specified culture media, turbidity in the broth media usually indicated contamination. This test is performed on the end – product and is one of the quality control tests specified for release of a batch of sterile product. The sterility test cannot be used to demonstrate the sterility of the entire batch but it may assist in identifying a non–sterile batch of a product.

4.11.2 Sterility Test Facilities

Sterility testing should be performed under aseptic conditions which are preferably consistent with the standard of clean room required for the aseptic manufacture of pharmaceutical products. Premises and equipment should be qualified according to the relevant principle of installation qualification & operational qualification (IQ/ OQ).

The sterility test should be conducted within a class A Laminar air flow cabinet located within a class B clean room, or in an isolator that need not be located within a controlled environment.

Air supplied to the environment should be provided through terminal HEPA filters. There should be a pressure differential of not less than 10 to 15 Pascals (guidance value) between each of the areas i.e., ambient / air lock and air lock / test room. Entry to the clean room should be via an air lock in which operators are required to change into a clean room garments. Protective garments should be changed for each work session or at least once a day if justified from the results of microbiological monitoring and validation studies.

Clean room fitting such as power outlets and light fittings should be flushed with the wall or ceiling surfaces and sealed to prevent entrainment of unclean air. Surfaces should be smooth and impervious to the cleaning agents used. Ultraviolet lamps may be fitted with in pass-through cabinets.

Outer surfaces of samples and equipment entering the testing suite should be disinfected, preferably with a sporicidal agent. Disinfectants used for cleaning should be free of microbiological contamination, which may be achieved through aseptic filtration or use of a product-compatible terminal sterilization method.

Environmental monitoring should be performed under operational (dynamic) conditions either within the isolator or in the laminar air-flow and associated background areas. This includes a combination of air and surface.

Sample methods, such as:

- Active air sampling
- Settle (exposure) plates
- Surface contact (RODAC) plates, swabs or flexible films.
- Operators gloved hand plates.

4.11.3 Tests for Sterility

Principle: Tests for Sterility are applied to substances or preparations which are required to be sterile, according to the pharmacopoeial standards. However, a satisfactory result only indicates that no contaminating microorganism has been found in the sample examined in the conditions of the test.

Very low levels of contamination cannot be detected on the basis of random sampling of a lot. Moreover, if contamination is not uniform throughout the lot, random sampling cannot detect contamination with any certainty. Compliance with the test for sterility alone cannot therefore provide absolute assurance of freedom from microbial contamination. Greater assurance of sterility must come from reliable manufacturing procedures and compliance with good manufacturing practice.

Precautions against microbial contamination

The test for sterility is carried out under aseptic conditions.

The test environment has to be adapted to the way in which the sterility test is performed.

The precautions taken to avoid contamination and they do not affect any micro-organisms which are to be revealed in the test.

The working conditions are monitored regularly by appropriate sampling of the working area and by carrying out appropriate controls.

Culture media and incubation temperatures

Media for the test may be prepared as described below or equivalent commercial media may be used, provided that they comply with the growth promotion test.

Fluid thioglycollate medium is primarily intended for the culture of anaerobic bacteria; however, it will also detect aerobic bacteria.

Soya-bean casein digest medium is suitable for the culture of both fungi and aerobic bacteria.

Fluid Thioglycollate Medium Composition

L-Cystine	0.5 g
Agar	0.75 g
Sodium chloride	2.5 g
Glucose monohydrate/anhydrous	5.5/5.0 g
Yeast extract (water-soluble)	5.0 g
Pancreatic digest of casein	15.0 g
Sodium thioglycollate or	0.5 g
Thioglycollic acid	0.3 mL
Resazurin sodium solution (1 g/l of resazurin sodium), freshly prepared	1.0 mL
Water R	1000 mL
pH after sterilization	6.9 - 7.3.

Mix the l-cystine, agar, sodium chloride, glucose, water-soluble yeast extract and pancreatic digest of casein with the water R and heat until solution is effected. Dissolve the sodium thioglycollate or thioglycollic acid in the solution and, if necessary, add sodium hydroxide (1 mol/L) VS so that, after sterilization, the solution will have a pH of 6.9-7.3. If filtration is necessary heat the solution again without boiling and filter while hot through moistened filter paper. Add the resazurin sodium solution, mix and place the medium in suitable vessels, which provide a ratio of surface to depth of medium such that not more than the upper half of the medium has undergone a colour change, indicative of oxygen uptake at the end of the incubation period. Sterilize using a validated process. If the medium is stored at a temperature between 2°C and 25°C in a sterile, airtight container. If more than the upper one-third of the medium has acquired a pink colour, the medium may be restored once by heating the containers in a water-bath or in free-flowing steam until the pink colour disappears and cooling quickly, taking care to prevent the introduction of non-sterile air into the container. Do not use the medium for a longer storage period than has been validated.

Fluid thioglycollate medium is to be incubated at 30-35°C.

For products containing a mercurial preservative that cannot be tested by the membrane-filtration method fluid thioglycollate medium incubated at 20-25°C may be used instead of soya-bean casein digest medium provided that it has been validated as described in growth promotion test.

- **Alternative Thioglycollate Medium**

  Where prescribed or justified and authorized, the following alternative thioglycollate medium might be used. Prepare a mixture having the same composition as that of the fluid thioglycollate medium, but omitting the agar and the resazurin sodium solution, sterilize as directed above. The pH after sterilization is 6.9–7.3. Heat in a water-bath prior to use and incubate at 30–35 °C under anaerobic conditions.

Soya-bean Casein Digest Medium Composition

Table 4.4

Pancreatic digest of casein	17.0 g
Papaic digest of soya-bean meal	3.0 g
Sodium chloride	5.0 g
Dipotassium hydrogen phosphate	2.5g
Glucose monohydrate/anhydrous	2.5/2.3 g
Water R	1 000 mL
pH after sterilization 7.1–7.5.	

Dissolve the solids in water R, warming slightly to effect solution. Cool the solution to room temperature. Add sodium hydroxide (1 mol/L) VS, if necessary, so that after sterilization the solution will have a pH of 7.1–7.5. Filter, if necessary, to clarify, distribute into suitable vessels and sterilize using a validated process. Store at a temperature between 2 °C and 25 °C in a sterile, well-closed container, unless it is intended for immediate use. Do not use the medium for a longer storage period than has been validated.

Soya-bean casein digest medium is to be incubated at 20–25 °C.

The media used comply with the following tests:

These tests are carried out before or in parallel with the test on the product to be examined.

Sterility: Incubate portions of the media for 14 days. No growth of micro-organisms occurs.

Growth promotion test of micro-organisms: Test each batch of ready-prepared medium and each batch of medium prepared either from dehydrated medium or from ingredients. Suitable strains of aerobes, anaerobes and fungi, micro-organisms are indicated in Table 4.1.

Inoculate portions of fluid thioglycollate medium with a small number (not more than 100 CFU) of the following micro-organisms, using a separate portion of medium for each of the following species of microorganism: *Clostridium sporogenes*, *Pseudomonas aeruginosa*, *Staphylococcus aureus* given Table 4.5. Inoculate portions of soya-bean casein digest medium with a small number (not more than 100 CFU) of the following micro-organisms, using a separate portion of medium for each of the following species of microorganism: *Aspergillus brasiliensis*, *Bacillus subtilis*, *Candida albicans*. Incubate for not more than 3 days in the case of bacteria and not more than 5 days in the case of fungi.

Seed-lot culture maintenance techniques (seed-lot systems) are used so that the viable micro-organisms used for inoculation are not more than five passages removed from the original master seed-lot.

The media are suitable if a clearly visible growth of the micro-organisms occurs.

Table 4.5 Strains of the test micro-organisms suitable for use in the Growth promotion test and the Method suitability test

Aerobic bacteria	
Staphylococcus aureus	ATCC 6538, CIP 4.83, NCTC 10788, NCIMB 9518, NBRC 13276
Bacillus subtilis	ATCC 6633, CIP 52.62, NCIMB 8054, NBRC 3134
Pseudomonas aeruginosa	ATCC 9027, NCIMB 8626, CIP 82.118, NBRC 13275
Anaerobic bacterium	
Clostridium sporogenes	ATCC 19404, CIP 79.3, NCTC 532, ATCC 11437, NBRC 14293
Fungi	
Candida albicans	ATCC 10231, IP 48.72, NCPF 3179, NBRC 1594
Aspergillus brasiliensis	ATCC 16404, IP 1431.83, IMI 149007, NBRC 9455

Method Suitability Test

This kind of test will help us to know whether product under test posseses any antimicrobial action or not. In case the product contains antimicrobial activity procedure should be modified. **Membrane filtration.** After transferring the content of the container or containers to be tested to the membrane add an inoculum of a small number of viable micro-organisms (not more than 100 CFU) to the final portion of sterile **diluent** used to rinse the filter. The flow chart of this test is shown in Fig. 4.16.

Direct Inoculation. After transferring the contents of the container or containers to be tested to the culture medium add an inoculum of a small number of viable micro-organisms (not more than 100 CFU) to the **medium**.

In both cases use **the same micro-organisms** as those described above under Growth promotion test of aerobes, anaerobes and fungi. Perform a growth promotion test as a positive control. Incubate all the containers containing medium for not more than **5** days.

If clearly **visible growth** of micro-organisms is obtained after the incubation, visually comparable to that in the control vessel without product, either **the product possesses no antimicrobial activity** under the conditions of the test **or such activity** has been satisfactorily **eliminated**. The test for sterility may then be carried out **without further modification.**

If clearly **visible growth is not obtained** in the presence of the product to be tested, visually comparable to that in the control vessels without product, **the product possesses antimicrobial activity** that has not been satisfactorily eliminated under the conditions of the test. **Modify the conditions** in order to eliminate the antimicrobial activity and repeat the method suitability test.

This method suitability is performed:

(a) when the test for sterility has to be carried out on a new product;

(b) whenever there is a change in the experimental conditions of the test.

The method suitability may be performed simultaneously with the Test for sterility of the product to be examined.

Test for sterility of the product to be examined

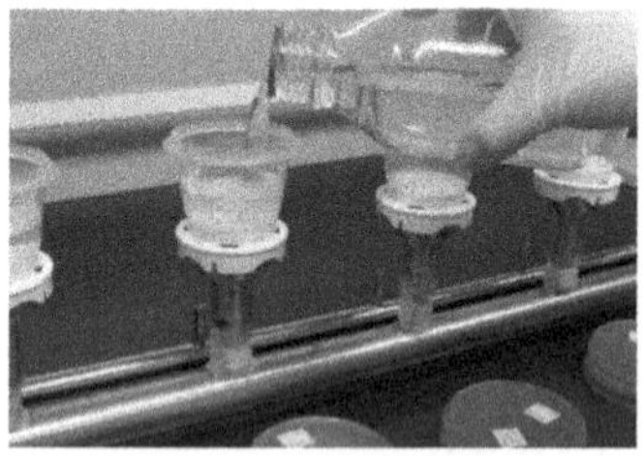

The test may be carried out using the technique of membrane filtration or by direct inoculation of the culture media with the product to be examined. Appropriate negative controls are included.

Conditions to use membrane filtration method

The product is filterable aqueous preparation,

Alcoholic or oily preparations

Preparations miscible with or soluble in aqueous or oily solvents

Solvents used in the preparations do not have an antimicrobial effect in the conditions of the test.

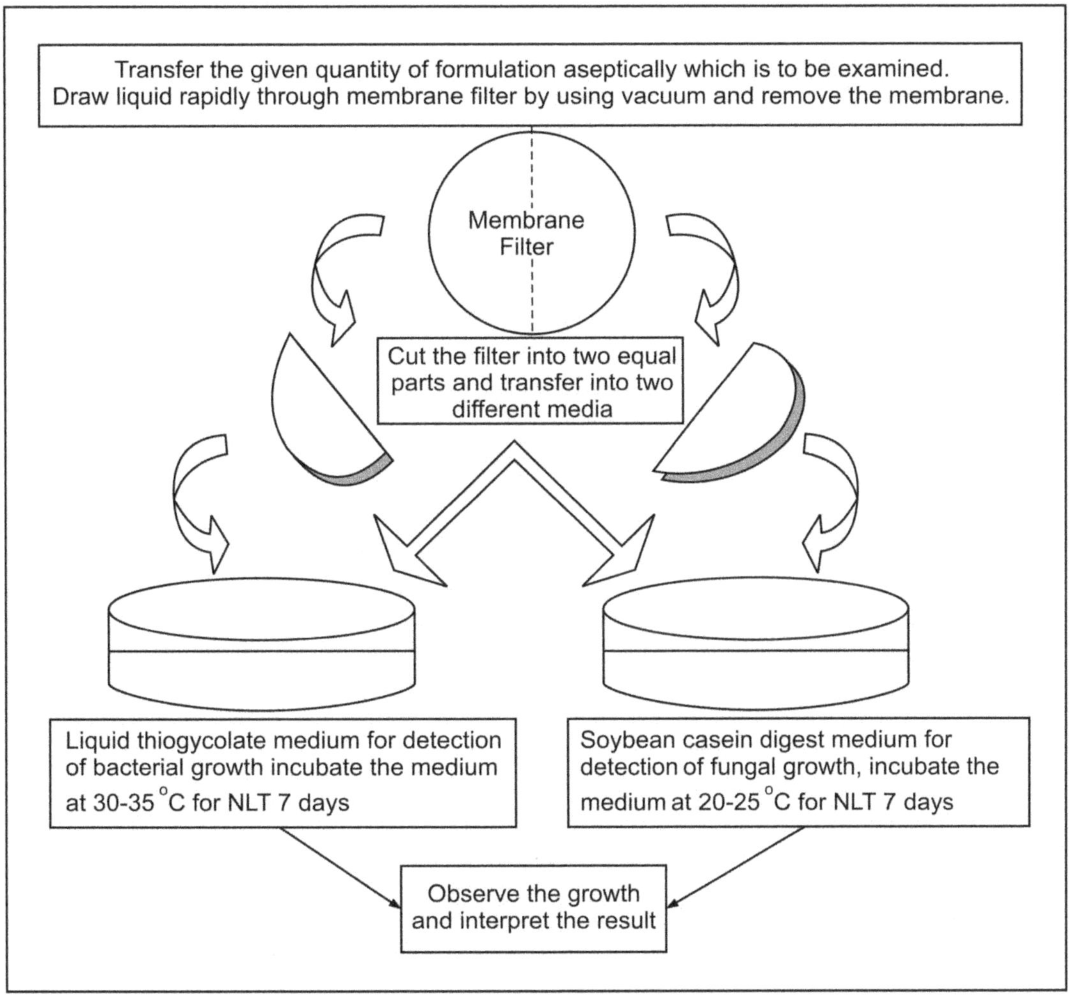

Fig. 4.16 Test for sterility procedure flow chart

Membrane filtration: Membrane filters about 50 mm in diameter having a nominal pore size not greater than 0.45 μm whose effectiveness to retain micro-organisms that has been established must be used.

Cellulose nitrate filters, for example, are used for aqueous, oily and weakly alcoholic solutions. Cellulose acetate filters, for example, for strongly alcoholic solutions.

Specially adapted filters may be needed for certain products, *e.g.*, for antibiotics.

The diameter of the membrane filter is crucial, if different diameter are used the volumes of the dilutions and the washings should be adjusted accordingly.

The filtration apparatus and membrane are sterilized by appropriate means.

The apparatus is designed so that the solution to be examined can be introduced and filtered under aseptic conditions;

The operation must permit the aseptic removal of the membrane for transfer into the medium or incubation suitability after adding the medium to the apparatus itself.

***Aqueous solutions*:** Appropriately transfer a small quantity of a suitable, sterile diluent such as a 1 g/L neutral solution of meat or casein peptone pH 6.9-7.3 onto the membrane in the apparatus and filter. (The diluent may contain suitable neutralizing substances and/or appropriate inactivating substances for example in the case of antibiotics).

Transfer the contents of the container or containers to be tested to the membrane or membranes, (if necessary after diluting to the volume used in the method suitability test with the chosen sterile diluent, but in any case using not less than the quantities of the product to be examined, prescribed in Table 4.6).

Table 4.6 Minimum Quantity to be used for each Medium

Quantity Per Container	Minimum quantity to be used for each medium unless otherwise justified and authorized
Liquids	
•less than 1 mL	The whole contents of each container
•1-40 mL	Half the contents of each container but not less than 1 mL
•greater than 40 mL and not greater than 100 mL	20 mL
•greater than 100 mL	10% of the contents of the container but not less than 20 mL
Antibiotic liquids	1 mL
Insoluble preparations, creams and ointments to be suspended or emulsified	Use the contents of each container to provide not less than 200 mg
Solids	
•less than 50 mg	The whole contents of each container
•50 mg or more but less than 300 mg	Half the contents of each container but not less than 50 mg
•300 mg–5 g	150 mg
•greater than 5 g	500 mg

Filter immediately. (If the product has antimicrobial properties wash the membrane not less than three times by filtering through it each time the volume of the chosen sterile diluent used in the method suitability test).

Do not exceed a washing-cycle of five times 100 mL per filter, (even if during method suitability it has been demonstrated that such a cycle does not fully eliminate the antimicrobial activity).

Transfer the whole membrane to the culture medium or cut it aseptically into two equal parts and transfer one half to each of two suitable media.

Use the same volume of each medium as in the method suitability test.

Alternatively transfer the medium onto the membrane in the apparatus.

Incubate the media for not less than 14 days.

Soluble Solids

Use for each medium not less than the quantity prescribed in Table 4.2 of the product

Dissolve the product in a suitable solvent such as the solvent provided with the preparation, water for injections R, sodium chloride (9 g/L) *TS or peptone (1 g/L) TS1

Finally proceed with the test as described above for aqueous solutions using a membrane appropriate to the chosen solvent.

*Pharmacopoeial Test Solutions

Oils and oily solutions: Use for each medium not less than the quantity of the product prescribed in Table 4.5.

Oils and oily solutions of sufficiently low viscosity may be filtered without dilution through a dry membrane.

Viscous oils may be diluted as necessary with a suitable sterile diluents such as isopropyl myristate R shown not to have antimicrobial activity in the conditions of the test.

Allow the oil to penetrate the membrane by its own weight then filter, applying the pressure or suction gradually.

Wash the membrane at least three times by filtering through it each time about 100 mL of a suitable sterile solution such as peptone (1 g/L) TS1 containing a suitable emulsifying agent at a concentration shown to be appropriate in the method suitability test (for example polysorbate 80 at a concentration of 10 g/L).

Transfer the membrane or membranes to the culture medium or media or vice versa as described above for aqueous solutions and incubate at the same temperatures and for the same times.

Ointments and creams. Use for each medium not less than the quantities of the product prescribed in Table 4.5.

Ointments in a fatty base and emulsions of the water-in-oil type may be diluted to 1% in isopropyl myristate R as described above, by heating, if necessary, to not more than 40°C.

In exceptional cases it may be necessary to heat to not more than 44°C.

Filter as rapidly as possible and

Proceed as described above for oils and oily solutions.

Direct inoculation of the culture medium: Transfer the quantity of the preparation to be examined prescribed in Table 4.5 directly into the culture medium so that the volume of the product is not more than 10% of the volume of the medium, unless otherwise prescribed.

If the product to be examined has antimicrobial activity carry out the test after neutralizing this with a suitable neutralizing substance or by dilution in a sufficient quantity of culture medium.

When it is necessary to use a large volume of the product it may be preferable to use a concentrated culture medium prepared in such a way that it takes account of the subsequent dilution.

Where appropriate and concentrated medium may be added directly to the product in its container.

Oily liquids: Use media to which have been added a suitable emulsifying agent at a concentration shown to be appropriate in the method suitability of the test, for example, polysorbate 80 at a concentration of 10 g/L.

Ointments and creams: Prepare by diluting to about 1 in 10 by emulsifying with the chosen emulsifying agent in a suitable sterile diluent such as peptone (1 g/L) TS1.

Transfer the diluted product to a medium not containing an emulsifying agent.

Incubate the inoculated media for not less than 14 days.

Observe the cultures several times during the incubation period.

Shake cultures containing oily products gently each day. However when fluid thioglycollate medium is used for the detection of anaerobic micro-organisms, keep shaking or mixing to a minimum in order to maintain anaerobic conditions.

Observation and Interpretation of Results

At intervals during the incubation period and at its conclusion examine the media for macroscopic evidence of microbial growth.

If the material being tested renders the medium turbid so that the presence or absence of microbial growth cannot be readily determined by visual examination, 14 days after the beginning of incubation transfer portions (each not less than 1 mL) of the medium to fresh vessels of the same medium and then incubate the original and transfer vessels for not less than 4 days.

If no evidence of microbial growth is found the product to be examined complies with the test for sterility.

If evidence of microbial growth is found the product to be examined does not comply with the test for sterility, unless it can be clearly demonstrated that the test was invalid for causes unrelated to the product to be examined.

Do not repeat the test unless it can be clearly shown that the test was invalid for causes unrelated to the preparation under examination.

The test may be considered invalid only if one or more of the following conditions are fulfilled:

(a) The data of the microbiological monitoring of the sterility testing facility show a fault;
(b) A review of the testing procedure used during the test in question reveals a fault;
(c) Microbial growth is found in the negative controls;
(d) After determination of the identity of the micro-organisms isolated from the test, the growth of this species or these species may be ascribed unequivocally to faults with respect to the material and/or the technique used in conducting the sterility test procedure.

If the test is declared to be invalid, it is repeated with the same number of units as in the original test.

If no evidence of microbial growth is found in the repeat test the product examined complies with the test for sterility. If microbial growth is found in the repeat test the product examined does not comply with the test for sterility.

Minimum number of items to be tested

The minimum number of items to be tested in relation to the size of the batch is given in Table 4.7.

Table 4.7 Minimum Number of items to be Tested

Number of items in the batch*	Minimum number of items to be tested for each medium, unless otherwise justified and authorized**
Parenteral preparations	
Not more than 100 containers	10% or 4 containers whichever is the greater
More than 100 but not more than 500 containers	10 containers
More than 500 containers	2% or 20 containers (10 containers for large-volume parenterals) whichever is the less
Ophthalmic and other non-injectable	
Not more than 200 containers	5% or 2 containers whichever is the greater
More than 200 containers	10 containers
If the product is presented in the form of single-dose containers, apply the scheme shown above for preparations for parenteral use	
Bulk solid products	
Up to 4 containers	Each container
More than 4 containers but not more than 50 containers	20% or 4 containers whichever is the greater
More than 50 containers	2% or 10 containers whichever is the greater

Adapted from the Fourth Supplement 2014; to the Fourth Edition of *The International Pharmacopoeia*

*If the batch size is not known, use the maximum number of items prescribed.

**If the contents of one container are enough to inoculate the two media, this column gives the number of containers needed for both the media together.

Aseptic techniques are defined as a set of procedures carried out to obtain an environment with minimal contamination from pathogenic microorganisms. These procedures are carried out under controlled conditions. The main goal of aseptic technique is to provide protection against infections.

4.12 Design of Aseptic Area

General Requirements

1. *Site of premises*: Aseptic area should be designed at a site away from stairs, lift shafts, corridors and general manufacturing area as these areas are capable of providing routes by which microorganisms may travel. Each stage of the production should be carried out in separate rooms of aseptic area. Store rooms should be adjacent to aseptic area where all sterile equipments and products can be stored.
2. *Size of premises*: Aseptic area should be large and spacious by which overall effect of microorganisms can be reduced which ultimately results in minimal contamination.
3. *Windows*: Large windows with transparent glass are suitable for aseptic area. Windows should remain closed and ventilation should be provided artificially by air filtration system. These type of windows are used to prevent heat loss from glass material.
4. *Doors*: Entrance should have double doors with an air-lock system. In this way, air entering from outside into the aseptic area can be prevented. High speed roll-up doors, sliding doors,
5. *Floors, walls and bench tops*: The floor, walls and bench tops should be, Easy to clean, smooth with no cracks and pores, impervious to cleaning agents like disinfectants and chemically resistant to solvents, dyes, strong acids or alkalies.

   Floor should be made up of the following materials, Terrazzo, Linoleum and plastics. Terrazzo is hard, durable long-lasting surface with excellent chemical resistance and very expensive to install

   Walls and ceiling should have surfaces made up of, Tiles that are smooth, non-absorbent in nature, Glass paint, Plastic laminate.
6. *Tops of working bench*: The tops of the working benches should be made up either of the Stainless steel or plastic laminates. Stainless steel often used throughout the facility because of its appearance, durability, smoothness, and resistance to rust, peeling and shedding

   Environmental monitoring in aseptic area: air controlling in the aseptic areas is done using laminar air flow systems.

Laminar air flow systems are generally of three types:

1. Vertical flow system
2. Horizontal flow system and
3. Wall to floor flow system

1. **Vertical flow system:** This system consists of false floor & ceiling. The air is filtered through pre-filters, electrostatic filters and HEPA filters in sequence. These 3 filters are placed in false ceiling. From the false floor, a small portion of filtered air is recirculated in to false ceiling through a recirculation duct

Advantages: The operating area is provided with exhaust filters which remove the remaining portion of the air. This provides protection to the operator. It is more preferable when compared to horizontal flow systems.

Disadvantages: It is an expensive system as it requires double installation of HEPA filters.

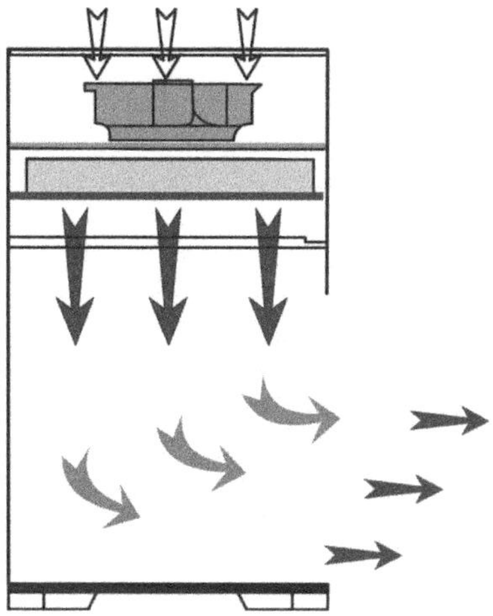

Fig. 4.17 Vertical flow system

2. **Horizontal flow system:** In this system, the air is filtered through prefilters, HEPA filters which are placed in lateral walls. Air is recirculated through punched plate wall or recirculation duct. Achievement of complete sterile conditions is not possible because the airflow is not focused on working area.

   The drawback of this system is during the handling of materials like antineoplastic drugs, this system fails to provide protection to the operator.

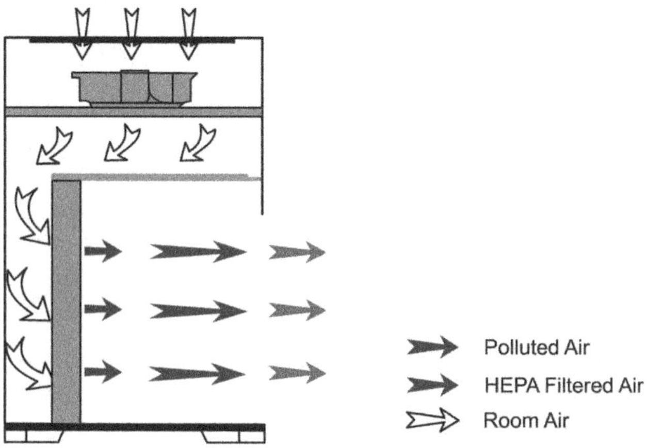

Fig. 4.18 Horizontal flow system

3. **Wall to floor system:** In this system, the filtered air enters from the lateral wall with an inclined flow towards the floor. This system offers high aseptic conditions but it is expensive.

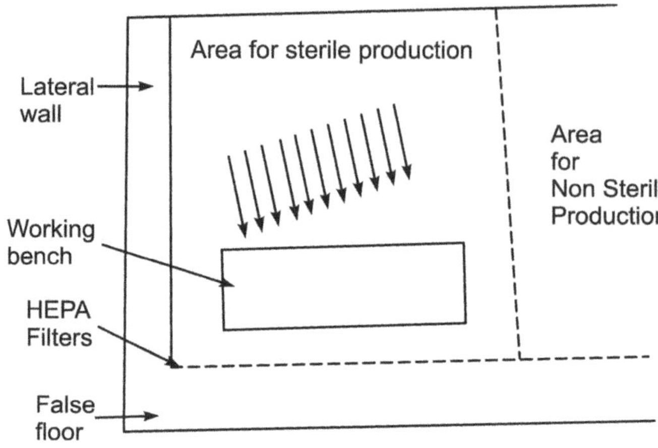

Fig. 4.19 Wall to floor system

4.12.1 Contamination sources in Aseptic Area and Prevention Methods

There are several sources of contamination such as process equipment, personnel and surfaces. Biological contaminants are ubiquitous. Microorganisms such as bacteria or fungi roam free in most environments and can cause disease. A major goal of aseptic applications, including surgery, pharmaceutical compounding or medical implant packaging is to *prevent* contaminants. Contaminants can be grouped into two categories, particulate (non-viable) or microbial (viable), and neither type may be visible to the naked eye.

Sources of contamination in Aseptic Area

Microbial and particulate contamination sources in the cleanroom include humans, air, surfaces, water, and the components used to manufacture the product. Humans are the main source of cleanroom contamination. People can also expel contaminants by talking, sneezing, and coughing, even while wearing a mask and depending upon the type of mask and other factors, not all particulate contaminants may be blocked.

The process of product contamination is influenced by many factors. Contamination can be introduced by materials, water, the degree of human contact, and the manufacturing environment. People and their specific activities may have direct contact with the product.

Contaminated work surfaces, tools, and fixtures can provide a direct transfer of contamination to the product

Control of Contaminants in the Aseptic Area

Each individual step in the entire biomanufacturing process, from the raw materials at the start to the final finished product, should be examined for potential risks. An approach used to examine the steps in a process is called the Hazard Analysis and Critical Control Points (HACCP).

Control through Facility Design

Aseptic area is a place where an attempt is made to limit, control, and eliminate the amount of airborne contamination. Many contaminants are continuously generated within a cleanroom by people, processes, equipment, and the facility, which are then transferred through the flow of air. Eliminating these contaminants is a function of appropriate facility design

Control through Air Supply

Cleanrooms used for aseptic processing require High Efficiency Particulate Air (HEPA) filters. HEPA filters are used to supply clean air to controlled areas such as cleanrooms. HEPA filters remove 99.97 percent of the particles suspended in air that are 0.3 microns or larger in size

Additional ways by which to maintain this environment include specific construction materials, air classifications, pressure differentials, airlocks, restricted entry, and flow of people and materials.

Control through Sterilization of Components and Equipment

The components and equipment used in aseptic biomanufacturing must be sterilized. Sterilization methods vary based on the material of the components to be sterilized. Commonly used methods for sterilization of biopharmaceuticals include: dry heat, gamma irradiation, ethylene oxide, Vaporized Hydrogen Peroxide (VHP)

Control by Aseptic Gowning

Wearing clean, sterilized clothing is necessary to protect the product and critical surfaces from contamination. Aseptic gowns, consisting of a gown, mask, gloves, goggles, and boots, cover all or most of a person. Individuals working within cleanrooms must be properly trained on aseptic gowning. The apparel provides a barrier between the individual wearing it and the sterile components and products; however, aseptic gowning does not provide 100 percent protection. Microorganisms have the ability to penetrate woven or non-woven fabrics to emerge into the surrounding air, thus proper gowning reduces but does not eliminate microorganisms shed by people in cleanrooms.

Control through Aseptic Techniques

Every activity that is done for aseptic processing should be performed with the mindset of reducing the probability of risk to the lowest-acceptable level.

Aseptic technique guidelines when working under a Biological Safety Cabinet

When working with a biological safety cabinet (BSC) as part of the aseptic process, it is important to understand the associated guidelines and limitations of their use.

BSCs and cleanrooms are categorized as Class 100 environments. This means that one cubic foot of air may have no more than 100 particles of 0.5 microns or larger. The critical surfaces in the aseptic processing area in the biological safety cabinet must see the first air from the HEPA filter.

Control by Cleaning and Disinfection

Cleaning

Cleaning is used to remove contaminants and residues that can interfere with the effectiveness of disinfectants. Proper cleaning is important for a successful disinfection. Cleaning does not have to be performed at the same frequency of disinfection. An example of a four-step cleaning process of a surface involves:

1. Scrubbing the surface with a mop or wipe and using a detergent solution
2. Rinsing the surface before the surface dries
3. Collecting any remaining liquid on the surface by wiping or vacuuming
4. Allowing the surface to dry then disinfecting

Disinfection

A disinfectant is defined as a chemical agent used on surfaces that destroys disease-causing microorganisms. Each type of disinfectant is also categorized by its use and the microorganisms against which itis effective: bacterial agents, fungicidal agents (fungi), virucidal agents (destroy/inactivate viruses), sporicidal agents (bacterial and fungal spores), and bacteriostatic agents (prevent the growth of bacteria but do not necessarily kill them). Solutions of these disinfectants must be sterile when used in Class 100 and Class 10,000 area classifications. Examples of disinfectants are sodium hypochlorite (halogen), 70% isopropyl alcohol (IPA), and peracetic acid (peroxygen).

Clean Room Classification

Typically used in manufacturing or scientific research, a clean room is a controlled environment that has a low level of pollutants such as dust, airborne microbes, aerosol particles, and chemical vapors. To be exact, a clean room has a controlled level of contamination that is specified by the number of particles per cubic meter at a specified particle size. The ambient air outside in a typical city environment contains 35,000,000 particles per cubic meter, 0.5 mm and larger in diameter, corresponding to an ISO 9 clean room which is at the lowest level of clean room standards.

Clean Room Overview

A clean room is any given contained space where provisions are made to reduce particulate contamination and control other environmental parameters such as temperature, humidity and pressure. The key component is the High Efficiency Particulate Air (HEPA) filter that is used to trap particles that are 0.3 micron and larger in size. All of the air delivered to a clean room passes through HEPA filters, and in some cases where stringent cleanliness performance is necessary, Ultra Low Particulate Air (ULPA) filters are used.

Personnel selected to work in clean rooms undergo extensive training in contamination control theory. They enter and exit the clean room through airlocks, air showers and/or gowning rooms, and they must wear special clothing designed to trap contaminants that are naturally generated by skin and the body.

Clean room garments include boots, shoes, aprons, beard covers, bouffant caps, coveralls, face masks, frocks/lab coats, gowns, glove and finger cots, hairnets, hoods, sleeves and shoe covers. The type of clean room garments used should reflect the clean room and product specifications. Low-level clean rooms may only require special shoes having completely smooth soles that do not track in dust or dirt. However, shoe bottoms must not create slipping hazards since safety always takes precedence. A clean room suit is usually required for entering a clean room. Class 10,000 clean rooms may use simple smocks, head covers, and booties. For Class 10 clean rooms, careful gown wearing procedures with a zipped cover all, boots, gloves and complete respirator enclosure are required.

Clean room Air Flow Principles

Clean rooms maintain particulate-free air through the use of either HEPA or ULPA filters employing laminar or turbulent air flow principles. Laminar air flow systems are typically employed across 100% of the ceiling to maintain constant, unidirectional flow. Laminar flow criteria is generally stated in portable work stations (LF hoods), and is mandated in ISO-1 through ISO-4 classified clean rooms.

Proper clean room design encompasses the entire air distribution system, including provisions for adequate, downstream air returns. In vertical flow rooms, this means the use of low wall air returns around the perimeter of the zone. In horizontal flow applications, it requires the use of air returns at the downstream boundary of the process. The use of ceiling mounted air returns is contradictory to proper clean room system design.

Clean Room Classifications

Clean rooms are classified by how clean the air is. In Federal Standard 209 (A to D) of the USA, the number of particles equal to and greater than 0.5mm is measured in one cubic foot of air, and this count is used to classify the clean room. This metric nomenclature is also accepted in the most recent 209E version of the Standard. Federal Standard 209E is used domestically. The newer standard is TC 209 from the International Standards Organization. Both standards classify a clean room by the number of particles found in the laboratory's air. The clean room classification standards FS 209E and ISO 14644-1 require specific particle count measurements and calculations to classify the cleanliness level of a clean room or clean area. In the UK, British Standard 5295 is used to classify clean rooms. This standard is about to be superseded by BS EN ISO 14644-1.

Clean rooms are classified according to the number and size of particles permitted per volume of air. Large numbers like "class 100" or "class 1000" refer to FED_STD-209E, and denote the number of particles of size 0.5 mm or larger permitted per cubic foot of air. The standard also allows interpolation, so it is possible to describe e.g. "class 2000."

Small numbers refer to ISO 14644-1 standards, which specify the decimal logarithm of the number of particles 0.1 µm or larger permitted per cubic metre of air. So, for example, an ISO class 5 clean room has at most 105 = 100,000 particles per m^3.

Both FS 209E and ISO 14644-1 assume log-log relationships between particle size and particle concentration. For that reason, there is no such thing as zero particle concentration. Ordinary room air is approximately class 1,000,000 or ISO 9.

ISO 14644-1 Cleanroom Standards

Class	Maximum particles/m^3						FED STD 209E equivalent
	> = 0.1 µm	> = 0.2 µm	> = 0.3 µm	> = 0.5 µm	> = 1 µm	> = 5 µm	
ISO 1	10	2					
ISO 2	100	24	10	4			
ISO 3	1,000	237	102	35	8		Class 1
ISO 4	10,000	2,370	1,020	352	83		Class 10
ISO 5	100,000	23,700	10,200	3,520	832	29	Class 100
ISO 6	1,000,000	237,000	102,000	35,200	8,320	293	Class 1000
ISO 7				352,000	83,200	2,930	Class 10,000
ISO 8				3,520,000	832.000	29,300	Class 100,000
ISO 9				35,200,000	5,320,000	293,000	Room Air

BS 5295 Cleanroom Standards

Maximum Particles/m^3					
Class	>=0.5 mm	> = 1 mm	>=5 mm	> = 10 mm	> = 25 mm
Class 1	3,000		0	0	0
Class 2	300,000		2,000	30	
Class 3		1,000,000	20,000	4,000	300
Class 4			20,000	40,000	4,000

4.13 Chemotherapy and Chemotherapeutic Agents

4.13.1 Chemotherapy

The treatment of a disease with a chemical substance is known as chemotherapy. In this, the chemical substances, used are called as chemotherapeutic agents.

- ♦ Chemotherapy has been practiced for centuries. Chemotherapy lead to 2 new discoveries.
  1. Sulfonamide compounds could be used successfully for the treatment of certain bacterial diseases.
  2. The discovery of a new and potent class of antibacterially active chemotherapeutic agents i.e., antibiotics.
- Europeans used quinine which is obtained naturally from cinchona tree to treat malaria as early as 1630. Syphilis is first disease treated by chemotherapeutic by Paul Ehrlich. The drug capable of curing disease without great danger to the patient was developed.

  Ehrlichs' compound has now been replaced by antibiotics.
- Gerhard Johannes Paul Domagk in 1939 showed the therapeutic value of sulfonamides that are especially useful in the treatment of infections caused by *Meningococci* and *Shigella*, respiratory infections caused by streptococci and staphylococci and urinary infections due to gram negative organism.

4.13.2 Chemotherapeutic Agents

Chemotherapeutic agents are the chemical substances used for the treatment of infectious diseases (or) diseases caused by the proliferation of malignant cells.

- ♦ Chemotherapeutic agents are prepared in laboratory or obtained from micro-organisms and some plants and animals.

- Naturally occurring substances are known as antibiotics. Some antibiotics are prepared commercially by microbial biosynthesis.
- Antitoxin and other substances produced by the bodies of infected animals are not considered to be chemotherapeutic agents.
- The compounds used for killing or inhibiting microbial growth are not classified as chemotherapeutic agents but as disinfectants, antiseptics or germicides.

Chemotherapeutic Agents must Satisfy the following Properties

- It should possess selective toxicity i.e., destroy or prevent the activity of a parasite without injuring the cells of the host or with any minor injury to its cells.
- It should be able to come in contact with the parasite by penetrating the cells and tissues of the host in effective concentrations.
- It should leave unaltered the hosts natural defense mechanisms such as phagocytosis and the production of antibodies.
- Antiseptics and germicides such as phenol, coal tar derivatives and many mercurial compounds are unsatisfactory as chemotherapeutic agents.
- Because germicides are not selective in their action on cells and they interface with phagocytosis, they do not penetrate cells and tissues and they do not come in contact with parasites and hence they are unsatisfactory as chemotherapeutic agents.

4.14 Action of Antimicrobial Drugs

Antimicrobial drugs are either bactericidal (they kill microbes directly) or bacteriostatic (they prevent microbes from growing).

1. Inhibition of Cell Wall Synthesis

- The cell wall of a bacterium consists of a micro molecular network called peptidoglycan. Peptidoglycon is found only in bacterial cell walls.
- Penicillin and certain other antibiotics prevent the synthesis of intact peptidoglycan, consequently, the cell wall is greatly weekened, and the cell undergoes lysis.
- Penicillin targets the synthesis process, only actively growing cells are affected by these antibiotics.
- Human cells donot have peptidoglycan cell walls, penicillin has very little toxicity for host cells.

2. Inhibition of Protein Synthesis

- Protein synthesis is a common feature of all cells, whether prokaryotic or eukaryotic, it is not a exact target for selective toxicity. However some differences exist between prokaryotes and eukaryotes regarding the structure of ribosomes.
- Eukaryotic cells have 80s ribosomes, prokaryotic cells have 70s ribosomes
- These difference in ribosomal structure accounts for the selective toxicity of antibiotics that affect protein synthesis
- Antibiotics targeting the 70s ribosomes can therefore have adverse effects on the cells of the host. Among the antibiotics that interface with protein synthesis are chloramphenical, erythromycin, streptomycin and the tetracyclines.
- Reacting with the 50s portion of the 70s prokaryotic ribosomes, chloromphenical inhibits the formation of peptide bonds in the growing polypeptide chain.
- Aminoglycosides, Tetracyclines – interfere with 30s ribosomes chloramphenicol, erythromycin, lincosamides – interface with 50s ribosome.
- Tetracyclines interface with the attachment of +RNA carrying the aminoacids to the ribosome, preventing the addition of aminoacids to the growing polypeptide chain.
- *Rickettsias* and *chamydias* are sensitive to tetracyclines.
- Aminoglycoside antibiotics, such as streptomycin and gentamicin, interface with the initial steps of protein synthesis by changing the shape of the 30s portion of the 70s prokaryotic ribosome.

3. Injury to the Plasma Membrane

- Polypeptide antibiotics, bring about changes in the permeability of the plasma membrane, these changes result in the loss of important metabolites from the microbial cell.
- Polymixin B causes disruption of the plasma membrane by attaching to the phospholipids of the membrane.
- Some antifungal drugs such as amphotericin B, miconzole, and ketoconazole are effective against a considerable range of fungal diseases. Such drugs combine with sterols in the fungal cell membrane to disrupt the membrane.
- Bacterial plasma membranes generally lack sterols, these antibiotics donot act on bacteria.
- Plasma membrane of animal cells do contain sterols, and Amphotericin B and Ketoconazole can be toxic to the host.
- Animal cell membrane have mostly cholesterol, against which the drug is most effective, so that the balance of the toxicity is title against the fungus.

4. Inhibition of Nucleic Acid Synthesis

A number of antibiotics interfere with the processes of DNA replication and transcription in micro-organisms.

- Rifampicin and Quinolones (ciprofloxacin) are more widely used in chemotherapy because they are more selectively toxic.

5. Inhibiting the Synthesis of Essential Metabolites

- A particular enzymatic activity of a microorganism cab be completely inhibited by a substance (antimetabolite) that closely resembles the normal substrate for the enzme.
- An example of competitive inhibition is the relationship between the antimetabolite sulphanilamide (a sulpha drug) and para – aminobenzoic acid.
- In many micro-organisms, PABA is the substrate for an enzymatic reaction leading to the synthesis of folic acid, a vitamin that function as a coenzyme for the synthesis of purine and pyrimidine bases nucleic acids and many aminoacids.
- In the presence of Sulhanilamide, the enzyme that normally PABA to folic acid combines with the drug instead of with PABA. This combination prevents folic acid synthesis and stops the growth of the micro-organisms.

4.15 Drug Resistance

It refers to unresponsiveness of a microorganism to an antimicrobial agent.

Bacterial become resistant to chemotherapeutic agents by four major mechanisms.

1. Destruction or inactivation of the drug (*e.g.*, β lactamaea)
2. Prevention of penetration to the target site within the microbe (a frequent mechanism for tetracycline resistance).
3. Alteration of the drug's target sites to make the microbe resistant to certain macrolide antibiotics.
4. Rapid efflux (ejection), which pumps the drug out of the cell before it can become effective.

   Variations on these mechanisms also occur. For example, a microbe could become resistant to Trimethoprim by synthesizing very large amounts of the enzymes against which the drug is targeted.

   - Polyene antibiotics like Amphotericin, Nystatin, Natamycin etc., become less effective when resistant organisms produce smaller amount of sterols against which the drug is effective.
   - Hereditary drug resistance is often carried by plasmids or by small segments of DNA called transposons that can jump from one piece of DNA to another.

- Some plasmids called resistance (R) factors often contain genes for resistance to several antibiotics.
- Strains of bacteria that are resistant to antibiotics are particularly common among hospital workers, where antibiotics are in constant use.

Natural Resistance: Some microbes have always been resistant to certain antimicrobial agents. They lack the metabolic process or the target site which is affected by the particular drug.

E.g., Gram- negative bacilli are normally unaffected by penicillin G or *M. tuberculosis* is insensitive to tetracyclines.

Acquired Resistance: It is the development of resistance by an organism due to the use of AMA over a period of time.

E.g., gonococci quickly developed resistance to sulphonamides.

Prevention of Drug Resistance

- No indiscriminate and inadequate or unduly prolonged use of antimicrobial agents should be made.
- Prefer rapidly acting and selective antimicrobial agents whenever possible.
- Use combination of antimicrobial agents whenever prolonged therapy is undertaken e.g., tuberculosis.

4.16 Biosafety Measures/Procedures

Biological safety is dependent on many proper practices and barriers, including:

1. Microbiological practices
    (a) Technical proficiency
    (b) Sterile technique
    (c) Washing hands
    (d) Good habits
2. Primary barriers
    (a) Biosafety cabinets
    (b) Personal protective equipment

Standard Microbiological Practices

The following standard and special practices, safety equipment, and facilities apply to agents assigned to Biosafety Level 1 (BSL-1).

1. Access to the laboratory is limited or restricted at the discretion of the PI when experiments or work with cultures and specimens are in progress.

2. Workers shall wash their hands after they handle viable materials, after removing gloves, and before leaving the laboratory.
3. Eating, drinking, smoking, handling contact lenses, applying cosmetics, and storing food for human use are not permitted in the work areas. Persons who wear contact lenses in laboratories should also wear goggles or a face shield.
4. Food is stored outside the work area in cabinets or refrigerators designated and used for this purpose only.
5. Mouth pipetting is prohibited.
6. Policies for the safe handling and disposal of sharps are followed.
7. All procedures are performed carefully to minimize the creation of splashes or aerosols.
8. Work surfaces are decontaminated at least once each day and again after any spill of viable material.
9. All cultures, stocks, and other regulated wastes are disposed of properly. Infectious waste requires decontamination before disposal by an approved decontamination method such as autoclaving.
10. Materials to be decontaminated outside of the immediate laboratory are to be placed in a durable, leak proof container and closed for transport from the laboratory. Materials to be decontaminated outside of the immediate laboratory are packaged in accordance with applicable local, state, and federal regulations before removal from the facility.
11. A biohazard sign must be posted at the entrance to a laboratory designated BSL-2 or higher. The sign or additional signage nearby should include the name of the agent(s) in use, the biohazard level, the name and phone number of the investigator, and emergency contact information.
12. An insect and rodent control program must be in effect.
13. A lab coat, gloves, and safety glasses must be worn when handling infectious materials.
14. The HAMM manual is available to lab staff.
15. Spills and exposures are reported immediately to the PI/LSC; large spills are reported to EH&S for assistance with clean-up.
16. Biosafety cabinets (BSCs) are used when there is potential for creating aerosols.
17. High concentrations or large volumes of infectious materials can be centrifuged outside the BSC only if the centrifuge tubes are sealed and opened inside a BSC.
18. Labeling done in accordance with biosafety guideline.

Aerosols

Aerosols are liquid droplets or solid particulates dispersed in air. Many aerosols are too small to see with the unaided eye and remain suspended for an extended period. The production of aerosols while handling infectious agents accounts for the greatest source of laboratory-acquired infections.

Generation of aerosols may be caused by using centrifuges, blenders, shakers, magnetic stirrers, sonicators, pipettes, vortex mixers, syringes and needles, freeze-dried samples, vacuum-sealed samples, mortars and pestles, culture tubes, inoculating floss, and separatory funnels.

Control of Aerosols

Perform activities in a biosafety cabinet.

1. Keep tubes stoppered when vortexing or centrifuging. Consider using tubes with screw-on tops.
2. If an aerosol has been created, leave the area and allow the droplets to settle. Place cloth soaked with disinfectant over work surface to deactivate droplets of infectious agents.
3. Slowly reconstitute or dilute contents of an ampule. Soaked gauze can be wrapped around ampoules while breaking or when stoppers are removed from tubes.
4. Mix solutions by discharging the secondary fluid down the side of the container as close as possible to the surface of the primary solution.
5. Allow inoculating needle to cool before touching biological specimens.

Pipetting

1. Mouth pipetting is forbidden.
2. No infectious mixture should be prepared by bubbling air through the liquid with the pipette.
3. No infectious materials should be forcibly discharged from pipettes.

Syringes and Needles

Avoid the use of syringes and needles when possible. Use the needle-locking type (Luer-lock) or a disposable syringe needle unit, or other safe sharps.

Used needles must not be resheathed, bent, broken, or removed from disposable syringes.

Needles and syringes must be disposed of in approved sharps containers. These are available at no charge through the Stockroom.

Disinfection and Sterilization: General Procedures

1. After each experiment, decontaminate work surfaces using appropriate disinfectant.
2. Disinfect countertops and equipment where biohazardous material is used frequently.

3. Decontaminate all infectious materials and contaminated equipment prior to their being washed, stored or discarded.
4. Use autoclavable or disposable materials whenever possible. Do not reuse disposable items.
5. When sharps containers are ¾-full, close lid and place in hall for pick-up. Housekeeping staff will collect sharps waste.
6. Housekeeping staff is not allowed entry into Biosafety Level 2 (and above) labs unless special arrangements have been made with the lab supervisor, who must ensure safe work practices are followed. BSL-2 lab staff is required to clean the lab and properly segregate all of the lab waste into the appropriate waste streams.

Essay Questions

1. Write a note on different disinfectant compounds along with their structure and modes of action
2. Explain the different tests for evaluating the effectiveness of disinfectants
3. Write a note on Antimicrobial action of drugs

Multiple Choice Questions

1. Ethyl alcohol concentrations effective against vegetative or nonspore forming cells is
   (a) 30-40% (b) 40-50%
   (c) 20-30% (d) 50-90%
2. One of the oldest and most effective germicidal agent used in the form of tincture
   (a) Iodine
   (b) chlorine
   (c) Fluorine
   (d) Bromine
3. Heavy metal effective against alage and moulds is
   (a) Silver
   (b) Mercury
   (c) Cadmium
   (d) Copper
4. Disinfectant used in fumigation of rooms and hospitals is
   (a) Acetaldehyde
   (b) Formaldehyde
   (c) Gluteraldehyde
   (d) Butyraldeyde
5. Simplest method of applying dry heat used in the sterilization of forceps, needles, scalpels is:
   (a) Flaming
   (b) Hot air sterilization
   (c) Incineration
   (d) Cauterization

Answers

1. (d) 2. (a) 3. (d)
4. (b) 5. (a)

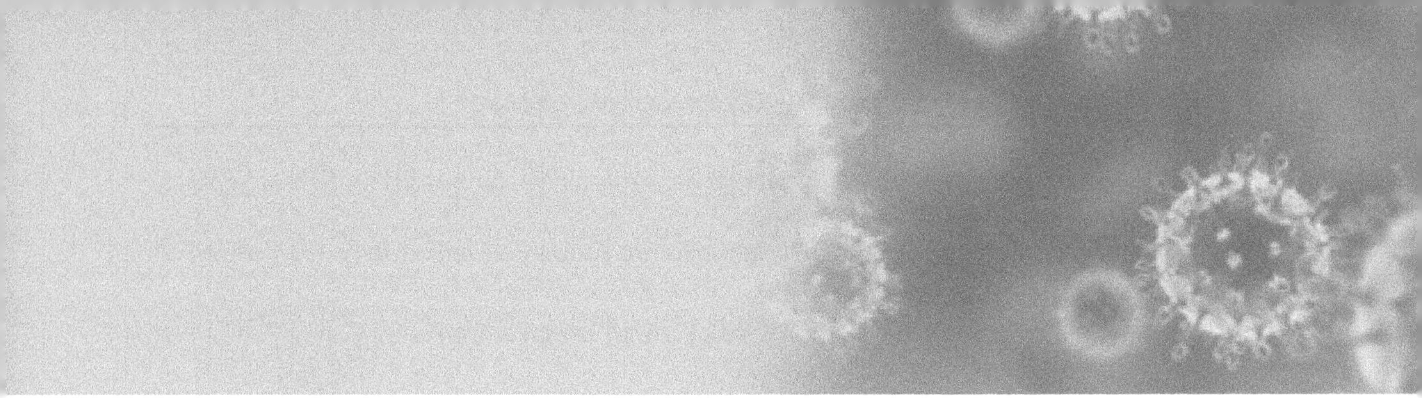

5 IMMUNOLOGY

LEARNING OBJECTIVES

After studying the chapter the students familiarize themselves with concepts in:

- *Understanding the attack of micro-organisms*
- *Understanding classification of Immunity*
- *Developing an insight in to structure and responses of an antibody*
- *Understanding the nature of vaccines and their applications*
- *Developing an insight into transmission of infections*
- *Understanding the nature of antigens*

5.1 Introduction

The term immunity refers to the general ability of a host to resist particular infection or disease by microorganism or other foreign substance. This term is derived from Latin term *immunis* meaning free of burden.

Types of Immunity

(a) Innate/Native immunity: Innate or Native immunity is the resistance to infections which an individual possesses by virtue of his genetic and constitutional make-up.

Innate immunity may be considered at the level of species, race or individual.

(i) Species: All human beings are totally unsusceptible to plant pathogens and too many animal pathogens such as Rinderpest virus or canine distemper virus.

- Typhoid fever is a serious disease in humans but mice are not affected.
- Man is susceptible to plague, but fowls are not.

- Micro-organisms that are pathogenic to humans do not affect fish or reptiles, and vice versa
- Frogs, being cold-blooded are resistant to anthrax unless they are warmed to 37 °C.
- If the body temperature of chickens is lowered from 39 °C to 37 °C, they become susceptible to anthrax.
- Most mammals are resistant to *Mycobacterium avium*, and the type of *mycobacterium* found in cold-blooded reptiles.
- Herbivorous animals are often resistant to diseases of carnivores and vice versa for a variety of reason.

(ii) Race: The people of Negroid origin in the USA are more susceptible to tuberculosis than the Caucasian race.

- Racial differences are known to be genetic in origin.
- African blacks have a high resistance to yellow fever but white men are very susceptible.
- Brahman cattle are resistant to the protozoan parasite responsible for tick fever in other breeds of cattle.
- Blacks show a relatively high resistance to tropical diseases such as malaria and yellow fever.
- Orientals exhibit a reduced susceptibility to syphilis.

(iii) Individuals

- In identical twins, leprosy is seen in only one of them.
- Some people are more resistant than others to cold and skin infections.

5.1.1 Acquired Immunity

The resistance that an individual acquires during life is known as acquired immunity. Acquired immunity is of two types, active and passive.

(a) Active immunity: The resistance developed by an individual as a result of antigenic stimulus. It is also known as active immunity.

(i) ***Natural acquired active immunity:*** It results from either a clinical or an apparent infection by a microbe.

A person who has recovered from an attack of measles develops natural active immunity.

(ii) ***After clinical infection:*** When a patient recovers from certain diseases he is left with a high degree of immunity.

In case of diphtheria, smallpox and poliomyelitis the immunity persists for life.

In case of influenza, pneumonia and gonorrhea, the immunity is of short duration.

(iii) ***After sub-clinical infection:*** Children in slum areas because of more frequent exposure to sub-infection often develop immunity to a variety of diseases more quickly than children in more affluent areas.

(iv) ***Artificial active immunity:*** It is the resistance induced by vaccines. Vaccines are preparation of live or killed micro-organisms or their products used for immunization. They stimulate the production of antibody.

5.1.2 Passive Immunity

The resistance that is transmitted passively to a recipient in a 'readymade' form is known as passive immunity. Here the recipient's immune system plays no active role, no antigenic stimulus; instead, performed antibodies are administered (Table 5.1).

(a) Naturally acquired passive immunity: It is the resistance passively transferred from mother to baby.

- In human infants, maternal antibodies are transmitted predominantly through the placenta, while in animals such as pigs, transfer of antibodies occurs mainly orally through the colostrum.

  e.g., Babies show high resistance to chicken pox, diphtheria, measles and scarlet fever and this is lost by the time the child is about 6 months old.

(b) Artificially produced passive immunity: It is the resistance passively transferred to a recipient by the administration of antibodies.

- The agents used for this purpose are hyper immune sera of animal or human origin, convalescent sera and pooled human γ-globulin. These are used for prophylaxis and therapy.
- Antisera of animal origin are now recommended only where human preparations are not available (antigasgangrene, antibotulinum sera; antivenins)
- Convalescent sera (sera of patients recovering from infectious diseases) contain high levels of specific antibody.
- Pooled human γ-globulin (γ-globulin from pooled sera of healthy adults) contain antibodies against all common pathogens prevalent in the region.
- Convalescent sera and pooled human gamma globulin were used for passive immunization against same virus infections.
- Human γ-globulin is also used in the treatment of patients with some immune deficiencies.

Table 5.1 Differences between Active and Passive Immunity

Active Immunity	Passive Immunity
Immunity effective only after lag period.	Immediate immunity
Immunological memory present	No memory
Not applicable in the immunodeficieny	Applicable in immunodeficiently
Negative phase may occur	No negative phase
Induced by infection or by immunogens	Readymade antibody transferred.
Active immunisation is used in prophylaxis. e.g., Diphtheria vaccine, tetanus vaccine, cholera, pertussis, plague, BCG, chicken pox vaccine, influenza vaccine	Passive immunisation is used in both prophylaxis and therapeutically *e.g.,* Diptheria antitoxin, Botulinum antitoxin, Gas – gangrene antitoxin Tetanus antitoxin
Booster effect on subsequent dose	Subsequent dose is less effective.
Produced actively by host's immune system	Received passively. No active host participation.

5.2 Immune Tolerance

- An antigenic molecule contains chemical grouping or antigenic determinants which, when introduced parenterally into the body, stimulates the production of an antibody.
- Some antigens may not induce antibodies but may sensitize specific lymphocytes leading to cell mediated immunity or may cause ***"immunological tolerance"***.
- The body must distinguish between "self" and "foreign", otherwise antibodies directed against its own antigen would destroy it.
- It can be said that an organism has a "tolerance" to its own antigens in that they do not provoke the immune responses. This importance was recognized by Paul Ehrlich where he called This term as "horroe and toxicus".
- The maintenance of the tolerant state required the continued presence of antigen, which was provided by the continued persistence of the A-line cells.
- Too much antigen is not desirable if one wishes to induce an immune response.
- Very small number of particles e.g., $10^6 \times 174$ bacteriophages can induce an immune response in guinea pigs.

5.2.1 Immune Response

The specific reactivity induced in a host by an antigenic stimulus is known as the immune response.

- Whenever cell is attacked with pathogen/antigen, immediate reactions occur in the organism (production of antibodies).

- In infectious diseases it is generally equated with protection against invading micro-organisms.
- Immune response includes reactions against any antigen, living or nonliving. It may lead to consequences that are beneficial, indifferent or injurious to the host.
- The immune response can be of two types.
  1. The humoral (antibody mediated) immunity
  2. The cellular (cell mediated) immunity.

5.3 Factors Influencing Infection

The ability of a pathogenic organism to cause infection depends on a number of factors.

(a) **Virulence:** (The degree of extent of pathogenicity): The virulence of many pathogenic bacteria is influenced by the presence or absence of a non-toxic polysaccharide material composing the capsule surrounding the cells.

Such capsules can prevent the engulfment and destruction of the bacteria by the phagocytic defense mechanisms of the body.

(b) **Exotoxins:** Some exotoxins have extraordinarily high potency, with only minute amounts being needed to kill animals.

An initial adherence of exotoxins by a particular region to tissue cells is an important first step in their toxic activity. Other regions or subunits of the toxin may have enzymatic activity that causes damage to the tissue cells.

(c) **Role of Bacteriophages and Plasmids:** Toxigenicity can be conferred on a bacterium as the result of acquiring a temperate bacteriophage that carries the gene for the toxin.

Bacteria can also become toxigenic by acquiring a plasmid that carries the gene for a toxin.

(d) **Streptolysin O (SLO) and Streptolysin S (SLS):** SLO is produced by *Streptococci pyogenes* and is inactivated by oxygen (hence the "O" in its name). The soluble toxin SLO penetrates the leukocyte from without damaging the membranes of cytoplasmic granules (lysosomes) within the cell. The powerful hydrolytic enzymes contained within the lysosomes are liberated into the cytoplasm and proceeds to destroy the phagocyte.

SLS is also produced by *S. pyogenes* and kills leukocytes in the same manner as SLO.

(e) **Direct Damage:** The pathogens use the host cell for nutrients and produce waste products. As pathogens metabolize and multiply in cells, the cells usually rupture. Many microbes are released when the host cell ruptures. Following their release pathogens that ruptures cells can spread to other tissues in even greater numbers.

Some bacteria can induce host epithelial cells to engulf them by a process that resembles phagocytosis. These pathogens can disrupt host cells as they pass through and can then be extruded from the host cells by a reverse phagocytosis process, enabling them to enter other host cells.

e.g., E.coli, Shigella, Salmonella and *Niggeria gonorrhea.*

Some bacteria can also penetrate host cells by excreting enzymes and by their own motility; such penetration can itself damage the host cell.

Most damage by bacteria however is done by toxins

5.4 General Resistance of the Host against Infection or Host Defense

The body has a number of lines of defense against infection:

(i) Prevention of Entry: This is achieved by the design of body structures, by the impermeability to micro-organisms of the intact and healthy skin and mucosa, by competition from the natural microbial flora of the host, by the antimicrobial activities of the secretions bathing the surfaces of the body.

The mucus covering of mucous membranes collects and retains micro-organisms and then action of cilia in the respiratory tract, aided by coughing and sneezing or peristaltic activity in the gut, removes them from the body.

The fatty acids in the skin, the pH of the gastric juices, the enzyme lysozyme in tears and sweat all inhibit or destroy micro-organisms.

(ii) Phagocytosis: Organisms that manage to invade the tissues are attacked by cells known as phagocytes which have the ability to engulf inert or living material, a process known as phagocytosis.

There are two types of phagocytes:

(a) *Fixed*: These belong to the reticulo-endothelial system of cells that line blood spaces in various parts of the body, including the spleen and liver. They are known as macrophages.

They ingest micro-organisms, amoeba waste from the blood as it passes.

(b) *Wandering*: The most important of these is the neutrophil type of polymerphonuclear leucocytes.

It moves about in the blood and in response to inflammatory changes caused by the presence of micro-organisms in the tissues, mobilizes at the site of infection, passes out of the capillary walls and attacks the invaders.

The leucocytes, like the fixed macrophages engulf the organisms and render them harmless. Together with large number of fellow leucocytes that are destroyed in the attack, contribute to the formation of pus.

In some cases, *e.g.*, with capsulated and other pathogens of high virulence, the phagocytes may be chemotactically repelled, leaving the organisms free to cause disease.

(iii) Enzymes: The virulence of some bacteria is thought to be aided by the production of extra cellular enzymes and related substances.

(a) Coagulase (a protein enzyme produced by several *micro-organisms* that enables the conversion of fibrinogen to fibrin in blood) are produced by some members of the genus *Staphylococcus*, they may be involved in the walling off process in boils produced by *Staphylococci*.

(b) Human body form clots to isolate the microbial infections. But bacterial kinases are the enzymes produced by bacteria to breakdown fibrin and then digest clots.

e.g., Fibrinolysin (Streptokinase) Staphylokinase

(c) Hyaluronidase is another enzyme secreted by certain bacteria, such as *streptococci*. It hydrolyses hyaluronic acid, a type of polysaccharide that holds together certain cells of the body particulate cells in connective tissue. It is involved in the tissue blackening of infected wounds and to help the microorganism spread from its initial site of infection.

Clostridium that causes gas gangrene also produces hyaluronidase.

(d) Collagenase produced by several species of *Clostridium* facilitates the spread of gas gangrene. Collagenase breaks down the protein collagen, which forms the connective tissue of muscles and other body organs and tissues.

As a defense against adherence of pathogens to mucosal surfaces, the body produces a class of antibody called IgA antibodies. There are some pathogens with the ability to produce enzymes, called IgA proteases that can destroy these antibodies penetration into the host cell cytoskeleton.

The microbes produce surface proteins called invasins that rearrange nearby acting filaments of the cytoskeleton. For example, when *S.typhimurium* makes contact with a host cell, invasions of the microbe cause the appearance of the host cell plasma membrane to resemble the splash of a drop of a liquid hitting a solid surface. This effect, called membrane ruffling is the result of disruption in the cytoskeleton of the host cell.

(iv) Dome of Host Cell: When a microorganism invades a body tissue, it initially encounters phagocytes of the host. If the phagocytes are successful in destroying the invader, no further damage is done to the host. But if pathogen overcomes the host's defense, then the microorganism can damage host cells in four basic ways.

1. By using the host's nutrients.
2. By causing direct damage in the immediate vicinity of the invasion.

3. By producing toxins, transported by blood and lymph, that damage sites are removed from the original site of invasion.
4. By hypersensitivity reactions inducing using the host's nutrients

(v) Siderophores: (Greek: "iron carrier") are small, high-affinity iron chelating compounds secreted by micro-organisms such as bacteria, fungi and grasses. Iron is required for the growth of most pathogenic bacteria; by siderophore receptors on the bacterial surface iron is received and brought into the bacterium. Siderophores are amongst the strongest soluble Fe^{3+} binding agents known.

Most of the iron is tightly bound to iron transport proteins, such as lactoferrin, transferrin, and ferritin as well as haemoglobin. In order to obtain free iron, some pathogens secret proteins called siderophores. These siderophores take the iron away from iron-transport proteins by binding the iron even more tightly.

5.5 Requirements for Immunogenicity

(i) Foreignness: The most important features of an immunogen is that an effective immunogen must be foreign with respect to the host. The adaptive immune system recognizes and eliminates only foreign (nonself) Agglutinogens.

Self Ags are not recognized and thus individuals are tolerant to their own self molecules, even though these molecules have the capacity to act as immunogens in other individuals of the same species.

(ii) Size: The second requirement for being immunogenic is that the compound must have a certain minimal Molecular weight. There is a relationship between the size of immunogen and its immunogenicity.

In general, small compounds with a Molecular weight (molecular weight) <1000 Da (*e.g.*, Penicillin, aspirin) are not immunogenic

(iii) Chemical Complexity: The third characteristic necessary for a compound to be immunogenic is a certain degree of chemical complexity.

e.g., homopolymers of amino acids or sugars are seldom good immunogens regardless of their size.

Similarly, a homopolymer of poly-r-D-glutamic acid (the capsular material of *Bacillus anthracis*) with Mw of 50,000 dalton is not immunogenic.

Virtually all proteins are immunogenic.

(iv) Dosage and route of Administration: Insufficient dose of Ag may not stimulate an immune response either because the amount administered fails to activate enough lymphocytes or because such a dose renders the responding cells unresponsive.

Besides the need to administer antigen there should an amount of Ag to induce an immune response, the number of doses administration also affects the outcome of the immune response generated.

The route of administration also affect the outcome of the immunization because this determines which organs and cell populations will be involved in the response, immunogens can be administered through a number of common routes-intravenous, intradermal, subcutaneous, intramuscular. Ags administered via the most common route namely, subcutaneously, generally elicit the strongest immune responses.

5.6 Non-Specific Immunity

5.6.1 Cell Tissues and Organs

Of the immune system show non specific or innate resistance. Cell types associated with Host show resistance to infection. Cellular activity responsible for phagocytosis and other aspects of nonspecific and specific resistances is carried on the following diverged groups of blood cells. (Table 5.2).

Table 5.2 Functions of Cellular Tissues and Organs in Immunity

S.No	Cell type	Location	Derivation	Description and Function
1.	Leukocytes (a) nuclear polymorpho granulocytes. 1. Neutrophils 2. Eosinophils 3. Basophils	Peripheral blood	Bone marrow stem cells	Classified according to structure and affinity for dyes. Labar nuclei and abundant cytoplasmic granules. No dye preference; Phagocytic Stain with eosin, an acid dye; phagocytic stain with basic stain bind IgE and produce histamine.
	(b) Lymphocytes		Lymphoid organs, bone marrow stem cells.	Smaller than monocytes larger nucleus; scanty cytoplasm; form T and B cells; Non phagocytic.
	(c) Monocytes		Bonemarrow stem cells	larger than granulocyte single horse shoe-shape or oval nucleus; few cytoplasmic granules; phagocytic.

Table 5.2 ***Contd...***

S.No	Cell type	Location	Derivation	Description and Function
2.	Plasma cells	Lymphoid organs (lymphnodes, spleen, thymus)	From B lymphocytes	Produce antibodies eccentric nucleus; non phagocytic.
3.	Macrophages (a) wandering 1. Alveolar 2. peritoneal (b) Fixed 1. Histiocytes 2. Kupffer cells	Other tissues Lung Abdomen Connective tissue Liver	Transformed from monocytes	Numerous cytoplasmic granules; phagocytic

5.6.2 Phagocytosis (Macrophage Activation)

Phagocytosis is defined as the receptor-mediated engulfment of large (≥0.5 μm) particles into plasma membrane-derived vacuoles called phagosomes. Following scission from the plasma membrane, the phagosomes undergo a maturation process, sequentially fusing with endosomes and lysosomes, ultimately becoming phagolysosomes highly acidic and hydrolase-rich organelles that degrade the internalized particles.

Phagocytosis is phylogenetically the oldest defense mechanism in animals. Phagocytic cells are the mononuclear macrophages (of blood and tissues) and the polymorpho nuclear microphages. The primary function of macro phages is phagocytosis.

- Phagocytosis refers to ingestion of micro-organisms or any particulate material by a cell. The primary function of macrophages is phagocytosis.
- It originates in protozoa as a combined mechanism for nutrition and defense, along the course of evolution, the phagocyte lost its tropic functions with the development of digestive enzymes.
- The phagocytes are of two types, granulocytes (microphages) and monocytes (macrophages).
- When a microbe infects granulocytes (neutrophils), monocytes move from site and are called macrophages.
- The blood macrophages are the largest of the lymphoid cells found in peripheral, blood (12-15 μm). The tissue macrophages are larger (15-20 μm)
- Mononuclear macrophage cells originate in the bone marrow from precursor cells and become monocytes in about 6 days.
- Monocytes in circulation have approximate half life of 3 days.

5.6.3 Inflammation

Inflammation is a non specific defense for the body, the symptoms are the same for a wide variety of injuries, inoculations and infections. Inflammation proceeds in three basic stages.

1. Vasodilatation and increased leakage from capillaries
2. Migration of phagocytes to the site of inflection
3. Tissue repair

Vasodilatation and increased capillary leakage represent one of the first issue responses after a trauma. The dilation of blood vessels in the vicinity of an injury increases local blood flow. Reddening of the skin causes swelling and fluid leakage through the enlarged vessels and into damaged tissues. The increased flow also brings more defensive cells and chemicals to injury while carrying of toxins, microbes, cellular debris and dead cells.

Several chemicals contribute to vasodilatation including histamine, kinins and prostaglandins. Histamine is released from injured mast cells in tissues. Kinins attract phagocytes. Prostaglandins are hormone like fatty acids released from damaged plasma membranes. They intensify the effect of histamine and kinins. Prostaglandins also stimulate phagocyte migration and cause pain, bringing and infection to conscious awareness.

Phagocyte migration involves neutrophils and macrophages that collect at the scene of an infection, typically within an hour after inflammation starts. They find the site of infection by following a tract of kinin chemical signals.

Monocytes arrive within several hours and are transformed into macrophages as they enter the tissue spaces. In addition to engulfing microbes and debris, macrophages remove dead neutrophils from the initial defensive response.

Tissue repair occurs once the invaders and the damaged tissues have been cleared away. New cells that are produced by mitosis replace damaged fibers and other structures.

5.7 Physical and Mechanical Barriers

Physical and Mechanical Barriers, along with the host's secretions, are the first line of defense against micro-organisms. Protection of the most important body surfaces by these mechanisms is discussed next.

(a) Skin: The intact skin contributes greatly to non specific host resistance. It forms a very effective mechanical barrier to microbial invasion. Its outer layer consists of thick, closely packed cells called kerantinocytes, which produce keratins. Keratins are selenoproteins that make up the main components of hair, nails and the outer skin cells. These outer skin cells shed continuously removing any grime or microorganism that manage to adhere to their surface.

Here they encounter a specialized set of cells called skin-associated lymphoid tissue (SALT). The major function of SALT is to confine microbial invaders to the area immediately underlying the epidermis and to prevent them from gaining access to the blood stream.

(b) **Mucous membrane:** The mucous membrane of the respiratory digestive and urogenital system withstand microbial invasion because the intact stratified squamous epithelia and mucous secretions from a protective covering that resists penetration and traps many micro-organisms. One antibacterial substance in these secretions is Lysozyme, which acts on bacteria by hydrolyzing glycosidic linkages in the cell wall mucopeptides; they also contain significant amounts of the iron-binding protein, lactoferrin. Lactoferrin is realized by activated microphages. Mucous membrane also has a specialized immune barrier called mucous-associated lymphoid tissue (MALT).

(c) **Respiratory system:** Microbes smaller than 10 μm often pass through the nasal cavity and are trapped by the mucociliary blanket that coats the mucosal surfaces of lower portions of the respiratory system. The trapped microbes are transported by ciliary action. That moves them away from the lungs. Microorganism that succeed in reaching the alveoli of lungs encounter a population of fixed phagocytic cells called alveolar macrophages; these cells can ingest and kill most bacteria by phagocytosis.

(d) **Gastrointestinal tract:** The very acidic gastric juice (pH 2 to 3) is sufficient to destroy most organisms and their toxins although exceptions exist (protozoan cysts, *Helicobacter pylori*, *clostridium* and *staphylococcus* toxins). Peristalsis and the normal loss of columnar epithelial cells act in concert to purge intestinal microorganism. The mucous membrane of the intestinal tract contain cells. These cells produced Lysozyme and a set of peptides called cryptins. Cryptins are toxic for some bacteria.

(e) **The genitourinary tract:** The flushing action of the slightly acidic urine maintains sterility of both male and female urethra semen is believed to contain antibacterial substances. The acid reaction of the vaginal secretion in female due to fermentation of glycogen by *lactobacillus* (normal flora) is markedly bactericidal towards most pathogenic organisms.

(f) **The eye:** The conjunctiva is is kept moist by the continuous flushing action of tears from the lacrymal glands. Tears contain lysozyme; lactoferrin and sIgA thus provide physical and chemical protection.

5.8 Chemical Mediators

(a) **Antimicrobial peptides:** The cationic peptides role is biological is their ability to damage bacterial plasma membrane. They alter membrane permeability by electrostatic interactions with membranes which cause the formation of ionic pores and or transient gaps. Three classes of cationic peptides are cathelicidin, defensins and histatin

(b) Bacteriocins: Many of the bacteria that are part of the normal microflora synthesize and release toxic proteins (eg: colicin, staphylococcin) called bacteriocins that are lethal to other strains of the same species as well as other bacterial species.

(c) Complement: The complement system is composed of a large number of serum proteins that play a major role in the animals' defensive immune response. Most complement components present in the serum are functionally inactive forms as proenzymes or zymogens. Complement activation pathways involves the activation of one component that triggers the activation of the next component in the sequence.

Upon activation, individual components are split into fragments, designated by lower-case letters. The larger fragments bind to the target near the site of activation and the smaller fragments diffuse from the site and can initiate localized inflammatory responses. There are three pathways of complement activation; the classical, alternative, and lectin path.

(d) Cytokines: Cytokines are required for immunoregulation of both specific and non specific immune responses.

Cytokines are classified into four types of cytokine families

(i) Chemokines
(ii) Hemato poietins
(iii) Interleukins
(iv) Tumor necrosis factor (TNF Family)

(e) Interferon (IFN): Interferons are small proteins produced by normal eukaryotic cells in response to viral infection or double-stranded RNA's (viral or synthetic). Interferons lack virus specificity since they donot react directly with the virion but instead induce the host cell to synthesize a non specific antiviral protein. Thus human interferon was most effective in protecting human cells and purified interferons are stable at low pH in tissue fluids. There are two types interferons i.e., IFN α and IFNγ.

Types IFN α and IFNγ antiviral activity, antiproliferative; stimulates macrophage activity; increases MHC class I protein expression on cells; regulates the development of the specific immune response.

IFNγ activation of T cells, macrophages, nuetrophils and NK cells; antiviral activity, antiproliferative; increases MHC class I and class II molecule expression on cells.

Interferons are a group of related low molecular weight, regulatory cytokines produced by certain eukaryotic cells in response to a viral infection.

Interferons α/β

- Antiviral activity
- Antiproliferative
- Stimulates macrophage activity
- Increases MHC class I protein expression on cells
- Regulates the development of specific immune response

Interferon-γ

- Activation of T cells, macrophages, neutrophils and Nk cells.
- Antiviral and anti-proliferative activities
- Increased class I and II MHC molecule expression on various cells.

(f) **Acute-Phage Proteins**

Microphages release cytokines (IL – 1, IL – 6, IL – 8, TNF – α, etc) upon activation by bacteria, which stimulate the liver to rapidly produce acute-phage proteins.

Acute phage proteins are C-Reactive protein (CRP), Mannose-binding lectin (MBL), and Surfactant Protein, A (SP-A) and D (SP-D) all of which can bind to bacterial surfaces and act as opsonins.

SP- A, SP – D and Clq are "collectins" - Proteins composed of a "collagen" like pattern connected by α-helices to globular "lectin" binding sites. Thus these proteins protect host tissues by binding to and assisting in the removal of bacteria.

(g) **Natural Killer Cells:** Recently, a sub population of lymphocytes has been discovered which are referred to as null cells. Null cells generally possess surface receptors for immunoglobulin; reports are conflicting as to whether they have complement receptors. The best-defined null cells are known as natural killer (NK) cells. They can kill cellular targets without prior exposure (immunization) to antigens of the target cells. Thus they can directly kill tumor cells and virally infected cells without ingesting them.

5.9 Specific Immunity

5.9.1 Antigens (Ags)

***Antigen*:** Those substances that can induce a specific immune response and specifically bind products of immune response *in vitro* or *in vivo*.

e.g., Antigen, Tolerogen, and Allergen.

e.g., Bacteria, Viruses, tumor cells, tissue from donor, actually, some of the proteins of these substances are the actual antigens.

An antigen is any agent capable of binding specifically to components of the immune response, such as the B cell receptor (BCR) on B-lymphocytes and soluble antibodies.

The ability of a compound to bound with antibodies and with cells of immune system is refers to antigenicity. There is functional distinction between the term antigen and immunogens.

An immunogen is any agent capable of inducing an immune response and is therefore immunogenic. The distinction between the terms is necessary because there are many compounds that are incapable of inducing an immune response, yet they are capable of binding with components of the immune system that have been induced specifically against them. Thus all immunogens are Ags, but not all Ags are immunogens.

5.9.2 Structure of Antigen

Antigen is composed of two parts one is hapten and another is carrier. Hapten only possess immunoreactivity whereas carrier enhances the immunogenicity of hapten.

Immunogens possess both characteristics like immunoreactivity and enhancing the immunogenicity.

Hapten +carrier $\rightarrow$ complete antigen (immunogens)

5.9.3 Classification of Antigens

(i) **According to immunogenicity of Antigens**
- (a) Antigen
- (b) Hapten

(ii) **According to the dependence of T cells:*** when Ags induce humoral immune response
- (a) TD-Ag (thymus dependent Ag)
- (b) TI-Ag (thymus independent Ag)

(iii) **According to source of antigen**
- (a) Xenoantigen
- (b) Alloantigen
- (c) Autoantigen

(iv) **Heterophile antigens (Forssman antigen):** The common antigen existing different species.

5.9.4 Important Antigens in Medicine

(i) **Pathogens and their products**
Pathogens: such as bacteria et al.
Surface antigen: "Vi" Ag
Somatic Ag: "O" Ag
Flagellar Ag: "H" Ag
Pilus Ag

(ii) **Exotoxin and toxoid**

(iii) **Heterophile Ag (Forssman Ag):** common Ags shared by different species

(iv) **Alloantigen:**
1. Antigens of red blood cell
2. ABO system (blood typing very important in transfusion Rh system (in Chinese >99%RH+)
3. HLA system (Human leukocyte antigen) relate to transplantation very important in immune regulation

(v) **Autoantigen:** Release of sequestered Ag
Change of molecular structure of auto-tissues

5.10 Haptens

Hapten also spelled haptene, small molecule that stimulates the production of antibody molecules only when conjugated to a larger molecule, called a carrier molecule. The term *hapten* is derived from the Greek *haptein*, meaning "to fasten." Haptens can become tightly fastened to a carrier molecule, most often a protein, by a covalent bond. The hapten-carrier complex stimulates the production of antibodies, which the unbound hapten cannot do and becomes immunogenic.

Many drugs that cause allergic reactions, such as penicillin, act as haptens. When injected or ingested, penicillin reacts chemically with proteins in the body to form a hapten-carrier complex that can lead to the life-threatening syndrome called anaphylaxis.

5.11 Immunogenicity

5.11.1 Recognition of Foreignness

The most important features of an immunogen is that an effective immunogen must be foreign with respect to the host. The adaptive immune system recognizes and eliminates only foreign (nonself) Ags.

Self Ags are not recognized and thus individuals are tolerant to their own self molecules, even though these molecules have the capacity to act as immunogens in other individuals of the same species

5.11.2 Class I MHC

Except non-nucleated cells (RBC) all cells use class I MHC molecules. This system contains a complex of two protein chains

1. alpha chain contains α_1, α_2, α_3 functional domains
2. β_2-microglobulin chain

The α_3 domain is attached to the plasma membrane by a short amino acid sequence that extends into the cell interior, while the rest of the protein protrudes to the outside. The β_2-microglubulin and α_3 segment are noncovalently associated with one another and are close to the plasma membrane. The α_1 and α_2, domain lie to the outside and form the antigen-binding pocket.

5.11.3 Class II MHC

These molecules are also transmembrane proteins consisting of α and β chains. Both chains combine to form a three dimensional protein pocket, the antigen-binding pocket, into which a nonself peptide fragment can be captured for presentation to other cells of immune system.

5.11.4 T-cells (T-lymphocytes)

T-lymphocytes arise in the bone marrow unlike B cells, which mature within the bone marrow, T-cells migrate to the thymus gland to mature. During its maturation within the thymus, the T-cells comes to express an unique antigen-binding molecule, called the T-cell receptor, on the membrane. T-cell donot make Abs but perform various effector-functions when Apc bring Ags into the secondary lymphoid organ. T-cells helps in eliminating Aps, cancer cells, virus-infected cells or grafts which have altered self-cells.

T-cells express distinct membrane molecules. On the basis of presence of one or the other of two membrane molecules. CD^+_4 and CD^+_8; there are two sub-population of helper T-cells-T-helper (T_4) cells (carries CD^+_4 membrane glycoprotein on their surfaces) and T-cytotoxic (T_c) cells carries CD^+_8 membrane glycoprotein on surfaces.

In addition, all T-cell subpopulations express the T-cell receptor that includes CD_3. The ratio of CD_4^+ and CD_8^+ T cells us approximately 2:1 in normal human peripheral blood, but it may be significantly diseases.

Cytotoxic T cells provide protection against intracellular pathogens such as viruses and some bacteria and parasites that multiply in the host-cell cytoplasm, where they are sheltered from attack by Abs. They provide this protection by killing the infected cell before the microbes can proliferate and escape from the infected cell to infect neighboring cells. Helper T cells are crucial for defense against both extracellular and intercellular pathogens. They help stimulate B cells to make Abs that inactivate or eliminate extra cellular pathogens and their toxic product. They also activate macrophages to destroy any intracellular pathogen multiplying within the microphages phagosomes and they help activate cytotoxic T cells to kill infected target cells.

5.11.5 Cellular Immune Response

It is a specific immune response that does not involve antibodies or complement but rather involves the activation of macrophages, natural killer cells, antigen-specific cytotoxic T-lymphocytes, and the release of various cytokines in response to an antigen.

Cell mediated immunity (CMI) protects the body from activating macrophages and natural killer cells, enabling them to destroy intracellular pathogens.

CMI Participates in the rejection of homografts and grafts versus host reaction.

It mediates the pathogenesis of delayed (type 4) hypersensitivity.

It provides immunological surveillance and immunity against cancer.

5.11.6 Mechanism of Cell Mediated Immunity

- The T cells are very specific to only a specific antigen.
- Unlike B cells, the T-cells do not respond to antigens. It responds to the antigens present on cell surfaces
- Before showing the responses, the antigens on cell surfaces need to be processed by the antigen the MH
- T-cells recognize the antigen only when it is in close association of an MHC antigen.
- An APC cell secretes interleukin-1 when stimulated by an antigen.
- Interleukin-1 is a monokine, a biologically active substance secreted by macrophages that activates the T-cells.
- The activated T-cells in turn secrete Interleukin-2 and surface receptors for interleukin-2 which binds the former.

- After the surface receptor binds to the interleukin-2, the T-cells start proliferating and differentiating into different types of effector cells, cytotoxic T-cells killer cells, natural killer cells and activated macrophages.

The first description of cell mediated immunity was that the specific lymphocytes recognize the relevant antigen or cell and transform into cytotoxic T-lymphocytes.

All the cells are produced from bone marrow but they are developed in thymus called T-cells

Based on the function T-cells are divided into:

(i) **T-Helper cells:** They contain a surface antigen which provides a vigorous immune response. Some helper T cells provide T dependent antigens to B – cells, and some others (eg: delayed hypersensitivity T-cells) are associated with certain allergic reactions and rejection of transplanted tissues.

- When the antigen interacts, the delayed hypersensitivity T-cells secret lymphokines that recruit defense cells like macrophages.

(ii) **Suppressor T-cells:** They check the conversion of B-cells into plasma cells as well as the T-cells.

- They check the immune response, and help the body to develop tolerance.
- Both helper cells and suppressor T-cells are known as regulatory T-cells as they regulate the immune response of the body against the antigens.

5.11.7 Cytotoxic T-cells

They destroy the target cells eg: transplanted tissue, cancer cells, viral and bacterial infections etc.

- Viruses and some of the bacteria multiply within the host cells, and, therefore, they rescue from the attack of antibodies. Hence, the cytotoxic T-cells recognize their antigens on the surface of host cells that produce viruses and destroy them.
- Cytotoxic T-cells come in the contact of host cells; release a protein (perforin) that makes a pore in the target cell which finally is destroyed.

5.11.8 Killer Cells

Some of the effector cells pose cytotoxic effect and, therefore, called the killer cells.

- The killer cells contain the receptors, which combine with Fc region of antibodies.

5.12 Chronology of Discoveries that Contributed to Immunological Techniques

1798	-	First demonstration of vaccination smallpox vaccination (Edward Jenner)
1890	-	Demonstration of antibody activity against diphtheria and tetanus toxins. Beginning of humoral theory of immunity. (Emil von Behring) and (Shibasaburo Kitasato)
1900	-	Antibody formation theory (Paul Ehrlich)
1938	-	Antigen-Antibody binding hypothesis (John Marrack)
1948	-	Antibody production in plasma B cells
1959 to 1962	-	Discovery of antibody structure (Gerald Edelman and Rodney Porter independently)
1960	-	Radioimmunoassay was first described in a scientific paper by Rosalyn Sussman Yalow and Solomon Berson published in 1960
1961 -1962	-	Discovery of thymus involvement in celluler immunity (Jacques Miller)
1966	-	A technique to prepare something like immunosorbent to fix antibody or antigen to the surface of a container was published by Wide and Jerker Porath in 1966
1971	-	Peter Perlmann and Eva Engvall at Stockholm University invented ELISA
1975	-	Generation of the first monoclonal antibodies (George Kohler and Cesar Milstein)

5.13 Antibodies (Abs)

B-cells or B-Lymphocytes (Fig. 5.1): (*Lympha* water and *cyte* cell) *lymphocytes require* a specific antigen to bind to a surface receptor the B-cell receptor on B cells so that cellular activation can occur. After B cells reach maturity within the bone marrow, they circulate in the blood and disperse into various lymphoid organs, where they become activated. The activated B cell is called a plasma cell and it begins to secrete large quantities of glycoproteins called antibodies.

Immature lymphocytes (lymphoblasts) produced in bone marrow that travel to the thymus for maturation become T cells. Those that remain and mature in bone marrow become B cells. Once mature, T and B lymphocytes migrate through the body in the circulatory system as part of the immune system (Fig. 5.1).

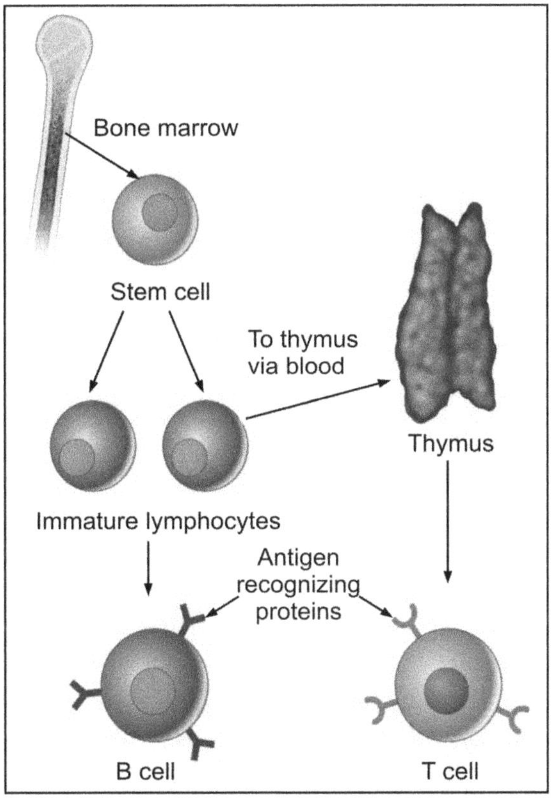

Fig. 5.1 B cell & T cell formation

5.13.1 Antibody Mediated Immunity

- The Humoral immune response is the aspect of immunity that is mediated by secreted antibodies produced in the cells of the B-lymphocyte (B cell).
- Secreted antibodies bind to antigens on the surfaces of invading microbes (such as viruses or bacteria).
- Humoral immunity is so named because it involves substances found in the humus, or body fluids.
- Humoral immunity participates in the pathogenesis of immediate (types 1, 2 and 3) hypersensitivity and certain autoimmune diseases.

5.13.2 Chemical Nature of Antibodies

- ***Antibodies***: They are proteins found in the blood serum and related fluids produced in response to antigens.

- The antibody will react specifically with the inducing antigen but its presence may or may not be related to the immune status of the host.
- Antibodies may be separated from other serum proteins by specific methods involving reaction with the antigen responsible for their induction, or by non-specific methods based on the physical and chemical properties of the antibody molecule.
- Each protein is composed of different amino acids, the total net charge on the proteins would be different and this would determine their rate of migration in an electric field.
- The four major plasma protein groups include:
  1. The fast moving albumin and
  2. The three globulin groups include α, β, γ respectively.

  The globulins which showed antibody activity were found to be primarily in the gamma fraction and secondarily in the slow-moving β globulins.

  The primary importance was the realization of the basic unit of all antibody molecules which is a four polypeptide chain arrays.

5.13.3 Structure of Antibody

Ab molecules are inverted-γ-shaped structures, made up of two identical heavy and two identical light polypeptide chains held together by disulphide (S-S) bonds. The longer chains are called 'heavy' (H) and the shorter ones 'light' (L) chains.

Each L chain is attached to the H chain by a disulphide bond. The two symmetrical chains are held together by one to five s-s (disulphide) bonds, depending on the types of Ig.

The Ab chains are structurally and antigenically distinct and contain constant and variable regions based on the structure of constant region of heavy chains, gamma (γ), Mu (μ), alpha (α), delta (δ) and epsilon (ε), Igs are classified into IgG, IgM, IgD and IgE respectively (Fig. 5.2).

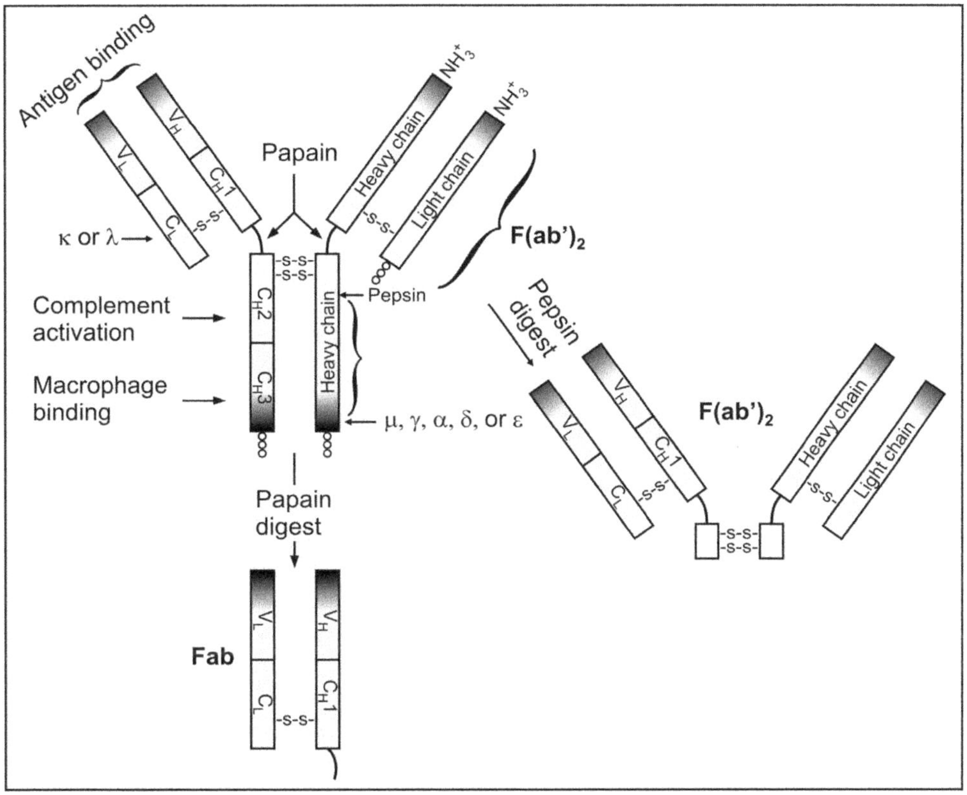

Fig. 5.2 Schematic representation of an Antibody Molecule

The L chains exists, its two forms Kappa (κ) and lambda (λ). Each immunoglobulin molecule shows either two kappas or two combinations. The light chains are named kappa and lambda after Korngold them. The kappa chains are preponderant in most of the immunoglobulins. κ and λ chains are present in a ratio of about 2:1 in any one individual.

- Antibodies table 5.3 (Immunoglobulins, Ig) are proteins derived from the 'immunoglobulin supergene'.

Table 5.3 An overview of Antibody Molecules Classes and Subclasses

Antibody	**Human and Mouse**			
	Light Chain	**Subtype**	**Heavy Chain**	
IgA	κ or λ	IgA_1	α_1	
	κ or λ	IgA2	α_2	
IgE	κ or λ	None	ε	

Table 5.3 *contd...*

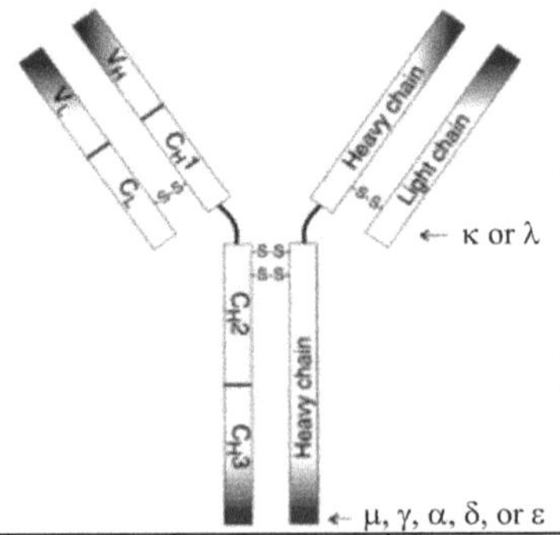

IgD	κ or λ	None	δ			
IgM	κ or λ	None	μ			
IgG	κ or λ	IgG_1	γ_1	κ or λ	IgG_1	γ_1
	κ or λ	IgG_2	γ_2	κ or λ	IgG_{2a}	γ_{2a}
	κ or λ	IgG_3	γ_3	κ or λ	IgG_{2b}	γ_{2b}
	κ or λ	IgG_4	γ_4	κ or λ	IgG_3	γ_3

- One end of the Ig binds to antigens (the F_{ab} portion, so called because it is the fragment of the molecule which is antigen binding), and the other end which is crystallizable, and therefore called F_c, is responsible for effectors functions.
- Each immunoglobulin contains 4 polypeptide chains.
- Shorter ones are called light chains (made up of 107 amino acids)
- Big ones are called heavy chains (made up of 214 amino acids)
- Light chains and heavy chains are joined by one inter disulphide bond.
- Light chains exist in two classes, λ (lambda) and κ (kappa). Each antibody molecule has either λ(lambda) or κ (kappa) light chains, not both.
- The light chain (L) has a molecular weight of approximately 25,000 Daltons.
- The heavy chain has a molecular weight of 50,000 D.
- IgA exists in monomeric and dimeric form.
- IgM exists in pentameric form; molecular weight is 900,000 k D.
- The links between monomers are made by a J chain.
- The heavy and light chains consist of amino acid sequences. In the regions concerned with antigen binding, these regions are extremely variable, whereas in the other regions of the molecule, they are relatively constant. Thus, each heavy and each light chain possesses a variable and constant region.
- Light chains and heavy chains are polypeptide chains. They show polarity.
- Heavy chains have 1-13 inter disulphide bonds only to show flexibility called as Hinge region or neck region.
- Trace amount of carbohydrates like fructose and mannose found in the hinge region.
- If papain and pepsin are used immunoglobulin breaks into two parts.

One half – F_c (fragment crystallisable)

Another half – F_{AB} (fragment antigen binding)

- The region of antibody reacting with antigen called prototype/antibody determinant region.

5.13.4 Production of Antibodies

The production of antibodies consists of three steps:

1. The entry of the antigen, its distribution and fate in the tissues and its contact with appropriate immunocompetent cells. (The afferent limb).
2. The processing of antigen by cells and the control of the antibody forming process (central functions)
3. The secretion of antibody, its distribution in tissues and body fluids and the manifestations of its effects (efferent limb)

***Antibody production follows a characteristic pattern consisting of*:**

(a) A lag phase, the immediate stage following antigenic stimulus during which no antibody is detectable in circulation.

(b) A log phase in which there is a steady rise in the titer of antibodies.

(c) A plateau of steady state when there is equilibrium between antibody synthesis and catabolism.

(d) The phase of decline during which the catabolism exceeds the production and the titer falls.

Antibodies are globulin proteins (proteins that have a compact, globular form) – therefore, we have come to use the term immunoglobulins (Ig) for Abs.

Abs are made in response to an antigen and can recognize and bind to the Ag. Bacterium or virus may have several epitopes that cause the production of different Abs.

Each antibody has at least two identical sites that bind to the epitope. These sites are known as antigen binding sites. The number of Antigen-binding sites on an Ab is called the valence of that Ab.

e.g., As most humans have two binding sites; they are bivalent.

5.13.5 Primary and Secondary Responses

***Primary responses*:** The term primary response refers to the antibody response to an initial antigenic stimulus.

- The primary response is slow, sluggish and short-lived, with a long lag phase and low titer of antibodies that does not persist for long.
- The antibody formed in the primary responses is predominantly IgM.

Secondary response: It is the response to subsequent stimuli with the same antigen.

- The secondary response is prompt, powerful and prolonged, with a short or negligible lag phase and a much higher level of antibodies.
- The antibody formed in the secondary response is IgG.
- A single injection of an antigen helps more in sensitizing or priming the immune competent cells producing the particular antibody than in the actual elaboration of high levels of antibody.
- Effective levels of antibody are usually induced only by subsequent injections of the antigens. It is for this reason nonliving vaccines are given multiple doses of active immunization.
- The first injection is known as the priming dose and subsequent injections as booster doses.
- When an antigen was injected into an animal already carrying the specific antibody in circulation, a temporary fall in the level of circulating antibody occurs due to the combination of the antigen with the antibody. This has been called the negative phase.

5.13.6 Immunoglobulin Classes

The simplest and most abundant Igs are monomers, but they can also assume some differences in size and arrangement.

The five classes of Igs are designated IgG, IgA, IgM, IgD and IgE, each class has a different role in the immune response. Molecules of IgA and IgM are aggregated to two or five monomers respectively that are joined together. Thus, each of these isotypes occupies a particular site in the body and has a particular role in defending the body against extracellular pathogens and their toxic products. Antibodies can accomplish this by direct interactions with pathogens or their products, for example by binding to active sites of toxins and neutralizing them or by blocking their ability to bind to host cells through specific receptors. When antibodies of the appropriate Isotype bind to antigens, they can activate the *classical pathway* of complement, which leads to the elimination of the pathogen by the various mechanisms. Soluble immune complexes of antigen and antibody also fix complement and are cleared from the circulation via complement receptors on red blood cells. Most classes of *antibody* are distributed by diffusion from their site of synthesis, but specialized transport mechanisms are required to deliver antibodies to luminal epithelial surfaces, such as those of the lung and intestine. The distribution of antibodies is determined by their Isotype, which can limit their diffusion or enable them to engage specific transporters that deliver them across epithelia.

5.13.6.1 IgG: (γ)

IgG is the major serum Ig making up 85% of the total amount in adults. IgG antibodies are large molecules of about 150 kDa composed of four peptide chains. It is a tetrameric quaternary structure. (Table 5.4).

Table 5.4 Receptors for IgG

Receptor	Present on	Interacts with
Fcr R_1 (CD 64)	Monocytes Neutrophils	IgG_1, IgG_3, IgG_4
Fcr R_2 (CD 32)	Neutrophils Eosinophils	IgG_1, IgG_3
Fcr R_3 (CD 16)	Neutrophils NK cells	IgG_1, IgG_3

As an IgG molecule has got two identical antigen binding sites, it is called divalent.

IgG participates in most of the immunological reactions such as precipitation, complement fixation and neutralization of toxin and viruses.

It is the only immunoglobulin that passes through placenta and provides natural passive immunity to newborn. Ig is not formed in the foetus in any significant amount.

IgG has a longest half life amongst all the Igs which is about 23 days.

In the human IgG molecule, the heavy chain (gamma chain) exists in four different forms and on this basis IgG has been classified as IgG_1, IgG_2, IgG_3 and IgG_4, which can be identified with specific antisera able to detect differences in the Fc fragment of the heavy chains

In human serum, the four IgG subclasses are distributed as IgG_1 (65%), IgG_2 (23%), IgG_3 (8%) and IgG_4 (4%).

Immunological response to bacterial polysaccharide is predominantly made by the IgG_2 production.

IgG is one of the major activators of classical complement pathway, particularly IgG_1 and IgG_3.

IgG has cellular receptors – Fcr R_1, Fcr R_2, Fcr R_3 which bind, recruit and activate cells such as polymorphous, macrophages and NK cells, FcR receptor is also responsible for active process of placental transfer from mother to foetus.

5.13.6.2 Immunoglobulin A

IgA is the principal Ig that appears in the seromucous secretions such as milk, saliva, tears, nasal fluids sweat, colostrums and in secretions of respiratory, intestinal and genital tracts.

Their content in serum is about 150-250 mg/100 mL and constitutes about 10 to 13% of serum Ig.

The molecular weight of IgA monomer is 1, 50,000 Daltons or 150 kD, sedimentation coefficient is 6.85, and half life is 6-8 days. Since IgA molecules express morphological diversity in different locations, the secretory IgA is much larger than serum IgA.

IgA is largely synthesized locally by plasma cells and only a little amount may be derived from serum. IgA production requires B cells help and special mucosal stimulation to promote production of secretory IgA.

IgA is dimerised within the epithelial cells of glands. Intestines and the respiratory tract with a cysteine rich polypeptide called J (joining) chaining.

The linkage occurs between J chains and Fc fragment. The dimeric IgA combines with another protein. Secretory component, synthesized by local epithelial cells and then the complex is transported across the cytoplasm and secreted into body fluids.

Although IgA does not fix complement, but it is capable of activating the alternate complement pathway and is also an effective opsonin with $F_{ca}R$ on monocytes and neutrophils.

5.13.6.3 IgM

Antibodies of the IgM class make up 5 to 10% of the Abs in serum.

IgM forms polymers where multiple immunoglobulins are covalently linked together with polypeptide "J" chain and disulfide bonds, mostly as a pentamer but also as a Hexamer. IgM has a molecular mass of approximately 970 kDa (in its pentamer form).

The large size of the molecule prevents IgM from moving about as freely as IgG does so IgM Abs generally remain in blood vessels without entering the surrounding tissue.

IgM is the predominant type of antibody involved in the response to the ABO blood group antigen on the surface of red blood cells.

It is effective in aggregating Ags and in reactions involving complement, and it can enhance the ingestion of target cells by phagocytic cells, as does IgG.

IgM offers protection against *"bacteraemia"*, its deficiency may lead to septicemia.

IgM is particularly important for immunity against the polysaccharide Ags present on the exterior of pathogenic bacteria.

IgM also promotes phagocytosis and bacteriolysis through its complement activation activity.

5.13.6.4 Immunoglobulin D

IgD is the least well characterized of the immunoglobulins from functional aspect. IgD was first detected by Rose and Fahey (1965) in myeloma protein. It is a 7s monomer present is a concentration of about 3 mg/100mt serum (less than 1% serum AgIG) and mostly intravascular in distribution.

Nearly all the IgD is present, together with IgM, on the membranes of a proportion of unstimulated B lymphocytes of blood and serve as recognition receptors for Ags. It has a monomeric structure similar to that of IgG. Their function is to signal the B cell to start antibody production upon antigen binding.

5.13.6.5 Immunoglobulin E

IgE is discovered by Ishizaka (1996) in serum of patients with certain types of allergies. Based upon the observation that allergic responses typically affect the skin, gut, and respiratory tract, the major sites of parasitic invasion, it is thought that IgE evolved as a defense against parasitic infestation. Helminthes stimulate a vigorous IgE production, including parasite-specific IgE antibody.

They play a very key role in early recognition of foreign material ("gate keeper function") or a general potentiating of the immune system response by the improved antigen presentation. Actually, allergy triggered by IgE may be considered a beneficial function of the host; the typical allergic reactions of mucus secretion, sneezing, itching, coughing, bronchoconstriction, tear production, inflammation, vomiting and diarrhea are all mechanisms that expel allergenic proteins from the body.

IgE is a 8s molecule with a short half life of 2.3 days. It constitutes less than 1% of the total immunoglobulin.

Although IgE is typically the least abundant isotype-blood serum IgE levels in a normal ("non-atopic") individual are only 0.05% of the Ig concentration.

Clearly bound to Fc receptor on most cells and found in insignificant amount in normal serum.

IgE molecules bind tightly by their Fc regions to receptors on mast cells and basophils, specialized cells that participate in allergic reactions shown in Fig. 5.3.

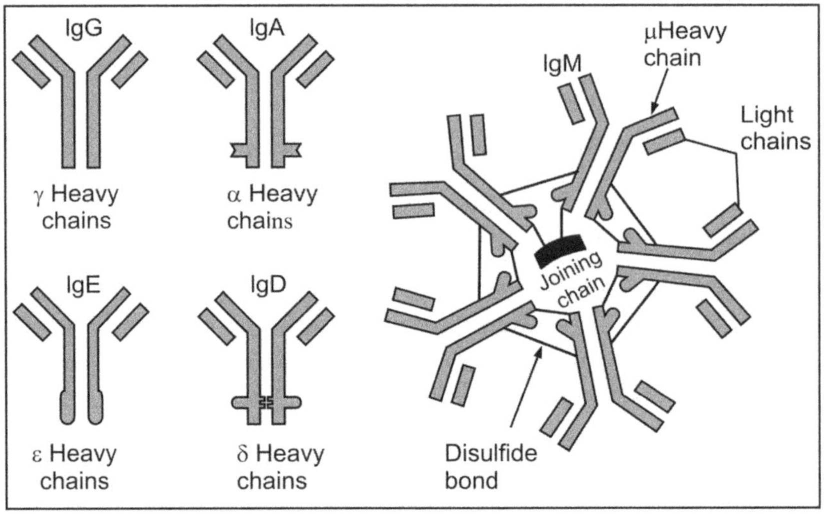

Fig. 5.3 Figures of different immunoglobulins

5.14 Antigens-Antibody Reactions

- The antigen-antibody reaction depends on non-covalent interactions including hydrogen bonds, ionic bonds, hydrophobic interactions and Vander Waals interactions.
- Antigen-antibodies combine with each other specifically and in observable manner.
- The reactions between antigens and antibodies serve several purposes.
  1. In the body, they form the basis of antibody mediated immunity in infectious diseases, or of tissue injury in some types of hypersensitivity and auto immune diseases.
  2. In the laboratory, they help in the diagnosis of infections, and of noninfectious antigens such as enzymes.
  3. These reaction can be used for detection and quantification of either antigens or antibodies.

Features of Antigen-Antibody Reaction

1. **Affinity:** Antibody affinity is the strength of the reaction between a single antigenic determinant and a single combining site on the antibody. It is the sum of the attractive and repulsive forces operating between the antigenic determinant and the combining site of the antibody.

2. **Avidity:** Avidity is a measure of the overall strength of binding of an antigen with many antigenic determinates and multivalent antibodies. Avidity is influenced by both the valence of the antibody and the valence of the antigen.
3. **Specificity:** Specificity refers to the ability of an individual antibody combining site to react with only one antigenic determinant or the ability of a population of antibody molecules to react with only one antigen.
4. **Cross reactivity:** Cross reacting refers to the ability of an individual antibody combining site to react with more than one antigenic determinant or the ability of a population of antibody molecules to react with more than one antigen.
   - There is no denaturation of antigen or antibody during the reaction.
   - Both antigens and antibodies participate in the formation of agglutinates or precipitates.

   Antigen-Antibody reactions conducted in vitro are known as serological reactions.

5.14.1 Precipitation Reactions

The reaction of soluble antigens with IgG or IgM antibodies to form large interlocking aggregates is called precipitation reaction.

- The precipitations formed by antibodies are known as precipitins.
- The precipitation reactions occur in two stages
- Rapid interactions within a second between antigen and antibodies and formation of complex.
- Slow rate of reaction completing even within a few minutes or hours and forming lattices from antigen-antibody complexes.
- When antibodies and antigens are in proper ratio, precipitation reactions normally occur.
- When there is excess amount of either of two, no visible precipitate is formed. One can produce the optimal ratio of these two by putting antigens and antibody adjacent to each other and waiting for their diffusion together.
- In precipitation test, a precipitation ring appears which display the creation of optimal ratio. This zone is known as zone of equivalence precipitation can take place in liquid media or in gel.

Mechanism of Precipitation

According to lattice hypothesis concept, multivalent antigens combine with bivalent antibodies in varying proportion, depending on the antigen-antibody ratio in the reacting mixture.

Precipitation results when a large lattice is formed consisting of alternating antigen and antibody molecules. This is possible only in the zone of equivalence.

In the zones of antigen or antibody excess, the lattice does not enlarge, as the valenceis of the antibody and the antigen are fully satisfied.

Application of Precipitation Reaction

The precipitation test may be carried out as either a qualitative or quantitative test.

- It is very sensitive in the detection of antigens and as little as 1 mg of protein can be detected by precipitation tests.
- It finds forensic application in the identification of blood and seminal stains, and in testing for food adulterants.

The following types of precipitation and flocculation tests are in common use.

1. **Ring test:** This is the simplest type of precipitation test, consists of layering the antigen solution over a column of antiserum in a narrow tube.
   - A precipitate forms at the junction of the two liquids.

   e.g., Ascoli's themo precipition test, grouping of streptococci by the Lancefield technique.
2. **Slide test:** When a drop each of the antigen and antiserum are placed on a slide and mixed by shaking, floccules appear.

   E.g.: VDRL test for syphilis
3. **Tube test:** A quantative tube flocculation test is employed for the standardisation of toxins and toxoids.
   - Serial dilutions of the toxin/toxoid are added to the tubes containing a fixed quantity of the antitoxin. The amount of toxin or toxoid that flocculates optimally with one unit of the antitoxin is defined as an LF dose.

   E.g.: Kahn test for syphilis.
4. **Immuno diffusion (precipitation in gel):** Immuno diffusion tests are performed in a gelled agar medium.
   - The reaction is visible as a distinct band of precipitation, which is stable and can be stained for preservation.
   - Immuno diffusion also indicates identity, cross reaction and nonidentity between different antigens.

Different modifications of the test are available

1. **Single diffusion in one dimension:** The antibody is incorporated in agar gel in a test tube and the antigen solution is layered over it.
   - The antigen diffuses downward through the agar gel, forming a line of precipitation that appears to move downwards. This is due to the

precipitation formed at the advancing front of the antigen, and is dissolved as the concentration of antigen at the site increases due to diffusion.

- The number of bands indicates the number of different antigens present.

2. **Double diffusion in one dimension:** The antibody is incorporated in gel, the column of plain agar in placed above it.
   - The antigen is layered on top of this.
   - The antigen and antibody move towards each other through the intervening column of plain agar and form a band of precipitate where they meet at optimum proportion.
3. **Single diffusion in two Dimensions:** The antiserum is incorporated in agar gel poured in flat surface.
   - The antigen is added to the wells cut on the surface of the gel. It diffuses radially from the well and forms ring shaped bands of precipitation concentrically around the well.
   - The diameter of the halo gives an estimate of the concentration of the antigen.
   - This method is employed for the estimation of the immunoglobulin classes in sera and for screening sera for antibodies to influenza viruses, among others.
4. **Double diffusion in two dimensions:** In test wells are cut, into which a purified antiserum (a serum containing antibodies) is added, and to each surrounding well, soluble form of test antigens are added.
   - Thereafter, a line of visible precipitate is formed between the wells where after diffusion optimal ratio of antigen-antibody is formed.
   - Through this test the presence of antibodies in the serum against more than one antigen at a time can be demonstrated.
   - We can also find out the identical, partially identical and different types of antigens through this test.
   - A special variety of double diffusion in two dimensions is the Elek test for toxigenicity in *Diphtheria bacilli*.
   - When *Diphtheria bacilli* are streaked at right angles to a filter paper strip carrying the antitoxin implanted on a plate of suitable medium, arrowhead shaped lines of precipitation appear on incubation, if the bacillus is toxigenic.
5. **Immunoelectrophoresis:** This method involves the electrophoretic separation of a composite antigen in its constituent proteins, followed by immune diffusion against its antiserum, resulting in separate precipitin lines.

- The technique is performed on agar or agarose gel, on a slide, with an antigen well and antibody trough cut on it.
- Antigen well filled with human serum.
- Serum separated by electrophoresis
- Antiserum trough filled with antiserum to whole human serum.
- Serum and antiserum allowed to diffuse into agar.
- Precipitin lines form for individual serum proteins.
- It is useful for testing the normal and abnormal proteins in serum and urine.

5.14.2 Electroimmunodiffusion

The development of precipitin lines can be speeded up by electrically driving the antigen and antibody.

Methods Include

1. Counter immunoelectrophoresis (counter current immunoelectrophoresis)
2. One dimensional single electro immunodiffusion (rocket electrophoresis)

1. **Counter Current Immuno Electrophoresis:** (counter immunoelectrophoresis (CIE)) antibody in a gel, but also uses electrophoresis for their rapid movement.
   - The principle of CIE is based on the movement of antigens and antibodies to opposite poles after applying electric current in buffers of correct electric strength and pH, because some of the antigens and antibodies have the opposite charges.
   - If a reaction occurs, a precipitation line appears within an hour.
   - By using this method protein can be separated within an hour.
   - CIE is useful for the diagnosis of bacterial meningitis and the other diseases.
2. **One dimensional single electro immunodiffusion (rocket electrophoresis):**
   - In this method the antiserum to the antigen to be quantitated is incorporated in agarose and gelled on the glass slide.
   - The antigen, in increasing concentrations, is placed in wells punched in the set gel.
   - The antigen is then electrophoresed into the antibody containing agarose
   - The pattern of immunoprecipitation resembles a rocket hence the name rocket electrophoresis.
   - The main application of this technique is for quantitative estimation of antigens.

5.14.3 Agglutination Reaction

Agglutination is the process of linking together of antigens by antibodies and the formation of visible aggregates given in Fig. 5.4.

- Agglutination reaction involve particulate antigens i.e., soluble antigens adhering to particles.
- Agglutination reactions are very sensitive, readable and available in several varieties.

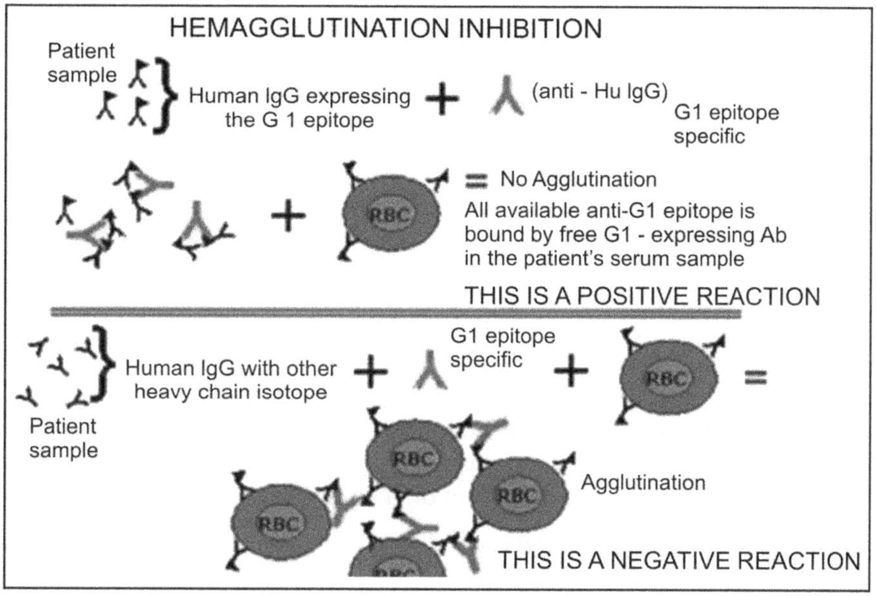

Fig. 5.4 Hemagglutination results

1. ***Direct Agglutination Test***
   - Direct agglutination test diagnoses antibodies against a large number of cellular antigens such as RBC's, bacteria and fungi.
   - This test is carried out in plastic microtiter plates that have several small shallow wells. Each well acts as small test tube.
   - Each well contains an equal amount of particulate antigen (eg., RBC's) but the amount of antibodies in the serum is serially diluted in successive wells so that their concentration may be half of the previous well.
   - If one starts with more antibodies, more dilutions will be required to lower the amount to a point at which agglutination does not occur. This is the measure of titer or concentration of serum antibody.

- In a positive reaction, agglutination occurs, and sufficient antibodies are present in the serum to link the antigen together. This results in the formation of antibody-antigen mat which sinks to bottom of well.
- In the negative reaction, agglutination does not occur and insufficient antibodies are present to cause the linking of antigens.

2. ***Indirect (passive) Agglutination Tests*:** These types of diagnostic tests are very rapid particularly for the detection of streptococci.
    - If the antigen are adsorbed onto particles (e.g., RBC, latex beads), soluble antigens can respond to agglutination test.
    - Antibody reacts with the soluble antigen adhering to the particles.
    - Therefore, the particles agglutinate with each other as these do in the direct agglutination tests.
    - The Weil-Felix reaction for serodiagnosis of typhus fever is a heterophile agglutination test and is based on the sharing of a common antigen between typhus *rickettsiae* and some strains of proteus bacilli.

5.14.4 Complement Fixation Test (CFT)

A group of 20 or more serum proteins are collectively known as complement. The complement system is an enzyme cascade. During reaction, the complement binds to antigen-antibody complex and is used up or fixed.

The phases in the complement cascade are

- Recognition,
- Activation amplification
- Membrane attack

Complement Action Steps:

- Lysis of foreign cells
- Increased vascular permeability
- Lysis of bacteria
- Neutrophil activation and chemotaxis
- Mast cell degranulation
- Smooth muscle contraction
- Localization of complexes in germinal centers
- Opsonization and phagocytosis of bacteria.
- This process of complement fixation may be used to measure even very small amount of antibody that does not produce a visible reaction such as precipitation or agglutination. Therefore, it is necessary to use indicator system.

- The test requires patient's serum, test antigen, complement from Guinea pig and antibodies of sheep RBC's to determine whether sheep RBC's may be lysed by Guinea pig complement.

The test is accomplished in two stages:

Stage 1: The patient's serum is heated at 56 °C for 30 minutes so that the complement should be inactivated.

- The heated serum is diluted and then added to known amount of specific antigen and complement.
- The test antigen may correspond to the diseases.

E.g., If a patient is suffering from a disease caused by *streptococci* the test antigen would be streptococcal antigen.

If the patient's serum contains antibodies against *streptococci*, the test antigen will form complement sequence. This mixture is again incubated for about 30 minutes. At this point, no antigen-antibody reaction occurs

Stage 2: The complement fixed by antigen-antibody reaction is detected by an indication system. This system consists of sheep RBC's containing specific antibodies attached to their surfaces.

- When these are added to complement, haemolysis of RBC's occur that impart changes in colour of the mixture. This shows that the complements have not been fixed during the first stage; therefore, these become available to cause haemolysis. This indicates that the patient has no streptococcal pneumonia.
- However, if the Guinea pig complements are destroyed, they would not be able to cause the lysis of RBC's.
- If the complements are fixed (by antigen-antibody reaction) during the first stage, this indicates that the patient has the infection of streptococci.
- The classical example of CFT is the Wassermann reaction, a method for the serodiagnosis of syphilis.
- The test consists of two steps.
- In the **first step**, the inactivated serum of patient is incubated at 37 °C for one hour with the Wassermann antigen and a fixed amount (two units) of Guinea pig complement.
- If the serum contains syphilitic antibody, the complement will be utilized during antigen antibody interaction.
- If the serum does not contain the antibody, no antigen-antibody reaction occurs and the complement will be left intact.
- The **second step** includes the testing for complement in the post incubation mixture this will indicate whether the serum had antibodies or not.

- This is followed by adding sensitized cells (sheep erythrocytes coated with 4MHD hemolysin), and incubating at 37 °C for 30 minutes.
- Lysis of the erythrocytes indicates that complement was not fixed in the first step and therefore, the serum did not have the antibody (–ve CFT).
- Absence of erythrocyte lysis indicates that the complement was used up in the first step and, therefore the serum contained the antibody (+ve CFT)

Indirect complement fixation test: The test is set up in duplicate and after first step, the standard antiserum known to fix complement is added to one set.

- If the test serum contained antibody, the antigen would have been used in the first step and therefore the standard antiserum added subsequently would not be able to fix complement therefore in the indirect test, haemolysis indicates a positive result.

Coagulating complement absorption test: For systems which do not fix guinea pig, an alternating method is the coagulating complement absorption test. (Fig. 5.5 & Table 5.5(a), (b) & (c)).

- This uses horse complement which is non hemolytic. The indicator system is sensitized sheep erythrocytes mixed with bovine serum.
- Bovine serum contains a β-globulin component called conglutinin, which acts as antibody to complement.
- Therefore conglutinin causes agglutination of sensitized sheep erythrocytes (conglutination) if they have combined with complement.
- If the horse complement had been used up by the antigen-antibody interaction in the first step, agglutination of sensitized cells will not occur.

Table 5.5(a) Complement Fixation Assay Test Phase

Complement Fixation Assay Test Phase	
Positive serum- Antibodies	**Negative serum- no Antibodies**
Antigen	Antigen
Complement	Complement
AG-AB complex formed	No Ag-Ab complex
Complement used up	Complement NOT used up

Table 5.5(b) Complement Fixation Assay Indicator phase

Complement Fixation Assay Indicator phase	
Positive Test phase - No complement	Negative test phase- Complement
Indicator system, Sheep RBCs, Anti sheep RBCs	Indicator System- Sheep RBCs, Anti Sheep RBC's
Result-NO LYSIS of RBCs. CLOUDY	Result- LYSIS of RBCs, CLEAR

Table 5.5(c) Advantages and Disadvantages of CFT

Advantages of CFT	Disadvantages of CFT
Reagents easily available	Indirect test
Semi quantitative or quantitative	Need adequate controls
Wide application	Reagents unstable
Extensively sensitive	Quantitation time consuming
	Cannot be automated

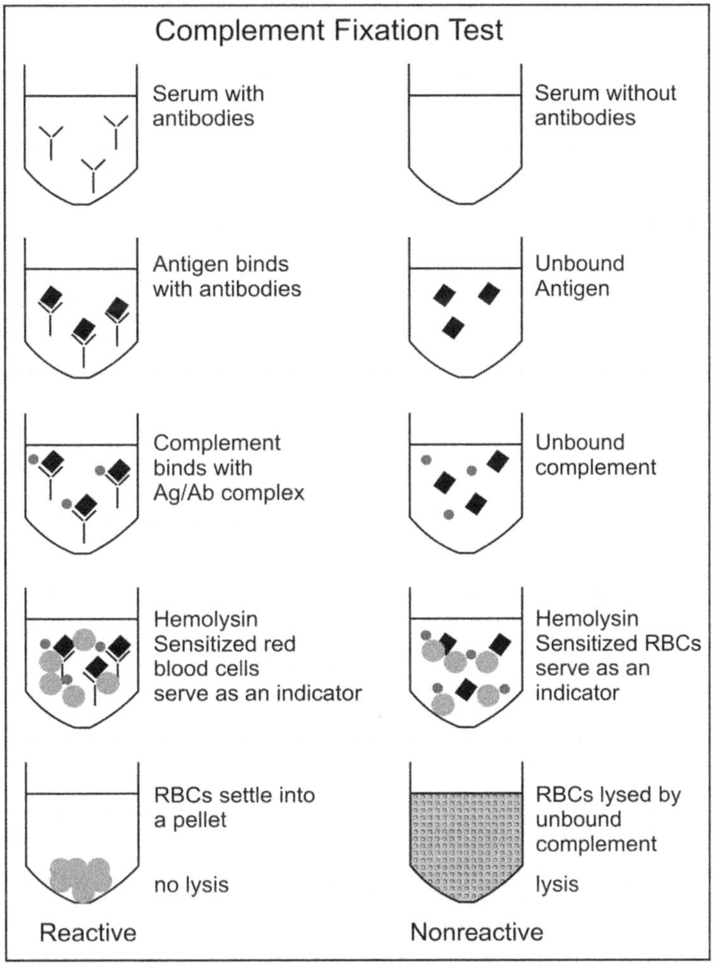

Fig. 5.5 Complement fixation test

5.14.5 Opsonisation

The name 'opsonin' was given to a heat liable substance present in fresh normal sera, which facilitated phagocytosis. This factor was subsequently identified as complement.

- Opsonisation is a phenomenon of adsorption of certain antibodies or complement ($c_3 - c_5$ complex) especially c_{3b} onto the surface of foreign material that result in stimulation in phagocytosis.
- Opsonization is also known as immune adherence.
- Opsonization is also one of the main antigen-antibody reactions associated with humoral antibodies.
- The two main opsonins (complement and certain antibodies) stimulate phagocytosis.
- The complement stimulates T-cells to process for cell mediated immunity and release histamine from leukocytes, which in turn increases the capillary permeability and smooth muscle contraction.
- 'Opsonic index' is used to study the progress of resistance during the course of disease.
- Opsonic index is defined as the ratio of the phagocytic activity of the patient's blood for a given bacterium, to the phagocytic activity of blood from a normal individual.
- It was measured by incubating fresh citrated blood with the bacterial suspension at 37 °C for 15 minutes and estimating the average number of phagocytosed bacteria per polymorphonuclear leukocyte (phagocytic index) from stained blood films.

5.14.6 Radioimmuno Assay (RIA)

- A variety of tests have been devised for the measurement of antigen and antibodies using labeled reactants.
- The term binder-ligand assay has been used for these reactions.
- The substance whose concentration is to be determined is termed as analyte or ligand. The binder protein which binds to the ligand is called the binder.
- RIA permits the measurement of analyte up to pictogram (10^{-12} gm) quantities.
- RIA has versatile applications in various areas of biology and medicine, including the quantitation.
- There are two methods of measuring RIA: the liquid phase and the solid phase RIA's.

1. **Liquid phase RIA:** The liquid phase RIA is based on competitive binding of radiolabelled antigen and unlabelled antigen, to a high affinity antibody.
    - The antigen labeled with ^{125}I is mixed with such a concentration of antibody that can just saturate the antibody.

- Therefore, the increasing amount of antigen (unlabelled) of unknown concentration is added.
- The two types of antigens now compete for available sites of the antibody.
- The antibody does not differentiate the labeled antigen from unlabelled one.
- Upon gradually increasing concentration of unlabelled antigen, the labeled antigen could be displaced from the binding sites available on antibody.
- The labeled antigens are made free in the solution.
- The amount of labeled antigen in solution is measured, and the concentration of unlabelled antigen can be determined.

2. **Solid phase RIA:** In solid phase RIA, either antigen or antibody is immobilized on a solid phase matrix. It is simple and easy in handling as compared to liquid phase RIA.

5.14.7 Neutralization Reaction

The neutralization reactions are the reactions of antigen-antibody that involve the elimination of harmful effects of bacterial exotoxins or a virus by specific antibodies.

- These neutralizing substance i.e., antibodies are known as antitoxins.
- This specific antibody is produced by a host cell in response to a bacterial exotoxin or corresponding toxoid (inactivated toxin).
- The antitoxin reacts with exotoxin and neutralizes it.
- These antitoxins can be artificially induced in animals such as horses.
- Thus, the antitoxin of animal sources in turn can be injected into human who provides a passive immunity against a toxin present in human body produced by the pathogen causing diphtheria, tetanus etc.
- Neutralization of animal viruses can be demonstrated in three systems - animals, eggs and tissue culture.

Toxin neutralization: Bacterial toxins are good antigens and induce the formation of neutralising antibodies which are important in protection against and recovery from diseases such as diphtheria and tetanus.

- Neutralisation tests in animals consist of injecting toxin-antitoxin mixtures and estimating the least amount of antitoxin that prevents death or disease in the animals.

5.14.8 Enzyme Immuno Assays (EIA)

The term enzyme immunoassay is used for all assays based on the measurement of enzymes labeled antigen, hapten or antibody.

EIA's are of 2 basic types: homogeneous and heterogeneous.

In homogeneous EIA, there is no need to separate the bound and free fractions so that the test can be completed in one step, with all reagents added simultaneously.

The EIA test can be used only for assay of haptens such as not microbial antigens and antibodies.

e.g., Enzyme multiplied immunoassay technique (EMIT), is simple method for small molecule drugs such as opiates, cocaine, and barbiturates amphetamine in serum.

Heterogeneous EIA requires the separation of the free and bound fraction either by centrifugation or by absorption on solid surfaces and washing.

It is therefore a multi step procedure, with reagents added sequentially.

e.g., ELISA

5.14.9 Enzyme Linked Immunosorbent Assays (ELISA)

ELISA Principle Basis and Extension

Enzyme-linked Immunosorbent Assays (ELISAs) combine the specificity of antibodies with the sensitivity of simple enzyme assays, by using antibodies or antigens coupled to an easily-assayed enzyme.

ELISAs can provide a useful measurement of antigen or antibody concentration. There are two main variations on this method: The ELISA can be used to detect the presence of antigens that are recognized by an antibody or it can be used to test for antibodies that recognize an antigen.

A general ELISA is a five-step procedure:

1. Coat the microtiter plate wells with antigen;
2. Block all unbound sites to prevent false positive results;
3. Add primary antibody (e.g., rabbit monoclonal antibody) to the wells;
4. Add secondary antibody conjugated to an enzyme (e.g., anti-mouse IgG);
5. Reaction of a substrate with the enzyme to produce a colored product, thus indicating a positive reaction.

There are many different types of ELISAs. One of the most common types of ELISA is "sandwich ELISA".

Buffer Preparation

1. Bicarbonate/carbonate coating buffer (100 mM):

   Antigen or antibody should be diluted in coating buffer to immobilize them to the wells:

   - 3.03 g Na_2CO_3
   - 6.0 g $NaHCO_3$
   - 1000 ml distilled water,
   - pH 9.6

2. PBS:

   - 1.16 g Na_2HPO_4
   - 0.1 g KCl
   - 0.1 g K_3PO_4
   - 4.0 g NaCl (500 ml distilled water)
   - pH 7.4

3. Blocking solution:

   - Commonly used blocking agents are 1% BSA, serum, non-fat dry milk, casein, gelatin in PBS.

4. Wash solution:

   - Usually PBS or Tris -buffered saline (pH 7.4) with detergent such as 0.05% (v/v) Tween20 (TBST).

5. Antibody dilution buffer:

   - Primary and secondary antibody should be diluted in 1x blocking solution to reduce non-specific binding.

Protocol of sandwich ELISA test:

1. Before the assay, both antibody preparations should be purified and one must be labeled.
2. For most applications, a polyvinylchloride (PVC) microtiter plate is best; however, consult manufacturer guidelines to determine the most appropriate type of plate for protein binding.
3. Bind the unlabeled antibody to the bottom of each well by adding approximately 50 μL of antibody solution to each well (20 μg/mL in PBS). PVC will bind approximately 100 ng/well (300 ng/cm^2). The amount of antibody used will depend on the individual assay, but if maximal binding is required, use at least 1 μg/well. This is well above the capacity of the well, but the binding will occur more rapidly, and the binding solution can be saved and used again.
4. Incubate the plate overnight at 4 °C to allow complete binding.

5. Wash the wells twice with PBS. A 500 mL squirt bottle is convenient. The antibody solution washes can be removed by flicking the plate over a suitable container.
6. The remaining sites for protein binding on the microtiter plate must be saturated by incubating with blocking buffer. Fill the wells to the top with 3% BSA/PBS with 0.02% sodium azide. Incubate for 2 h to overnight in a humid atmosphere at room temperature.
7. **Note:** Sodium azide is an inhibitor or horseradish peroxidase. Do not include sodium azide in buffers or wash solutions if an HRP-labeled antibody will be used for det*ection.*
8. Wash wells twice with PBS.
9. Add 50 µL of the antigen solution to the wells (the antigen solution should be titrated). All dilutions should be done in the blocking buffer (3% BSA/PBS). Incubate for at least 2 hr at room temperature in a humid atmosphere.
10. Wash the plate four times with PBS.
11. Add the labeled second antibody. The amount to be added can be determined in preliminary experiments. For accurate quantitation, the second antibody should be used in excess. All dilutions should be done in the blocking buffer.
12. Incubate for 2 hr or more at room temperature in a humid atmosphere.
13. Wash with several changes of PBS.
14. Add substrate as indicated by manufacturer. After suggested incubation time has elapsed, optical densities at target wavelengths can be measured on an ELISA plate reader.

    Note: Some enzyme substrates are considered hazardous, due to potential carcinogenicity. Handle with care and refer to Material Safety Data Sheets for proper handling precautions.

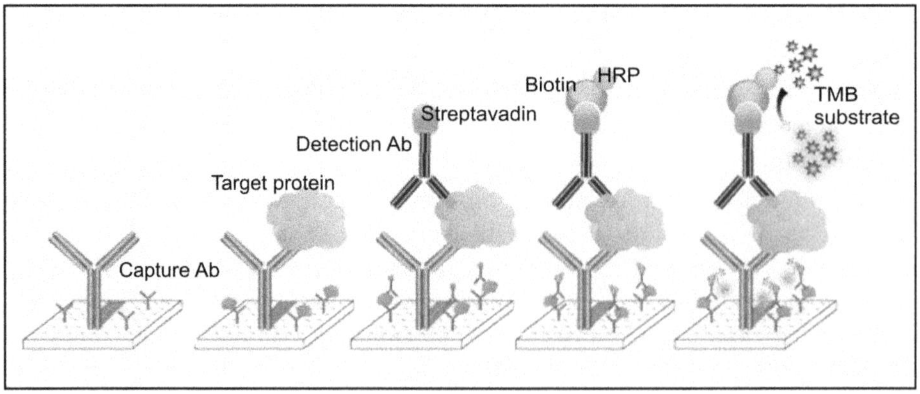

Fig. 5.6 ELISA Test

5.15 Classification of Vaccines

Vaccines are preparations of antigenic substances that are administered for the purpose of inducing in the recipient a specific and active immunity against the infective agent or toxin produced by it.

Bacterial Vaccines: Bacterial vaccines are either sterile suspensions of live or killed bacteria or sterile extracts of derivatives of bacteria. Most vaccines against bacterial infections are effective at preventing disease Reactions can occur after vaccinations Vaccines are available against tuberculosis, diphtheria, tetanus, pertussis, *Haemophilus influenzae* type B, cholera, typhoid, and *Streptococcus pneumoniae*.

Bacterial toxoides: Bacterial toxoids are toxins or material derived therefrom, the toxicity of which has been reduced to a very low level or completely eliminated by chemical or physical means without destroying their immunizing potency. Examples are Tetanus toxoid, Botulism toxoid.

Viral and rickettsial vaccines: Viral and rickettsial vaccines are suspensions of viruses or rickettsiae and are prepared from infected tissues or blood obtained from artificially infected animals, from cultures in fertile eggs, or from cell or tissue cultures. Examples of viral vaccines are Hepatitis A & B vaccines, Influenza vaccine, MMR vaccine, Poliomyelitis vaccine, rabies vaccine, rotavirus vaccine, Yellow fever vaccine etc. and *Rickettsia rickettsii* vaccine is an example of rickettsial vaccine.

Antisera (Immunosera): Antisera are native (unconcentrated) sera or preparations from native sera containing specific immunoglobulins that have prophylactic or therapeutic action when injected into persons exposed to or suffering from a disease caused by a specific micro-organism. Examples are snake venom antiserum, scorpion venom antiserum, tetanus immune-human globulin etc.

There are several different types of vaccine available and with new technology, there will be further additions. The body response to a vaccine depends on the type of vaccine being administered. The more similar a vaccine is to the natural disease, the better the immune response to the vaccine.

5.15.1 The following is the fate of most Vaccines Injected Directly into Muscle Tissue

1. Vaccine antigen disassociates from adjuvant (i.e. Aluminum hydroxide).
2. Cells of the non-specific immune system (i.e. Macrophages and dendritic cells) recognize the antigen as foreign and engulf it. These cells then chop the antigen into smaller fragments and display these on their cell surfaces.

3. The dendritic cells move through the lymphatic system to a local lymph node where specific T cells and B cells, which recognize the fragments of antigen generates a specific immune response.
4. Other components in the vaccine such as the adjuvant and preservative, if present, are absorbed into the blood where they circulate and are excreted in the stools and urine.

5.15.2 There are Two Basic Types of Vaccines based on the Properties of Antigens

(i) Live attenuated Vaccines
(ii) Inactivated Vaccines.

The characteristics of live and inactivated vaccines are different, and these characteristics determine how the vaccine is used.

Live Attenuated Vaccines: are produced by modifying a disease-producing ("wild") virus or bacteria in a laboratory. The resulting vaccine organism retains the ability to replicate (grow) and produce immunity, but usually does not cause illness. Live attenuated vaccines include live viruses and live bacteria. Reduction of virulence is known as attenuation and can be achieved by passage through unfavorable hosts, repeated cultures in artificial media, growth under high temperature or in the presence of weak antiseptics, desiccation, or prolonged storage in culture.

Properties of Live Attenuated Vaccines

Live vaccines are derived from "wild," or disease-causing, virus or bacteria.

These wild viruses or bacteria are attenuated, or weakened, in a laboratory, usually by repeated culturing.

Unlike live antigens, inactivated antigens are usually not affected by circulating antibody.

Inactivated vaccines may be given when antibody is present in the blood (*e.g.*, In infancy, or following receipt of antibody-containing blood products).

Inactivated vaccines always require multiple doses. In general, the first dose does not produce protective immunity, but only "primes" the immune system. A protective immune response develops after the second or third dose.

The immune response to an inactivated vaccine is mostly humoral, little or no cellular immunity results.

Antibody titers against inactivated antigens diminish with time. As a result, some inactivated vaccines may require periodic supplemental doses to increase, or "boost," antibody titers.

Examples of currently available inactivated vaccines are limited to inactivated whole viral vaccines (influenza, polio, rabies and hepatitis A). Whole inactivated bacterial vaccines include Pertussis, Typhoid, Cholera, and Plague. "Fractional" vaccines include subunits (Hepatitis B, Influenza, Acellular Pertussis), and Toxoids (Diphtheria, Tetanus).

- The measles vaccine used today was isolated from a child with measles disease in 1954.
- Almost 10 years of serial passage on tissue culture media were required to transform the wild virus into vaccine virus.
- Live attenuated vaccines must replicate (grow) in the vaccinated person.
- A relatively small dose of virus or bacteria is given to stimulate an immune response.
- Anything that either damages the live organism in the vial (e.g., Heat, light), or interferes with replication of the organism in the body (circulating antibody) can cause the vaccine to be ineffective.
- They are generally effective with one dose, except those administered orally.

  Disadvantages: Live attenuated vaccine virus could theoretically revert back to its original pathogenic (disease-causing) form. This is known to happen only with live (oral) polio vaccine.
- Due to interference from circulating antibody to the vaccine virus, active immunity may not develop from a live attenuated vaccine.
- Antibody from any source (e.g., transplacental, transfusion) can interfere with the growth of the vaccine organism and lead to a poor response or no response to the vaccine (also known as vaccine failure).
- May cause severe or fatal reactions as a result of uncontrolled replication (growth) of the vaccine virus, with immunodeficient persons (e.g., From leukemia, treatment with certain drugs, or HIV infection).
- The measles vaccine virus seems to be more sensitive to circulating antibody. Polio and rotavirus vaccine viruses are least affected.
- They are labile, and can be damaged or destroyed by heat and light.
- They must be handled and stored carefully.

Examples of currently available live attenuated viral vaccines include Measles, Mumps, Rubella, Varicella, Yellow fever, Influenza (intranasal) and Oral polio vaccine. Bacterial vaccines include BCG and Oral Typhoid vaccine.

5.15.2.1 Inactivated Vaccines

These vaccines can be composed of either whole viruses or bacteria, or fractions of either: Fractional vaccines are either protein-based or polysaccharide-based. Protein-based vaccines include toxoids (inactivated bacterial toxin), and subunit or subvirion products.

Most polysaccharide-based vaccines are composed of pure cell-wall polysaccharide from bacteria. Conjugate polysaccharide vaccines are those in which the polysaccharide is chemically linked to a protein. This linkage makes the polysaccharide a more potent vaccine.

These vaccines are produced by growing the bacteria or virus in culture media, then inactivating it with heat and/or chemicals (usually formalin). In the case of fractional vaccines, the organism is further treated to purify only those components to be included in the vaccine (e.g., The polysaccharide capsule of *pneumococcus*). Inactivated vaccines are not alive and cannot replicate. The entire dose of antigen is administered in the injection. These vaccines cannot cause disease from infection, even in an immune deficient person.

Polysaccharide Vaccines

Polysaccharide vaccines are a unique type of **inactivated subunit vaccine** composed of long chains of sugar molecules that make up the surface capsule of certain bacteria. Pure polysaccharide vaccines available include: pneumococcal, meningococcal, and *Salmonella typhi*. The immune response to a pure polysaccharide vaccine is typically T-cell independent, which means that these vaccines are able to stimulate B-cells without the assistance of T-helper cells.

Properties of polysaccharide vaccines

T-cell independent antigens, including polysaccharide vaccines, are not consistently immunogenic in children < 2 years of age.

Young children do not respond consistently to polysaccharide antigens, probably because of immaturity of the immune system. Repeated doses of most inactivated protein vaccines cause the antibody titer to go progressively higher, or "boost."

Repeat doses of polysaccharide vaccines do not cause a booster response.

Antibody induced with polysaccharide vaccines has less functional activity than that induced by protein antigens, because the predominant antibody produced in response to most polysaccharide vaccines is IgM and little IgG is produced.

Conjugate Vaccines

In the late 1980s, it was discovered that the problems with polysaccharide vaccines could be overcome through a process called conjugation. Conjugation changes the immune response from T-cell independent to T-cell dependent, leading to increased immunogenicity in infants and antibody booster response to multiple doses of vaccine.

Examples of conjugated polysaccharide vaccine were for *Haemophilus influenza type b (Hib)*.

Also now available are conjugate vaccines for pneumococcal disease and meningococcal disease.

Recombinant Vaccines

Vaccine antigens may also be produced by genetic engineering technology. These products are sometimes referred to as recombinant vaccines. There are four genetically-engineered vaccines that are currently available:

- Hepatitis B vaccines are produced by insertion of a segment of the hepatitis B virus gene into the gene of a yeast cell. The modified yeast cell produces pure hepatitis B surface antigen when it grows.
- Human papillomavirus vaccines are produced by inserting genes for a viral coat protein into either yeast (as the hepatitis B vaccines) or into insect cell lines. Viral-like particles are produced and these induce a protective immune response.
- Live typhoid vaccine (Ty21a) is *Salmonella typhi* bacteria that have been genetically modified to not to cause illness.
- Live attenuated influenza vaccine (LAIV) has been engineered to replicate effectively in the mucosa of the nasopharynx but not in the lungs.

5.16 Vaccine Preparations

5.16.1 Polio Vaccine

Vaccine: Vaccines are preparations of live or killed micro-organisms or their products used for immunization.

- Sabin polio vaccine is an example of live attenuated vaccine preparation.
- Salk polio vaccine is an example of killed vaccine preparation.
- Salk's killed polio vaccine is a formalin inactivated preparation of the three types of poliovirus grown in monkey kidney tissue culture. Standard virulent strains are used.
- The three types of polioviruses are grown separately in monkey kidney cells.
- Viral pools of adequate titer are filtered to remove cell debris and clumps, and inactivated with formalin (1:4000) at 37 °C for 12-15 days.
- Stringent tests are carried out to ensure complete inactivation and freedom from extraneous agents.
- The three types are then pooled and after further tests for safety and potency, issued for use.
- Killed vaccine is given by injection. It is therefore called inactivated or injectable poliovaccine.
- Three doses given 4-6 weeks apart constitute the primary vaccination, to be followed by a booster six months later.
- The first dose should be given to babies after the age of six months to ensure that immune response is not impaired by residual maternal antibodies.

- Immunity can be sustained by booster doses every 3-5 years thereafter.
- An enhanced potency IPU produced in human diploid cells induces better seroconversion following two subcutaneous doses, 4-8 weeks apart.
- A third dose may be given 6-12 months later

Live Polio Vaccine (Sabin's Polio Vaccine)

- Sabin's vaccine strains were developed by plaque selection in monkey kidney tissue culture.
- Attenuated strains for live vaccine should possess the following criteria
  1. Should not be neurovirulent as tested by intraspinal inoculation in monkeys.
  2. Should be able to set up intestinal infection following feeding and should induce an immune response.
  3. Should be stable and should not acquire neurovirulence after serial enteric passage.
  4. Should possess stable genetic characteristics (markers) by which they can be differentiated from the wild virulent strains.

Live polio vaccine is administered orally and is therefore known as oral polio vaccine (OPV)

- It is prepared by growing the attenuated strains in monkey kidney cells.
- Very stringent precautions are taken to ensure freedom from extraneous agents like SV40 and B virus.
- After tests for neurovirulence, genetic stability and potency, the vaccine is issued either in the monovalent or trivalent form, in pleasantly flavored syrup.
- The use of molar $MgCl_2$ or sucrose stabilizes the vaccine against heat inactivation, particularly under tropical conditions.
- The vaccine is usually given in the trivalent form, it can be given to young infants, as the maternal antibody has little effect on intestinal infection.
- Theoretically, a single dose is sufficient to establish infection and immunity but in practice three doses are given at 4-8 week intervals, to ensure that all three types of the vaccine virus multiply in the intestine.
- The shelf life of the vaccine at 4-8 °C is four months and a + – 20 °C is two years.

5.16.2 BCG Vaccine

BCG, the tuberculosis vaccine, is an attenuated strain of *M.bovis*.

- Immunoprophylaxis is by intradermal injection of the live attenuated vaccine developed by Chalmette and Guerin (1921), the Bacillus Chalmette Guerin or BCG.

- Injection of BCG in animals induces self limit infection, with multiplication and dissemination of the bacillus in different organs and production of small tubercles.
- Within a few weeks the bacilli stop multiplying although they survive in the tissues for long periods. This gives rise to delayed hypersensitivity and immunity.
- BCG vaccine be administered to babies by intradermal injection on the deltoid immediately after birth, or as early as possible thereafter, before the age of 12 months.
- The vaccine need not be administered after the age of two years.
- BCG induces a nonspecific stimulation of the immune system providing some protection against leprosy and leukemia.
- BCG grows under high bile salts and the gene responsible for causing infection is inactivated.

5.17 Bacterial Toxins

There are two kinds of Bacterial toxins.

1. ***Exotoxins*:** So-called because they diffuse freely through the bacterial cell wall into the medium in which the organisms are growing.
2. ***Endotoxins*:** So-called because they are retained within the bacteria and are freed only when the cells die and start to disintegrate.

5.17.1 Exotoxins

They have the following characteristics:

(i) They are the products of the metabolism of actively growing bacteria.

(ii) They are produced mainly by Gram +ve bacteria.

(iii) They are water soluble and can pass into the surrounding medium. This provides a means of separating toxin from the cells, since the latter can be removed on a bacteria – proof filter through which the toxin containing medium will pass.

(iv) Chemically, they are high molecular weight proteins and some are enzymes, they are relatively thermostable and lose activity at about 60 °C.

(v) They are extremely toxic to the body. *Botulinus toxin*, produced by clostridium botulinum, an organism responsible for a food poisoning, is the most toxic substance known.

When exotoxin producing bacteria grow in the body the toxins are carried in the blood stream to all parts, the most serious consequences of infection are due to the effects of the toxins rather than the damage to the tissues invaded by the bacteria. *e.g.,* In diphtheria, the causative organism grows in the throat producing a membrane that may cause asphyxiation.

The general effects of exotoxins are often caused on the nervous system and the heart. *e.g.,* Tetanus exotoxin is neurotoxin and causes severe muscular spasms.

Other toxins cause death of tissues (neuro toxins) intestinal damage (enterotoxins), haemolysis, haemolysins, destruction of WBC (leucocidins).

Exotoxin producing bacteria include clostridium botulinum, clostridium tetani (tetanus) clostridium perfringens, septicum, welchii (gas gangrene) and coryne bacterium diphtheriae (diphtheria).

Exotoxins are soluble, heat-labile proteins that are usually released into the surroundings as the bacterial pathogen grows given in Table 5.6.

- In genral, exotoxins are produced by gram-positive bacteria, although some gram-negative bacteria also make exotoxins.
- Exotoxins are usually synthesized by specific bacteria that often have plasmids or prophages bearing the toxin genes.
- They are associated with specific diseases and often are named for the disease they produce (eg., the diptheria toxin)
- Exotoxins are among the most lethal substances known; they are toxic in mocrogram-per-kilogram concentrations (eg., *batulinum toxin*), but are typically heat labile, inactivated at 60-80 °C.
- Exotoxins are proteins that exert their biological activity by specific mechanisms.
- As proteins, the toxins are highly immunogenic and can stimulate the production of neutralizing antibodies called antitoxines.
- The toxin proteins can also be inactivated by formaldehyde, iodine and other chemicals to form immunogenic toxoids (for e.g., tetanus toxoid)
- The tetanus vaccine is a solution of tetanus toxoid.
- Exotoxins can be grouped into four types based on their structure and physiological activities.
    1. One type is the AB toxin, which gets its name from the fact that the portion of the toxin (B) that binds to a host the enzyme activity that causes the toxicity.
    2. A second type, which also may be an AB toxin, consists of those toxins that affect a specific host site (nervous tissue neurotoxins), the intestine (enterotoxins), general tissues (cytotoxins) by acting extracellular or intracellular on the host cells.
    3. A third type does not have separable A and B portions and acts by disorganizing host cell membranes. Examples include the leukocidins, hemolysins and phospholipases
    4. A fourth type is the superantigen that acts by stimulating T cells directly to release cytokines.

5.17.2 Endotoxins

They have the following characteristics

(i) They are structural elements of bacteria.

(ii) They are contained in most bacterial cells but greatest amounts are found in Gram –ve bacteria.

(iii) They are not excreted into the surrounding medium and are liberated only when the cells die or disintegrate.

(iv) They are complexes of phospholipid, polysaccharide, protein, most of them are thermostable.

(v) They are much less toxic.

(vi) Endotoxin producing bacteria include *Vibrio chlolerae* (cholera), *Pasteurella pestis* (plague), *Salmonella typhi* (typhoid), *Salmonella paratyphi* (p-typhoid), *Bordetella pertussis* (whooping cough).

- Gram-negative bacteria have *Lipopolysaccharide* (LPS) in the outer membrane of their cell wall that, under certain circumstances, is toxic to specific hosts. This LPS is called an endotoxin because it is bound to the bacterium and is released when the microorganism lyses given in Table 5.6.
- Bacterial endotoxins are
  - (a) Heat stable
  - (b) Toxic (nanogram amounts)
  - (c) Weakly immunogenic
  - (d) Generally similar, despite source
  - (e) Usually capable of producing general systematic effects: fever (pyrogenic), shock, blood coagulation, weakness, diarrhoea, inflammation, intestinal haemorrhage with endotoxins resulted in complications-even death-to patients.
- Endotoxins can be problematic for individuals and firms working with cell cultures and genetic engineering. The result has been the development of sensitive tests and method to identify and remove these endotoxins.
- Most firms have set a limit of 0.25 endotoxin units, 0.025 ng/mL, or less as a release standard for their drugs, media or products.
- Endotoxins can initially activate Hageman factor (blood clotting factor XII), which in turn activates up to four humoral systems: coagulation, complement, fibrinolytic, and kininogen systems.
- Removal of endotoxins presents more of a problem than their detection.
- Those present on glassware or medical devices can be inactivated if the equipment is heated at 250 °C for 30 minutes.

Table 5.6 Differences between Exotoxin and Endotoxin

Exotoxin	Endotoxin
Excreted by organisms	Integral part of cell wall
Excreted by both Gram positive and Gram-negative bacteria	Found mostly in Gram-negative bacteria
Chemically polypeptide	Lipopolysaccharide complex
Relatively unstable, heat labile (60 °C)	Relatively stable, heat tolerant
Highly antigenic, neutralized by antitoxin	Weakly immunogenic, antibodies are antitoxic
Can be toxoid	Cannot be toxoid
Highly toxic, fatal in µg quantities	Moderately toxic
Usually binds to specific receptors	Specific receptors not found
Not pyrogenic usually	Fever by induction of interleukin1 (IL-1) production.
Located on extra chromosomal genes (e.g. plasmids)	Located on chromosomal genes

5.17.3 Toxoids

The toxoids, used as vaccines are toxins that have been incubated with formalin. This treatment completely destroys their toxic properties without causing significant loss of antigenic qualities.

Toxoids are of three types:

(i) Diphtheria vaccine

(ii) Tetanus vaccine

(iii) Staphylococcus toxoid

5.17.3.1 Diphtheria Vaccine

Preparation of Toxin

A suitable strain of *Corynebacterium diphtheria* is grown on a liquid medium and must not be made with broth prepared from horse muscle.

Horse muscle must not be used because the presence of horse protein in the toxin and toxoid preparation made from it, might sensitize the recipient to horse serum and make dangerous the subsequent injection of sera, which are made in horses.

After incubation under optimal conditions until toxin production has reached a satisfactory level, the bulk of organisms are removed on paper pulp and the filterate is sterilized using fibrous pads or ceramic candles.

Conversion of Toxin to Toxoid

Formaldehyde solution (formalin) is added and the mixture incubated at 37°C until the toxicity has been removed which takes 2-3 weeks. The resulting material is known as Formal toxoid (FT).

It was an excellent antigen but it often causes severe reactions in adults.

5.17.3.2 Preparation of other forms of Toxoid

(i) Toxoid – antitoxin floccules (TAF): If suitable amounts of toxoid and antitoxin are mixed, floccules are obtained that contain almost all the antigenic activity and when separated, washed are free from contamination with broth and metabolites. This product is known as toxoid anti toxin floccules and causes fewer reactions.

Neutralized product has no significant activity because neither toxoid nor antitoxin is damaged when they combine. Therefore, the combination can dissociate under suitable conditions.

e.g., after the floccules have been injected into the body, leaving the toxoid free to stimulate antibody production.

Therefore the following method of preparation is used:

80 units of antitoxin are added to 100 units of toxoid i.e., the toxoid is slightly neutralized.

After leaving for about three weeks to allow the floccules to form and settle, the supernatant liquid is decanted.

The floccules are then washed with saline, by decantation, until the washings are colorless and resuspended in saline containing a bactericide.

Advantages

1. It is especially valuable for adults, who are much more sensitive than young children to the reaction causing constituents of immunological preparation.
2. It is a weaker antigen; therefore two doses must be given because it contains diphtheria antitoxin, which is made from horse serum.

Disadvantages

Slight risk of sensitization.

(ii) Alum Precipitated toxoid (APT): This preparation from slow absorption of precipitated toxoids from the site of injection and slow excretion from the body led to increased antigenic activity. Its development was made to make purer toxoids.

High quality of formal toxoid is treated with charcoal to remove

(a) colouring matter

(b) non-specific impurities that might cause reactions.

After filtration, to remove charcoal, a suitable concentration of alum is added. This reacts with bicarbonate phosphate and protein impurities in the toxoid to produce a precipitate containing $Al(OH)_2$ phosphate. The toxoid is adsorbed onto this mineral carrier.

The precipitate is washed and suspended in saline containing a bactericide provides a depot in tissues from which the antigen is slowly released to give a prolonged stimulus.

Advantages

1. APT produces much higher antibody levels than FT and TAF and therefore two doses are sufficient.
2. It is free from sensitizing horse protein and contains toxoid of improved purity.

Disadvantages

1. Adults and older children may show local reactions to the carrier.
2. There is a slight risk of provoking paralytic poliomyelitis in the limb in which the injection is given.
3. Inspite of its high efficiency it has been largely replaced by combined prophylactics because they are more convenient.

(iii) Purified Toxoid Aluminium Phosphate (PTAP): The main difference between PTAP and APT is that it contains a much purer form of toxoid. This is obtained:

(a) by using a semi-synthetic medium in the preparation of the toxin, to exclude as much non-specific material as possible.

(b) by a complicated purification of the toxoid involving the use of $Mg(OH)_2$ to precipitate colour, phosphate and some protein, ammonium sulphate and cadium chloride as protein precipitants.

The separation of much of the unwanted protein reduces the reactions, but also removes the impurities that give a precipitate with alum.

Therefore it is necessary to use a preformed carrier i.e., pure hydrated aluminium phosphate.

Advantages

1. PTAP is an excellent antigen due to its depot effect.
2. Toxoid is very pure and can be freeze dried.
3. It is very stable.
4. The production of batches of uniform potency is greatly facilitated.

Disadvantages

1. It carries the small risk of provocative poliomyelitis.

(iv) **Purified Diphtheria Formal Toxoid in combined Prophylactics:** The Ministry of Health recommends that children should be immunized against four infectious diseases (diphtheria, tetanus, pertussis and poliomyelitis) during the first year of life.

It is customary to use a combined vaccine containing either diphtheria, tetanus and pertussis antigens or these 3+ poliomyelitis antigens.

Purified diphtheria formal toxoid (FT) can be used successfully in these preparations because it is less active alone than any of the three adsorbed forms its effect is potentiated by the presence of dead pertussis bacteria which appear to act like alum salts, as an adjuvant.

5.17.3.3 Tetanus Toxoid

- A sterile preparation of the formaldehyde-treated products containing growth of *Clostridium tetani.*
- It contains a non-phenolic preservative. It should be stored 2 ° to 8 °C and not be allowed to freeze.
- A sterile preparation of plain tetanus toxoid precipitated or adsorbed by alum, aluminum hydroxide or aluminum phosphate adjuvant.

Tetanus is caused by *Clostridium tetani*, an anaerobic gram-positive, endospore forming rod.

- Prevention of tetanus involves the use of the tetanus toxoid.
- The toxoid, which incorporates an adjuvant (aluminium salts) to increase its immunizing potency, is given routinely with diphtheria toxoid and pertussis vaccine.
- An initial dose is normally administered a few months after birth, a second dose 4 to 6 months later, and finally a reinforcing dose 6 to 12 months after the second injection.
- Another booster is given between the ages of 4 to 6 years.
- For many years, booster doses of tetanus toxoid were administered every 3 to 5 years.
- However, that practice has been discontinued since it has been shown that a single booster dose can provide protection for 10 to 20 years.
- Serious hypersensitivity reactions have occurred when too many doses of toxoid were administered over a period of years.
- Booster doses are generally given when an individual has sustained a wound infection and only if it has been 10 or more years since the previous dose.
- Control measures for tetanus are not possible because of the wide dissemination of the bacterium in the soil and long survival of its spores.
- Prevention depends on active immunization with toxoid, proper care of wounds contaminated with soil, prophylactic use of antitoxin

5.18 General Methods of Immunization

Immunization results in the demonstrable presence of protective levels of antibodies. Vaccination is a form of immunization. It is the immunization that is responsible for the complete eradication of smallpox from India. The agents or products through which immunization is achieved are called immunization agents.

Active immunization is the process of increasing resistance to infection whereby micro-organisms or products of their activity act as antigens and stimulates certain body cells to produce antibodies with a specific protective capacity. It is a slow-process dependent upon the rate at which the antibody formation takes place. Biological products comprising vaccines and toxoids confer active immunity.

Passive immunization, which results in immediate protection of short duration, may be achieved by the administration of the antibodies themselves. Biological products comprising human immune sera and animal immune sera confer passive immunity.

Expanded program on Immunization (EPI): In 1974 the World Health Assembly adopted a resolution creating the EPI, the aim of which was to provide immunization against target diseases (diphtheria, measles pertussis, poliomyelitis, tetanus, and tuberculosis) for all children throughout the world.

Table 5.7 Indian Medical Association Recommended Immunization Schedule followed in India

Sl No.	Age	Disease	Vaccination	Remarks
1.	At birth	Hepatitis B	Hep B vaccine -I	
2.	At birth	Polio	Oral PV 0 dose	
3.	Birth to 6 weeks	Tuberculosis	BCG	
4.	4 -6 Weeks	Hepatitis B	Hep B Vaccine -II	
5.	6 Weeks	Diphtheria, Pertussis Tetanus, Polio	DPT-I OPV -I	
6.	10 weeks	Diphtheria, Pertussis Tetanus, Polio Hepatitis B	DPT-II OPV-II Hep B Vaccine iii*	*Delhi Govt recommendation
7.	14 Weeks	Diphtheria, Pertussis Tetanus, Polio	DPT-III OPV- III Hep B vaccine IV*	*Delhi Govt recommendation
8.	24 Weeks	Hepatitis B	Hep B Vaccine III*	*IAP (Indian Academy of Pediatrics) recommendation
9.	9 -12 Mths	Polio Measles	OPV-IV Measles	
10.	15-18 months	Mumps, Measles Rubella	MMR*	

Table 5.7 *Contd...*

Sl No.	Age	Disease	Vaccination	Remarks
11.	18 months	Diphtheria, Pertussis Tetanus, Polio	DPT –Booster I OPV –V	*Recommended by Delhi Govt and IAP only
12.	24 months	Typhoid	Typhoid*	*IAP recommendation
13.	4-5 Yr	Diphtheria, Pertussis Tetanus, Polio	DPT Booster – II OPV -VI	

5.19 Immunological Diagnostic Tests

5.19.1 Mantoux Test

Persons infected with *M. tuberculosis* develop cell-mediated immunity because the bacteria are phagocytosed by macrophages. This immunity involves sensitized T cells and is the basis for the tuberculin skin test. In this test a purified protein derivation (PPD) of *M.tuberculosis* in person has had tuberculosis, or was exposed to *M.tuberculosis* sensitized T cells react with these proteins and a delayed hypersensitivity reaction occurs within 48 hours; this positive skin reaction appears as an indurations (hardening) and reddeining of the area around the injection site. In a young person, a positive skin test could indicate active tuberculosis. In older persons, it may result from previous disease, vaccination or a false positive test.

In both cases, x-rays and bacterial isolation are completed to confirm the diagnosis.

- Laboratoory diagnosis of tuberculosis is by visualization of the acid-fast bacterium, chest x-ray, commercially available DNA probes, and the Mantoux or tuberculin skin test.

5.19.2 Schick Test

Schick test measures the level of immune system of a person to the infection of diphtheria. When testing the status of immunity, a small amount of diphtheria exotoxin is inoculated in the skin of a person. Depending on the ability and quantity of antitoxin, positive or negative responses develop.

- If serum antitoxin in body would be in sufficient amount to neutralize the exotoxin, no visible reaction will occur.
- In control, when serum antitoxin is in insufficient amount the exotoxin will damage the tissue at the site where incision was made, and will produce a swollen and reddish area which is converted into brown within 4 or 5 days. This shows that the immune response is not present to a satisfactory level.

5.19.3 Dick Test

This test is a method of determining susceptibility to scarlet fever by injection into the skin of 0.1 cubic centimeter of scarlet fever toxin. A reddening of the skin in an area over 10 millimeters (0.4 inches) in diameter within about 24 hours indicates a lack of immunity to the disease. The test was developed in 1924 by the U.S. physicians George and Gladys Dick.

5.19.4 Schultz-Charlton Test

A skin test for the diagnosis of scarlet fever performed by the intracutaneous injection of human scarlet fever immune serum; In 1918, Schultz and Charlton first reported that the intracutaneous injection of from 0.5 to 1 cc. of normal or scarlet fever convalescent serum would blanch (make white or pale by extracting colour) the rash of scarlet fever at the site of injection. A positive reaction consists of blanching of the rash in the area surrounding the point of injection. They also showed that the blanching substance was present in serum taken after the fourteenth day of scarlet fever, but that serum taken earlier in the disease did not have blanching power.

5.19.5 Widal Test

Widal test is a reaction involving the agglutination of typhoid bacilli when they are mixed with serum containing typhoid antibodies from an individual who has typhoid fever.

5.20 Hypersensitivity

The term hypersensitivity refers to the injurious consequences in the sensitized host, following contact with specific antigens.

- Hypersensitivity is concerned with what happens to the host as a result of the immune reaction.
- Hypersensitivity reactions can be divided into four types: type I, type II, type III and type IV, based on the mechanisms involved and time taken for the reaction.

5.20.1 Type I Hypersensitivity

(Anaphylactic, IgE or regain dependent):

- Antibodies ('cytotropic' IgE antibodies) are fixed on the surface of tissue cells (most cells and basophiles) in sensitised individuals.
- The antigen combines with the cell fixed antibody, leading to release of pharmacologically active substances (vasoactive amines) which produce the clinical reaction.
- Type I hypersensitivity is also known as immediate anaphylactic hypersensitivity.

- In this type of hypersensitivity the 1° immune response will be normal effect is seen only in 2° immune response.
- Instead of IgA or IgD culprit antibody such as IgE is released.
- IgE will also attack phagocytic cell of the host and degranulation occurs.

Mechanism of Anaphylaxis

- IgE molecule are bound to surface receptors on mast cells and basophils.
- These cells carry large number of such receptors called F_c ER receptors, analogous to TCR receptors on T cell surface.
- IgE molecules attach to these receptors by their F_c end.
- The antigen molecules combine with the cell bound IgE, bridging the gap between adjacent antibody molecules.
- This cross-linking increases the permeability of the cells to calcium ions and leads to degranulation, with release of biologically active substances contained in the granules.
- The manifestations of anaphylaxis are due to pharmacological mediators, which are of two kinds.
- Primary mediators which are preformed contents of mast cell and basophil granules (histamine, serotonin, eosinophil chemotactic factor, haparin etc)
- Secondary mediators which are newly formed upon stimulation by mast cells, basophils and other leucocytes (slow reacting substance of anaphylaxis, prostagladins, platelet activating factor and cytokines such as IL3, IL4, IL5, IL6, Gm-csF)

Anaphylactoid Reaction: Intravenous injection of peptone, trysin and certain other substances provokes a clinical reaction resembling anaphylactic shock. This is termed 'anaphylactoid' reaction'.

- Type I hypersensitivity reaction usually takes 15-30 minutes from the time of exposure to the antigen.

e.g., weeze (whistling sound during night times)
Asphyxia (breath lessness)
Asthma
Vomiting
Diarrhoea

5.20.2 Type II Hypersensitivity

- These reactions involve a combination of IgG (or rarely IgM) antibodies with the antigenic determinants on the surface of cells leading to cytotoxic or cytolytic effects.

- Examples are lysis of red cells caused by antierythrocyte antibodies in autoimmune anemia's and hemolytic disease of the newborn.
- The reaction time is minutes to hours.
- Alternatively a free antigen or hapten may be absorbed on cell surfaces.
- Subsequently reaction of the combined antigen or hapten with its corresponding antibody leads to cell damage.
- In some Type II reactions, the antibody combines with cell surface receptors and disrupts normal function, either by uncontrolled activation (eg: Graves diseases) or by blocking (eg: *Myasthenia gravis*)
- Diagnostic tests include detection of circulating antibody, the tissues involved and the presence of antibody and complement in the lesion (biopsy) by immunofluorescence.
- Treatment involves anti-inflammatory and immunosuppressive agents.

5.20.3 Type III Hypersensitivity

- Type III hypersensitivity is also known as immune complex hypersensitivity.
- The reaction may be general (eg: serum sickness) or may involve individual organs including skin (e.g., systemic lupus erythematosus, Arthus reaction), kidneys (e.g., lupus nephritis), lungs (e.g., Aspergillosis), joints (e.g., rheumtoid arthritis) or other organs.
- The reaction may take 3-10 hours after exposure to the antigen (as in Arthus reaction).

Arthus reaction: Arthus (1903) observed that when rabbits were repeatedly injected subcutaneously with normal horse serum, the initial injections had no local effect but with later injections, there occurred intense local reaction consisting of edema, indurations and haemorrhagic necrosis. This is known as the Arthus reaction and it's a local manifestation of generalised hypersensitivity.

- The tissue damage is due to formation of antigen-antibody precipitates causing complement of antigen-antibody of inflammatory molecules activation and release of inflammatory molecules.
- The Arthus reaction can be passively transferred with sera containing precpitating antibodies (IgG, IgM) in high *titres*.
- Serum sickness: This is a systemic form of Type III hypersensitivity
- This appeared, 7-12 days following a single injection of a high concentration of foreign serum such as the diphtheria antitoxin.

- The pathogenesis is the formation of immune complexes (consisting of the foreign serum and antibody to it that reaches high enough titers by 7-12 days) which get deposited on the endothelial lining of blood vessels in various parts of the body, causing inflammatory infiltration.

Treatment includes anti-inflammatory agents.

5.20.4 Type IV Hypersensitivity

- Type IV hypersensitivity is also known as cell mediated or delayed type hypersensitivity.
- The classical example of this hypersensitivity is tuberculin (montoux) reaction which peaks 48 hours after the injection of antigen (PPD or old tuberculin).
- The lesion is characterized by indurations and erythema.
- In delayed hypersensitivity, the interaction between antigens and T-cells occur.
- The reaction is not induced by circulating antibodies but by sensitised T cells (Tdth, Th1, Th2, Tc) which, on contact with the specific antigen, release cytokines that cause biological effects on leucocytes, macrophages and tissue cells.
- Delayed hypersensitivity cannot be passively transferred by serum but can be transferred by lymphocytes or the transfer factor.
- Two types of delayed hypersensitivity are recognized the tuberculin (infection) type and the contact dermatitis type.

Tuberculin (Infection) Type

- When a small dose of tuberculin is injected intradermally in an individual sensitised to tuberculoprotein by prior infection or immunisation, an indurated inflammatory reaction develops at the site within 48-72 hr.
- In unsensitised individuals, the tuberculin injection provokes no response.
- The tuberculin test therefore provides useful indication of the state of delayed hypersensitivity (cell mediated immunity) to the bacilli.

Contact Dermatitis Type

- Delayed hypersensitivity sometimes results from skin contact with a variety of chemical – metals such as Nickel and chromium, simple chemicals like dyes, picrylchloride, dinitrochlorobenzene, drugs such as penicillin and toiletries.
- Sensitisation is particularly liable when contact is with an inflamed area of skin and when the chemical is applied in an oily base.

- Antibiotic ointments applied on patches of dermatitis frequently provoke sensitisation.
- The substances involved are in themselves not antigenic but may acquire antigenicity on combination with skin proteins.
- Sensitisation requires percutaneous absorption.
- Langerhans cells of the skin capture locally applied hapten, along with the modified tissue proteins, and migrate to the draining lymph nodes where they present the processed antigen along with MHC molecules to T cells.
- The sensitised T cells travel to the skin site, where on contacting the antigen they release various lymphokines.
- Contact with the allergen in a sensitised individual leads to ' contact dermatitis', the lesions varying from macules and papules to vesicles that break down, leaving behind raw weeping area typical of acute eczematous dermatitis.
- Hypersensitivity is detected by the 'patch test'
- The allergen is applied to the skin under an adherant dressing.
- Sensitivity is indicated by itching appearing in 4-5 hours, and local reaction which may vary from erythema to vesicle or blister formation, after 24-28 hours.

5.21 Allergenic Extracts

Allergenic extracts comprise a large group of products that are unique compared to other biologics and conventional pharmaceuticals.

- A specific license is required for their manufacture, and they are available mainly from specialty companies.
- Allergenic extracts are relatively crude drugs by contemporary standards.
- Allergenic extracts are concentrated solutions or suspensions of allergens used for the diagnosis and treatment of allergic diseases.

Handling

- Allergenic extracts usually are designated as being aqueous or glycerinated products.
- Normal saline or similar isotonic electrolyte solution is the diluent.
- The preparations are normally buffered to pH 8 and contain phenol (0.4%) as a preservative.
- The most common measures of allergenic potency are by weight/volume and the protein nitrogen unit.
- Weight/volume is the weight of allergic substance extracted pre volume of extracting fluid.

For example: A 1: 50 extract is prepared by extracting 1 g of substance with 50 mL of solvent and decimal dilutions of this extract provide 1:500, 1:5000 etc concentrations.

- One protein nitrogen unit represents 0.01 mcg of total protein nitrogen in the product.
- A typical allergenic substance contains multiple allergenic molecules and epitopes of varying potency, and there is significant chemical and biological variation with different lots of the substance.
- The potency of these products is expressed in terms of allergy units or bioequivalent allergy units.

5.21.1 Examples of Allergenic Extracts

1. ***Pollen extract***: Pollen is a fine yellowish powder that is transported from plant to plant by the wind, by birds, by insects or by other animals. The spread of pollen helps to fertilize plants and can mean misery for seasonal allergy with symptoms like sneezing, nasal congestion, runny nose, watery eyes, itchy throat and eyes wheezing etc., Some of the plants producing such allergic pollens from which allergenic extracts are prepared are Alfalfa, barley, canary grass, dandelion, eucalyptus, hazelnut, juniper, mustard, palm, ryegrass, etc.
2. ***Fungal extract***: Airborne fungal spores occur in greater concentrations than pollen grains. Immunoglobulin E-specific antigens (allergens) on airborne fungal spores induce type I hypersensitivity (allergic) respiratory reactions in sensitized atopic subjects, causing rhinitis and/or asthma. Some of the fungal and mould extracts used are *Alternaria, candida, epidermaphyton, fusarium, mucor, penicillium species, rhizopus, sacchromyces* etc.
3. ***Dust extracts***: Dust allergies may trigger asthma symptoms, such as wheezing, coughing, tightness in the chest and shortness of breath. Dust Allergy symptoms are sneezing, runny or stuffy nose, and red, itchy or teary eyes wheezing, coughing, tightness in the chest and shortness of breathe Itching. Some of the dust allergy triggers are dust mites, Cockroaches, Mold, Pollen, Pet hair, feathers etc.
4. ***Insect allergen extracts***: The insect allergy occurs due to bite, sting, and inhalation of insect parts mainly of the order –*Hymenoptera*. For biting insects, the optimal allergens source may be the salivary glands. Some examples of allergic insect extracts are Fire ant, black ant, housefly, wasps, yellow jacket bee, hornet, fire ant, honeybee, moth, mites, mosquitoes, fruitfly, cockroach, caddis fly, etc.
5. ***Food allergy***: Food allergy is an immune-based disease. A group of the eight major allergenic foods is often referred to as the Big-8 and comprises milk, eggs, fish, crustacean shellfish, tree nuts, peanuts, wheat and soybean. The symptoms of food allergy are asthma, rhinitis, headache, urticaria etc.

6. ***Seasonal Allergies***: Spring Allergies: As the trees start to bloom and the pollen gets airborne, allergy sufferers begin their annual ritual of sniffling and sneezing in spring.

   Summer Allergies: Many of the allergic triggers that can make us miserable in the spring persist into summer.

   Fall Allergies: The allergy triggers might be slightly different, but they can be just as misery-inducing as the flower pollen that fills the air in the spring and summer.

   Winter Allergies: Allergic reactions, mainly due to cold weather, mainly affecting skin and lips.
7. ***Pet Allergies***: Allergy to proteins and glycoproteins from animal sources is an important public health problem affecting both children and adults. Some of the pets causing allergic reactions are dogs, cats,etc.
8. ***Latex Allergy***: Type IV hypersensitivity are due to latex additives. Allergic reactions to latex may be serious and can very rarely be fatal. People who are at higher risk for developing latex allergy include Health care workers and others who frequently wear latex gloves, people who have had multiple surgeries such as children with spina bifida, People who are often exposed to natural rubber latex, including rubber industry workers etc.,
9. ***Drug Allergy***: In Drug allergy, the reaction is triggered by certain medicaments like penicillin, Aspirin and other NSAIDs such as Ibuprofen, Anticonvulsants, and drugs related to Monoclonal antibody therapy, Chemotherapy etc. Patch tests help to confirm the etiology of the cutaneous adverse drug reactions involving delayed hypersensitivity mechanisms.
10. ***Miscellaneous inhalant extracts***: Besides above sources, there are number of other miscellaneous substances causing allergies like Hairs from various sources such as human, camel, cat, rabbit fur, wool, Bird feathers such as from chicken, pigeon, duck etc. and Algae, gum acacia, jute, silk, tobacco etc.

Essay Questions

1. Write a note on classification of Immunity
2. Write a note on nature of vaccines and their applications
3. Explain the transmission of infections

Multiple Choice Questions

1. Bright field microscope provide magnification of about
   (a) 1000 × 2000
   (b) 500 × 1000
   (c) 2000 × 4000
   (d) 5000 × 10000
2. Which amongst the following micro-organisms causes dust borne infection
   (a) Mycobacterium tuberculosis
   (b) Pnuemococcal pneumonia
   (c) Nisseria gonorrohea
   (d) Strptococcus pygogenes

3. Infection of the blood is caused by which of the following micro-organisms
   (a) Shigella
   (b) salmonella
   (c) Nesseria
   (d) Erysipelas

4. Which amongst the following microorganism adheres to epithelial cells of the small intestine
   (a) E.coli strains
   (b) Nesseria gonorrhoe
   (c) Vibrio cholera
   (d) Streptococcus pygogenes

5. Which of the following is an example of live vaccine
   (a) Oral polio vaccine-sabin
   (b) injectable polio vaccine-salk
   (c) Hepatitis vaccine
   (d) Bcg vaccine

6. Which amongst the following is the first synthesized antibody
   (a) IgG
   (b) IgA
   (c) IgD
   (d) IgM

Answers

1. (a)	2. (c)	3. (c)
4. (a)	5. (a)	

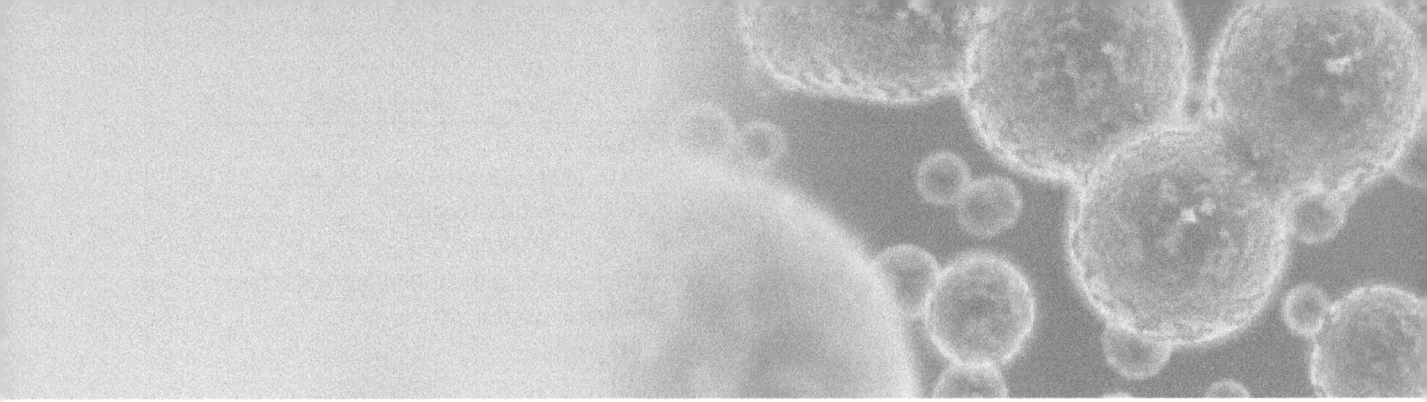

6 Bacterial Genetics

LEARNING OBJECTIVES

After studying the chapter the students familiarize themselves with concepts in:

- *Determining recombination in bacteria*
- *Understanding bacterial genetics*
- *Understanding various features of spontaneous mutations*
- *Various detection and isolation of mutants*
- *Understanding various mechanisms of mutations*

6.1 Introduction

Genetic recombination can be referred as the exchange of genetical material between two double strand molecules with identical (a) very similar sequences. In bacteria the genetic information is preserved in a single chromosome and in minichromosome called episomes and plasmids. The chromosome of *Escherichia coli* is a double stranded DNA circle of about 5 million base pairs encoding approximately 5,000 genes. Because there is only one chromosome, each gene (with occasional exceptions) is present in only one copy. Bacteria reproduced by simple fission results in distribution of their genetic material to the two progeny cells equally. They are haploid; a multinucleate do not go through mitotic and meiotic cycle like in eukaryotes. One important consequence of having a haploid genome is that genetic changes have an immediate effect on the phenotype or properties of the bacterial cell.

Bacterial variation can also occur by **horizontal transfer** of genetic material from one cell to another. Consider two cells from different populations: bacterium B has features distinct from those of bacterium A. There are three possible mechanisms for transferring a trait from B to A:

1. **Transformation**, release and uptake of naked DNA from one bacterium (the donor cell) to another bacterium (the recipient cell);
2. **Transduction**, packaging and transfer of bacterial DNA from a donor cell, to recipient cell by bacteriophage, and
3. **Conjugation**, bacterial mating in which cells must be in contact, through a specialized sex pilus.

For all three processes, the transferred DNA must be stably incorporated into the genetic material of the recipient bacterium.

This can occur in two ways:

(i) **Recombination (Table 6.1)**, or integration of the transferred DNA into the bacterial chromosome; or

(ii) **Establishment of a plasmid**, i.e., the transferred material essentially forms a minichromosome capable of autonomous replication.

Mutation and gene transfer work together to accelerate the rate of bacterial evolution. The spontaneous changes required to produce a new function (*e.g.*, antibiotic resistance) may occur at a low frequency. However, once the function has developed, it can readily spread to other bacterial populations. The limitation is the probability and efficiency of gene exchange between different bacteria. Under certain conditions, gene exchange is very efficient.

Table 6.1 Criterion

Recombination Process	Cell Contact Required	Sensitive to DNase
Transformation	No	Yes
Transduction	No	No
Conjugation	Yes	No

6.2 Criteria for Determining the Mode of Recombination in Bacteria

6.2.1 Transformation (Gene Exchange between Bacteria)

In 1928 Griffith, an English health officer discovered transformation process initially in pathogenic strains of *Streptococcus pneumonia*. He injected a mouse with a mixture consisting of a few rough (non capsulated and non pathogenic) pneumococci and large number of heat killed smooth (capsulated pathogenic) cells.

He showed that injecting into mice a mixture of heat killed virulent (smooth) *S. pneumoniae* with a live attenuated (rough) strain led to the development of a live virulent strain, which ultimately killed the mouse. Avery, MacCleod and McCarty purified the transforming substance and identified it as DNA. This experiment was the first to demonstrate that DNA was the genetic material. It was also the first discovery of gene transfer between bacteria. Since then, other bacteria, including certain species of *Haemophilus*, *Bacillus*, *Actinobacillus*, and *Neisseria*, have been found to be naturally transformable. These bacteria have developed highly specialized functions that will bind DNA fragments and transport them into the cell.

Griffith also showed that the transforming factor could be passed from the transformed cells to their progeny and thus had the characteristic of gene.

These mechanisms can be quite distinct. In the case of *Bacillus subtilis*, any DNA can be taken up.

Bacillus and *Streptococcus* unwind the DNA and transport only a single strand.

In contrast, *Haemophilus*, *Actinobacillus*, and *Neisseria* require a specific sequence to be present on the DNA fragments and transport double-stranded DNA fragments. Transformable organisms take up DNA when they are in a **competent** state.

In *Bacillus*, this state is triggered by small diffusible molecules whose concentration indicates when the culture has reached a certain density.

In *Haemophilus*, competence is induced by nutritional starvation. These signals somehow trigger the expression of proteins that enable the cells to bind and take up DNA.

In nature, the DNA to be taken up is thought to be released into the environment by lysis of bacterial cells.

Transformation is probably the least efficient mechanism of gene transfer because naked DNA is sensitive to nucleases in the environment.

In the laboratory, mutant strains can be transformed to wild type by the addition of purified DNA extracted from a wild type strain. The process depends on the DNA and is sensitive to the addition of DNAse.

The ability to introduce DNA into bacterial cells in the laboratory is the basis for "reverse genetics," in which a gene is first cloned, mutated *in vitro*, and reintroduced into the bacterial cell to study the resulting phenotype.

Natural Transformation

Cells that are in a state in which they can be transformed by DNA in their environment are said to be the competent. In significant number of bacteria, entry into the competent state is encoded by chromosal genes and signaled by certain environmental conditions.

Such bacteria are now capable of undergoing natural transformation. For example, certain species of *Haemophilus*, *Bacillus*, *Actinobacillus* and *Neisseria*, have been found to be naturally transformable.

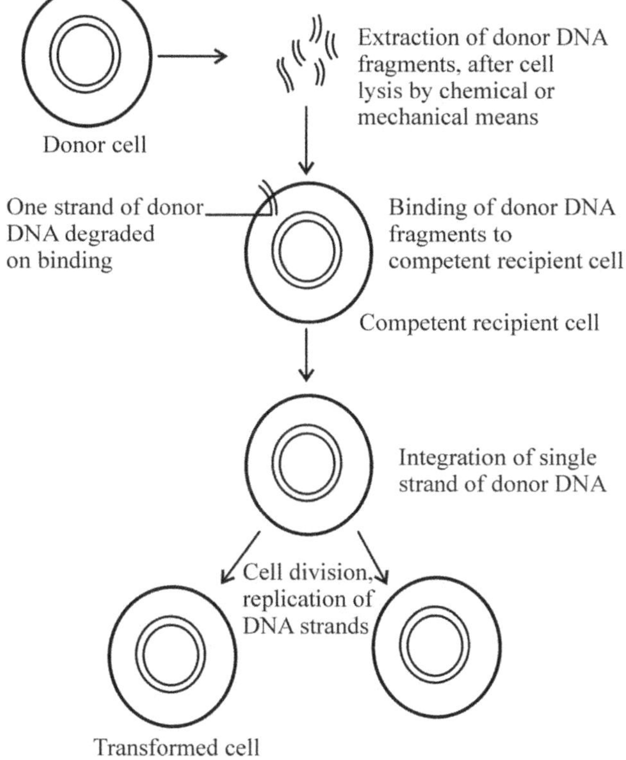

Fig. 6.1 Principal steps in bacterial transformation

Artificial Transformation

Bacteria which do not become competent under ordinary conditions of culture, they can made competent by artificial treatments such as exposure of cells to high concentrations of divalent cations like $CaCl_2$ such systems of transformations have been termed as artificial transformation. Some organisms that are not naturally transformable, like *E. coli*, can be made competent for transformation by treating the cells with $CaCl_2$ or placing them in an electric field (electroporation).

Mechanism for Bacterial Recombination

Inside the recipient cell the donor DNA fragment is positioned alongside the recipient DNA in such a way that homologous genes are adjacent.

Enzymes act on the recipient DNA, causing nicks and excision of a fragment. Then the donor DNA is integrated into the recipient chromosome in place of the excised DNA. The recipient cell then becomes the recombinant cell because its chromosome contains DNA of both the donor and the recipient cell. (The excised DNA pieces from the recipient chromosome are probably broken down by specific enzymes.)

Generally the process of transformation involves the following stages:

1. Reversible binding of ds-DNA molecule to cell surface through receptor site.
2. Irreversible uptake of DNA of donor.
3. Conversion of ds-DNA of donor to SS-DNA by nucleolytic degradation of one strand.
4. Integration of a part of all single strands of donor DNA into the chromosome of recipient cell.
5. The segregation and phenotypic (a set of observable characteristics) expression of integrated donor gene or genes in the recombinant cell i.e., transformed cell.

Transformation process can be occurred without cell contact. It is DNAse sensitive recombination process. This process occurs in absence of DNAse in the medium. These two criteria helps in differentiating process from other two i.e., transduction and conjugation.

In bacterial recombination, cell do not fuse, and usually only a portion of the chromosome from the donor cell (male) is transferred to the recipient cell (female). The recipient cell thus becomes a merozygote, a zygote that is a partial diploid. Once merozygote transformation has occurred, recombination can take place.

Applications of transformation: The utilization of bacterial transformation in medicine, particularly in the pharmaceutical industry is an exciting development that has led to the fast and efficient production of many drugs needed by society. By placing certain suitable bacteria into a bath of calcium chloride, scientists have been able to artificially stimulate the bacteria to uptake certain chosen genes and then incorporate them into their genomes. This transgenic bacterium, if the process was successful, can then express the foreign genes by the production of proteins, and mass produce them because of their ability to speedily and exactly clone themselves. In one example, an E-coli bacterium was stimulated to uptake and incorporates into its genome the human gene for the production of insulin. So instead of painstakingly harvesting small amounts of insulin from hogs, insulin can now be mass produced by the transgenic bacterium. Other examples of important drugs that are produced utilizing the bacterial ability of transformation include human growth hormone, erythropoietin, a drug used to stimulate red blood cell production in people suffering from anemia, tissue plasminogen activator, which is used to dissolve blood clots, as well as several others.

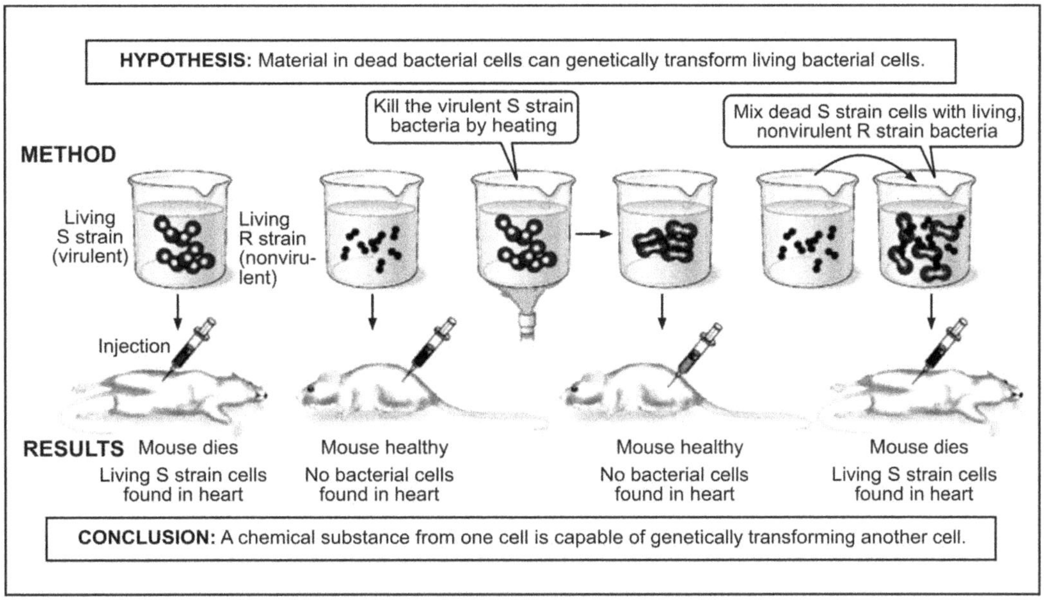

Fig. 6.2 Demonstration of genetic transformation

Pollution control is a major concern in the world today because of earth's limited resources. But, there is an effective and natural way to help do away with pollution, and this process is called bioremediation. Bioremediation is the utilization of some types of transgenic bacteria, fungi, normal bacteria, and/or other microbes to decompose many forms of garbage and to break down petroleum products. An example of an instance where a transgenic bacterium was utilized in the fight against pollution is seen in the breakdown of naphthalene, an environmental pollutant found in many artificially created soils, by the genetically altered pseudomonas fluorescence. This bacterium was stimulated to uptake the gene for fluorescence so that as it broke down the naphthalene it would produce light in proportion to the amount of chemical it had broken down, thus allowing scientists to monitor the efficiency of the process. A more famous example involving the use of transgenic bacteria genetically engineered for the breakdown of hydrocarbons in oil was seen in their use in the Exon-Valdez oil spill.

6.2.2 Bacterial Conjugation

Because lacking of knowledge of any mating system in bacteria, it was impossible to explore the system experimentally to Luria and Delbruck (1943) who had demonstrated that bacteria have a stable hereditary system. The first demonstrate of recombination in bacteria was achieved by Lederberg and Tatum in 1946 in a brilliant and remarkable experiment that opened the door to a whole new world of microbiology.

Conjugation in bacteria must be quite rare. Since it was not found by anybody (in spite of many attempts), so few possible recombinants were selected from a large population.

Two different auxotrophic (an organism having a growth requirement of specific nutrients not necessarily in the parental strain) strains of *E.coli* were combined and allowed to mate. Then combined cultures were plated on a minimal medium, which can grow only phototrophs (the organisms that can synthesize all their aminoacid requirements). Phototrophic colonies were grown, then it was understood that growth of phototrophic bacteria is because of recombination between the auxotroph.

Polyauxotrophs (mutants with more than one nutritional requirement) were used so that back mutation or spontaneous reversion to the wild type would not occur to confuse the results. The photrophs which arose could not have arisen by the phenomenon of transformation. It is experimentally proved that bacterial recombination by conjugation is indeed a true sexual process. It is apparent that mating or conjugation in *E.coil* is radically different from sexual mating in higher organisms. It is not a reproductive process that occurs regularly at each generation. It does not involve meiosis since bacterial cells are haploid, or dies if it involve the fusion of gametes.

It involves the transfer of some DNA from one cell to another followed by separation of the mating pair of cells. In conjugation it is possible for large segments of the chromosome, and in special cases the entire chromosome is transferred.

Sex factors: There is a sexual differentiation in *E.coli*; in other words, different mating types of the bacterium exist. Male cells contain a small circular piece of DNA, which is in the cytoplasm and not part of the chromosome, called the sex factor or F factor (fertility factor).

These cells are referred to as F (+) and are donors in mating. Female cells lack this factor and are labeled F(-). They are recipient cells.

Crosses between two F(-) strains do not yield recombinants. However, in F (+) x F (-) crosses, the male replicates its sex factor, and one copy of it is almost always transferred to the female recipient. The F (-) cell is converted to an F(+) cell) (Fig. 6.3) and is itself capable of serving as a donor. So as long as the cell grows the conjugation process can continue in an infectious way with repeated transfer of the sex factor. The transfer of the factor is independent of the transfer of chromosomal genes.

F factor DNA is only sufficient to specify about 40 genes which control sex factor replication and synthesize sex pili. F factor DNA replicates independently of the F (+) donor cell's normal chromosome. The transfer of the F factor is also independent.

Sex pili seem to act to bind an F (-) cell to an F (+) cell, pulling the F(-) cell into close contact. Sex pili are tubules through which DNA passes from a F (+) to a F (-) cell during conjugation, although the DNA may be passed from one cell to another at sites of contact between them.

6.2.2.1 Extra Chromosomal Genetic Elements (Plasmids)

In addition to the normal DNA chromosome, extra chromosomal genetic elements are often found in bacteria. These elements are called plasmids and are capable of autonomous replication in the cytoplasm of the bacterial cell.

Plasmids are circular pieces of DNA that extra genes. Some plasmids are capable of either replicating autonomously or integrating into the bacterial DNA chromosome and are called episomes. Thus the F factor of *E.coli* was called an episome because it can alternately exist in the F (+) of Hfr (high frequence recombination, or Hfr strains) state.

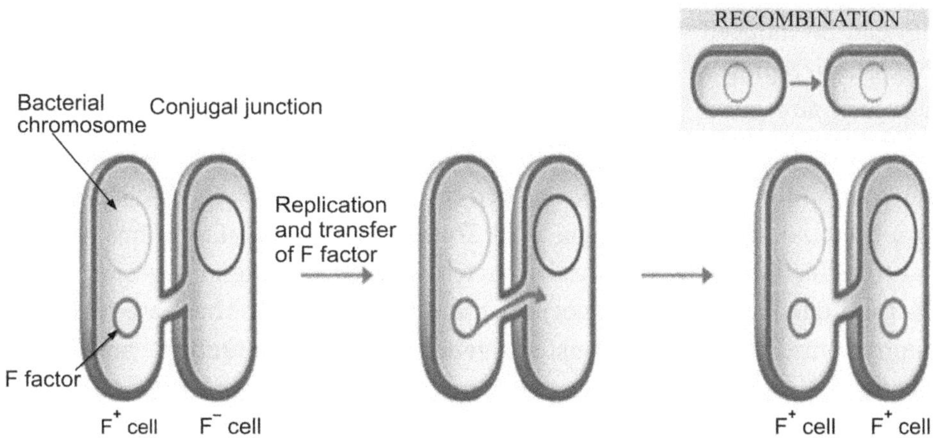

(a) When an F factor (a plasmid) is transferrred from a donor (F^+) to a recipient (F^-), the F^- cell is converted to an F^+ cell.

Fig. 6.3 Bacterial conjugation

Applications of Bacterial Conjugation

Bacterial conjugation is a mechanism for horizontal DNA transfer with potential for universal DNA delivery. The conjugal machinery can be separated into three functional modules: the relaxosome, the coupling protein and a type IV protein secretion system. Module interchangeability among different conjugative systems opens up the possibility of "à la carte" engineering of DNA delivery into virtually any cell type.

6.2.3 Transduction

Bacteriophages have the ability to transfer genes from one bacterial cell to another, a process known as transduction.

Most bacteriaphages, the virulent phages, undergo a rapid lytic growth cycle in their host cells. They inject their nucleic acid, usually DNA, into the bacterium, where it replicates rapidly and also directs the synthesis of new phage proteins. Within 10 to 20 min, the new DNA combines with the new proteins to make whole phage particles, which were released by destruction of the cell wall and lysis of the cell.

However, some bacterial viruses, the temperature phages, which ordinarily do not lyse the cell, carry DNA that can behave as a kind of episome in bacteria; like other episomes, such as the F factor, these viral genomes can become integrated into the bacterial genome; they are then known as prophages. Bacteria that carry prophages (lysogenic bacteria) can be induced with ultraviolet light and other agents to make the prophages start to replicate rapidly and go through a lytic growth cycle, resulting in lysis of the cell with release of new phage particles.

Phages particles may become filled with cell chromosomal DNA or a mixture of chromosomal and phages DNA. Such aberrant phages can attach to other bacteria and introduce bacterial, rather just phage, DNA from one cell to another. Thus we can define bacterial transduction as the transfer by bacteriophages, serving as a vector, of a portion of DNA from one bacterium (a donor) to another (a recipient). There are two varieties of bacteriophage-mediated gene transfer: **generalized transduction** and **specialized transduction**.

Generalized transduction occurs as a result of the lytic cycle. In the process of packaging bacteriophage DNA, the head structures of some bacteriophages will package random fragments of the bacterial chromosome. Thus, the lysate contains two kinds of particles that differ only in the kind of DNA they contain. Most of the particles contain viral DNA. When these inject their DNA, the lytic cycle will repeat and new bacteriophage particles will be produced. A small fraction of the particles, possibly as high as 1%, contain fragments of the bacterial chromosome in place of the bacteriophage DNA. When one of these particles injects its DNA into the cell, the cell is not killed. The newly introduced DNA contains only bacterial genes and is free to recombine with the chromosome. Some transducing bacteriophages can introduce 100-200 kilobases of DNA. Because the bacterial fragments that are packaged are essentially random, virtually any bacterial gene of the bacterial chromosome can be transduced (hence, the term "generalized" transduction). Entire plasmids can be transduced by phages. Some plasmids, notably those encoding antibiotic resistance in *staphylococci* have evolved signals to allow efficient packaging by phage particles and subsequent transfer by transduction. Another element **pathogenicity island**, in the *Staphylococcus* chromosome which codes for toxic shock toxin senses the presence of an infecting phage, excises, replicates, and is efficiently packaged.

Transducing particles, like bacteriophage particles, are stable in the environment for long periods of time. Thus, bacterial genes can be stored in the environment and transduction of a bacterial cell may occur long after the original bacterial population was lysed by the bacteriophage infection. Studies on dissemination of antibiotic resistance have revealed generalized transduction to be a significant mechanism of gene transfer in nature.

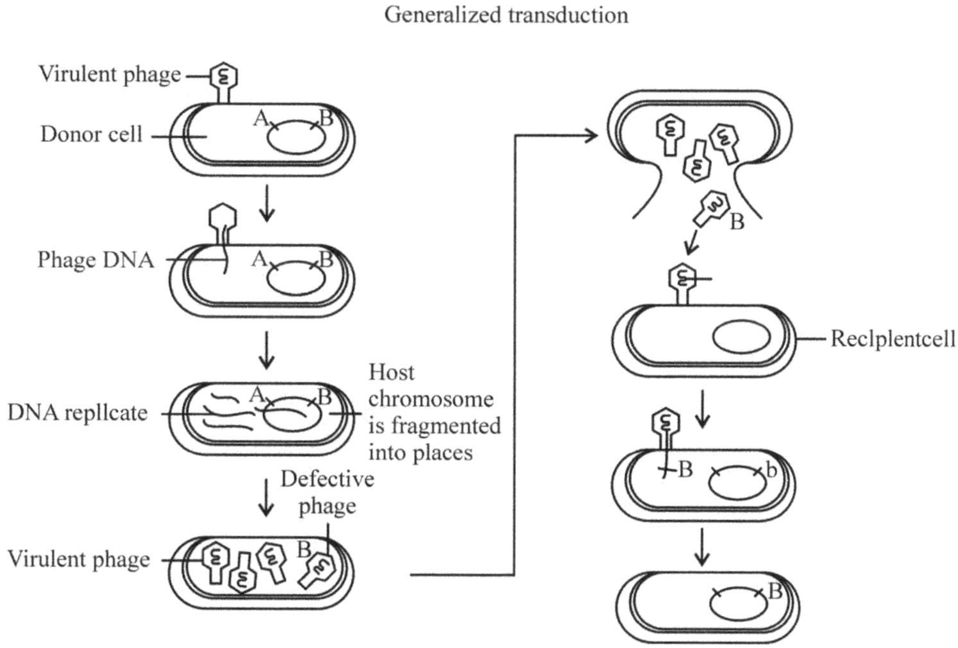

Fig. 6.4 Generalized transduction

Specialized transduction requires a temperate bacteriophage. In this class of transduction, a bacterial gene becomes associated with the bacteriophage genome (e.g. by recombination). When such a bacteriophage lysogenizes a new bacterial host, it brings with it the associated bacterial gene. Because it is a bacterial gene, its expression is not turned off by the bacteriophage repressor that inhibits expression of the lytic functions. A well known example is the b phage of *Corynebacterium diphtheriae*, which carries the gene for diphtheria toxin. Cells of *C. diphtheriae* that are non-lysogenic for the bacteriophage are incapable of causing diphtheria. *C. diphtheriae* cells that carry the b phage in the chromosome express the gene for diphtheria toxin and produce disease. Other examples include changes in the O-antigens of *Salmonella*, antibiotic resistance genes, erythrogenic toxin in *Streptococcus pyogenes*, the tissue destroying a-toxin of *Staphylococcus aureus*, enterotoxin of *E. coli,* cholera toxin of *Vibrio cholerae*, and neurotoxin by *Clostridium botulinum*. Such alterations of the properties of a bacterial cell by lysogeny with a temperate bacteriophage are known as lysogenic conversion shown in Fig. 6.6.

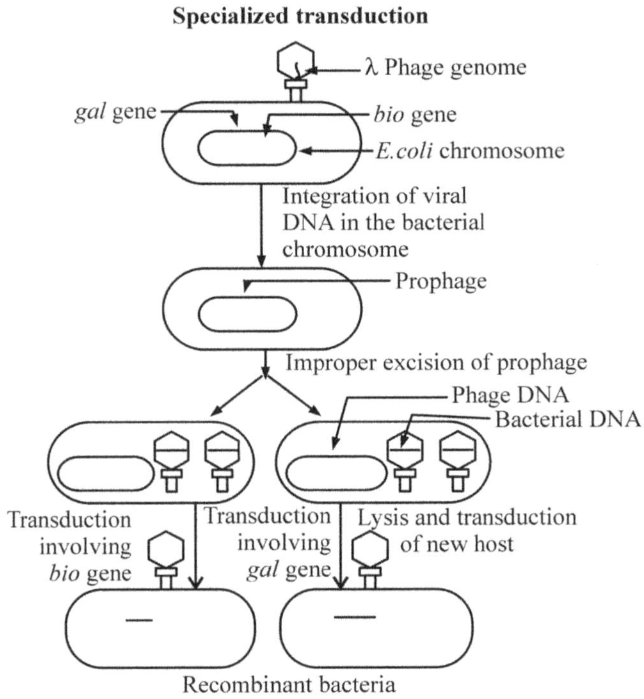

Fig. 6.5 Specialized transduction

6.2.3.1 Transduction - Uses in Research

Generalized transducing viruses are the most useful in mapping bacterial chromosomal genes. Since the amount of DNA that is packaged by the virus is determined by the size of the head of the virus, each viral particle holds the same amount of DNA. The initial cutting of the host chromosome is a random event, giving all genes approximately the same probability of being packaged and transferred. Each piece of DNA that is packaged will be the same length, meaning that the closer together two genes are, the higher the probability that the two genes will be present on the same fragment of packaged DNA. In other words, the closer together the genetic markers are, the higher the frequency of co-transduction. Therefore the distance between closely linked chromosomal genes can be calculated by measuring the frequency that two genes or genetic markers are co-transduced.

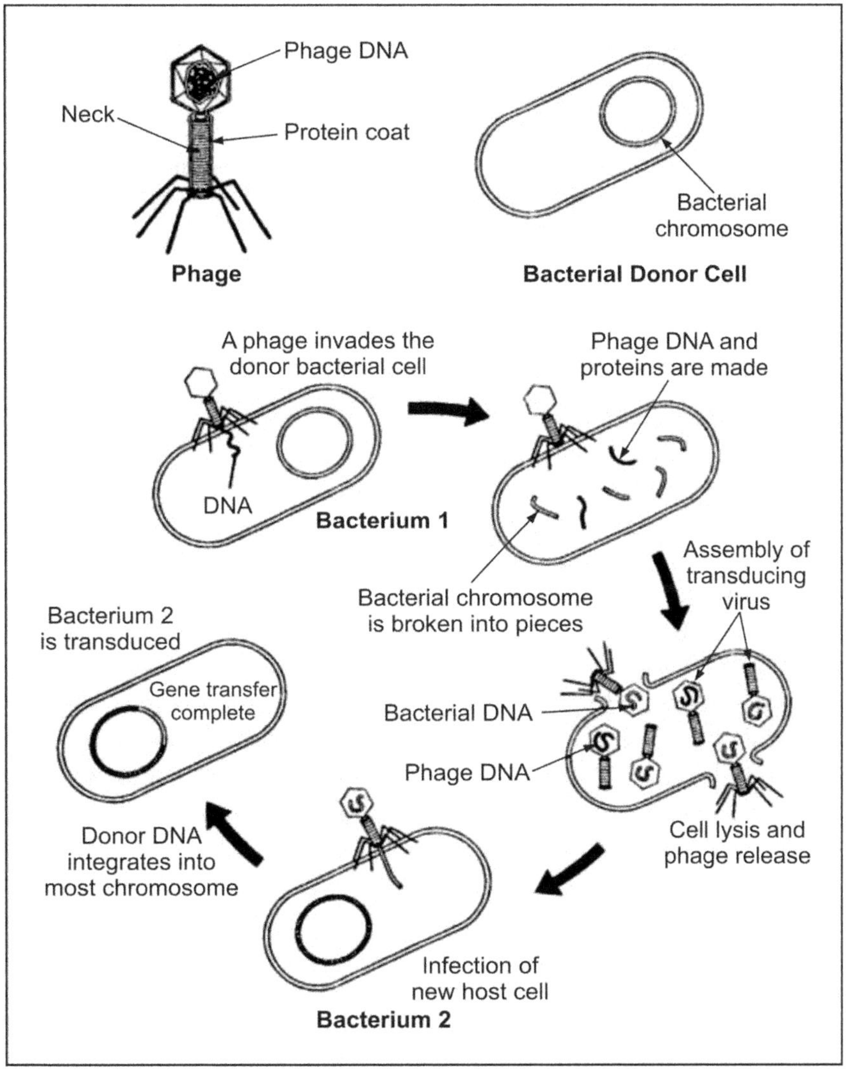

Fig. 6.6 Transduction

6.3 Bacterial Genetics

6.3.1 Mutagenesis

Genetics includes the study of the inheritance (heredity) and the variability of the characteristics of an organism. Inheritance is based on genes that are faithfully transmitted from parents to offspring during reproduction. Nevertheless, "mistakes" the changes in the genetic material do occur. Such sudden, heritable change in the genetic material are called mutations.

In 1880s, for the first time Hugo de Vries (1848-1935), a Dutch botanist, one of the independent rediscoveries of Mendelism, put forward his views regarding the formation of new species in 1901. He used the term mutation to describe the phenotypic changes in evening primrose, *Oenothera lamarckiana.*

The term mutation is derived from the Latin word *mutare* means to change.

Mutation refers to any heritable change in nucleotide sequence of a gene of the organisms irrespective of altered phenotypic expression of characters of the organisms.

When a bacterial cell divides, the two daughter cells are generally indistinguishable. Thus, a single bacterial cell can produce a large population of identical cells or clone. On solid medium, a clone is manifested as an easily isolated colony. Occasionally, a spontaneous genetic change occurs in one of the cells. This change (**mutation**) is heritable and passed on to the progeny of the variant cell to produce a **subclone** with characteristics different from the original (**wild type**) parent. This is termed **vertical inheritance**. If the change is detrimental to the growth of the cell, the subclone will quickly be overrun by the healthy, wild type population. However, if the change is beneficial, the subclone may overtake the wild type population. This is an example of how evolution is directed by **natural selection**.

The term mutation refers both to the change in the genetic material and to the process by which the change occurs. These changes are associated with the two fundamental properties of the cell (or) organism, namely the genotype and the phenotype.

The genotype refers to the genetic constitution of the cell. The phenotype is the expression of the genotype in observable properties characteristics of the cell (or) organism. The genotype of a culture of cells remains relatively constant during the growth. However, it can change by mutation. This change can result in an alteration in the observable properties (or) phenotype of the cells.

Spontaneous Mutations occurs without known cause, they are resulting from an inherent low level of metabolic errors that is mistakes during DNA replication. Induced mutations are resulting from exposure of organisms to mutagenic agents such as ionizing radiations and various chemicals that react with DNA. Spontaneous mutations occur infrequently, although the observed frequencies vary from gene to gene and from organism. Treatment with mutagenic agents can increase mutation frequencies by orders of magnitude.

Mutagens: Mutagens are chemical (or) physical agents that increase the frequency at which mutations occur during the growth of culture.

Mutation that occurs due to physical agents is called physical mutagenesis, if it is due to chemical agents then it is referred as chemical mutagenesis. These mutagens act in one (or) the other of two quite different ways.

1. Some Chemical mutagens become associated with the DNA that are called intercalating agents (or) some incorporated into it called base analogues.
2. A large variety of other mutagens are reacting mutagens which react chemically with DNA – usually with one of its purine (or) pyrimidine bases.

6.3.2 Chemical Mutagens

Class	Example
Aziridines	Ethyleneimine
Mustard-I[st] mutations identified	N_2 mustard, sulphur mustard
Epoxides	Ethyleneoxide, diepoxybutane
Miscellaneous	Hydroxylamine

DNA repair mechanisms: DNA damage can occur by UV radiation, x-rays and certain chemicals. Cells contain specific enzymes which can repair damaged DNA.

- Many kinds of bacterial cells and yeasts have been shown to possess an efficient photo reactivating mechanism for repairing damages caused by UV radiation.
- Photoreactivation occurs when cells exposed to lethal doses of UV light are immediately exposed to visible light. A special enzyme designated PRE, induced by visible light, splits or unlinks the dimers formed because of exposure to UV light and restores the DNA to its original state.

Excision repair: Some bacteria have enzymes called endonucleas and exonucleases that excise or cut out a damaged segment of DNA.

- Enzymes such as polymerases and ligases, repair the resulting break by filling in the gap and joining the fragments together. This mechanism is termed as excision repair.

SOS repair: SOS (save our soul) repair is a by-pass repair system. It is also called emergency repair. The process by which *E.coil* repairs large amounts of DNA damage is called inducible or SOS repair. This process is not a single discrete mechanism but includes diverse responses such as the ability to repair pyrimidine dimers, to induce various prophages, to shut off respiration, and to delay septum formation during cell division. The process is a very efficient one; however, it tends to insert mismatched bases and thus is error prone and introduces additional mutation.

Intercalating agents: These are planar molecule and can insert between the stacked pairs of bases in the core of DNA molecule. Such incorporation distorts the backbone of the double helix results in frame – shift mutations when the distorted helix is replicated.

Base analogues: Mechanism of mutagenic action of base analogues can be illustrated by considering example of 2-aminopurine which is commonly used mutagen. In its usual amino form it pairs with thyme and in imino form it pairs with cytosine. Thus it usually has paring properties like adenine, but the probability of its being in the imino form is greater.

6.3.3 Physical Mutagens

Mutations also results from ionizing and non-inoizing radiations. H. J. Muller was the person who first demonstrated that mutation could be induced by an external factor. Examples for ionizing radiations are penetration into living tissues. The high energy rays collide with the atoms and cause the release of electrons, leaving positively changed free radicals (or) ions. These ions in turn collide with other molecules, causing the release of further electrons. The net result is that a "core" of ions is formed. This process of ionization is induced by X-rays, protons and neutrons as well as alpha, beta and gamma rays replaced by radioactive isotopes of the elements ^{32}P,^{35}S and cobalt-90.

Mechanism of X-rays (Ionizing radiations)

These ionizing radiations produce gross changes in structure of the chromosome. These changes in chromosome structure result from breaks in chromosome caused by ionizing radiations. For example X-rays causes breakage of covalent bonding.

Ultra-Violet Radiations

In contrast to X-rays, they do not pocess sufficient energy to induce ionization. However they are readily absorbed by purines and pyrimidines which then enter a more reactive (or) excited state. Because of their lower energy they penetrate tissues slightly, only the surface layers of cells in muticellular organisms.

The maximum absorption of UV by DNA is at wavelength of 254 nm. The principal damage caused by UV light is the formation of pyrimidine dimers, the most common being thymine dimers between adjacent bases which causes a distortion of DNA helix.

6.3.4 Occurrence of Mutations

Mutations most commonly occur during DNA replication. The occurrence of mutation may be spontaneous or induced.

Spontaneous mutations: This type of mutation is commonly referred as Naturally occurring mutation. The best example for spontaneous mutation is Tautomerism (changing from one form to another, keto – enol and vice versa).

Induced mutations: Any agent that increases the mutation rate is called as mutagen. Mutations obtained by the use of a mutagen are said to be induced.

- The major effect of UV light is to cause the formation of dimers by cross linking between adjacent pyrimidine, especially thymine, residues in DNA. These cross linked residues disrupt the normal process of replication.
- When X rays interact with DNA, the result is usually a break in the phosphodiester backbone of the nucleic acid.

6.3.5 Features of Spontaneous Mutations

Mutations can arise for number of reasons

1. Errors in DNA replication
2. Physical damage of DNA
3. Chemical damage
4. Recombination and transposition.

One main cause of spontaneous mutations results from the fact that bases can exist as different forms called tautomers, which are capable of forming different base pairs. During replication, adenine, which normally base-pairs with thymine in its normal amino form, switches to its rate imino form (tautomerism) and base pairs with cytosine instead of thymine. If this error is not repaired before the next round of replication the A-T base pair will change to a G-C base pair.

Adenine Base Tautomerization Adenine

(aminoform) (iminoform)

Base-pairs with thymine Base-pairs with cytosine

Adenine changes from amino to imino form reverts to aminoform

Fig: Spontaneous mutations of as A-T base pair to G-C as result of adenine base tautomerization.

6.3.6 DNA Repair Mechanisms

Damaged DNA resulted due to the mutations can be repaired by three mechanisms.

1. Photoreactivation (PR)
2. Excision repair
3. Post replication recombination repair

1. Photo reactivation mechanism used in breaking of thymine dimers resulted from UV induced mutions. PR involves an enzyme that splits the thymine dimers by binding in the presence of visible light, specifically light within the blue region of the spectrum.

2. Endonuclease catalyses the first step, they recognizes the thymine dimers & cleaves the posphodiester backbone of the DNA strand containing the dimmer at a site near the damage. An Exo-nuclease then removes a segment of strand adjacent to the Endo-nuclease including dimmer. A DNA polymerase (DNA poly I) then fills the gap using complementary strand as a template. At last DNA ligase then catalyzes closer of final phosphor-diester linkage between adjacent nucleotides.
3. The third type of dark repair of UV damage involves both replication and recombination, that is why it is called a post replication recombination repair. When DNA molecules containing thymine dimers are replicated, gaps are formed in the nascent complementary strands opposite the dimers because DNA polymerases cannot use the distorted strands of a template. After a lag due to the thymine dimmer blockage replication is reinitiated at secondary initiation sites beyond the dimmer. This results in progeny double helices with thymine dimers in one strand and gaps in the complementary strand. If these two "sister" chromosomes recombine such that the dimers and gaps end up in one chromosome and the intact undamaged segments end up in the other chromosome, the latter will be functional and produce viable cell.

6.3.7 Types of Mutations

Two common types of mutations (Fig 6.7) are point mutations and frameshift mutations.

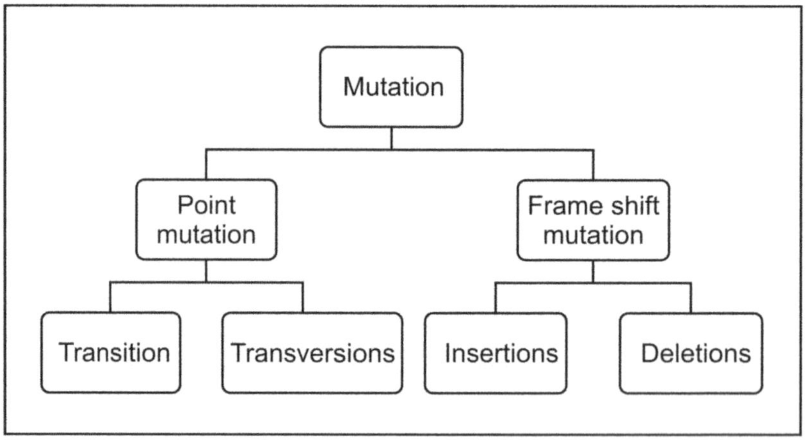

Fig. 6.7 Classification of mutations

1. **Point Mutations:** Point mutations occur as a result of the substitution of one nucleotide for another in the specific nucleotide sequence of a gene.

   Transition: Mutations resulting from tautomeric shifts in the bases of DNA involve the replacement of purine in one strand of DNA with the purine and the replacement of pyrimidine in the complementary strands with other pyrimidine. Such base pair substitutions are called transitions. The substitution of one purine for another purine or one pyrimidine for another pyrimidine is termed as Transition shown in Fig. 6.7.

Transversion: The replacement of a purine by a pyrimidine, or vice versa is termed as Transversion.

This base-pair substitution may result in one of three kinds of mutations affecting the translation process.

(i) Missense mutation

(ii) Nonsense mutation

(iii) Neutral mutation

Missense mutation: The altered gene triplet produces a codon in the mRNA which specifies an aminoacid different from the one present in the normal protein. This mutation is called as missense mutation. *Ex*: Sickle cell anaemia.

Nonsense mutation: This type of mutation occurs due to incomplete protein synthesis i.e., premature termination of protein formation during translation. As a result of this mutation an incomplete polypeptide is formed which is nonfunctional.

Neutral mutation: The altered gene triplet produces a mRNA codon which specifies the same amino acid because the codon resulting from mutation is a synonym for the original codon this is a neutral mutation.

2. **Frameshift Mutations:** They involve the addition (or) deletion of one (or) few base pairs. Base pair additions and deletions are combinedly referred to as frameshift mutations. These mutations alter the reading frame of all base-pair triplets in the gene.

   In prokaryotes large proportions of spontaneous mutations are occurring and they are found to be single base pair insertions (additions) and deletions rather than base-pair substitutions.

   These mutations result from an addition or loss of one or more nucleotide in a gene and are termed insertion or deletion mutation respectively. This results in a shift of the reading frame.

   - Frame shift mutations generally lead to nonfunctional proteins, because, entirely new sequence of amino acids is synthesized from a frame shift reading of the nucleotide sequences of mRNA shown in Fig. 6.8.

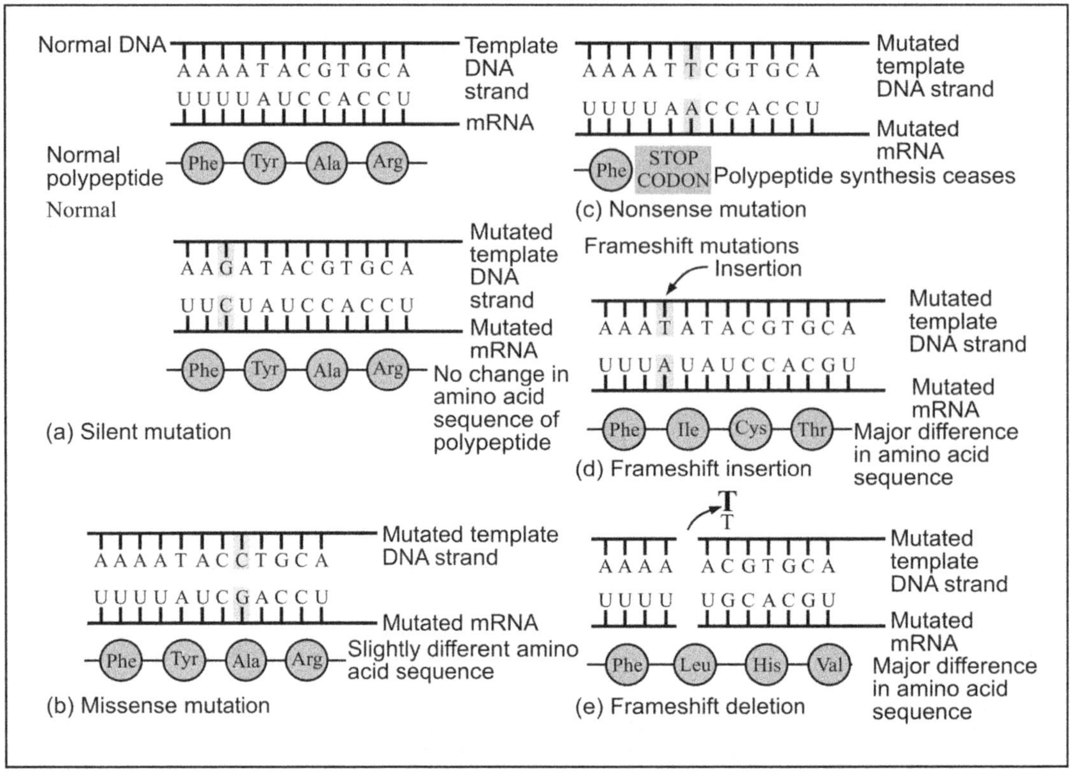

Fig. 6.8 Different of types of mutations

6.3.8 Detection and Isolation of Mutants

Mutation occurring in micro-organisms can be detected and efficiently isolated from the parent organisms of other mutants. Awareness of wild type characters of an organism is essential for studying mutation so that mutants can easily be detected. Since, mutations are rare about one per 10^7 to 10^{11} cells, it is very important to have a very sensitive detection system so that the rare mutant may not be missed from detection.

Some of the methods of detection have been described as below.

6.3.8.1 Replica Plating Technique

This technique is used to detect auxotrophic mutants which differentiates between mutants and wild type strains on the basis of ability to grow in the absence of an amino acid. Isolation of a leucine auxotroph through replica plating follows the following steps

(i) Generates the mutants by treating a culture with a mutagen.

(ii) *e.g.*, nitrosoguanidine

(iii) Inoculate a plate containing complete growth medium and incubate it at proper temperature. Both wild type and mutant survivors will form colonies on the complete medium. This plate containing complete medium is called masterplate.

(iv) Prepare a piece of sterile velvet (Fig. 6.9) and gently press on upper surface of master plate to pick up bacterial cells from each colony. As pressed on master plate, again gently press the velvet on replica plates containing complete medium in one set and lacking only leucine in the other set. Thus, the bacterial cells are transferred in replica plates in the same position as in master plate.

(v) Incubate the plates and compare the replica plates with master plate for the bacterial colony not growing on replica plate. The leucine auxotrophs (Leu^-) will not grow on replica plates devoid of leucine. Isolate and culture Leu^- cells growing on complete medium.

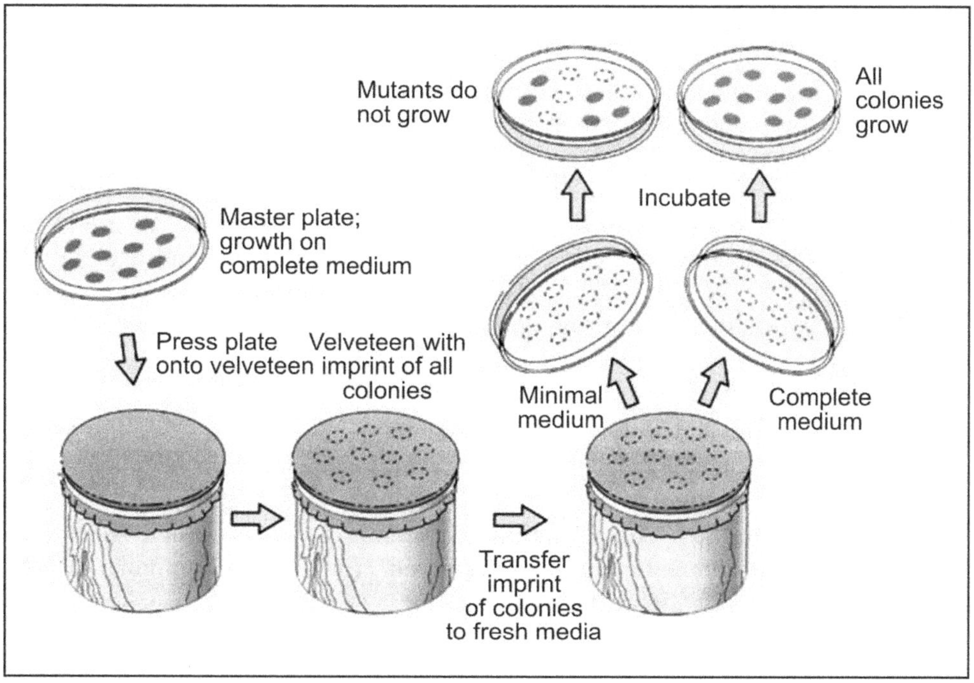

Fig. 6.9 Replice plating technique for isolation of mutants

Replica plating can also be used to isolate the temperature sensitive mutants. It involves by forming colonies at 30 °C and then transferring these colonies on two plates, one incubated at 30 °C and the other at 42 °C. The colony which grow at 30 °C and absent at 42 °C certainly consist of temperature sensitive mutant.

6.3.8.2 Resistance Selection Method

It is the other approach for isolation of mutants. Generally the wild type cells are not resistant either to antibiotics or bacteriophages. Therefore, it is possible to grow the bacterium in the presence of the agent (antibiotics or bacteriophage and 100k for survivors). This method is applied for islolation of mutants resistant to any chemical compounds that can be amended in agar, phage resistant mutants.

6.3.8.3 Substrate Utilization Method

This method is employed in the selection of bacteria. Several bacteria utilize only a few primary carbon sources. The cultures are plated onto a medium containing an alternate carbon sources. Any colony that grows on medium can use the substrate and are possibly mutants. These can be isolated.

Sugar utilization mutants are also isolated by means of colour indicator plates. A popular medium (EMB agar) is used for this purpose. EMB agar contains two dyes eosin and methylene blue in the medium. Colour of these dyes is sensitive to pH. This medium also contain lactose sugar as carbon source and complete mixture of aminoacids. Therefore, both lactose wild type (Lac^+) and lactose mutant (Lac^-) cells can grow and form colonies on EMB agar plates. The Lac^+ cells catabolize lactose and secrete acids, therefore, local pH of the medium decreases. This results in staining of colony to dark purple. On the other hand, Lac^- cells are unable to utilize lactose and use some of the aminoacids as carbon source. After utilization of aminoacid, possibly ammonia is produced that increases the local p^H and decolourizes the dye resulting in white colony.

6.3.8.4 Carcinogenicity Test

This method is based on detecting potential of carcinogens and testing for mutagenicity in bacteria. Ames et al. (1973) developed a method for deletion of mutagenicity of carcinogens which is commonly known as Ames test. It is widely used to detect the carcinogens. The Ames test is a mutational reversion assay in which several special strains of *salmonella typhimurium* are employed. Each strain contains a different mutation in the operon of histidine biosynthesis.

The Ames test employs the following steps:

(i) Prepare the culture of *salmonella* histindine auxotrophs (His^-)

(ii) Mix the bacterial cells and test substance (mutagen) in dilute; molten the top agar with a small amount of histidine in one set, and control with complete medium plus large amount of histidine.

(iii) Pour the molten mix on the top of minimal agar plates and incubate at 37°C for 2-3 days. Until histidine is depleted all the His^- cells will grow in the presence of test mutagens. When histidine is completely the original wild type characters) will grow on agar plate. The number of spontaneous reverants is low, whereas the number of reverants induced by the test mutagen is quite high. To estimate the relative mutagenicity of the mutagenic substance the visible colonies are counted and compared with control. The high number of colonies represents the greater mutagenicity.

A mammalian liver extract is added to the above molten top agar before plating. The extract converts the carcinogens into electrophilic derivatives which will soon react with DNA molecule. In natural way this process occurs in mammalian system when foreign substances are metabolized in the liver does, therefore, the liver extract is added to this test, just to promote the transformation shown in Fig. 6.10.

The Ames test has now been used with thousands of substances and mixtures such as the industrial chemicals, food additives, pesticides, hairdyes and cosmetics.

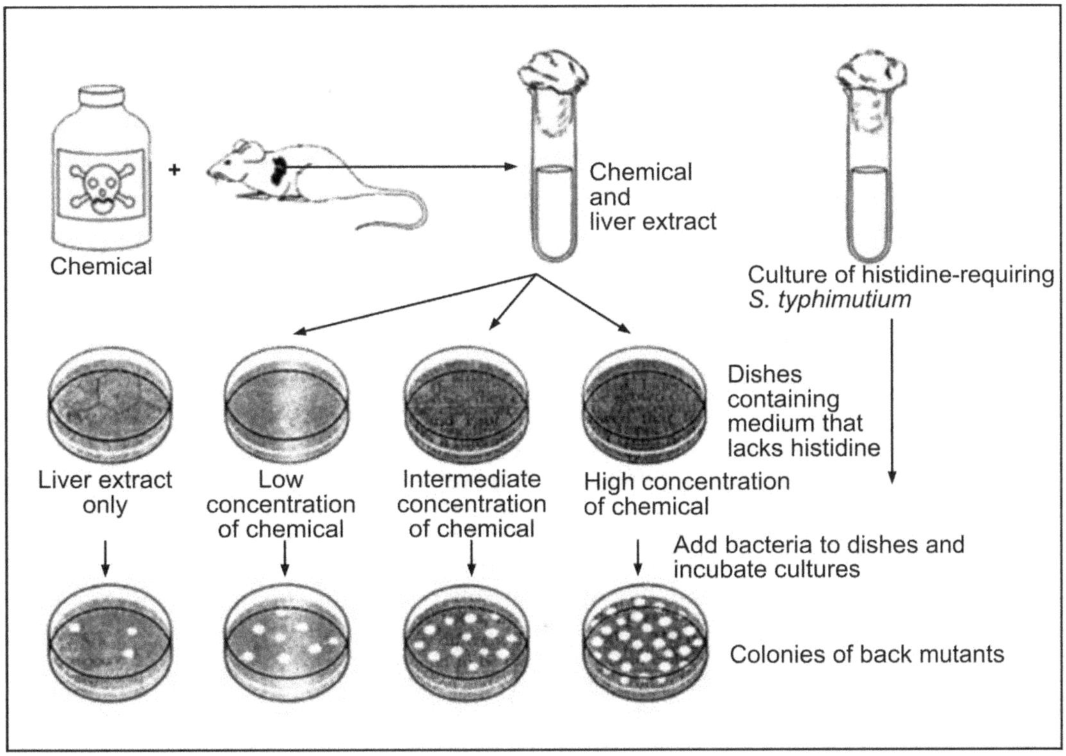

Fig. 6.10 The ames test

6.4 DNA Replication

Bacteria are almost always haploid, which means that their chromosomes are unpaired. In contrast, most eukaryotic cells are diploid, they have paired homologous chromosomes which may be heterozygous (carry different alleles or genus occupying the same relative locus on homologous chromosomes) shown in Fig. 6.8.

- All bacteria have their genetic loci in a single linkage group; that is, they have a single chromosome per genome.
- The chromosome of a typical bacterium is a circular double stranded DNA molecule; that is, the double helix for a complete genome has no free ends.
- The circular chromosome is further twisted on itself in the bacterial cell to form a supercoil.
- It has an approximate molecular weight of 2.5×10^9 Daltons and has about 4×10^6 base pairs.

There are three general methods of replication of the DNA molecule.

Theta (θ) mode: The replication of a circular DNA molecule is initiated at a certain point called the origin, which is specific for each bacterial species.

- Replication proceeds in two directions around the chromosome, leading to the formation of a "bubble" which increases in size as replication proceeds. This mode is called theta because intermediate structures resemble the Greek letter θ.
- In this process, a circular parental chromosome is replicated to two circular daughter chromosomes, in each of which one strand of the parental DNA molecule is conserved and a complementary strand is newly synthesized.

Sigma (σ) or "Rolling circle" mode: Replication begins with the cleavage of phosphodiester bond in one strand of the circular DNA molecule to produce a nick with 3' – OH and 5' – po_4 ends on that strand.

- The complimentary circular strand then serves as template for the synthesis of a new strand. As this strand grows at the 3' – OH end, the 5' – po_4 end of the some strand is displaced to form a "tail" on the circle.
- As the replication proceeds, a circular parental molecule is converted to two daughter molecules, one circular and the other linear. This mode is called sigma because intermediate structures have the Greek letter σ conformation.
- The sigma mode of DNA molecule replication is carried out by some bacteriophages, such as λ and $\phi \times 174$ whose progeny viral DNA is linear.

Linear mode: All eukaryotic organisms and some viruses have linear DNA molecules. Replication of these chromosomes is initiated at specific sites by the formation of replication bubbles.

- Small viral linear DNA molecules may have only one point of initiation points per molecule.
- Large DNA molecules of eukaryotes may have hundreds of initiation points per molecule.

- A replication bubble grows in size as DNA replication (Fig. 6.11) proceeds from the point of initiation. Adjacent bubbles fuse to form larger ones as replication proceeds.
- Upon completion of replication, two linear double-helical daughter molecules are formed from one linear parental molecule.
- Prokaryotes replicate their DNA from one origin or growing point per molecule while eukaryotes replicate from many origins per molecule.
- Replication may occur in either a unidirectional or bidirectional manner from each origin.

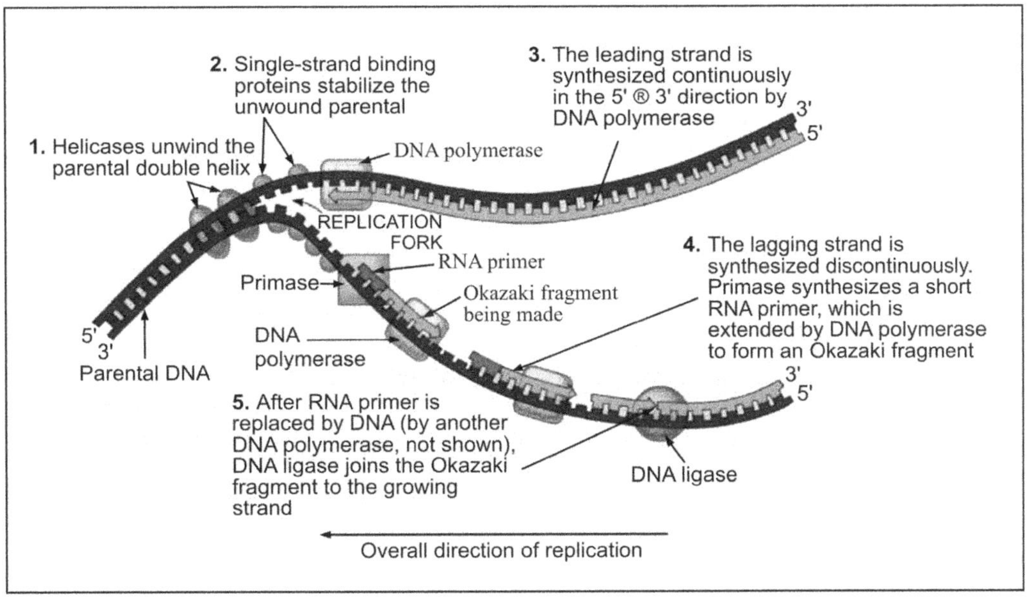

Fig. 6.11 A Summary of DNA replication

Events at the growing point (Replication Fork)

- At the growing point both DNA strands are duplicated.
- Prokaryotic DNA strands are synthesized at the rate of about 1000 nucleotides per second, at a replication fork.
- Eukaryotic DNA strands are synthesized more slowly at about 100 nucleotides per second.
- Many enzymes are involved in this synthesis; they are helix-unwinding protein (ATP-dependent), a helix-destabilizing protein, and a helix-relaxing protein (DNA gyrase). These enzymes participate on opening the parental DNA helix, a head of the replication fork.
- DNA replication is discontinuous, that is, the strands are replicated in small fragments called "Okazaki" fragments, in the 5'-3' direction.

- Initiation of DNA replication requires a primer, a short sequence of RNA that is synthesized by RNA polymerase and is complementary to the DNA which serves as a template.

6.5 Transcription (RNA Synthesis)

DNA itself cannot directly order for the synthesis of aminoacids but forms its transcripts first which is then translated into protein. For the first time in 1958 F. crick suggested that there is unidirectional flow of information from DNA to RNA to protein.

This sequential transfer of information from DNA to protein via RNA is known as central dogma.

- The tRNA, mRNA and rRNA are involved in the process of transcription. However an enzyme transcriptase i.e. DNA-dependent RNA polymerase is required for the synthesis of RNA by using ribonucleotide triphosphates i.e., ATP, GTP, CTP and UTP.
- The synthesis of RNA is different from that of DNA in the following features.
  - (i) Only one of the two strands of any given segment of DNA serves as the template.
  - (ii) Only specific, relatively short lengths of DNA are transcribed i.e., and RNA chain is a transcript of a short section of DNA.
- Transcription is the first step in gene expression. The process involves separation of the two DNA strands, one of which serves as a template for the synthesis of a complementary strand of mRNA by DNA-dependent RNA polymerse.

Transcription stages: Transcription involves 3 steps shown in Fig. 6.9.

1. Initiation
2. Elongation
3. Termination

Initiation: The enzyme RNA polymerase plays a key role in recognition and binding of initiation site. Transcription initiated at specific sites on the bacterial chromosome that are defined by short sequences of bases of DNA called promoters. RNA polymerase binds to the promoter over a relatively long region intending from approximately 45 base pairs upstream from the point at which transcription is transcription/mRNA synthesis.

Elongation: once initiated σ factor is released and binds to another core enzyme.

- When both core enzyme and sigma particle are combined there it is called as holoenzyme.

Termination: Termination of mRNA synthesis is also at specific regulatory sequences of DNA nucleotides along the DNA molecule which are recognized by the RNA polymerase. Furthermore, a tetrameric protein factor called the rhofactor binds to RNA polymerase and promotes its termination.

There are two types of mechanisms that brings about termination.

(i) Rho-independent termination

(ii) Rho-dependent termination.

Rho-independent termination: The Rho-independent signal for termination is recognized by DNA itself. RNA forms a hair pin loop like structure.

Rho-dependent termination: This termination requires the Rho protein encode by rhogene. The Rho factor is a hexamer. Rho factor moves along RNA from its binding site to the enzyme RNA polymerase. The movement is facilitated by the hydrolysis of ATP that provides energy, which is required for the separation of core enzyme, RNA.

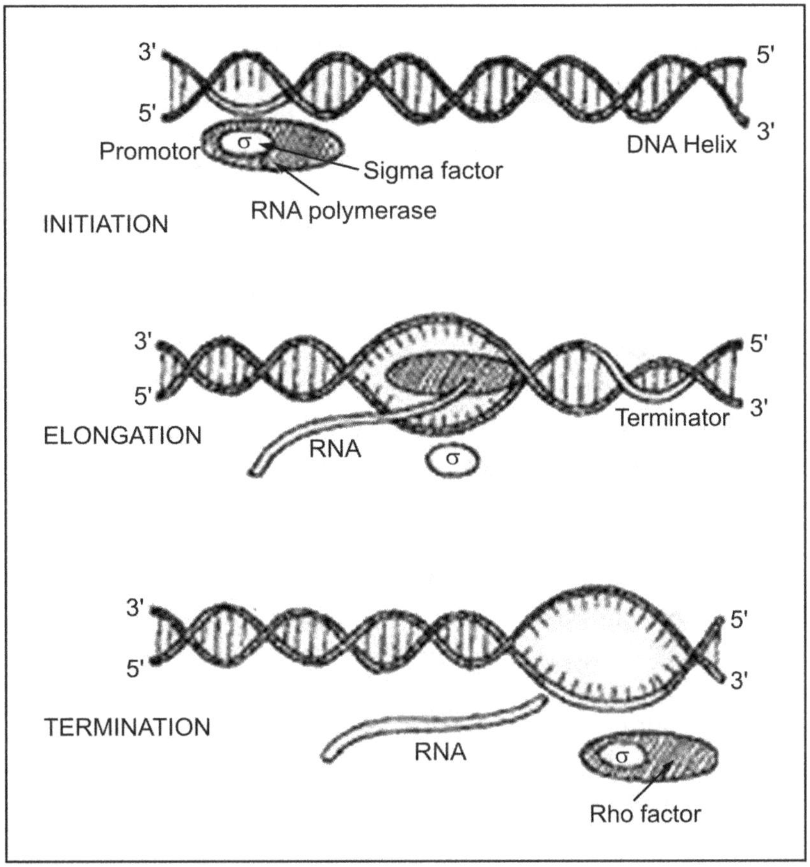

Fig. 6.12 Summary of RNA synthesis

6.6 Translation

Translation is the process in which the genetic information present in the mRNA molecule directs protein synthesis. mRNA has codons, capable of specifying a particular aminoacid. All the three types of RNAs are involved in protein synthesis in the following main steps:

(i) Activation of aminoacids

(ii) Transfer of aminoacid to tRNA

(iii) Assembly of the protein chain on the Ribosome.

(i) Activation of aminoacids: In protein synthesis only L-aminoacids take part. The D-aminoacids are screened from the all 20 aminoacids. Each aminoacid has a specific aminoacyl tRNA synthetase and a specific tRNA. The aminoacids are activated by aminoacyl-tRNA synthetase. This activation reaction requires energy in the form of ATP.

The activated aminoacid remains tightly bound to the enzyme after activation.

(ii) Transfer of aminoacid to tRNA: The process of transfer of activated aminoacids to tRNA is called charging of tRNA. This reaction is catalyzed by the enzyme that was originally bound to the aminoacid.

The tRNA function in protein synthesis is to carry aminoacids and recognize codons in mRNA.

Clover leaf model of t-RNA

- Ist arm called acceptor arm. It accepts the aminoacids.
- IInd called D arm/DHU arm (digydroxy uridine)
- IIIrd arm called anticodon arm which specifically recognizes the complementary codon in mRNA for a specific aminoacid.
- IVth arm called variable arm. It has no particular shape and function.
- Vth arm is called Tψc (Thymine, pseudouridine and cytosine). Thymine is an exception because RNA has oracil in the place of Thymine.

(iii) Assembly of the protein chain on the ribosome: The ribosome is the site of protein synthesis. Its rRNA is transcribed from certain portions of DNA by the same energy requiring process used for synthesis of mRNA and tRNA.

The ribosomes of E.coil have been studied extensively and have been found to consist of two subunits, which are identified by a sedimentation constant (s) and determined by ultracentrifugation studies. The larger subunit is a 50s particle, while the smaller unit is a 30s particle. Ribosomal subunits may associate or dissociate with each other. The association of 30s and 50s submit to form a 70s ribosome shows that the sedimentation behavior of the 70s ribosomes is not a simple addition of the units of the smaller particles. Each subunit is made up of ribosomal RNA molecule and numerous proteins.

6.6.1 Steps of the Synthesis of a Protein Chain on a Ribosome

Step 1: A ribosome binds to one end of a mRNA molecule at a specific site.

Step 2: A charged tRNA carrying the first aminoacid molecule then attaches to the chain-initiating codon(x) of the mRNA.

Step 3: Another tRNA carrying the second aminoacid binds at the next codon(y).

Step 4: The amino group of the aminoacid on the second tRNA reacts with the active terminal carboxyl group on the aminoacid of the first tRNA is then to form a dipleptide; the first tRNA is then released. The mRNA is moved along the ribosome to position the next codon(z) in readiness for the tRNA carrying the third aminoacid.

A single molecule of mRNA is long enough for several ribosomes to read the molecule at the same time. When a number of 70s ribosomes are actively engaged in protein synthesis on a strand of mRNA, this is called polysome.

6.7 Gene Regulation

The DNA of a microbial cell consists of genes, a few to thousands, which do not express at the same time. At a particular time only a few genes express and synthesize the desired protein. The other genes remain silent at this moment and express when required.

- Requirement of gene expression is governed by the environment in which they grow. This shows that the genes have a property to switch on and switch off.
- 20 different aminoacids constitute different proteins. All are synthesized by codons. Therefore, synthesis of all the aminoacids requires energy which is useless because all the aminoacids constituting proteins are not needed at a time. Hence, there is need to control the synthesis of those aminoacids which are not required. Therefore, a control system is operative which is known as "Gene regulation".
- There are certain substrates called inducers that induce the enzyme synthesis.

For example, if yeast cells are grown in medium containing lactose, an enzyme lactase, is formed. Lactase hydrolyses the lactose into glucose and galactose. In the absence of lactose, lactase synthesis does not occur. This shows that lactose induces the enzymes lactase. Therefore, lactase is known as inducible enzyme.

6.7.1 The Lac Operon

For the first time Jacob and Monod (1961) gave the concept of operon model to explain the regulation of gene action.

An operon is defined as several distinct genes situated in tandem (an arrangement in which a team of machines, are lined up one behind another, all facing in the same direction) all controlled by a common regulatory region. Commonly an operon consists of repressor, promoter, operator and structural gens. The message produced by an operon is polycistronic because the information of all structural genes resides on a single molecule of mRNA.

- The lactose utilizing system (Fig. 6.13) consists of two types of components; the structural genus (lac z, lac y and lac A) the products of which are required for transport and metabolism of lactose and the regulatory genes (lac I, lac O, lac P). These two components together comprises of the lacoperon.

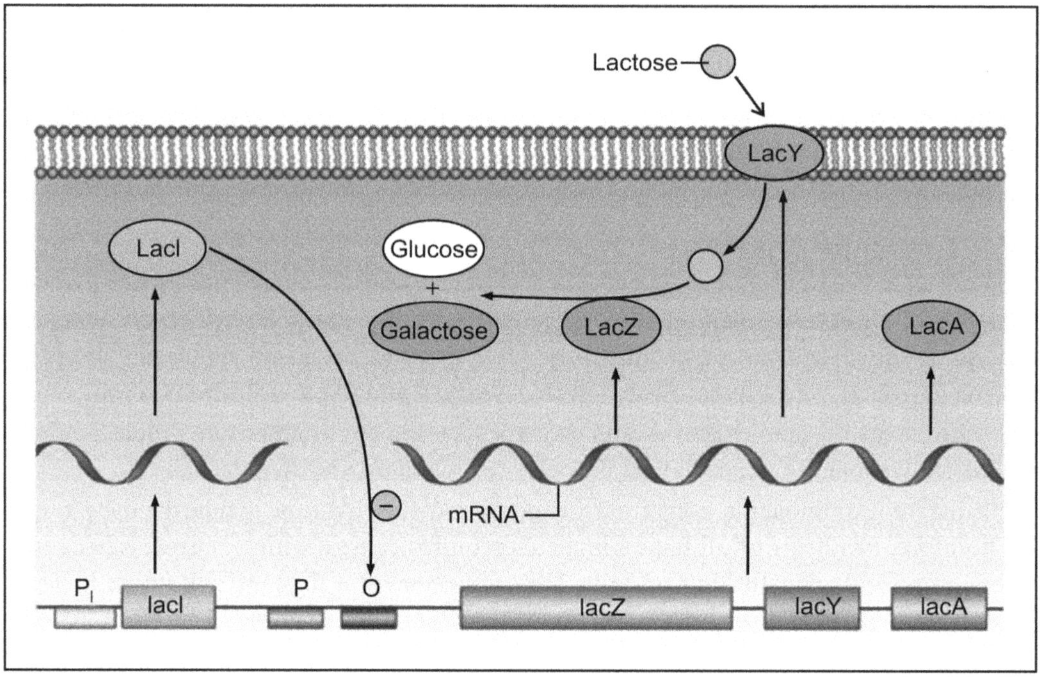

Fig. 6.13 Gene regulation by lac operon

The regulation of lacoperon of E.coil has the following:

(i) Structural genes: The lactose operon of *E.coil* is composed of three structural z, y and A. 'Z' gene transcribes mRNA for a single long polypeptide chain to form the enzyme b-glactosidase. This enzyme catalyses the hydrolysis of lactose in glucose and galctose. 'y' gene transcribes the mRNA that translates the permease protein. The enzyme permease facilitates the lactose to enter inside the bacterium.

'A' gene specifies the enzyme transcetylase.

(ii) **Operator gene:** Operator lies immediately left to the structural gene. When the operator is 'on', the structural gens can't function. Operator is the target for the attachment of repressor protein produced by the regulator gene. The base pairs in the operator region are palindrome i.e., show two fold symmetry from a point. The repressor proteins bind to the operator and form an operator-repressor complex which in turn physically blocks the transcription of z, y and A genes by preventing the release of RNA polymerase to begin transcription.

(iii) **The promoter gene:** The actual site of transcription initiation is known as promoter region. It is left the operator region. mRNA transcription by the RNA polymerase. This enzyme first along the operator region and structural genes, like operators the promoter region consists of palindromic sequence of nucleotides.

(iv) **The repressor (Regulator) gene:** The regulator gene transcribes the mRNA for the protein called repressor. This lac repressor regulates the expression of structural genes by binding the operator region. In the absence of lactose, repressor binds to the operator and blocks the path of RNA polymerase and presents the expression of structural genes.

6.7.1.1 Positive Regulation of the Lac Operon-Catabolic Control

Positive control of enzyme synthesis is said to occur when an association between a protein and a part of the regulatory region of an operon is essential for expression of related structural genes in the operon. Expression of the lac operon is inhibited when a more efficient source of energy, such as glucoses is present in the medium. The presence of glucose results in a decreased concentration of intracellular cyclic Amp. Cyclic Amp is necessary for the efficient expression of the lac operon since it activates the catabolite gene activator protein (Cap), which in turn activates transcription of lac mRNA by RNA polymerase at the promoter site.

Phenotypic Changes due to Environmental Alterations

Bacteria, like the cells of higher organisms, carry more genetic information-their genotype-than is utilized or expressed at any one time. The extent to which this information is expressed depends on the environment. A facultative anaerobic bacterium will produce different end products of metabolism, depending on the presence or absence of oxygen during growth. The presence or absence of oxygen determines which enzymes function and which donot. The outstanding feature of a phenotypic change due to environment is that it involves most of the cells in the culture. A phenotypic change of this type is not inherited: rather, it occurs when some condition of the environment changes. A return to the original phenotype occurs when the original environmental conditions are restored.

Genotypic changes: The genotype of a cell is determined by the genetic information contained in its chromosome. The chromosome is divided into genes.

- A gene is a functional unit of inheritance. It specifies the information of a particular polypeptide as well as various type of RNA.
- Each gene consists of hundreds of nucleotide pairs.
- Any gene is capable of changing or mutating to a different form so that it specifies information of an altered or new protein which may in turn change the characteristics of the cell.

For example, the substitution of even one aminoacid among several hundred in a polypeptide chain may cause the protein to be non functional.

- A mutation is a change in the nucleotide sequence of a gene. This gives rise to a new genetic trait, or a changed genotype.
- A cell or an organism which shows the effects of a mutation is called a mutant. Thus we occasionally see sudden changes in familiar plants and animals.
- In nature, mutations are rare events which occur at random and arise spontaneously with no regard to environmental conditions.

6.7.2 Tryptophan Operon

Operon is the coordinated unit of genetic expression in bacteria. The *trp* operon is an operon a group of genes that are used, or transcribed, together that codes for the components for production of tryptophan. The *trp* operon is present in many bacteria, but was first characterized in *Escherichia coli.* The operon is regulated so that when tryptophan is present in the environment, the genes for tryptophan synthesis are not expressed. It was an important experimental system for learning about gene regulation, and is commonly used to teach gene regulation.

- Tryptophan is an aromatic amino acid and is required for the synthesis of all proteins that contain tryptophan.
- The 20 common amino acids are required in large amounts for protein synthesis, and E.coil can synthesize all of them.
- The genes for the enzymes needed to synthesize a given amino acid are generally clustered in an operon and are expressed whenever existing supplies of that amino acid are inadequate for cellular requirements.
- When the amino acid is abundant, the biosynthetic enzymes are not needed and the operon is repressed.
- The *E.coil* tryptophan (trp) operon includes five genes for the enzymes required to convert chorismate to tryptophan.

- The five structural genes are [trp E, trp D, trp C, trp B, trp A] and the regulatory elements – primary promoter (trp p), operator (trp O), attenuator (trp a), secondary internal promoter (trp P_2) and terminator (trp t)
- The five structural genes of tryptophan operon code for three enzymes (two enzymes contain two different subunits) required for the synthesis of tryptophan from chorismate.
- The mRNA from the trp operon has a half-life of only about 3 min, allowing the cell to respond rapidly to changing needs for this amino acid.

6.7.2.1 Tryptophan Operon Regulation by a Repressor

- The trp repressor is a homo dimer, each subunit containing 107 amino acid residues.
- When tryptophan is abundant it binds to the Trp repressor, causing a conformational change that permits the repressor to bind to the trp operator and inhibit expression of the trp operon.
- The trp operator site overlaps the promoter, so binding of the repressor blocks binding of RNA polymerase.
- Once again, this simple on/off circuit mediated by a repressor is not the entire regulatory story. Different cellular concentrations of tryptophan can vary the rate of synthesis of the biosynthetic enzymes over a 700-fold range.

Attenuator as the second control site for tryptophan operon (Fig. 6.14)

- The trp operon attenuation mechanism uses signals encoded in four sequences within a 162 nucleotide leader region at the 5' end of the mRNA, preceding the initiation codon of the first gene.
- Within the leader lies a region known as the attenuator, made up of sequences 3 and 4. These sequences base-pair to form a G $\equiv$ C-rich stem-and-loop structure closely followed by a series of U residues.
- The Attenuator structure acts as transcription terminator.
- Sequence 2 is an alternative complement for sequence 3.
- If sequence 2 and 3 base pair, the attenuator structure cannot form and transcription continues into the trp biosynthetic genes, the loop formed by the pairing of sequences 2 and 3 does not obstruct transcription.
- Regulatory sequence 1 is crucial for the tryptophan sensitive mechanism that determines whether sequence 3 pairs with sequence 2 (allowing transcription to continue) or with sequence 4 (attenuating transcription).
- Formation of the attenuator stem-and loop structure depends on events that occur during translation of regulatory sequence 1, which encodes a leader peptide (so called because it is encoded by the leader region of the mRNA) of 14 amino acids, two of which are Trp residues.

- When Tryptophan concentrations are high, concentrations translation to proceed rapidly past the two Trp codons of sequence 1 and into sequence 2, before sequence 3 is synthesized by RNA polymerase.
- In this situation sequence 2 is covered by the ribosome and unavailable for pairing to sequence 3 when sequence 3 is synthesized; the attenuator structure (sequence 3 and 4) forms and transcription halts.
- When tryptophan concentrations are low, however, the ribosome stalls at the two Trp codons in sequence 1, because charged tRNA Trp is less available. Sequence 2 remains free while the sequence 3 is synthesized, allowing these two sequences to base-pair and permitting transcription to proceed.
- When tryptophan levels are high, the ribosome quickly translates sequence 1 (open reading frame encoding leader peptide) and blocks sequence 2 before sequence 3 is transcribed. Continued transcription leads to attenuation at the terminator-like-structure formed by sequences 3 and 4 incomplete.

When tryptophan levels are low, the ribosome pauses at the Trp codons in sequence 1. Formation of paired structure between sequences 2 and 3 prevents attenuation, because sequence 3 is no longer available to form the attenuator structure with sequence 4.

- Two polycistronic mRNAs are produced from tryptophan operon one derived from all the five structural genes and the other obtained from the last three genes.
- Besides acting as a core pressor to regulate trp operon, tryptophan can inhibit the activity of the enzyme anthranilate synthetase.

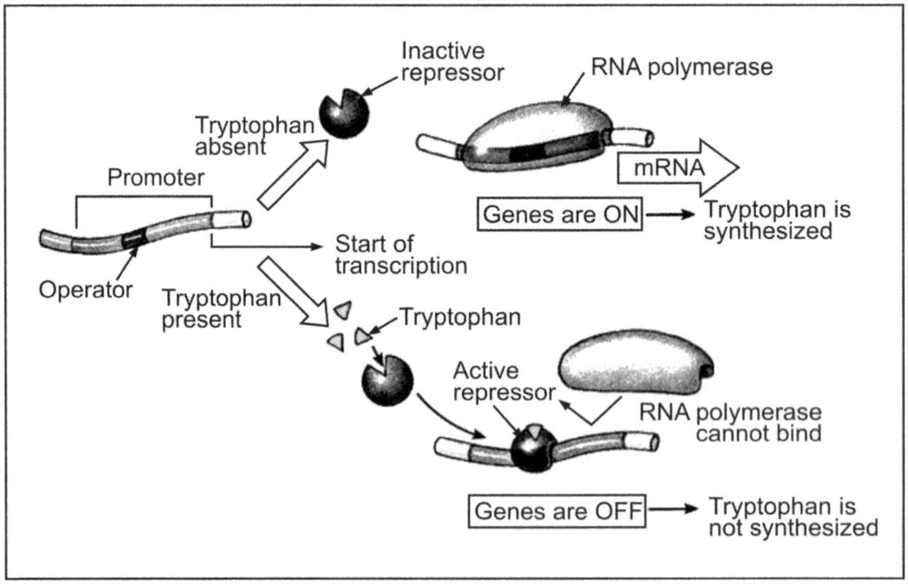

Fig. 6.14 Gene regulation by tryptophan operon

6.8 Phase Variation

Phase variation is defined as the random switching of phenotype at frequencies that are much higher (sometimes >1%) than classical mutation rates.

Phase variation contributes to virulence by generating heterogeneity; certain environmental or host pressures select those bacteria that express the best adapted phenotype

Phase variation is a method for dealing with rapidly varying environments without requiring random mutation employed by various types of bacteria, including *Salmonella* species.

It involves the variation of protein expression, frequently in an on-off fashion, within different parts of a bacterial population.

Although it has been most commonly studied in the context of immune evasion, it is observed in many other areas as well.

Salmonella use this technique to switch between different types of the protein flagellin. As a result, flagella with different structures are assembled.

Once an adaptive response has been mounted against one type of flagellin, or if a previous encounter has left the adaptive immune system ready to deal with one type of flagellin, switching types renders previously high affinity antibodies, TCRs and BCRs ineffective against the flagella.

The flagellar antigens of most ***salmonellae*** exist in one of two phases, phase 1 and phase 2.

Phase 1 antigen is more specific and is shared by a few species only and designated as a, b, c, d etc., upto z, and after z as z_1 z_2 z_3 up to z_{14}.

Phase 2 antigen is nonspecific or group phase and is shared by several unrelated species of *salmonellae.*

It is always necessary to identify antigenic factor of flagella in phase 1 and sometimes in phase 2 and for which a culture in the alternative phase has to be produced. This is done by passing the bacteria through a Craigie's tube, containing homologous phase antiserum incorporated in agar.

V→ w Variation

- The virulence of *Salmonella typhi* is associated with the presence of the Vi antigen

  Fresh isolates of *S.typhi* with Vi antigen are generally inaggulutinable by O – antiserum because Vi antigen completely masks the O antigen (**O antigen** (Ger. *ohne Hauch,* without film), the antigen that occurs in the bodies of bacteria).
- These are called v forms.
- The V forms are only agglutinable by Vi antiserum.
- Organisms lose their Vi antigen either partially or completely after repeated subculture in the laboratory.

- With partial loss of Vi antigen, *S .typhi* are agglutinable by both O and Vi antisera and these intermediate forms are called Vw forms.
- When there is complete loss of Vi antigen, the strain is agglutinable only by O – antiserum. These are called w form.

The Vi antigen of *S. paratyphi* and *S. Dublin* generally cannot completely mask the O antigen.

S-R Variation

The smooth to rough variation occurs due to mutation and is associated with

(a) Change of colonial morphology from smooth to rough.

(b) Loss of O antigen and virulence of the strain. It can be avoided by maintaining laboratory cultures in Dorset's egg medium or by lyophilisation.

- Only *Rickettsiae* show phase variation.
- The freshly isolated organisms are in phase I and on repeated passage on yolk sac they attain phase II.
- Unlike other *Rickettsial* species, *Coxiella burnetii* contain two distinct plasmids.

Essay Questions

1. Write a note bacterial genetics
2. Explain the features of spontaneous mutations
3. Write a note on isolation of mutants

Multiple Choice Questions

1. The transfer of DNA from donor call to recipient call through specialized sex pilus is called
   (a) Transduction
   (b) Transformation
   (c) conjugation
   (d) Transcription
2. Sickle cell anemia is an example of
   (a) Missense mutation
   (b) Nonsense mutation
   (c) Natuiral mutations
   (d) Point mutations
3. Which of the following belongs to Azridines class of chemical mutagens
   (a) Hydroxyl amine
   (b) Ethyleneimine
   (c) diepoxybutane
   (d) ethyleneimine
4. All eukaryotic organisms have which mode of the DNA replication
   (a) Theta mode (b) Linear mode
   (c) Sigma mode (d) Rolling mode
5. The Regulator Gene Transcribes the mRNA for the protein called
   (a) Repressor gene (b) Operator gene
   (c) Structural gene (d) Promoter gene

Answers

1. (c)	2. (a)	3. (d)
4. (b)	5. (a)	

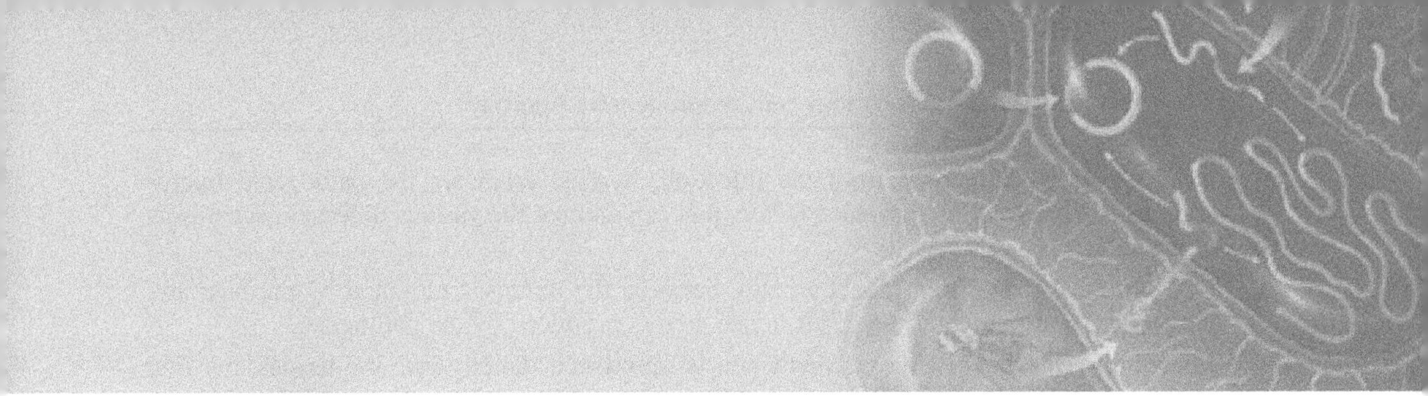

7 EPIDEMIOLOGY OF DISEASES

LEARNING OBJECTIVES

After studying the chapter the students familiarize themselves with concepts in:

- *Understanding the activity of various disease causing agents*
- *Understanding Epidemiology of various micro-organisms*
- *Delving an insight into various modes of pathogens actions*
- *Understanding various diagnostic procedures of the specific pathogens through various culture findings*
- *Identifying the various treatment strategies and prevention of the pathologic invasion of the microbes*

7.1 General Principles of Infection

Infectious diseases occur as a result of interaction between pathogenic microorganism and the host.

All the infectious diseases begin at some surface of the host whether it be the external surfaces such as the skin and conjunctiva or internal surfaces such as mucus membranes of the respiratory tract, intestine or urogenital tract.

In most infectious diseases the pathogenic microorganism penetrates the body surface and gains access to the internal tissues.

In some kind of infections, the pathogens may remain localized near its point of entry into the body and in other kinds; it may be transported to some other body site.

Some pathogens may cause generalized infections, in which microorganism becomes widely distributed and grows throughout the body and some are capable to grow within the cells of the host causing severe disruption of normal physiological processes.

In other infections the pathogen may grow extracellularly.

If a host is to recover from the infection, it must eradicate the pathogenic micro-organisms which exhibit virulence factors that can combat the various defense mechanisms of the host.

Thus, an infection represents a battle between the defenses mounted by the host and the particular armamentarium of virulence factors produced by the pathogens.

Microbial adherence: Unless a pathogen is introduced directly into the tissues, the first step of infection is usually adherence or attachment of the pathogen to some surface of host.

Moreover, the attachment is selective i.e., various pathogens attach only to certain tissues.

E.g.:

1. *Neisseria gonorrhoeae* cause gonorrhea adhering specifically to epithelial cell layer of human cervix, urethra and conjuctiva by means of pili and avoids being washed away by the flow of mucus or tears.
2. *E.coli* strains cause "scours" a diarrheal disease of new born pigs also possess pili that allow bacteria firmly to attach to the mucosal lining of the small intestine.
3. *Vibrio cholera* causes cholera adhering to the epithelial cells of the small intestine of the humans.

Certain proteins located on the outer surface of the bacterial cell wall have been shown to be essential for the initiation of infections.

E.g.: Streptococcus pyogenes causes streptococcal sore throat attaches specifically to the epithelial cells of throat by means of cell wall proteins called M proteins.

Table 7.1 Types of Infections

Term	Definition	Example
Acute	Has a short duration and relatively severe course	*Streptococcal pharyngitis*
Chronic	Has a long duration	TB
Fulminating	Occurs suddenly and with severe intensity	Cerebrospinal meningitis caused by *N.meningitidis*
Localized	Restricted to a limited area of the body	Urinary tract infection caused by *E.Coli*
Generalized	Affects many or all parts of the body	Blood infections such as typhoid fever
Mixed or polymicrobial	More than one kind of micro- organism contributes to the infection.	Gas gangrene, in which a combination of *clostridium* species may occur.
Primary	An initial localized infection that decreases resistance and thus paves intrusion by the same microorganism or other organism.	Viral influenza
Secondary	Infection that is established after a primary infection has caused a decreased resistance	*Pneumococcal pneumonia* following viral influenza.

7.1.1 Transmission of Diseases

The causative agents of disease can be transmitted from the reservoir of infection to a susceptible host by *three methods*

1. Contact Transmission of Disease
2. Vehicle Transmission of Disease
3. Vectors Transmission of Disease

7.1.2 Contact Transmission of Disease

- Spread of an infectious agent by person to person contact
- They are of three types:
  - (i) Direct contact transmission
  - (ii) In Direct contact transmission
  - (iii) Droplet transmission

(i) Direct contact transmission or person-to-person transmission: Close or intimate contacts that results in the spread of infectious agents or direct contact transmission refers to close contact that results in exposure to skin and body secretions no intermediate object is involved.

The most common forms of direct contact transmission are touching, kissing and sexual intercourse. Among the disease that can be transmitted by direct contact are viral respiratory tract disease, staphylococcal infections, hepatitis-A, measles, scarlet fever and sexually transmitted diseases (syphilis, gonorrhea and genital herpes)

Direct contact is also one way of spreading AIDS and infectious mononucleosis.

Potential pathogens can also be transmitted by direct contact from animals or animal products to humans

e.g.: Rabies and Anthrax.

(ii) Indirect contact transmissions: When the agent of disease is transmitted from its reservoir to a susceptible host by means of a nonliving object.

The general term for any nonliving object involved in the spread of infection is a fomites.

e.g., Handkerchiefs, towels, bedding, diapers, drinking cups, togs, moneys and thermosters.

- Contaminated syringes, serve as fomites in the transmission of AIDS and hepatitis.

(iii) **Droplet transmission:** Transmission of infectious agents in droplets from respiratory secretions by coughing, sneezing or talking, is another form of contact transmission. They travel less than meter from the reservoir to host.

In one sneeze, 20,000 droplets may be produced.

The best examples are tuberculosis influenza, pneumonia and pertussis (whooping cough).

7.1.3 Vehicle Transmission of Disease

The transmission of a pathogen by an inanimate reservoir or transmission of disease agents by a medium, such as water, food or air; other media include blood and other body fluids, drugs and intravenous fluids.

- Water borne transmission: Pathogens are usually spread by water contaminated within treated or poorly treated sewage. Diseases transmitted via this route include cholera, waterborne shigellosis and leptospirosis.

Food borne transmission: Pathogens are generally transmitted in food that are incompletely cooked, poorly refrigerated or prepared under unsanitary conditions.

Food borne pathogens cause disease such as food poisoning and tape worm infestation.

Airborne transmission: To the spread of agents of infection by droplet nuclei in dust that travel more than 1 meter from the reservoir to the host.

For example microbes are spread by droplets, which may be discharged in a fine spray from the mouth and nose during coughing and sneezing.

These droplets are small enough to remain airborne for prolonged periods.

The viruses that cause measles and the bacterium that causes tuberculosis can be transmitted through airborne droplets. Dust particles can harbor various pathogens. *Staphylococci* and *streptococci* can survive on dust and be transmitted by the air borne route.

Spores produced by certain fungi are also transmitted by the airborne route and can cause such disease as "histoplasmosis", "coccidioidomycosis" and "blastomycosis".

7.1.4 Vectors Transmission of Disease

An arthropod can carry disease-causing organism from one host to another. Animals also can carry pathogens from one host to another.

Arthropod vectors transmit diseases by 2 general methods.

A. Mechanical transmission B. Biological transmission

7.1.4.1 Mechanical Transmission

It is the passive transport of the pathogens on the insect's feet or the body parts.

If the insect makes contact with a host's food, pathogens can be transferred to the food and later swallowed by the host.

e.g.: House lice, for instance, can transfer the pathogens typhoid fever.

7.1.4.2 Biological Transmission

It is an active process and is more complex.

The arthropod bites an infected person or animal and ingests some of the infected blood.

The pathogens then reproduce in the vector and the increase in the number of pathogens increase the possibility that they will be transmitted to another host.

Some parasites reproduce in the gut of the arthropod; this can be passed with feces. If the arthropod defecates or vomits while biting a potentials host, the parasite can enter the wound.

Other parasites reproduce in the vectors gut and migrate to the salivary gland; these are directly infected into bile. Some protozoa and helminthic parasites use the vector as a host for a developmental stage in their life cycle.

7.2 Carrier, Vectors, Reservoirs

Carrier

The commonest source of infection for humans is humans themselves. The parasite may originate from a patient or a carrier. A carrier is a person who harbors the pathogenic microorganism without suffering from only ill effect because of it. Definitions of some important carriers:

Healthy carrier is one who harbors the pathogens but who displays no symptoms of the disease and capable of transmitting the pathogens, while

Convalescent carrier is one who has recovered the pathogen in his body but still capable of transmitting the pathogens to others.

Temporary carrier state lasts less than six months.

Chronic carrier may last for several years and sometimes even for the rest of one's life.

Paradoxical carrier refers to a carrier who acquires the pathogen from another carrier.

Reservoirs

Many pathogens are able to infect both human beings and animals. Animals may, therefore act as sources of human infection. Such animals serve to maintain the parasite in nature and act as the reservoirs of human infections. They are therefore called reservior hosts. Infectious diseases transmitted from animals to human beings are called zoonoses. Zoonotic diseases may be bacterial (plague from rats), viral (Rabies from dogs) proto zoal (toxo plasmosis from cats), helminthic (hydatid disease from dogs) and fungi (zoophilic dermatophytes from cats and dogs).

Vectors

Blood sucking insects transmit pathogens to human beings. The diseases so caused are called arthropod borne disease. Insects such as mosquitoes, ticks, mites, flies, fleas and lice that transmit infections are called "vectors". Such vectors are called mechanical vectors in other instances; the pathogen multiplies in the body of the vector, often undergoing part of its development at cycle in it. Such vectors are termed biological vectors. The interval between the times of entry of pathogen into the vector in the vector becoming infective is called the extrinsic incubation period.

Besides acting as vectors, some insects may also act as reservoir hosts. Infection is maintained in such insects by transovarial (certain arthropod vectors they transmit disease-causing bacteria from parent arthropod to offspring arthropod) or transstadial passage (passage of a microbial parasite, such as a virus or rickettsia, from one developmental stage (stadium) of the host to its subsequent stage or stages, particularly as seen in mites).

Arthropod Vectors

Some disease producing organisms are transmitted by insects (*e.g.*, Flies and Mosquitoes) and other arthropods (*e.g.*, Flexs and Ticks).

In certain cases the vectors simply act as accidental carriers of the organisms from filth to food or to the human host. In this way, plague and typhoid fever are transferred by fleas and house-flies respectively.

In other cases, the micro-organisms are transmitted by blood-sucking arthropods and spend part of their life cycle in the vector.

E.g., Transmission of malaria by Anopheles mosquito

Transmission of yellow fever by *Aedes albopictus* mosquito,

Sleeping sickness by the tsetse fly and

Murine typhus by rat fly

7.3 Microbial Attack

Many of the properties contributing to microbial pathogenicity and virulence are unclear or unknown, but if the microbe over powers the host defenses, disease results. To cause disease, most pathogens must gain access to the host adhere, to host tissues, penetrate or evade host defenses and damage the host tissues. However some microbes cause disease by accumulations of microbial waste products but not by direct damage of host tissue.

When micro-organisms invade the body and cause damage to the tissues, infection is said to have occurred. Diseases produced by micro-organisms are called infectious diseases.

(i) Physical contact with a diseased person or animal: As the casual organisms have only a brief existence outside the human body; venereal diseases are almost contracted in this way.

e.g., Rabies is transferred to man through the bite of an infected dog.

Strict precautions are essential for the protection of hospital medical staff, who are at particular risk when treating patients with infectious diseases.

(ii) Droplet infection: Coughing, sneezing and even quiet talking may cause expulsion from the respiratory tract few fine droplets containing micro-organisms which may be inhaled by individuals nearby.

It is by above mechanism that respiratory diseases are often transmitted. *e.g.*, whooping cough, influenza.

(iii) Dust-borne infection: Some disease producing bacteria remain alive for long period in the dried condition and contaminated dust stirred up by cleaning processes may infect wounds or be inhaled.

e.g., Mycobacterium tuberculosis.

(iv) Contact with contaminated articles: Clothes, bedding, hand kerchiefs, towels, toys and other items recently contaminated by a diseased person are sources of infection, either through contact or via the microbe laden particles discharged from them into air by movement.

(v) Hand infection: The hands are a major potential means by which micro-organisms from saliva, nasal mucus, skin infection and even feces are transmitted to other individuals and food.

7.3.1 Entry of Micro-organisms

Portals of Entry: The portals of entry for pathogens are mucous membrane, skin and direct deposition beneath the skin or membranes (parenteral route).

(i) **Mucous membranes:** Many bacteria and viruses gain access to the body by penetrating mucous membranes lining the respiratory tract, genitourinary tract and conjunctiva.

Diseases that are commonly contracted via respiratory tract include the common cold, pneumonia, tuberculosis, influenza, measles and small pox.

Most micro organisms can gain access to the gastrointestinal tract in food and water via contaminated finger. Most micro-organisms that enter the body in these ways are destroyed by hydrochloric acid (HCl) and enzymes in the stomach or by bile and enzymes in the small intestine. Those that survive can cause disease. Microbes in the GIT can cause poliomyelitis, hepatitis A, typhoid fever, amoebic dysentery, giardiasis, shigellosis (bacillary dysentery) and cholera. These pathogens are then eliminated with feces and can be transmitted to other hosts via contaminated water, food or fingers.

The genitourinary tract is a portal of entry for pathogens that are contacted sexually. Some microbes may penetrate an unbroken mucous membrane; others require a cut or abrasion of some type.

Examples: HIV, genital warts, Chlamydia, herpes, syphilis, and gonorrhea.

(ii) **Skin:** The skin is one of the largest organs of the body in terms of surface area and offers important defense against disease. Unbroken skin is impenetrable by most micro organisms. Some micro organisms gain access to the body through openings in the skin, such as hair follicles and sweat gland ducts. Some fungi grow on the keratin in skin or infect the skin itself.

(iii) **The parenteral route:** Other micro-organisms gain access to the body when they are deposited directly into the tissue beneath the skin or into mucous membranes when these barriers are penetrated or injured.

This route is called the parenteral route. Punctures injections, bites, cuts, wounds, surgery and splitting due to swelling or drying can all establish parenteral routes. HIV, the hepatitis viruses and bacteria that cause tetanus and gangrene can be transmitted parenterally.

(iv) **The preferred portal of entry:** Many pathogens have a preferred portal of entry that is a prerequisite to their being able to cause disease. If they gain access to the body by another portal, disease might not occur. For example, the bacteria of typhoid fever, *Salmonella typhi*, produce all the signs and symptoms of the diseases when swallowed (preferred route), but, if the same bacteria are rubbed on the skin (or only a slight inflammation) occurs. Some pathogens can initiate disease from more than one portal of entry. *e.g.*, *Yersinia pestis* (Plague), *Bacillus anthracis* (anthrax).

(v) **Numbers of invading micro-organisms:** If only a few microbes enter the body, they will probably overcome by the host's defenses. However if large numbers of microbes gain entry, the stage is probably set for disease. Thus, the likelihood of disease increases as the number of pathogens increases.

(vi) Adherence: The first step in initiation of infection is usually adherence or attachment of the pathogen to some surface of the host. The attachment between pathogen and host is accomplished by means of surface molecules on the pathogen called adhesins or ligands that bind specifically to complementary surface receptors on the cells of certain host tissues. Adhesins may be located on a microbe's glycocalyx or on other microbial surface structures, such as pili/fimbriae and flagella.

The majority of adhesins on the micro-organisms studied so far are glycoproteins or lipoproteins. The receptors on host cells are typically sugars, such as mannose.

Nisseria gonorrhea, the causative agent of gonorrhea, adheres specifically to the epithelial cell layer of the human cervix, urethra and conjunctiva by means of pili and thus avoids being washed away by the flow of mucus or tears.

Escherichia also possess pili that allow the bacteria to attach firmly to the mucosal lining of the small intestine, *Vibrio cholera* adheres to the epithelial layer of the small intestine of humans.

Streptococcus pyogenes, the causative agent of streptococcal sore throat, attaches specifically to the epithelial cells of the throat by means of cell wall proteins called M proteins.

Treponema palladium, the causative agent of syphilis uses its tapered end as a hook to attach to host cells.

(vii) Adherence of viruses: The surface of influenza virus particles is studded with hemagglutinin spikes that can cause attachment of the viruses to specific muco protein receptors on the surface of host cells.

Epithelial: Polio virus attach to lipid and glycoprotein containing receptors on host cells of intestinal tract and central nervous system and subsequent infection of the latter can lead to paralysis.

Attachment by degrading protective mucus layers of mucous membranes and allowing viral attachment to the underlying epithelial cell is with the help of neuraminidase spikes of virion.

(viii) Penetrate host defenses: Although some pathogens can cause damage on the surface of tissues, most must penetrate tissues to cause disease. The following are factors that contribute to the ability of bacteria to invade a host.

(a) Capsules: Some bacteria make glycocalyx material that forms capsules around their cell walls; this property increases the virulence of the species. The capsule resists the host's defenses by impairing phagocytosis. The chemical nature of the capsule appears to prevent the phagocytic cell from adhering to the bacterium.

Examples of capsulated bacteria:

Streptococcus pneumoniae	-	Pneumococcal pneumonia
Klesbiella pneumoniae	-	Pneumonia

Haemophilus influenzae	-	Pneumonia and meningitis (children)
Bacillus anthracis	-	Anthrax
Yersinia pestis	-	Plague

Capsules are not the only cause of virulence. Many non-pathogenic bacteria produce capsules and the virulence of some pathogens is not related to the presence of a capsule.

(b) **Cell wall Components:** Chemical constituents of the cell walls contribute to virulence.

Name of the organism	Chemical substance	Available	Mechanisms
Streptococcus pyogenes	M-protein Heat resistant and acid resistant protein	Cell surface and fimbriae	Mediates attachment of the bacterium to epithelial cells of the host and helps bacterium resist phagocytosis by WBC
Nisseria gonorrhoeae	Opa protein	Outer membrane	Following attachment by both Opa and fimbriae, the host cell takes in the bacteria
M.tuberculosis	Waxy lipid (mycolic acid)	Cell wall	Resisting digestion by phagocytes

7.4 Events in Infection following Penetration

(i) **Growth in underlying tissues:** Whether the means of penetration of a body surface by a microorganism is passive (any mechanically caused breach in the body surfaces can introduce pathogens directly into the underlying tissue) or active (pathogen own mechanism of adherence and penetration), the microbes multiply, resist the defense mechanisms of the host and begins to cause tissue damage.

In some infections the micro-organisms may simply grow in the tissue in which it finds itself, causing localized infections.

e.g,: Abscess caused by *Staphylococcus aureus* a swollen area of cavity in the tissue containing the *Staphylococci*, numerous white blood cells (that collectively form a pasty mass called pus) and dead disintegrating tissue cells that have been killed by the toxins elaborated from the *Staphylococci*.

In other infections the organism may not remain localized but may spread through the tissues. An example is the anaerobic bacterium *Clostridium perfringens* which cause the wound infection gas gangrene. Initiation of gas gangrene depends on the occurrence of anaerobic conditions in the wound, as occurs in crushed tissue of clotted blood. As *C. perfringens* begins to grow, the bacteria releases toxins that kill some of the surrounding healthy tissue. By this means the *clostridia* can quickly invade the entire length of a muscle. Amputation of an effected limb is often the only way to stop the spread of *C. perfringens* to the rest of the body.

(ii) Infection of the lymphatic system: Many pathogenic micro-organisms can spread from the initial site of infection to the lymphatic system. It leads to a bacterium and generalized infection. The organisms may then pass via the lymphatic vessels to a regional lymph mode, there they multiply and then pass to the thoracic duct, which empties lymph into the venous blood circulation via the subclavian vein. Thus the organisms reach the heart and ultimately are eventually distributed throughout the body.

e.g., Erysipelas, an inflammatory disease of the skin caused by *S. pyogenes*

Bubonic plague (lymph node become inflamed enlarged and sore when infected called bubo).

(iii) Infection of the blood: From the initial site of entry into the body by passive or active means, a pathogenic microorganism may be able to enter a blood capillary or venule and thereby gain direct access to the blood vascular system, causing a bacteremia (presence of bacteria in the blood). Once in the blood stream the organism can be carried to various parts of the body and cause localized infections.

e.g., *Neisseria meningitidis* present in the nosopharynx can reach the meninges (membranes that cover the brain and spinal cord) by means of a transient bacteremia and can thereby cause severe meningitis. *Spirochetes* of the green *leptospira* can reach the kidneys where they may eventually cause acute renal failure.

7.5 Different Diseases

7.5.1 Amoebiasis

Amoebiasis (Fig. 7.1) refers to infection caused by the amoeba *Entamoeba histolytica* which belongs to sarcodina group of protozoans which is a monogenetic organisms i.e., require only one host to complete the life cycle. Hence, it chooses humans as a definite host.

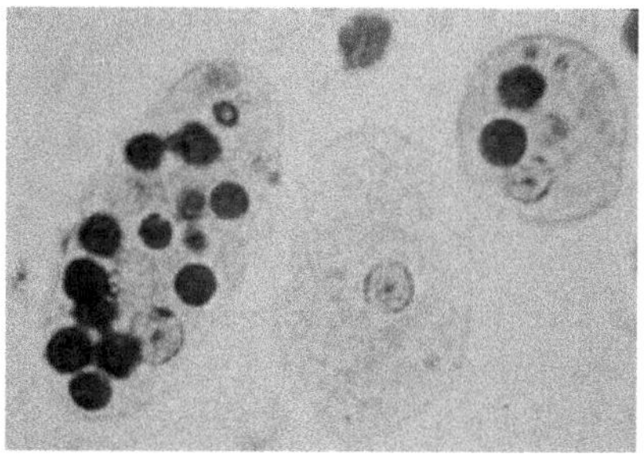

Fig. 7.1 Slide of amoebiasis infection

Morphology: It exists in three forms:

1. Trophozoite or magna form
2. Precystic or minuta form
3. Cystic form

1. **Trophozoite or magna form:** It is the most active motile and freely formed form which is pathogenic to human beings & seen in mucous and submucous layers of the large intestine of humans. The cytoplasm is differentiated into outer clear and non-granular ectoplasm and the central fluid granular endoplasm shown in Fig. 7.3.
2. **Pre cystic form:** It is a small spherical non motile and non feeding form which shows +ve absence of food vacuole irrespective of tropozoid form. Pre cystic form lives in the lumen of large intestine which is a non-pathogenic stage to man. But when the resistance of host's body is low it changes into magna form and invades the tissues of intestine.
3. **Cystic form:** Minute form undergoes encystation which becomes spherical surrounded by a highly resistant and refractive cyst wall. It contains one or two glycogen masses which will be acting as reserved food materials. It also contains chromatoid bodies which are made up of ribonucleo protein and the nucleus retains the characters of the trophozoite stage.

   Cyst is uninucleate where its nucleus is divided to form a binucleate and finally to tetranucleate or quadranucleate cyst shown in Fig. 7.2.

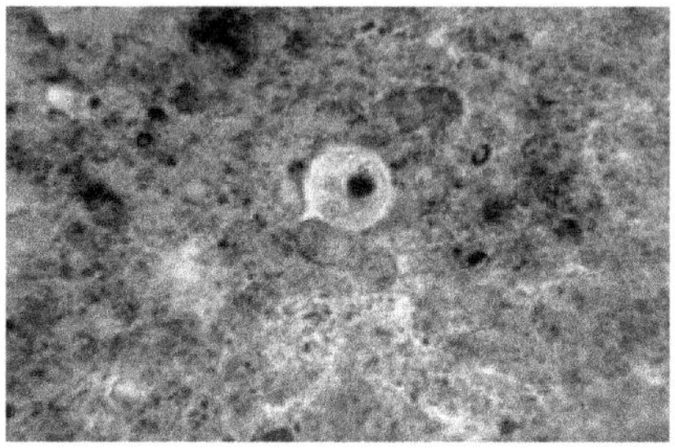

Fig. 7.2 Cystic forms of amoebiasis

Translation and Development

The parasite spreads through the contaminated water or food. The normal level of chlorine does not kill the amoeba. The cysts are not affected by the acid of stomach i.e HCl. Only the vegetative cells are destroyed. On the epithelial cell of the wall of large intestine the vegetative cells multiply. This results in severe dysentery where the faeces contain mucus and blood.

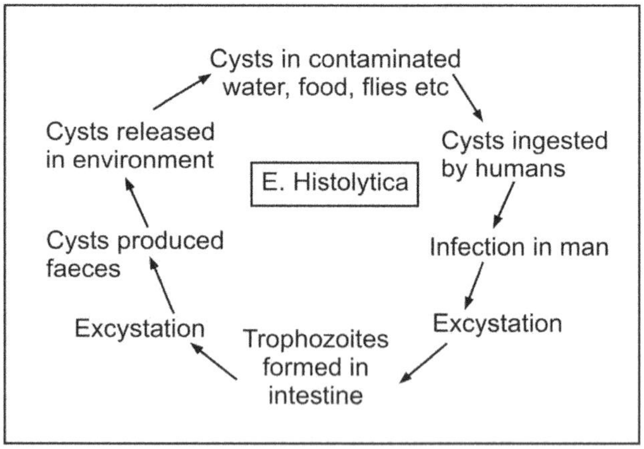

The pathogen feeds upon RBCs and damages the tissue of gastrointestinal tract. During severe cases, amoebae may enter the tissues of vital organs and cause abscess in liver, lungs, intestinal wall. The intestinal wall becomes perforated. The pathogen is identified by observing the amoebae in faeces and RBCs in trophozoites.

Clinical Features and Pathogenicity

The organism multiply by binary fission and spread radically outwards to form a flask shaped ulcers containing cellular debris, lymphocytes, blood corpuscles and bacteria. This causes the formation of abscesses in intestinal wall which further causes dissolution and necrosis of tissues by proteolytic enzymes "*Histolyne*" secreted by trophozoites.

As submucous layer is ruptured, ulcers burst with rupturing of blood capillaries which cause a condition called "Dysentery". "Amoebic dysentery" is characterized by intestinal inflammation, fever and loss of blood and mucous in fecal matter. If not treated well, trophozoites invades the liver, lungs and finally to brain resulting in the formation of abscesses.

The effected liver becomes enlarged which is called as "Amoebic hepatitis".

Diagnosis of human illness

- Asymptomatic human infections are usually diagnosed by finding cysts shed in the stool.
- In symptomatic infections, the motile form (the trophozoite) can often be seen in fresh feces.
- Serological tests are useful in detecting infection by *E. histolytica* if the organism goes extra-intestinal and in excluding the organism from the diagnosis of other disorders.
- Demonstration of Antibodies in the blood using ELISA test.

Treatment

- *E. histolytica* infections occur in both the intestine and in tissue of the intestine and/or liver.
- As a result, two different classes of drugs are needed to treat the infection, one for each location.
- Metronidazole or a related drug such as Tinidazole, Ornidazole, is used to destroy amoebae that have invaded tissue. These are rapidly absorbed into the blood stream and transported to the site of infection.
- Effective chemotherapeutic drugs are Metronidazole and Iodoquinol.

Prevention

- Protection of food by proper covering
- Purification of drinking water
- Proper disposal of sewage
- Following hygienic habits

7.5.2 Influenza (Viral Disease)

Influenza, commonly known as the **flu**, is an infectious disease that affects birds and mammals caused by RNA viruses of the family *Orthomyxoviridae*. The name influenza comes from the Italian word ***influenza*** which means "influence".

Symptoms: In humans, common symptoms of the disease are chills, fever, pharyngitis, muscle pains, severe headache, coughing, weakness and general discomfort.

- In more serious cases, influenza causes pneumonia.
- Influenza can produce nausea and vomiting especially in children.

Mode of Transmission: Influenza is transmitted from infected mammals through the air by coughs or sneezes, from infected birds through their droppings.

- Influenza can also be transmitted by saliva, nasal secretions, feces and blood.
- Infections also occur through contact with these body fluids or with contaminated surfaces.

Types of Influenza Virus

The influenza virus is an RNA virus of the family *Orthomyxoviridae*, which comprises five genera.

- Influenza virus A
- Influenza virus B
- Influenza virus C
- Isa virus
- Thogoto virus

Influenza Virus A

- Wild aquatic birds are the natural hosts for a large variety of influenza A.
- The type A viruses are the most virulent human pathogens among the three influenza types and cause the most severe disease.

Influenza Virus B: Influenza B virus almost exclusively infects human and is less common than influenza A.

The only animal known to be susceptible to influenza B infection is the seal.

Influenza Virus C: This virus generally infects humans, pigs and can cause severe illness and local epidemics.

It can cause mild diseases in children.

Prevention

Vaccination: Vaccination against influenza with an influenza vaccine is recommended for high-risk groups such as children and the elderly, or in people with asthma, diabetes or heart disease.

The most common method to produce influenza vaccine is by growing the virus in fertilized hen eggs. After purification, the virus is inactivated to produce an inactivated-virus vaccine.

Due to high mutation rate of the virus, a particular influenza vaccine usually confers protection for only a few years.

Infection Control

- Good personal health.
- Hygienic habits like hand washing etc.
- It is advisable for the people to cover their mouths while sneezing and to wash their hands regularly.

Alcohol is an effective sanitizer against influenza viruses, while 4° ammonium compounds can be used with alcohol to increase the duration of the sanitizing action.

Treatment

- People with flu are advised to drink plenty of liquids, take rest and avoid using alcohol, tobacco etc.
- Medications such as paracetamol is advised because it relieves the fever and muscle aches associated with the flu.
- Children and teenagers with flu symptoms should avoid taking aspirin during an influenza infection because it can lead to Reye's syndrome, a disease related to the liver.

Two Classes of Antiviral

1. **Neuraminidase inhibitors:** Antiviral drugs such as Oseltamivir and Zanamivir are neuraminidase inhibitors. These drugs are often effective against both Influenza A and B.
2. **M_2 Inhibitors (Adamantanes):** The antiviral drugs such as Amantadine and Rimantadine block a viral ion channel (m_2 protein) and prevent the virus from infecting cells. These drugs are ineffective against influenza B.

7.5.2.1 Human Swine Flu

Human swine flu is a highly contagious respiratory disease caused by a new strain of influenza virus. Symptoms of human swine flu include a fever (temperature over 38 °C), cough, sore throat, aches and tiredness. Human swine flu is also known as human swine influenza, influenza A (H_1N_1) virus or H1N1 influenza 09. The name 'swine flu' comes from a strain of the virus that is found in pigs. In 2009, a new strain of the swine flu virus that affects humans was identified. Cases of human swine flu have been confirmed in countries throughout the world.

Symptoms

The symptoms of human swine flu usually cause short-term illness similar to seasonal flu. Symptoms may include: High temperature, Cough, Sore throat, Body aches, Running nose, Headache, Chills, Fatigue, Diarrhea and vomiting (on occasions).

How the human swine flu virus is spread

The ways in which human swine flu can spread include:

- A person infected with human swine flu is contagious as long as they are showing symptoms and for upto three days from the start of antiviral treatment. Young children may be infectious for longer periods.
- A person caring for someone sick with human swine flu can become infected from inhaling infected sneeze or cough droplets. This is known as direct contact.
- The human swine flu virus can live for about two hours outside of the body. Infection can occur when a person touches a contaminated object (such as a dirty tissue) and then touches his or her own nose, eyes or mouth. This is known as indirect contact.
- In some cases, human swine flu is asymptomatic, which means the infected person feels fine and has no symptoms. However, they can still infect other people.

Pig farmers can be infected directly from infected pigs – for example, by handling sick pigs and not washing their hands. The swine flu virus is not spread through food products. It is safe to eat pork, bacon and ham. Eating properly handled and cooked pork and other pork products is safe.

Diagnosis methods may include

- Medical history
- Travel history
- Physical examination
- Nose and throat swabs (for laboratory analysis).

Self-care instructions for a person with human swine flu are the same as for seasonal flu:

- Drink plenty of fluids.
- Stay at home and get plenty of rest.

Treatment – Medication

An antiviral medication such as Oseltamivir (Tamiflu) can prevent the influenza virus from spreading inside your body, if started within 48 hours of the first symptoms. This may reduce the severity of symptoms and the time taken to recover from illness. Tamiflu can also be taken as a preventative measure if you have been in close contact with someone who is confirmed as having human swine flu (for example, if you share a house). Avoid unnecessary medication

Human swine flu vaccine: People from high risk groups are especially encouraged to have the human swine flu vaccine. These include:

- Pregnant women
- People with chronic health conditions such as asthma, heart and lung disease, cancer, obesity, diabetes, kidney disease, neurological disease and people with suppressed immune systems
- Children in special schools
- Healthcare workers
- Indigenous people
- Parents and guardians of infants under six months old.

7.5.3 Diphtheria (Bacterial Disease)

Diphtheria is a serious air-borne contagious disease caused by *Corynebacterium diphtheria* which is a gram+ve bacterium. It is an upper respiratory tract illness characterized by sore throat, low fever and an adherent membrane (a pseudo membrane) on the tonsils, pharynx.

Symptoms

- Fatigue, fever, a mild sore throat
- Children infected have symptoms that include nausea, vomiting, chills and a high fever. Patients experience neck swelling referred to as bull neck.

Mode of Transmission

- Transmitted by inhaling the respiratory droplets from an infected person.
- Transmitted through infected skin lesion.

Diagnosis

Diphtheria is diagnosed by culturing the bacterium and observation of pseudo membrane in throat. The bacteria produces dipheria toxin which is an exotoxin that causes an inflammation and grayish pseudo membrane on respiratory mucosa.

On physical examination one can observe characteristic grey membrane (pseudo membrane) in throat, swelling of neck or larynx.

Treatment

- Patients with severe cases should be given a diphtheria antitoxin. [Prepared from horse serum)
- Antibiotics are used in patients or carriers to eradicate *C. diphtheria* and prevent its transmission to others
- Antibiotics like Erythromycin, Procaine penicillin-G are used. Patients with allergies to Penicillin-G or Erythromycin can use Rifampicin or Clindamycin.

Prevention

- Diet should be given in the form of liquid to avoid inconvenience in swallowing.
- Schick test measures the level of immune system of a person to the infection of diphtheria.
- Active immunization with DPT vaccine.
- Measures should be taken to completely disinfect the patient's surroundings.

7.5.4 Infective Hepatitis

An acute but benign form of viral hepatitis caused by an RNA virus that does not persist in the blood serum and is usually transmitted by ingesting food or drink that is contaminated with fecal matter.

- The term viral hepatitis refers to a primary infection of the liver by any one of a heterogeneous group of "Hepatitis virus" which currently consists of type A, B, C, D, E and G.

Hepatitis A Virus (HAV): HAV is the only human *hepatitis virus* which can be cultivated *in vitro*. It has also been cloned. HAV is resistant to inactivation by heat at 60 °C for 1 hour, ether and acid at pH 2.0. HAV is a 27 nm non enveloped RNA virus belonging to picoma virus family. It was originally designated as 'Interovirus 72'. Hepatitis A (formerly known as infectious hepatitis) is a liver disease caused by the hepatitis A virus.

Mode of Transmission

The hepatitis A virus enters the body through the mouth and is passed in the stool (feces). The virus can then be carried on an infected persons hand and can be spread by direct contact, or by consuming food or drink that has been handled by the individual.

- It can be spread by drinking water that has been contaminated with improperly treated sewage.

- The virus multiplies in the intestinal epithelium and reaches the liver by hematogenous spread.

Symptoms

- Fatigue
- Poor appetite, fever and vomiting.
- Some people may develop jaundice.

Symptoms appear two to six weeks after exposure, but usually within three to four weeks.

Lab Diagnosis

- Diagnosis is usually detection of antibody.
- The virus can be visualized by IFM in fecal extracts.
- IgM Ab-HAV-Ab appears during the late incubation period.
- ELISA test is done for the detection of IgM and IgG antibodies.

Treatment

There are no special medicines or antibiotics that can be used to treat a person once the symptoms appear. Generally, bed rest and not drinking alcoholic beverages are recommended.

Prevention

- Improved sanitary practices
- Prevention of fecal contamination of food and water
- A medicine called gamma globulin or the hepatitis A vaccine is recommended.
- Hepatitis A vaccine is also used to stop the spread of infection.

7.5.5 Hepatitis B Virus (HBV)

It is also known as serum hepatitis. It is caused by hepatitis B virus. HBV is a 42 nm DNA virus with an outer envelope and a inner core, 27 nm in diameter, enclosing the viral genome and a DNA Polymerase.

- HBV is assigned to a separate family '*Hepana viridae*' because of its unique features.

Mode of Transmission

Hepatitis B is transmitted through:

- Contaminated needles and syringes

- By blood transfusion
- It is also transmitted through placenta and through sexual contact.

Clinical Features

- The incubation period is about 1-6 months.
- Hepatitis B infection is more harmful than Hepatitis A infection.
- Hepatitis B infection can lead to liver cancer.
- Extrahepatic complications like arthralgia, glomerulonephritis may occur.
- About 90-95% of adults with acute hepatitis B infection recover in 1-2 months of onset and eliminate the virus from the body within 6 months
- Mortality is about 0.5-2% but may be more in post-transfusion cases.

Pathogenesis

The pathogenesis of hepatitis appears to be immune mediated. Hepatocytes carry viral Ag dependent cell and cytotoxic T-cell attack. In the absence of adequate immune response, HBV infection may not cause hepatitis but may lead to carrier state. Therefore infants and immuno deficient persons are more likely to become a symptomatic carriers following infection.

Under the electron microscope sera from type B hepatitis patients show three types of particles. The most abundant form is a "Spherical particle", 22 nm in diameter.

- The second type of particle is filamentous or tubular with a diameter of 22 nm and of varying length.
- These two particles are antigenically identical and are surface components of HBV which are produced in great excess.
- The third type of particle is a double walled spherical structure, 42 nm in diameter. It is also known as "Dane particle" as it was first described by Dane.
- The envelope proteins expressed on the surface of the virion and the surplus 22 nm diameter, spherical and filamentous particle constitute the hepatitis B surface Ag.

HBS Ag consist of two major polypeptide one of which is glycolysated.

Resistance

- HBV is relatively heat stable virus. It remains viable at room temperature for long periods.
- Heating at 60 °C for 10 hours reduces infectivity by 100-1000 fold.
- It is susceptible to chemical agents exposure to hypochlorite (10,000 ppm available chlorine), glutaraldehyde inactivates infectivity, though HBS Ag may not be destroyed by sub treatment.

Diagnosis

- Detection of HBs Ag in blood, because HBs Ag is the first marker to appear in blood after infection.
- Presence of HBV DNA in the serum of infected person is other method for diagnosing HBV infection.
- HBC Ag provides information about relative infectivity. Its presence denotes high infectivity and its absence, along with the presence of anti-HBC, indicates low infectivity.
- Anti HBC is predominantly IgM, but after about 6 months it is mainly IgG. Selective test is done for IgM or IgG.

Prevention

- Screening of blood donors for Hepatitis B virus infection.
- Proper sterilization of needles and syringes.
- Immunization with Hepatitis B vaccine.

7.5.6 Tuberculosis

Tuberculosis is a communicable disease caused by bacteria called *Mycobacterium tuberculosis*.

Morphology: It is straight or slightly curved rod occurring in pairs or on small clumps which are gram+ve fungus like bacteria, non-motile, non-sporing saprophytic organism.

- They do not stain readily but once stained resist decolourisation therefore called acid fast bacilli. They can be stained by Ziehl Neelsen's stain

Symptoms

The symptoms of tuberculosis are:

- Prolonged cough
- Rise of temperature in the evening.
- Loss of weight
- Loss of appetite
- Night sweats
- Chest pain

Source of Infection

The main source of infection is the sputum of a patient suffering from tuberculosis.

Mode of Transmission

Tuberculosis is mainly an air borne infection. It is transmitted by droplet infection and droplet nuclei.

- It is transmitted by fomites such as dishes or other articles used by tuberculosis patients.
- Coming in contact with the sputum of tuberculosis patient.
- Poverty, over crowding and poor ventilation.
- Drinking unboiled milk of infected cow.

Cultured Characters

- Optimum temperature is 37 °C with a pH of 6.4 to 7.
- The selective media for the growth of tubercle organism is "Lowenstein Jensen medium" (LJ media) which contains mineral salt solution asparagine, malachite green where it forms dry, rough, irregular colonies with creamy white or yellowish colonies
- In liquid media growth begins at the bottom with the formation of a surface pellicle.

Pathogenesis

The essential pathology in tuberculosis is the production of a characteristic lesion i.e., tubercle which is composed of a peripheral zone of lymphocytes and fibroblasts in the infected tissues.

Tubercle lesions are of two types

1. Exudative which is an acute inflammatory reaction with accumulation of arema polymorphonuclear leucocytes
2. Productive which is a cellular type of lesion.

Primary tuberculosis leads to pneumonia which occurs about 3 to 8 weeks, from the time of infection and associated with tuberculin hypersensitivity. In majority of cases lesions heals spontaneously in 2 to 6 months leaving behind a calcified nodule.

Secondary tuberculosis follows shortly after primary tuberculosis but more commonly it arises from reactivation of dormant primary lesions many decades after initial infection.

Diagnosis

- Microscopic examination by performing gram staining where sputum is collected from laryngeal swabs or bronchial washings collected in the morning hours in a sterile container.
- Diagnosis can also be made by ELISA test or may be by polymerase chain reaction and ligase chain reaction can also be done.

- Identification is done by culturing the organisms on a suitable medium i.e., L J medium. Cultures are examined for growth after incubation at 37 °C for about 4 days.
  A –ve report is given if no growth occurs after 8-12 weeks. If any growth is seen it is smeared and tested by ZN staining.
- Smear preparation can also be done by ziehlneelsen's staining.
- Diagnosis can also be done by a specific method PETROFF's method, where the sputum is incubated with an equal volume of 4% NaOH solution at 37 °C for about 20 minutes. It is then centrifuget at 3000 rpm for 20 minutes and the sediment is with n/10 HCl used for smear, culture and animal inoculation methods.

Prevention

- Preventive treatment (chemoprophylaxis) with INH (Isoniazid) or INH plus Ethambutol.
- Treatment of infected patients with suitable drugs such as INH, Rifampicin and Streptomycin.
- Immunisation by BCG vaccine.

7.5.7 Gonorrhoea

Gonorrhoea is a sexually transmitted disease caused by Gonococci named *Neisseria gonorrhoeae*

Morphology: In smears from the urethral discharge in acute gonorrhea, the organism appears as a *diplococcus* with the adjacent concave, being typically kidney shaped.

- Gonococci possess pili on their surface. Pili facilitate adhesion of the cocci to mucosal surface and promote virulence by inhibiting phagocytosis.

Antigenic Properties

- Gonococci are antigenically heterogenous, they are capable of changing their surface structures *in vitro*.
- Pili which are hair like structures several micrometers long, act as virulence factor by promoting attachment to host cells.
- The tri-laminar outer membrane of gonococci contains many different proteins I is the major constituent and shows antigenic diversity.
- The outer membrane also contain lipopolysaccharide.

Symptoms

People with gonorrhoea are asymptomatic or have subclinical disease.

- Women may complain of vaginal discharge, difficulty urinating (dysuria), abnormal bleeding, projectile urination.
- Possibility of increased production of male hormones.

Mode of Transmission

- In most of the cases, gonorrhoea is transmitted by direct sexual contact.

Pathogenicity: The disease is acquired by sexual contact.

- The first step in infection is adhesion of gonococci to the urethra or other mucosal surfaces. Pili are involved in adhesion.
- The cocci penetrate through the intercellular spaces and reach the sub epithelial connective tissue by the third day after infection. The incubation period is 2-8 days.
- In women, the initial infection involves the urethra and cervix uteri.
- In men, the disease starts as an acute urethritis with a mucoprurulent discharge containing gonococci in large numbers.

Resistance

- The gonococcus is very delicate organism, readily killed by heat, drying and antiseptics. It is a strict parasite and dies in 1-2 hours in exudates outside the body. In cultures, the coccus dies in 3-4 days but survive in slant cultures at 35 °C if kept under sterile paraffin oil.

Diagnosis

- In women, besides the urethral discharge, cervical swabs should also be collected. This should be done carefully, using a speculum.
- Identification of gonococci in smears is done by fluorescent antibody techniques.
- Intracellular gram–ve diplococcic in stained smears provide an evidence of gonorrohea in men.
- In acute gonorrhoea, cultures can be obtained readily on Chocolate agar or Muller-Hinton agar incubated at 35-36 °C under 5-10% CO_2. The growth is identified by morphology and biochemical reactions.

Treatment

- Antibiotics that may be used to treat gonorrhoea include:
- Amoxicillin, Ampicillin, Azithromycin, Cefriaxone-125 mg single IM dose or Ciprofloxacin – 500 mg single oral dose, plus Doxycycline 100 mg twice daily for seven days.
- Sulphonamides are useful but resistance developed rapidly.

- Penicillin is ineffective at treating rectal gonorrhoea, this is because other bacteria within the rectum produce β-lactamases, that destroy penicillin. Very large doses of Penicillin were used.

Prevention and Control

- Detection of cases and tracing the contacts.
- Screening of special groups like army personnel, industrial workers, blood donors etc.
- Health education about sexually transmitted diseases and their problems.

7.5.8 Bacillary Dysentery

Bacillary dysentery is an infectious disease of the intestinal tract caused by bacteria *Shigella dysenteriae* of the genus *Shigella.*

Bacillary dysentery is associated with species of bacteria from the *Enterobacteriaceae* family.

- Dysentery is a clinical condition of multiple etiology, characterized by frequent passage of blood stained, mucoprurulent stools

Morphology

- *Shigellae* are short, gram–ve rods about 0.5 μm × 1-3 μm in size.
- They are non motile, non sporing and non capsulated, fimbriae may be present.

Symptoms

(A) In Acute bacillary dysentery

- Eating contaminated food
- Fever, abdominal pain, diarrhea, tenesmus and bloody purulent stools.

(B) Chronic bacillary dysentery

- Having past history of acute bacillary dysentery.
- Recurrent or persistent abdominal pain.
- Accompanied with diarrhoea or alternation of diarrhoea and constipation.
- blood-stained stools.

Source of Infection

The only source of infection are human beings or less often carriers.

Mode of Transmission

- Direct, through contaminated fingers
- Through fomites-such as door handles, water taps, lavatory seats.
- Through water
- Through contaminated food or drink
- Through flies which may transmit the infection as mechanical vectors.
- Shigellosis may occur in young male homosexuals as part of the gay bowel syndrome.

Antigenic Structure

- *Shigella* possess one or more 'major' antigens and a large number of 'minor' somatic 'o' antigens. Some possess k antigens.
- These are not relevant in typing but may sometimes interfere with agglutination by 'o' antisera.
- In general, the antigenic structure of *shigella* is simple, compared to the complex structure of *salmonella*.

Pathogenicity

- *Shigella* cause bacillary dysentery infection by ingestion.
- The minimum infective dose is low, as few as 10-100 bacilli being capable of initiating the disease, because they survive gastric acidity better than other entero bacteria.
- The bacilli infect the epithelial cells of the intestinal villi in the large intestine and multiply inside them, spreading laterally and penetrating into the lamina propria.
- Bacillary dysentery has a short incubation period (1-7 days, usually 48 hours)
- The severity of disease may vary from acute fulminating dysentery to mild diarrhoea.

Diagnosis

- Diagnosis is made by isolating the bacillus from feces.
- For inoculation it is best to use mucus flakes if they are present in the sample.
- Mac Conkey and DCA plates are incubated. After overnight incubation at 37 °C, the plates are inspected for nonlactose fermenting colonies, which are tested for motility and biochemical reactions.
- Identification is confirmed by slide agglutination with polyvalent and monovalent sera.

Treatment

- Replacement of lost fluids from the body.
- The choice of antibiotic should be based on the sensitivity of the prevailing strain.
- Multiple drug resistance plasmids are widely prevalent in shigellae.
- Fluroquinolones, doxycycline, ampicillin, ciprofloxacin are indicated.

Prevention and Control

- Improving personal and environmental sanitation.
- Consumption of contaminated food and water should be avoided.
- Antibiotics have no place in prophylaxis.
- No effective vaccine is available.

7.5.9 Tetanus

Tetanus is caused by *Clostridium tetani*. *C. tetani* is a gram+ve, anaerobic and spore forming bacterium, the endospores of which are found in soil, dust and faeces of many farm animals and humans.

- Tetanus is characterized by toxic muscular spasms, usually commencing at the site of infection.

Symptoms

- Lock jaw
- Muscular rigidity
- Painful spasm of voluntary muscles.

Mode of Transmission

- Transmission of the bacterium takes place through skin wound. The endospores enter in wounds/breaks caused in skin.
- The spores also enter through contaminated wounds, injury or abrasions. The injury may be trivial pin prick, puncture wounds, unsterile surgery etc.

Mechanism of action of Tetanospasmin

In the wound the neurotoxin, tetanospasmin, is released after the death and break down of bacteria. Tetanospasmin is an endopeptidase that breaks the synaptic vesicle membrane protein, synaptobrevin. This in turn inhibits exocytosis and release inhibitory neurotransmitters at synapses within the motor nerves of spinal cord. This results in stimulation of skeletal muscles that lose its control.

Tetanospasmin cause tension and twisting in skeletal muscles present around the wound. The jaw muscles become tight consequently, there develops trismus (lock jaw) which is an inability to open the mouth, due to spasm or contraction of master muscles.

Diagnosis

- Demonstration of *C.tetani* by microscopy, culture or by animal innoculation.
- Isolation is more likely from excised bits of tissue from the necrotic depths of wounds, than from wound swabs.
- The material is inoculated on one half of a blood agar plate.
- *C. tetani* produces a swarming growth which may be detected on the opposite half of the plate after 1-2 days incubation anaerobically.
- For identification and toxigenicity testing, blood agar plates having tetanus antitoxin spread over one half of the plate are used.
- The *C.tetani* strains are stab-inoculated on each half of the plate, which is then incubated anaerobically for two days. Toxigenic *C.tetani* strains show hemolysis around the colonies; only on the half without the antitoxin lysis is inhibited by antitoxin on the other half.

Immunisation and Control Measures

- Tetanus is prevented by using tetanus toxoid.
- The tetanus toxoid is a formaldehyde-treated toxin that is precipitated in the form of salt of aluminium to increase its immunizing potency.
- The tetanus toxoid is given with DPT programmes.
- After a few months of birth, initial dose is given.
- The second dose should be given after 4-6 months of the first dose.
- Finally, the reinforcing dose should be given 6 to 12 months after the second dose.
- Between the age of 4 to 6 years, a final booster is given.
- A single booster dose can provide protection for 10 to 20 years.
- Preventive measures must be adopted by active immunization with toxoid, prophylactic use of antitoxin and using penicillin.

Treatment

- Tetanus patients should be treated in hospitals, preferably in special units.
- Treatment consist of controlling spasms, maintaining airway by tracheostomy with intermittent positive pressure respiration and attention to feeding.
- Human TIG 10,000 IU suitably diluted may be given by slow IV infusion, followed if needed by another 5000 IU later.
- Antitoxin is of great value in treatment.

7.5.10 Polio (Poliomyelitis)

Poliomyelitis (Greek ***polios*** means gray and ***myelos*** means marrow or spinal cord), polio or infantile paralysis is caused by the poliovirus which is a member of family *picornavirus*.

Morphology: The virus is a spherical particle consisting of viral proteins arranged in icosahedral symmetry. The genome is SS RNA.

Resistance

- Polio virus is resistant to ether, chloroform, detergents and proteolytic enzymes of the intestinal contents.
- The organism is stable at pH of 3 wherein fecal matter it can survive for months at 4 °C and years at –20 °C.
- It is readily inactivated by heating at 55 °C for about 30 minutes.
- Chlorination destroys the virus but phenolic compounds are not effective.

Cultivation methods

- Inoculation can be done in monkey or may be in chick embryos.
- The virus grown readily in tissue cultures and also in primary monkey kidney cultures which are used for diagnostic culture and vaccine production.

Symptoms

- Fever, sore throat, headache, stiffness of neck.
- In few cases it leads to foot drop and flaccid paralysis of limbs.

Mode of Transmission

- Transmission occurs by fecal-oral route.
- Direct infection occurs through contaminated fingers.
- Indirect infection occurs through contaminated water, food and flies.

Pathogenicity

- The virus multiplies initially in the epithelial cells of the elementary canal and the lymphatic tissues, from the tonsils to the payer's patches.
- The organism then spreads to lymph nodes and enters into the blood stream causing minor or "primary viraemia".
- After further multiplication in the reticulo endothelial system the virus enters the blood stream again causing major or "secondary viraemia" and is carried to spinal cord and brain.

- In the CNS the virus multiplies selectively in the neurons destroying them causing degeneration of "Nissel bodies" with nuclear changes.
- Lesions are produced mostly in the interior parts of spinal cords causing paralysis.
- The incubation period of the organism is about 10 days which may range from 4 days to 4 weeks.

Prevention and Control

- Proper disposal of urine and faeces.
- Protection of water sources and supply of safe drinking water.
- Immunisation with Salk vaccine and Sabine vaccine. Salk vaccine is a killed vaccine it is administered by injection. Sabine vaccine is a live polio vaccine.

7.5.11 Typhoid

Typhoid (Greek ***typhoides*** means smoke) fever is caused by *Salmonella typhi.*

Morphology: *Salmonella* are gram –ve, rod shaped bacterium about 1-3 μm × 0.5 μm in size. They are motile with peritrichate flagella, except for one type, *Salmonella gallinarum-pullorum* which is always non-motile. Mutants of other types may sometimes be found, they do not form capsules or spores but may posses fimbriae.

Symptoms

- Continuous fever for 3-4 weeks. There is a stepwise increase.
- Severe headache, malaise
- Back pain.

Mode of Transmission: The source of infection are feces.

- It is mainly by contaminated water and food
- It is transmitted by fingers and flies.

Pathogenicity

S. typhi, after ingestion/drinking of water, colonies the small intestine, penetrate the epithelium and spread to lymphoid tissues, blood, liver and gall bladder.

Diagnosis

- Laboratory diagnosis is made by demonstrating the bacteria in stool, urine and blood.
- Serological test such as Widal test is done,.

Prevention and Immunisation

- Purification of drinking water and milk.

- Prevention of handling of food by carriers.
- Complete isolation of the carriers.
- Immunization can be done through administration of oral typhoid vaccine.

Treatment

- Use of antibiotics such as ceftizoxane, trimethoprim sulfamethoxazole or ampicillin.
- Drugs like chloramphenicol is also used.
- Use of vaccine for high risk individuals.

7.5.12 Cholera

Cholera (Latin ***chola*** means bile) has caused pandemics in Asia and Africa. It caused by a gram–ve, slightly curved, *Vibrio cholera*, that contains a single polar flagellum.

Structure of Vibrio Cholera

Vibrio Cholerae is a gram-negative bacterium that produces cholera toxin, an enterotoxin, whose action on the mucosal epithelium lining of the small intestine is responsible for the disease.

Symptoms

- Diarrhoea, which is watery and brown at first, but quickly, changes to large volumes of pale fluid stools (rise-water stools).
- Hypovolemic shock due to dramatic fluid loss from the continuous diarrhoea.
- Complications include muscular cramps, renal failure, pulmonary edema, cardiac arrhythmias.

Mode of Transmission

- It is transmitted by taking contaminated food and water by fecal material from patients or carriers.
- Direct person to person spread by contact may not be common but hand contamination of stored drinking water which is an important method of domestic spread of infection.

Pathogenicity

- Natural infection with cholera occurs only in humans not in animals.
- In human infection the vibrios enter orally through contaminated water or food.
- It adheres to the mucosa of small intestine and secretes a cholera toxin, choleragen.

- Choleratoxin is a protein. It possesses two functional units: an enzymatic subunit A and an intestinal receptor-binding subunit B.
- The subunit A acts as diphtheria toxin. It enters into the epithelial cells of intestine, binds to ADP-ribosyl group and activates the enzymes adenylate cyclase.
- Thus, choleragen induces the secretion of water and chloride ions and inhibits absorption of sodium ions. The patient loses water and electrolytes. This results in cramping of abdominal muscles, vomiting, fever and watery diarrhoea.
- During infection a person can lose 10-15 litres of fluid.
- Finally patients die due to loss of water and electrolytes and increased amount of blood proteins that leads shocks and collapse of circulatory system.

Cholera toxin increases skin permeability and it is also called as permeability factor. It can be demonstrated by the 'skin blueing test' when cholera toxin is injected intradermally in rabbit or guinea pigs and pantamine sky blue injected intravenously afterwards, the site of toxin injection becomes blue. Cholera toxin also is estimated by ELISA.

Diagnosis

- Stool, collected in the acute stage of the disease, before the administration of antibiotics, is the most useful specimen for laboratory diagnosis.
- Diagnosis of the bacterium is by culture from faeces, and agglutination reaction with specific antisera. The patients are immediately rehydrated with NaCl plus sucrose solution.
- On arrival in the laboratory, the specimens sent in enrichment media should be incubated for 6-8 hours including transit time.
- The specimens sent in holding media should be inoculated into enrichment media, to be incubated for 6-8 hours before being streaked on a selective and a non selective medium.
- Generally, the plates are examined after overnight incubation at 37 °C.

Immunity: In cholera, the vibrio remains confined to the intestine, where they multiply and elaborate the enterotoxin which is responsible for the disease.

- Immunity may be directed against the bacterium or against the toxin antibacterial or antitoxic.
- Immunity may be local, in the intestine or systemic, appearance of local antibodies in the intestine has been known for a long time. These are known as 'copro antibodies' as they appear in the feces. They consist of IgG, IgM and IgA.

Prophylaxis

- Prevention of the disease is straightforward if proper sanitation practices are followed.

- All materials (such as clothing and bedding) that come in contact with cholera patients should be sterilized in hot water using chlorine bleach if possible.
- Treatment of general sewage before it enters the waterways or underground water supplies.
- All water used for drinking, washing or cooking should be sterilized by boiling or chlorination in any area where cholera may be present.

Two types of oral vaccines have been tried.

1. Killed oral whole cell vaccines with and without the inclusion of the B subunit of cholera toxin
2. Live oral vaccines.

Treatment

- The treatment of cholera consists essentially of the prompt and adequate replacement of lost fluid and electrolytes.
- Oral administration of fluid containing glucose and electrolytes either alone or supplemented by I.V fluids is a highly successful and freely available method of treating cholera.
- Cereal based preparations are equally effective and usually more acceptable.
- The antibiotics recommended to patients are tetracycline, trimethoprim, sulfa-methoxazole or ciprofloxacin.

7.5.13 Filariasis

Filariasis is a parasitic and infectious tropical disease, that is caused by thread-like filarial nematodes worms. There are 9 known filarial nematodes which use human as the definitive host. These are divided into 3 groups according to the niche within the body that they occupy.

1. lympthatic filariasis – caused by *Wuchereria bancrofti*
Brugia malayi
Brugia timori
2. Subcutaneous filariasis – caused by *Loa loa*
Mansonella streptocerca
Onchocerca volvulus
Dracunculus medinenis
3. Serous cavity filariasis – caused by *Mansonella perstans*
Mansonella ozzardi

Symptoms

- Lymphangitis
- Lymphadenitis
- Elephantiasis of genitals, legs, arms.
- Pulmonary eosinophilia may be produced.
- Subcutaneous worms present with skin rashes, urticarial papules and arthritis

Vectors of Filariasis

- The vectors of W. bancrofti are *Culex, Anopheles and Aedes mosquitoes*.
- The vectors for B. malayi and B.timori are mansonia mosquitoes.

Mode of Transmission

Filariasis is transmitted by the bite of infected vector mosquitoes. The parasite is deposited near the site of puncture. It passes through the skin and reaches the lymphatic system.

Life Cycle of Human Filarial Nematode Worms

- It consists of five stages.
- After the male and female worm mate, the female gives birth to live microfilariae by the thousands.
- The microfilariae are taken up by the vector insect (intermediate host) during a blood meal.
- In the intermediate host, the microfilariae moult and develop into 3rd stage (infective) larvae.
- Upon taking another blood meal, the vector insect injects the infectious larvae into the dermis layer of our skin.

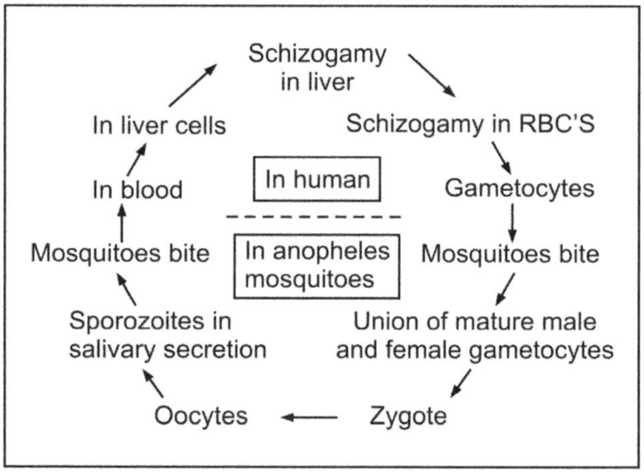

- After approximately one year the larvae moult through 2 more stages, maturing into to the adult worm.
- Individuals infected by filarial worms may be described as either "microfilaraemic" or "amicrofilaraemic" depending on whether or not microfilaria are found in their peripheral blood.

Diagnosis

- Filariasis is usually diagnosed by identifying microfilariae on a Giemsa stained thick blood film. Blood must be drawn at night, since the microfilaria circulate at night, when their mosquito vector is most likely to bite. Also, decreased peripheral temperature may attract more microfilariae.
- Polymerase chain reaction and antigenic assays are also available for making the diagnosis.
- X-ray can show calcified adult worm in lymphatics.
- DEC provocation test is performed to obtain satisfying number of parasite in day-time samples.

Treatment

- The recommended treatment for killing adult filarial worms in patients outside the United States is albendazole combined with ivermectin.
- A combination of diethyl carbomazine and albendazole is also effective.
- Doxycycline was suggested for treating elephantiasis.

Prevention and Control

- Vector control by using larvicides like abate and baytex
- Health education about good drainage, antimosquitoe measures and filariasis treatment.

7.5.14 Food Poisoning

Food poisoning is defined as acute gastro enteritis caused by ingestion of foods that contain germs like bad bacteria or toxins, which are poisonous substances. There are two types of food poisoning:

Food infection and food intoxicaction.

- Food infection refers to the presence of bacteria or other microbes which infect the body after consumption.
- Food intoxication refers to the ingestion of toxins contained within the food, including bacterially produced exotoxins, which can happen even when the microbe that produced the toxin is no longer present or able to cause infection.

Causes

- Food poisoning usually arises from improper handling, preparation or food storage.
- Food borne illness can also be caused by pesticides or medicines in food and naturally toxic substances like poisonous mushroom or reef fish.

- Food borne disease can also be caused by a large variety of toxins that affect the environment.

Symptoms

- Nausea
- Abdominal pain, vomiting, diarrhoea
- Gastroenteritis
- Fever, headache or fatigue.
- Food borne illness due to *campylobacter, yersinia, salmonella or shigella* infection is a major cause of reactive arthritis.
- Tetradotoxin poisoning from reef fish and other animals causes numbness and shortness of breath.

Incubation Period

The delay between consumption of a contaminated food and appearance of the first symptoms of illness is called the incubation period. This ranges from hours to days (rarely months or even years, such as in the case of creutzfeldt – Jacob disease)

Infectious Dose

The infectious dose is the amount of agent that must be consumed to give rise to symptoms of food borne illness and varies according to the agent and the consumer's age and overall health.

- In the case of salmonella, a relatively large inoculum of 1 million to 1 billion organisms is necessary to produce symptoms in health human volunteers.

Pathogenic Agents

- Bacteria are a common cause of food borne illness.
- The bacteria which can produce food poisoning are:
- *Compylobacter jejuni*
- *Clostridium perfringens*
- *Salmonella species*
- *E. coli*

Exotoxins: In addition to disease caused by direct bacterial infection, some food borne illnesses are caused by exotoxins which are excreted by the cell as the bacterium grows.

- *Clostridium botulinum* which is an anaerobic bacterium grows in improperly canned low-acid foods and produces botulin, a powerful paralytic toxin and causes a disease called botulism.
- *Staphylococcus aureus* produces a toxin that causes intense vomiting.

Mycotoxins and alimentary mycotoxicoses

- The term alimentary mycotoxicoses refers to the effect of poisoning by mycotoxins through food consumption.
- The common food borne mycotoxins include:

Aflatoxins: Originated from *Aspergillus flavus, Aspergillus parasiticus*. They are frequently found in tree nuts, peanuts, maize, sorghum and other oil seeds including corn and cotton seeds.

Diagnosis

- Examination of the sample of your stool and urine to test for possible germs that might have caused food borne illness.
- The type of treatment for food poisoning or food borne illness will depend on the specific germ.

Prevention and Control

- Wash fruits and vegetables well before eating them
- Only eat foods that are properly cooked
- Inspection of meat
- Pasteurisation of milk
- Protection and covering of food during processing and storage
- Check the expiry date on packaged foods
- Health education of food handlers and cooks about cleanliness.

7.5.15 Leprosy

Leprosy (Greek *Leprosei* means scaly, Scabby, rough) or Hansen's disease is a chronic infectious disease caused by mycobacterium leprae.

- It affects mainly skin, peripheral nerves and nasal mucosa but capable of affecting any tissue or organ.
- The disease may be classified into four types
    1. Lepromatous
    2. Tuberculoid
    3. Dimorphous and
    4. Indeterminate

Lepromatous Leprosy: In the infected individuals, who do not develop hypersensitivity, there occurs progressive form of disease which is known as lepromatous leprosy.

This type of leprosy is characterized by lepromas (tumour like growths) on the skin and along respiratory tract. Lepromin test is –ve

Tuberculoid Leprosy: It is mild, nonprogressive and associated with delayed type hypersensitivity reaction to antigen on the surface of *M.leprae*.

Dimorphous leprosy: Possess characteristics of both tuberculoid and lepromatous types.

Indeterminate: It is the early unstable tissue reaction which is not characteristic of either the lepromatous or the tuberculoid type. In many persons, the indeterminate lesions undergo healing spontaneously.

Epidemiology

- Leprosy is a contact disease that degenerates the tissues and deforms the body organs.
- Humans are the only reservoir of the disease.
- Very large numbers of bacilli are shed in the nasal secretions.
- Leprosy is now confined mainly, but not exclusively, to the under developed areas of the tropics and the southern hemisphere.

Symptoms

- The earliest symptoms of leprosy are slightly pigmented eruptions of skin which are several centimeter in diameter.
- Partial or total loss of cutaneous sensation in the affected area.
- Thickening of nerves.

Mode of Transmission

- Disease is transmitted to children when prolonged exposures to infected persons are made.
- Insect vectors may have a role in the transmission of leprosy
- Sometimes it is transmitted by droplet infection.

Immunity

- The type of leprosy in an individual is determined by the status of cell mediated immunity in that person. When it is adequate, the lesions are the tuberculoid type.
- When cell mediated immunity is deficient, the lepromatous type of disease develops.
- The macrophages are able to phagocytose the bacilli but instead of being destroyed, the bacilli proliferate inside the cells.
- Lepromatous patients are not more susceptible to viruses, parasites and other pathogens against which CMI is important

- The lymphocyte present in skin granulomas are almost exclusively CD_8^+ cells, in contrast to tuberculoid lesions which contain predominantly CD_4^+ cells.

Lepromin Test

- The only method for studying immunity in leprosy was a skin test for delayed hypersentivity.
- The lepromin test is not used to diagnose leprosy, nor does it indicate prior contact with the *lepra bacillus*.

The test is employed for the following purposes:

- To classify the lesions of leprosy patients. The lepromin test is +ve in tuberculoid, –ve in lepromatous and variable in dimorphous and indeterminate types of diseases.
- To assess the prognosis and response to treatment A positive reaction indicates good prognosis and a negative one bad prognosis.
- To assess the resistance of individuals to leprosy.

Diagnosis

Demonstration of acid fast bacilli in the lesions.

For routine examination, specimens are collected from the nasal mucosa, skin lesions and ear lobules.

Detection of antibody against *M. leprae*, phenolic glycolipid antigen has been claimed to be a specific diagnostic test.

- Ziehl-Neelsen stained smears of lepromatous nodules or skin scrapings show the acid fast bacilli as packed bundles.
- ELISA test is also an immunodiagnostic test for leprosy.

Treatment

- Multiple drug therapy is recommended in leprosy to avoid resistance.
- Dapsone was the first effective chemotherapeutic agent against leprosy.
- Ethionamide or propionamide can also be used along with Dapsone.
- Clofazimine is also effective against leprosy.
- An immunotherapeutic vaccine (mycobacterium w) developed at the National Institute of Immunology, New Delhi is claimed to enhance the effect of MDT.

Prophylaxis

- Prevention of contact between the patient and other normal persons, especially children.
- Case finding and adequate therapy have been the methods employed for prophylaxis.
- BCG vaccine was observed to induce lepromin positively and hence its use in the prevention of leprosy was suggested.

7.5.16 Syphilis

Syphilis is a contagious sexually transmitted disease caused by a spirochete, *Treponema pallidum*. Congenital syphilis is a disease which is acquired in uterus from the mother.

Morphology: It is a thin, desiccate, *Spirochete* with tapering ends, which is actively motile exhibiting rotation among the long axis backward and forward movements.

- These organisms can be seen by performing gram–ve staining or Indian ink preparation and also done by sliver impregnation method.

Mode of Transmission

- Sexual intercourse is the most common way of transmission.
- Contact of the bacteria.
- Congenital syphilis in the new born is caused by infection from the mother through the placenta.

Stages of Syphilis

In untrelated adults the disease occurs in the following three stages:

(i) Primary Syphilis

- In the primary stage incubation period is of about 10 days to 3 weeks.
- This stage is characterized by a small painless and reddened ulcer or chancre.
- Chancre has a hard ridge that looks as the infection site and consists of spirochetes.
- Disease is transmitted if contact with chancre is made during sexual intercourse.

(ii) Secondary Syphilis

The second stage is established within 2-10 weeks after the primary lesions.

- This stage is characterized by a skin rash.
- At this stage symptoms include loss of patches of hairs, malaise and fever.
- There are flat wart like lesions which are filled with spirochetes.

(iii) Teritiary Syphilis: After several weeks the disease becomes latent.

- During the latent period disease is not infectious except transmission from mother to foetus. This is called congenital syphilis.
- After several years a tertiary stage develops when secondary syphilis remains untreated.
- The symptoms include formation of degenerative lesions (gammas) in the skin, bone, cardiovascular and nervous systems.
- At this stage number of spirochetes is drastically reduced.
- This results in mental retardness, blindness, a "shuffle" walk leading to paralysis.

Resistance

- Inactivated by drying or by heat i.e., 41-42°C in one hour.
- Fomites are of little importance in the transmission of infection.
- It is inactivated by contact with O_2, distilled water, soap, antiseptics, and antibiotics.

Antigenic Structure

- Treponemal infection includes at least three types of Ab's, first is the regain Ab that react in the standard test for syphilis.
- The second in group Ag found in *Treponema pallidum*.
- The third Ag is a polysaccharide compound which shows species specific.

Pathogenicity

- Venereal syphilis is acquired by several content, where the organism enters the body through mucosa, abrasions or through skin.
- *Treponema pallidum* moves by axial filament and enters the body through mucus membrane or abrasion or wound.

Diagnosis

- Syphilis is diagnosed through clinical history, physical examination, immuno-fluorescence examination of fluid from lesions to observe typical mortality.
- The serological tests include:
  - (i) Test for monotreponemal antigen by VDRL (venereal disease laboratories test), RPR (Rapid plasma regain test), Complement fixation test or the Wassermann test.
  - (ii) Test for treponemal antibodies.
- Diagnosis can also performed by ELISA test or enzyme immuno assays.

Prevention and Control

- Public education
- Prompt treatment of new cases.
- Treatment of source of infection and contact
- Maintaining sexual hygiene
- Prophylaxis (condoms)

7.5.17 Malaria

Plasmodium is a common spore-forming protozoan parasite on human which causes malaria.

Four pathogenic species of plasmodium have been recognized:

- *P. falciparum*
- *P. malariae*
- *P. ovale*
- *P. vivax*
- *P. falciparum* is the most dangerous species followed by P. vivax.

Symptoms

- Chills and fever
- Anaemia
- Liver and spleen enlargement

Mode of Transmission

It is transmitted by the bite of female *Anopheles* mosquito which acts as a vector.

Life Cycle: The life cycle of *plasmodium* is very complex.

Malaria is associated with a mosquito vector, *Anopheles*. The mosquito carriers the inocula of *P. vivax* where it multiplies and produces the sporozoites. After mosquito bite, the sporozoites present in saliva are delivered in the blood of human. Thirty minutes after bite, the sporozoites enter in liver cells and undergo reproductive suchizogamy through a series of intermediate stages. At the last stage of schizogamy, a large number of merozoites are released in the blood stream. The merozoites are infectious which in turn infect the red blood corpuscles and under-go reproductive schizogamy. A large number of merozoites are released upon rupture of RBC's. The merozoites infect the other RBC's and renew the cycle. The infected RBC'S are disintegrated which release the toxic substances. The toxic substances induce the characteristic symptoms of malaria i.e., chills and fever. After reaching the body temperature up to 40 °C, fever subsides. However, due to break down of RBC's, the patient suffers from anaemia, liver and spleen enlargement. As per estimate 1% infected RBC's contain about 10,000 millions of parasite at a time in the blood of malaria patients. Rest of merozoites act as male or female gametocytes. Again the merozoites enter in the digestive tract of new mosquitoes when they bite the infected person. The merozoites multiply in digestive tract of mosquito, pass through reproductive cycle and form infective sporozoites.

Diagnosis

- Diagnosis of plasmodium can be made by taking out blood samples, preparation of smear and microscopic observations for the presence of parasite.

Treatment

- Quinine and derivatives of quinine eg., chloroquine, primaquine etc., have been used for several years.
- Chloroquine inhibits DNA replication at merozoite stage.
- Recently resistance to these drugs have been reported. Therefore, in recent years drug combinations has been recommended eg: Fansidar which is a combination of pyrimethamine and sulfadoxine.

Prophylaxis

- Destruction of mosquitoes by spraying DDT or kerosene.
- Prevention of mosquito bite by rubbing mosquito repellants or using mosquitoes nets.
- Hygienic measures like good drainage. This will prevent stagnation, where mosquitoes breed.

7.5.18 AIDS

Acquired immune deficiency syndrome is a disease of the human immune system caused by the human immuno deficiency virus (HIV).

Morphology

- HIV is a spherical virus, about 90-120 nm is size.
- The nucleocapsid has an outer icosahedral shell and an inner cone shaped core, the genome is diploid composed of two identical single stranded, positive sense RNA copies.
- In association with viral RNA is the reverse transcriptase enzyme, which is characteristic feature of retro virus.

- When the virus infects a cell, the viral RNA is transcribed by the enzyme, first into single stranded DNA and then to double stranded DNA which is integrated into the host cell chromosome,
- During viral replication, when the naked virus buds out through the host cell surface membrane, it acquires a lipoprotein envelope, which consists of lipid derived from the host cell membrane and glycoprotein which are virus coded.
- The major virus coded envelope proteins are the projecting knob like spikes on the surface and the anchoring transmem pedicles.
- The spikes constitute the major surface component of the virus which binds to the CDY repeceptors on susceptible host cells transmem pedicles.

Symptoms

- People with AIDS also have an increased risk of developing various cancers such as Kaposi's sarcoma, cervical cancer and cancers of immune system known as lymphomas.
- AIDS often have systemic symptoms of infection like fevers sweats, swollen glands, chills, weakness and weight loss.
- *Pneumocystis pneumonia* (PCP) or pneumocystosis is a form of pneumonia, caused by the yeast-like fungus *Pneumocystis jirovecii.*
- Gastrointestinal infections.
- Tumours and malignancies

Mode of Transmission

Infection is transmitted when the virus enters the blood or tissues of a person and comes into contact with a suitable host cell usage of contaminated needles and syringes blood contact through transfusion of contaminated blood and blood products. Intravenous drug users.

The receptor for the virus is the CDY Ag and therefore the virus may infect any cell bearing the CDY Ag on the surface. Lymphocyte some other immune cells possess the CDY Ag on the surface and so are susceptible to infection.

Clinical Features of HIV Infection

1. **Acute HIV infection:** within 3-6 weeks of infection with HIV about 50% persons experience low grade fever, malaise, headache, lymphadinopathy, sometimes with rash and arthropathy resembling glanular fever.
    - Tests for HIV Ab's are usually –ve at the onset of illness but become +ve during its course. Hence, this syndrome has been called "seroconversion illness". The pathogenesis of seroconversion illness is believed to be due to immune complexes as well as to the direct effects of viral multiplication.

2. **Asymptomatic or latent infection:** All persons infected with HIV, whether or not they experience seroconversion illness pass through a phase of symptom less infection which may last up to several years.
3. **Persistent Generalised lymphan:** This has been defined as the presence of enlarged lymph nodes, at least 1 cm in diameter, in 2 or more non contagious, extra lingual sites that persist for at least three months.
4. **AIDS related complex:** This group includes patients with considerable immunodeficiency suffering from various constitutional symptoms or minor opportunistic infections. The symptoms include:
   - Fatigue
   - Unexplained fever
   - Persistent diarrhoea
   - Loss of more than 10% of body weight
5. **AIDS:** This is the end-stage disease representing the irreversible breakdown of immune defence mechanisms, leaving the patient to progressive opportunistic infection.
   - The characteristic pathogen initially was *P. carinii* but now *M. tuberculosis*.

Gastro intestinal system: The mouth is often involved in AIDS, with thirst, gingivitis, kaposis sarcoma.

CNS: The typical CNS infection are toxoplasmosis, cryptococcops. Infections are also sent with CMV, herpes complex, mycobacteria, aspergillus of the CNS are common.

Malignancies: kaposis sarcoma was the characteristic lesions seen in male homosexuals. The other tumours commonly seen are lymphomas both the Hodgkin and non Hodgkin types.

Cutaneous: Besides kaposis sarcoma, herpes lesions, seborrheic dermatitis, pruigo are the common cutaneous lesions.

Dementia: HIV may cause direct cytopathogenic damage in the CNS. It can cross the BBB and cause encephalopathy leading to loss of higher functions.

Pediatric AIDS: Virus transmission may occur to the fetus in pregnancy as early as the first trimester. Many of the infected children may or may not survive for a year.

Children develop humoral immunodeficiency early, leading to recurrent bacteria infections, failure to thrive, chronic diarrhea etc.

Diagnosis

1. **Immunological tests:** The following parameters help to establish the immune deficiency in the HIV infection.
   (a) Total leukocyte and lymphocyte count to demonstrate leucopenia and a lymphocyte count usually below 2000/mm^3.

(b) T-cell subset assays: Absolute CDY^+ T cell count will be usually less than $200/mm^3$.
(c) Platelet count will show thrombocytopenia.
(d) Raised IgG and IgA levels.
(e) Diminished CMI as mediated by skin tests.
(f) Lymph node biopsy showing profound abnormalities.

2. **Tridot method:** Following a single massive infection as by blood transfusion, the virus Ags may be detectable in blood after about 2 weeks.
   - The major core Ag P^{24} is the earliest virus marker to appear in blood and the one tested for IgM Ab's appear in about 4-6 weeks to be followed by IgG Ab's.
   - The appearance of P^{24} antigenemia and virionea, followed by IgM Ab response coincide with the acute or seroconversion illness.
   - The P^{24} Ag capture assay (ELISA) which uses anti p^{24} Ab as the solid phase. The test is +ve in about 30% of HIV infected persons with prior dissociation of the Ag-Ab complex the +ve rate increase to about 50%.
   - The test is most useful in persons recently exposed to risk of infection in whom Ab test is –ve.
   - It is currently used for screening blood donars in the USA, along with HIV and ELISA.

Virus isolation: Once infected with HIV a person remains infected for life.

- The virus is present in circulation and body fluids, within lymphocytes, cell-free virus titres parallel P^{24} titres being bound during the asymptomatic period and again high towards the end.
- The virus is present in many parts of the body and can be isolated from peripheral lymphocyte.
- The technique of isolation is by co-cultivation of the patients lymphocyte with uninfected lymphocyte.
- Viral replication can be detected by demonstration of reverse transcriptase activity as well as Ag's on the system.
- Viral isolation is not suitable as a routine diagnostic test.
- The test will be +ve only in a proportion of persons infected with HIV.

Polymerase chain reaction

- PCR has become the gold standard for diagnosis in all stages of HIV infection.
- Two forms of PCR have been used, DNA PCR and RNA PCR.

- In the DNA PCR, peripheral lymphocytes from the subject are lysed and the proviral DNA amplified using primer pairs from relatively constant regions of HIV genome, generally from Gog and LTR regions.
- The test is highly sensitive, and can detect HIV proviral DNA at a frequency of one copy per 10,000 cells.
- A related test, HIV RNA PCR can be used for diagnosis as well as for monitoring the level of viremia.
- PCR tests are complex of cost up and are indicated only when other methods cannot give a definite results.

Diagnosis of HIV

The earliest test of HIV is a blood test in 1985. It was available to measure the antibodies to HIV which are the immune response to HIV. The most common method of diagnosis of HIV now is ELISA. If antibodies to HIV are found in ELISA, another technique is usually recommended to confirm the result, typically a test of western blot. However, antibodies to HIV typically develop within several weeks of infection. During this interval, if by the antibody test of ELISA or western blot, the result may show negative (the so called "window period"), while the virus of HIV does exist in a patient's body. In that case, the diagnosis test can be made by detection of the presence of virus in the blood rather than the antibodies, such as tests for HIV RNA or p24 antigen, or just use a HIV-1 p24 ELISA Pair Set. Recently, a new test has been approved that measures both HIV antibodies and p24 antigen, shrinking the duration of the window period from infection to diagnosis.

Prevention and Control

- Screening of blood donars for AIDS.
- Use of disposable syringes for injection.
- Use of contraceptive devices like nirodh.
- Health education about AIDS, its problem and methods of prevention.
- Screening of high risk groups like drug addicts.

Treatment

- Treatment with antiviral agents like azidothymidine. It is not a cure but it can prolong the life of the patient.
- Current treatment for HIV infection consists of highly active antiretroviral therapy or HAART.

- Typical regimens consist of two nucleoside analogue reverse transcriptase inhibitor. (NARTIs or NRTIS) plus either a protease inhibitor or a non-nucleoside reverse transcriptase inhibitor.
- Standard goals of HAART include improvement in the patient's quality of life, reduction in complications, and reduction of HIV viremia below the limit of detection.

7.5.19 Whooping Cough

It is an infectious disease caused by *Bordetella pertussis* (latin per means intensive, and tussis means cough). This disease is caused by a gram–ve bacterium.

It is highly contagious disease and affects the children first. About 95% population of the world is affected by whooping cough.

Symptoms

- Mild fever
- Irritating cough
- Cough occurs in series of paroxysms without breathing.

Mode of Transmission

- The bacterium is transmitted through droplets of infected persons and enter into the healthy one after inhalation. It is established from 7 to 14 days of infection.
- The bacterium is attached to the ciliated epithelia cells of upper respiratory tract.
- It produces an adherence factor called filamentous haemaglutinin that recognizes complementary molecule of the host cell.
- After being attached to the epithelium, the bacterium produces several toxins.
- These toxins develop the symptoms.
- The most important toxin is pertussis toxin. In its presence the tissues become susceptible to histamine and serotonin, and response of lymphocyte is increased.
- In addition, *B. pertussis* also produces an extracellular enzyme (adenylate cyclase) and a tracheal cytotoxin and a dermonecrotic toxin. These destroy the tissue of epithelium.
- Due to secretion of thick mucus the ciliary action is impeded and the ciliated epithelial cells die.

Diagnosis

Laboratory diagnosis of this bacterium includes

- Culture of the bacterium

- Fluorescent antibody
- Staining of smears from nasopharyngeal swabs
- Serological tests.

Prevention and Control

- Early diagnosis by bacteriological examination of nose and throat secretions.
- Active immunization with pertussis vaccine or DPT vaccine
- Passive immunization with hyper immune gamma globulin.
- The children of 2-3 years age are recommended for vaccination with DPT vaccine.

Treatment

The chemotherapeutic agents are chloramphenicol, tetracycline or erythromycin.

7.5.20 Rabies

Rabies (Latin *rabere* means madness) is caused by number of different strains of neurotropic viruses. Most of them belong to the genus *Lyssavirus* of the family *Rhabdoviridae.*

Morphology

The rabies virus is bullet shaped 180 × 75 nm, with one end rounded or conical and the other planar/concave. The lipoprotein envelope carries knob like species, composed of glycoprotein G.

Resistance

The virus is sensitive to ethonal, iodine preparations, 4° ammonium compounds, soap, detergents, lipid solvents such as ether, chloroform and acetone.

- It is inactivated by phenol, formalin.
- Thermal inactivation occurs in one hour at 50 °C and 5 minutes at 60 °C.
- It dies at room temperature.
- It can be preserved at –70 °C or lyophilisation for storage in dry ice.

Antigenic Properties

- The surface spikes are composed of glycoprotein G, which is important on pathogenesis, virulence and immunity.
- It mediates the binding of the virus to acetyl choline receptors in neural tissues induce haemagglutination, inhibiting (HI) and neuralging (protective) Ab's.
- It stimulates cytotoxic T-cell immunity

- The purified glycoprotein may therefore provides a safe and effective subunit vaccine.

Symptoms

- Symptoms begin after 2 to 16 weeks of exposure of virus
- Anxiety
- Irritability, depression, fatigue, loss of appetite, fever, and sensitivity to light and sound consequently, it results in paralysis.

Host Range and Growth Characteristics

Animals

- All mammals are susceptible to rabies infection.
- Cattle, faxes are highly susceptible.

  The rabies virus isolated from natural human animal infection is termed the "Street Virus" following inoculation by any route, it can cause, fatal encephalitis in lab animals after a long and variable incubation period of about 1-12 weeks.
- Intra cytoplasmic inclusion bodies (Negribodies) can be demonstrated in the brain of animals fusing can be demonstrated in the brain of animals dying of street virus infection.

Chick Embryo

The rabies virus can be grown in chick embroys. The usual mode of inoculation is into the yolk sac.

Tissue Culture

The rabies virus can grow in several and continuous cell cultures such as chick embryo.

Pathogenesis

- Human infection is usually caused by theof rabbit, dogs or other animals.
- When these animals bite humans or other healthy animals, viral particles are spread through saliva.
- Virus attaches to the plasma membrane of skeletal muscle cells by glycoprotein envelope spike. It enters the cell and multiplies. When in sufficient number, they enter the nervous system through unmyelinated motor and sensory terminals. They bind with the reported binding site (i.e., nicotinic acetylcholine receptor).

  Finally the virus reaches to the spinal cord and results in first specific symptoms (pain at wound site). As the virus dissenminates, a progressive encephalitis develops. Consequently, virus spreads throughout the body including saliva. In humans the incubation period is usually from 1-3 months, though it may be as short as 7 days or as long as three years. The incubation period is usually short in persons bitten on the face or head, and long in those bitten on the legs. This may be related to the distance the virus has to travel to reach the brain. The incubation period is generally shorter in children than in adult.

- The cause of disease in humans can be classified in four stages: prodome, dilute encephalitic phase, coma and death.
- The acute neurological phase usually begins with hyperactivity, which is characteristically intermittent with bizarre behaviour, agitation or seizures appearing between apparently normal periods such hypersensitivity may be spontaneous or precipitated by external stimuli. The pathogenic feature is difficulty in drinking, together with intense thirst.
- In dogs, the incubation period is usually 3-6 weeks but it may range from 10 days to a year. The initial signs are an alert, troubled air and a change in diposition with restlessness, skrapping at imaginary objects, licking or inawing at the site of the bite. After 2-3 days of this prodromal stage, the disease develops into either the furious or dumb type of rabies.
- In furious rabies, the dog runs biting without provocation and indiscriminately the lower jaw droops and saliva droops from the mouth.
- Paralysis, convulsions and death follow.
- The second type dumb rabies is the paralytic form in which the animal lies bundled, unable to feed.
- The dog may not bite but attempts to feed it are dangerous.

Diagnosis

- Rabies can be diagonised by observing the Negri bodies (mass of viruses or subunits of unassembled viruses) under light microscope.
- However, today diagnosis is done by direct immunofluorescent-antibody (DIFA) of brain tissue.
- Isolation of viral particles.
- Testing the Negri bodies
- Rapid enzyme-mediated immuno diagnosis test.

Following tests are done in the lab:

1. **Demonstration of rabies virus Ag by immunoflouroscence**
   - It is more sensitive test than the visualization of negri bodies. The advantage of this test is it will give immediate result. Examination of salivary gland by immunofluorescence is useful. It may indicate whether the animal was shedding the virus in saliva.

2. **Demonstration of Inclusion bodies**
   - Impression smears of the brain are stained by seller's technique, which has the advantage that fixation and staining are done simultaneously.
   - Negri bodies are seen as interacytoplasmic, round or oval, purplish pink structures with characteristic, basorphilic inner granules.
   - Negri bodies vary in size from 3-27 μm.
   - If the impression smears are –ve the tissue should be sectioned and stained by Griemsa or mann's method.
   - Failure to find Negri bodies does not exclude the diagnosis of rabies.

Prophylaxis

Prophylaxis is generally employed after exposure to infection and is therefore called antirabic treatment. This consists of local treatment, antirabic vaccines and hyperimmune serum.

Classification of Vaccines

Neural Vaccines: They are of following

1. ***Simple Vaccines*:** It is a 5% suspension of sheep brain infected with fixed virus and inactivated with phenol at 37 °C leaving no residual like virus.
2. ***Beta propiolactone Vaccines*:** This is a modification of simple vaccine in which beta propiolactone is used as the inactivating agent instead of phenol.
3. ***Infant brain vaccines*:** The encephalitogenic factor in brain tissue is a basic protein associated with myelin. It is scanty or absent in the non-myelenated neural tissue of new born animals.

Non-Neural Vaccines

1. ***Egg Vaccines*:** Duck egg Vaccine prepared from a fixed virus adapted for growth in duck eggs and inactivated with b-propiolactone was used but was discontinued.
2. ***Tissue Culture Vaccines*:** The first cell culture vaccine was the human diploid cell (HDC) vaccine developed by Koprowsky.
   - It is purified and concentrated preparations of fixed rabies virus.
3. ***Sub-Unit Vaccines*:** The glycoprotein subunit on the virus surface, which is the protectivating Ag, has been cloned and r.vaccines produced.

Vaccination Schedule: It includes three classes:

Class I

(a) Patients in whom the risk is estimated to be slight. These include: a-licks, including direct contact with saliva, fresh cuts or abrasion on all parts of the body except the head, face, neck or fingers.

(b) Licks on intact mucous membrane.
(c) Bites or Scratches which have raised the epidermis but have not drawn blood, on all parts of the body except the head, face, neck or fingers,
(d) Consumption of unboiled milk.

Class II

(a) Persons who are estimated to be at moderate risk.
(b) All bites or scratches on the fingers which are not lacerated, not more than half a cm long and have penetrated the true skin.
(c) Bites or scratches on all parts of the body except the head, face, neck or fingers.

Class III

(a) Person in whom the risk is estimated to be great. These include licks on definitely remembered fresh cuts or abrasions on head, face or neck.
(b) All bites or scratches on the head, face or neck.
(c) All bites or scratches on the fingers which are more than ½ cm long or have penetrated into the true skin.
(d) All bites penetrating the true skin and drawing blood, when there are 5 teeth marks or more.
(e) All bites on any part of the body causing extensive laceration.
(f) All jackal and wolf bites.
(g) Any class-II patient who has not received treatment within 14 days of exposure.

The recommended schedule of vaccination for the different classes is as follows:

	Simple Vaccine	BPL Vaccine
Class I	2 ml × 7 days	2 ml × 7 days
Class II	5 ml × 14 days	3 ml × 10 days
Class III	10 ml × 14 days	5 ml × 10 days

Prevention and Control

Prevention and control of rabies involve pre-exposure vaccination of dogs and cats and post exposure vaccination of humans.

Treatment

Until recently rabies was considered to be invariably fatal and no serious attempt at treatment was made, apart from sedation.

- It has odour from established rabies with intensive supportive case and management of complications.
- No, specific antirabies agent is available.

7.5.21 Plague

Plague occurs primarily in wild ground squirrels, chipmunks, mice and prairie dogs. The disease is caused by the gram-negative bacterium *Yersinia pestis*.

Symptoms: Fever, chills, headaches, extreme exhaustion, appearance of enlarged lymph nodes called buboes (bubonic plague)

- In 50 to 70% of the untreated cases, death follows in 3 to 5 days from toxic conditions caused by the large number of bacilli in the blood.

Mode of Transmission

- It is transmitted form rodent to human by the bite of on infected flea.
- Direct contact with infected animals or their products, or inhalation of contaminated airborne droplets.
- Initially spread by contact with flea-infested animals, *Y. pestis* can spread among people by airborne transmission.
- Once in the human body, the bacteria multiply in the blood and lymph.
- An important factor in the virulence of *Y. pestis* is its ability to survive and proliferate inside phagocytic cells rather than being killed by them.

Epidemiology of Plague

- The epidemiology of plague is complex. Plague is mainly a disease of wild rodents and is spread from animal to animal by fleas.
- Human plague epidemics follow a sequence of events.
- Domestic rats i.e., rats that share human habitations, contract plague via fleas from infected wild rodents.
- The blood of infected rats contains large numbers of plague bacilli.
- When a rat flea ingests this contaminated blood, the action of a bacterial coagulase may cause a clot to form in the insect's proventriculus. This blockage prevents the access of food to the midgut (stomach) of the insect, and a flea in this condition becomes very hungry.
- As the rat hosts die, the fleas leave the corpses and begin to attack human hosts.
- Because of the blockage of the proventriculus, the human blood that is ingested by a flea becomes mixed with *plague bacilli*.

Bubonic plague: The bubonic form is characterized by chills, fever, nausea, vomiting, general weakness and enlarged inflamed lymph glands (bubos).

- Once a human contracts bubonic plague, the disease can be transmitted from person to person via human fleas or human lice.
- In some bubonic plague, patients, the bacilli may reach the lungs and establish a pneumonia (pneumonic plague). This form of plague is highly contagious because it can be transmitted from person to person via aerosols and is no longer dependent on arthropods.

Diagnosis

- Direct microscopic examination.
- Culture of the bacterium.
- Serological tests.
- Identity confirmation of *Yersinia pestis* by PCR.

Treatment

Streptomycin is effective for treatment of plague.

Chloramphenicol or tetracycline can also be used.

Prevention

- Prevention of plague can be achieved by control measures.
- Control of plague depends first upon control and elimination of domestic rats and rat fleas.
- Other preventive measures include immunization grams and elimination of human fleas and lice.

Essay Questions

1. Write a note on activity of various disease causing agents.
2. Write a note on Epidemiology of various micro-organisms.
3. Explain the various modes of various modes of pathogens actions.
4. Explain the diagnostic procedures of the specific pathogens through various culture findings.
5. Write a note on various treatment strategies and prevention of the pathologic invasion of the microbes.

Multiple Choice Questions

1. The most active motile and freely formed pathogenic form to humans is
   (a) Trophozoid form
   (b) Precystic form
   (c) Cystic form
   (d) Minuta form
2. The virus which generally infects humans and pigs and can cause severe illness and local epidemics is
   (a) Influenza a virus
   (b) Influenza b virus
   (c) Influenza c virus
   (d) Influenza d virus

3. Neuraimidase inhibitors among the following are
   (a) Oseltamivir
   (b) Salanquir
   (c) Rotanavir
   (d) Lopinavir
4. Serum hepatitis is caused by
   (a) HAV (b) HBV
   (c) HCV (d) HDV
5. Subcutaneous filarisis is caused by
   (a) Wuchereria bancrofti
   (b) Mansonella streptocera
   (c) Brugia timori
   (d) Mansonella ozardi

Answers

1. (a)	2. (c)	3. (a)
4. (b)	5. (b)	

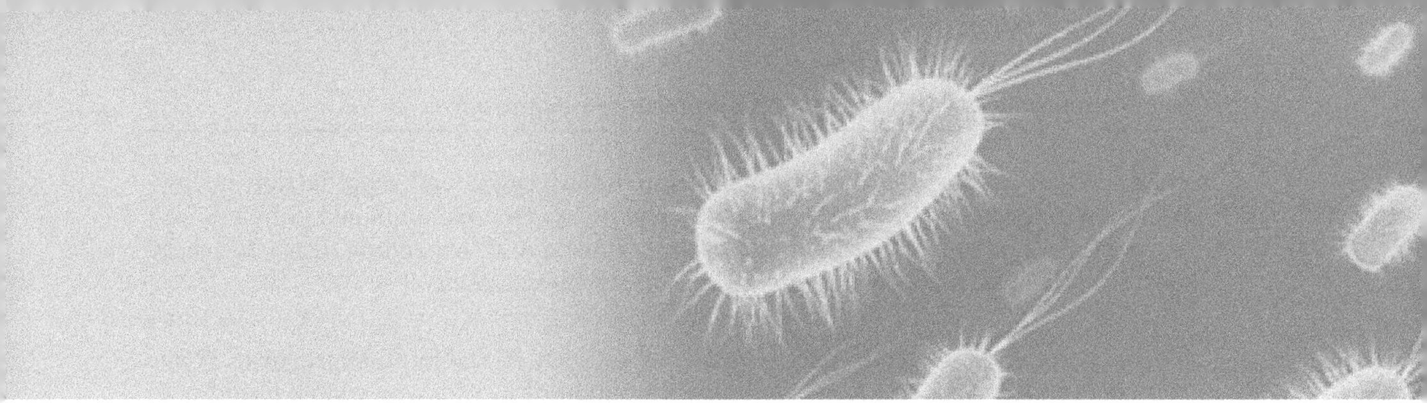

8 MICRO-ORGANISMS AND THEIR ENVIRONMENT

LEARNING OBJECTIVES

After studying the chapter the students familiarize themselves with concepts in:

- *Understanding the effect of Hydrostatic pressure on micro-organisms*
- *Understanding the effect of radiation action in the inactivation of micro-organisms*
- *Understanding osmosis in Preservation of foods from microbial contamination*
- *Understanding the role of oxygenases in inhibiting the growth of aerobic micro-organisms*
- *Developing an insight on the effects of vibration in causing fragmentation and lysis of micro-organisms by agitation.*
- *Understanding the Ionic effect and its mode of action in inhibiting the growth of micro-organisms*
- *Understanding the microbial adaptations to environmental conditions*

8.1 Microbial Growth in Natural Environments

Micro-organisms in a particular location are exposed to many overlapping gradients of nutrients and various other environmental factors. Micro-organisms will grow in 'microenvironments' until an environmental or nutritional factor limits growth. Liebig's law of minimum states that the total biomass of an organism will be determined by the nutrient present in the lowest concentration relative to the organisms requirements. Shelford's law of tolerance states that there are limits to environmental factors, below and above which a microorganism cannot survive and grow, regardless of the nutrient supply. Each organism has a specific temperature, pH, oxygen level and hydrostatic pressure to grow. The growth of a microorganism depends on both the nutrient supply and its tolerance of the environmental conditions. In response to low nutrient levels (oligotrophic environments) and intense competition, many micro-organisms become more competitive in nutrient capture and exploitation of available resources. Morphology of the organism can change in order to increase its surface area and ability to absorb nutrients. Micro-organisms can also undergo step by step shut down of metabolism except for housekeeping genes.

Natural substances can also directly inhibit microbial growth and reproduction in low-nutrient environments. These agents include phenolics, tannins, ammonia, ethylene etc. This may be a means by which micro-organisms avoid expending limited energy resources until an adequate supply of nutrients becomes available.

Growth of natural prokaryotic populations outside the laboratory can be determined by counting the number of viable micro-organisms present. A viable microorganism is one that is able to grow actively, resulting in the formation of a colony or visible turbidity in liquid medium. John R. Postgate of University of Sussex in England was one of the first to note that micro-organisms stressed by survival in natural habitats were sensitive to secondary stresses. Such stresses can produce viable micro-organisms that have lost the ability to grow on media normally used for their cultivation. To determine the growth potential of such microorganism, Postgate micro viability assay, in which micro-organisms are cultured in the thin agar film under a cover slip. The ability of a cell to change its morphology, even if it does not grow beyond the single stage indicates that the microorganism does show life signs.

The situation in natural environments with mixed populations is much more complex. Often only 1 to 10% of observable cells are able to form colonies. The microbiologist is attempting to grow micro-organisms that perhaps never have been cultured or characterized. At present, molecular techniques involving PCR amplification and small subunit ribosomal RNA analysis are increasingly used to analyze diversity of uncultured microbial population.

8.2 Different Factors that Affect the Microbial Growth

Temperature

- Oxygen
- Desiccation
- Extreme cold
- Ionic effect
- Electricity
- Osmotic pressure
- Radiant energy
- Hydrostatic pressure
- Mechanical impact
- Vibration

8.2.1 Temperature

Environmental temperature profoundly affects micro-organisms like all other organisms. The most important factor influencing the effect of temperature on growth is the temperature sensitivity of enzyme catalyzed reactions. Each enzyme has a temperature at which it functions optimally.

***At very low temperature*:** Microbial membranes solidify.

***At very high temperature*:** Lipid bilayer melts and disintegrates.

- When organisms are above their optimum temperature, both function and cell structure are affected. Microbial growth has a fairly characteristic temperature dependence with distinct cardinal temperature – maximum, optimum and minimum growth temperature. The optimum temperature ranges from 0 °C to 75 °C.
- Microbial growth occurs at temperatures extending from less than – 20 °C to over 120 °C.
- Some archea can grow up to 121 °C, the temperature normally used in autoclaves.
- The cardinal temperatures are not fixed; they also depend upon pH and available nutrients.
- Some fungi can grow at temperatures as high as 55 to 60 °C.
- Prokaryotes can grow at much higher temperature the eukaryotes.
- For example *Crithidia fasciculate*, a flagellated protist living in the gut of mosquitoes will grow in a simple medium at 22-27 °C. However it cannot be cultured at 33-34 °C without the addition of extra metals, amino acids, vitamins and lipids.
- Micro-organisms can be placed in various classes based on their temperature ranges.

The relation between temperature and growth is given in Fig. 8.1 and Fig. 8.5.

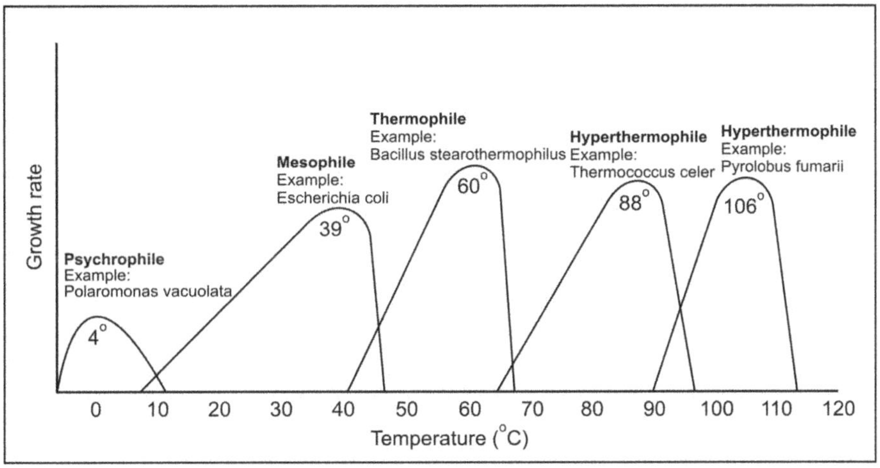

Fig. 8.1 The relations between temperature and growth

(a) ***Psychrophiles or cryophiles*:** These micro-organisms are numerically dominant in bottom sea sediments, sea ice, surface water and melt pools of the polar oceans. They grow well at 0 °C or lower and have an optimum temperature of 15 °C. Isolates from Arctic sediments (Knoblauch et al., 1999). Psychrophiles cardinal growth temperatures:

Minimum: at or below 0 °C

Optimum: 15 °C

Maximum: 20 °C

The micro-organisms with higher growth optimum and maximum were called Psychrotrophic. Now the term Psychotrophic is changed to Psychrotolerant. *e.g., Desulfobacter hydrogenophilus* (Widdel, 1987). Psychrophiles cover a wide range of phylogenetic diversity i.e., they have the representatives in important functional groups like methanotrophs, sulfate reducers and methanogens.

(b) ***Facultative Psychrophiles*:** They can grow at 0 to 7 °C and have an optimum temperature between 20 and 30 °C.

(c) ***Mesophiles*:** These are micro-organisms with growth optima around 20 to 45 °C.

(d) ***Thermophiles*:** They can grow at temperatures of 55 °C or higher and growth optima 55 and 65 °C. Most isolated Sulfate Reducing Bacteria (SRB) Beijerink, 1895.

(e) ***Hyperthermophiles*:** These grow at 90 °C or above and has growth optima between 80 °C and about 113 °C.

Differences between psychrophiles and psychrotolerants:

Psychrophiles

Psychrotolerants

(Permantly cold sediments)

(Moderate climate)

1. Exhibited constant fatty acid composition with high amounts of unsaturated or short-chain fatty acids.
2. These are "specialists "in a small temperature range, in which they probably outcompete mesophilic/psychrotolerant species.
3. Change the ratio of saturated, unsaturated and cyclopropane containg fatty acids with changing temperature via *de novo* synthesis.
4. These are "generalists", which probably outcompete psychrophiles in environments with changing temperatures

Cold adaptations of micro-organisms

- Effects on growth rate and growth yield
- Metabolic activity

- Protein flexibility and cold-adapted enzymes
- Protein synthesis and cold-induced proteins
- Effects on membrane and lipid structure

Most of the micro-organisms fall under mesophilic category

- The important adaptations that micro-organisms do at high temperature are stabilization of enzymes and nucleic acids and an increase in the melting point of lipids.
- With DNA, the stabilization can be accounted by an increase in the guanine plus cytosine content with their strong hydrogen bonding and a corresponding increase in adenine plus thiamine.
- Lipids of plants, animals and micro-organisms have long been known to vary in composition with the environment temperature. This is another essential adaptation.
- The organisms growing at lower temperature usually have their entire growth range shifted downward.
- It has been proved that protein synthesis both *in vivo* and *in vitro* is reduced when the temperature approaches the maximum. The same system appears to be limiting when tested at minimum temperature for growth.
- Temperature adaptation is possible in Sulfate Reducing Bacteria (SRB)
- Dissimilatory sulfate-reduction occurs between –1.8 °C (arctic sediment) and above 100 °C (Guaymas basin sediment) Fig. 8.4 shows different biomolecules in bacterial cell.

8.2.2 Hydrostatic Pressure

Most organisms on land or on the surface of water are always subjected to a pressure of 1 atm. The hydrostatic can reach 600 to 1100 atm in the deep sea. Despite these extremes, bacteria survive and adapt. Many are barotolerant. Some bacteria in the gut of deep sea invertebrates such as amphipods and holothurians are truly barophilic and grow more rapidly at high pressures (Ex. *Photobacterium, Shewanella, Colwellia*).

- Hydrostatic pressure has been shown to exert a marked effect on the growth of a number of representative species of bacteria. There are striking differences in the Hydrostatic pressure of surface waters and of water in oceanic depths. Hydrostatic pressure affects chemical equilibrium, which in turn, results in lowering the pH of seawater, resulting in a change in the solubility of nutrients such as bicarbonate, HCO_3^-. Growth of most of the species was visibly retarded by a hydrostatic pressure of 400 atm, and plate counts indicated that growth was slower and death faster at only 300 atm than at normal pressure. High hydrostatic pressures also inhibited the action of enzymes. Hydrostatic pressure increases with depth at the rate of 1 atm per

10 m. Barophilic micro-organisms are the organisms which cannot grow at normal atmospheric pressures, have been isolated from pacific trenches, where enormous hydrostatic pressure exist, and the pressure is measured in tons per square inch. Hydrostatic pressure of the deep sea is an important factor in the occurrence and growth of marine micro-organisms in this environment (Fig. 8.2).

- Haight and Morita reported that the enzyme aspartase isolated from *E.coil* also was inactivated by high pressures. *Escherichia coli* mutants resistant to inactivation by high hydrostatic pressure.
- In general, barophilic bacteria grow best at pressures slightly less than the pressure of the site from which they were isolated, and almost all must be grown under psychrophilic conditions (about 2 °C).
- ***Barophilic micro-organisms*** are adapted to high pressures e.g., higher amount of unsaturated fatty acids within their membrane, or modified enzymes.
- ***Adaptation of membrane lipids:*** Pressurized cultures show higher percentage of unsaturated fatty acids

Pressure

High pressures have an influence on:

- Boiling point and viscosity of water
- Membrane fluidity
- Stability of certain biomolecules

8.2.3 Desiccation

Desiccation of the microbial cell causes a cessation of metabolic activity, followed by decline in the total viable population. In general, the time of survival of micro-organisms after desiccation varies, depending on the following factors:

1. The kind of microorganism.
2. The material in or on which the organisms are dried.
3. The completeness of the drying process.
4. The physical conditions to which the dried organisms are exposed eg: light, temperature and humidity.

Species of Gram-negative cocci such as *Gonococci* and *Meningococcal* are very sensitive to desiccation; they die in a matter of hours.

- *Streptococci* are much more resistant.
- Viruses are usually found to be quite resistant to desiccation.
- The *Tubercle bacillus* dried in sputum remains visible for even longer periods of time.

- Dried spores of micro-organisms are known to remain viable indefinitely.
- In the process of lyophilization, organisms are subjected to extreme dehydration in the frozen state and then sealed in a vacuum. In this condition, desiccated (lyophilized) cultures of micro-organisms remain viable for many years. Spores are more resistant to desiccation than vegetative cells. Capsulated organisms are more resistant to drying than non-capsulated organisms. Organisms in the desiccated state are not capable of multiplication; moisture is necessary for this to occur. Young cells are more resistant to desiccation than old cells. Death of bacteria by dry heat is believed to be the result of desiccation followed by oxidation.

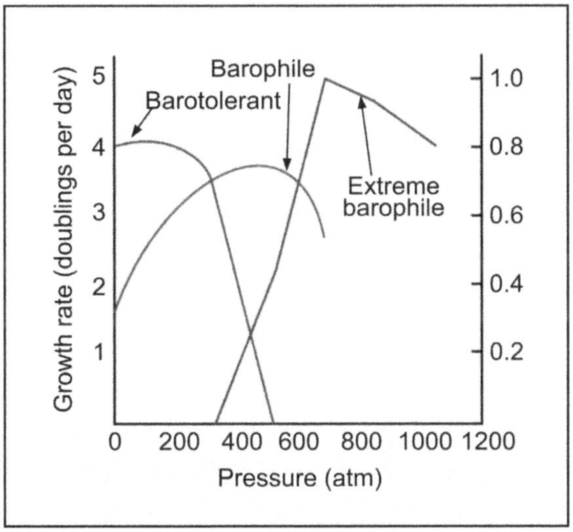

Fig. 8.2 The relations between pressure and growth rate

8.2.4 Osmotic Pressure

- Osmotic pressure refers to the pressure which develops when two solutions of different concentrations are separated by a semipermeable membrane. Passage of water; occur through the membrane, in the direction of the higher concentration. The trend is towards equalizing the concentration of solute on both sides of a membrane. The solute concentration within microbial cells is approximately 0.95%. If the cells are exposed to solutions with higher solute concentration, water will be drawn out of the cell. The process is called plasmolysis.
- The reverse process, that is passage of water from a low solute concentration into the cell, is termed plasmoptysis.
- In an extremely hypertonic environment due to the presence of these substances (salts and sugars) at high concentrations that enables water to leave the microbial cell precisely shown in Fig. 8.7.

- Preservation of food products like pickles, fruits by the use of high concentrations of salts and sugars which eventually exert their effects on account of the osmotic pressure.
- The fundamental principle of osmotic pressure is largely exploited in the prolonged preservation of food products.

Examples

(a) Concentrated salt solutions (Brine solution) may be used profusely in the preservation and cure of meats, fish, vegetables, pickles etc.

(b) Concentrated sugar solutions (sugar syrup) may be employed, extensively in the preservation of lime juice, fruits etc.

Zimmerman (1969) reported that dilute solutions of salts (0.017 N) did not cause cells of *Serratia marcescens* to lose water whereas stronger solutions (1.71 N) markedly reduced the weight and water content of centrifugally packed cells. He concluded that:

1. The cells lost weight and water to concentrated salt solutions through a non-osmotic competitive dehydration, causing shrinkage of the protoplasmic gel. The cell wall was too rigid to show any appreciable shrinkage. Therefore a space appeared between the cell wall and cytoplasmic membrane.
2. Cells may have equilibrated their water activity with that of their environment by two mechanisms, namely, the loss of water by plasmolysis or competitive dehydration, and alteration in cell permeability.
   - Scheie found cells of *E.coil* to be plasmolysed in sucrose solutions.
   - Bacteria are sensitive to osmotic effects but to a lesser extent than plant and animal cells.
   - A greater increase in the osmotic pressure of the surrounding solution is necessary before any destructive action on bacteria is observed.
   - The use of high osmotic pressure finds practical application in the preservation of some foods from attack by fungi.

8.2.5 Oxygen

- The importance of oxygen to the growth of an organism correlates with its metabolism. Almost all energy conserving metabolic processes involve the movement of electrons through an electron transport system. For chemotrophs, an externally supplied terminal electron acceptor is critical to the functioning of the electron transport system. The nature of the terminal electron acceptor is related to an organism's oxygen requirement.

- An organism which grows in the presence of atmospheric oxygen is an aerobe, whereas one that can grow in the absence of atmospheric oxygen is an anaerobe. All multicellular organisms are completely dependent on atmospheric O_2 for growth, they are obligate aerobes. Oxygen serves as the terminal electron acceptor for the electron transport chain in aerobic respiration.
- Aerobic eukaryotes employ oxygen in the synthesis of sterols and unsaturated fatty acids. Facultative anaerobes do not require oxygen for growth but grow better in its presence. In the presence of oxygen they use aerobic respiration.
- Aerotolerant anaerobes such as *Enterococcus faecalis* simply ignore O_2 and grow equally well whether it is present or not.

The Role of Oxygenases in Aerobic Micro-organisms

- Although the primary metabolic function of O_2 in strict aerobes is to serve as a terminal electron acceptor, it also serves as a co substrate for enzymes that catalyzes some steps in assimilation of aromatic compounds and alkanes. These enzymes are termed as oxygenases.

  e.g., Oxygenative ring cleavage of catechol, an intermediate in the assimilation of many aromatic compounds.

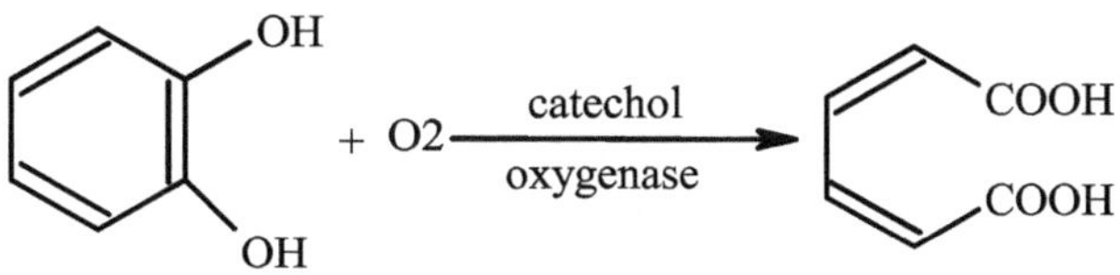

- Many aerobic *Pseudomonades* that are able to use aromatic compounds or alkanes as sole source of carbon and energy are called denitrifying bacteria.

  Oxygen accepts electrons and is readily reduced because its outer orbital electrons are unpaired

$$O_2 + e^- \rightarrow O_2^{\overline{\cdot}} \text{ (Superoxide radical)}$$

$$O_2^{\overline{\cdot}} + e^- + 2H^+ \rightarrow H_2O_2 \text{ (Hydrogen peroxide)}$$

$$H_2O_2 + e^- + H^+ \rightarrow H_2O + OH\cdot \text{ (Hydroxyl radical)}$$

  These products of oxygen reduction are extremely toxic because they oxidize and rapidly destroy cellular constituents. A microorganism must be able to protect itself against such oxygen products or it will be killed.

- Many micro-organisms possess enzyme that afford protection against toxic O_2 products.

- Obligate aerobes and facultative anaerobes usually contain the enzymes superoxide dismutase and catalase, which catalyze the destruction of peroxide radical and hydrogen peroxide.

$$2O_2^{\overline{\cdot}} + 2H^+ \xrightarrow{\text{superoxide dismutase}} O_2 + H_2O_2$$

$$2H_2O_2 \xrightarrow{\text{catalase}} 2H_2O + O_2$$

$$H_2O_2 + NADH + H^+ \xrightarrow{\text{peroxidase}} 2H_2O + NAD^+$$

- Aerotolerant micro-organisms may lack catalase but almost always have superoxide dismutase.
- The aerotolerant *Lactobacillus* uses manganous ions instead of superoxide dismutase to destroy superoxide radical.
- All strict anaerobes lack both enzymes or have them in very low concentrations and therefore cannot tolerate oxygen.

8.2.6 Effect of Vibration

Micro-organisms can be killed by agitation with various substances.

- Curar and Evans agitated bacterial and spore suspensions with glass beads, sand carborundum and obtained large reduction in viable counts.
- The cells were killed by fragmentation. Recovery was not possible unless damage was slight. It is reasonable to suppose that recovery occurs only when the nucleus or nuclear material remains uninjured.

8.2.7 Ionic Effect

Quaternary Ammonium Compounds

- Most compounds of the germicidal cationic detergent class are quaternary ammonium salts. The R_1 R_2 R_3 and R_4 groups are carbon groups linked to the nitrogen atom.
- The bactericidal power of the quaternaries is exceptionally high against gram +ve bacteria, they are also quiet active against gram – ve organisms.
- Quaternaries have been shown to be fungicidal as well as destructive to certain of the pathogenic protozoa. Viruses appear to be more resistant than bacteria and fungi.

Mode of Action

- A variety of damaging effects of quaternaries upon micro-organisms have been observed. These include denaturation of proteins, interference with glycolysis and membrane damage.

- Experimental evidence suggests that most likely site of the damage to the cell is the cytoplasmic membrane.
- Another important characteristic of quaternaries is the ability to manifest bacteriostatic action far beyond their bactericidal concentration.
- For example, the limit of bactericidal action for a given compound may be at a dilution of 1:30,000; yet it may be bacteriostatic in dilutions as high as 1:200,000. The action of these compounds demonstrates the need to distinguish between static and lethal activity in test procedures for the evaluation of disinfectants.

8.2.8 Radiant Energy

Electromagnetic radiations of various types have much impact in the environment. As the wavelength of electromagnetic radiation decreases, the energy of the radiation increases – gamma rays and X rays are much more energetic than visible light or infrared waves (Fig. 8.3). Sunlight is the major source of radiation on the earth. It includes visible light, ultraviolet radiation, infrared rays and radio waves. Most life is dependent on the ability of photosynthetic organisms to trap the light energy of the sun as visible light.

Many forms of electromagnetic radiation are very harmful to micro-organisms. Ionizing radiation, radiation of very short wavelength or high energy can cause atoms to lose electrons or ionize.

The two major forms of ionizing radiation, X rays which are artificially produced and gamma rays which are emitted during radioisotope decay. Low levels of ionizing radiation will produce mutations, higher levels are directly lethal.

Some prokaryotes like *Deinococcus radiodurans* and bacterial endospores are resistant and can cause a variety of changes in cells like; it breaks hydrogen bonds, oxidises double bonds, destroys ring structures and polymerizes some molecules. Oxygen enhances these destructive e effects, probably through the generation of hydroxyl radicals (OH.). Destruction of DNA is the most important cause of death of micro-organisms. Ultraviolet radiation kills all kinds of micro-organisms due to its short wavelength (approximately 10 to 400 nm) and high energy. The most lethal UV radiation has a wavelength of 260 nm, the wavelength most effectively absorbed by DNA. Formation of thymine dimmers in DNA is the primary mechanism of UV damage; these dimmers inhibit DNA replication and function. This damage is repaired by photo reactivation, where blue light is used by a photo reactivating enzyme (photolyase) to split the thymine dimmers. Dark reactivation, where a short sequence containing the thymine dimmers can also be excised and replaced in the absence of light. Damage can also be repaired by the recA protein in recombination repair and SOS repair.

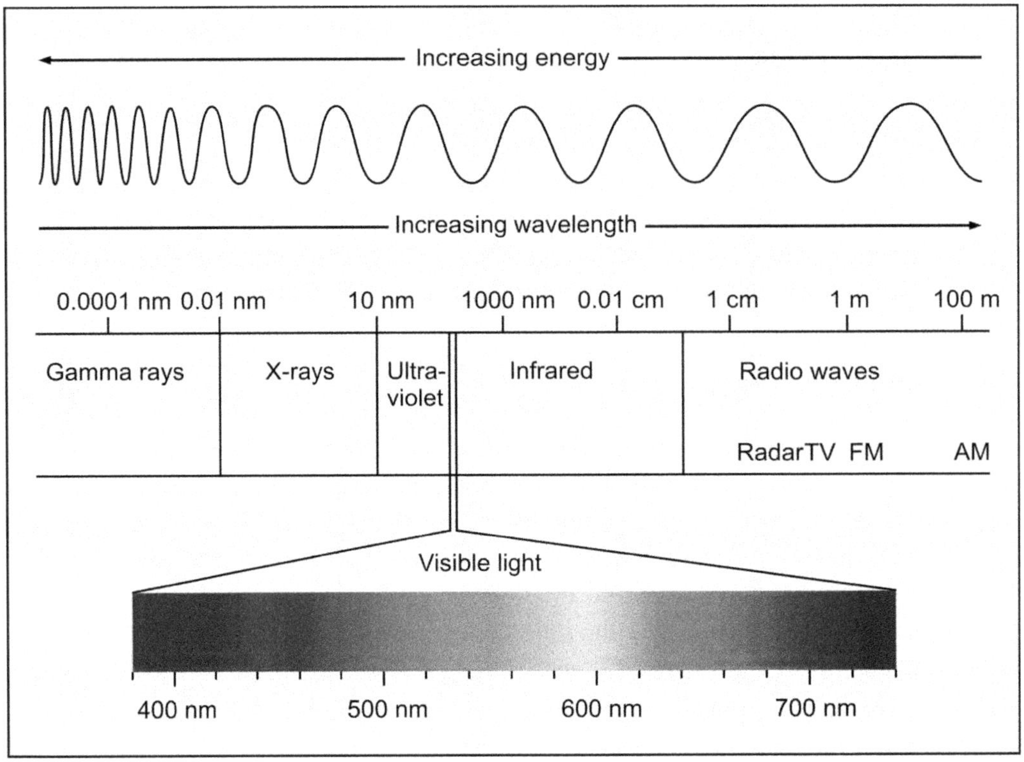

Fig. 8.3 Electromagnetic spectrum

Radiation energy is emitted in all directions from luminous bodies, radiographical tubes, particle accelerators, radioactive elements and fluorescent substances. Many forms of electromagnetic radiation are very harmful to micro-organisms. Inactivation of micro-organisms by UV radiation is principally a function of the radiant energy dose. The primary mechanism of microbial inactivation is the creation of thymidine dimers in DNA, which prevents replication. The most lethal UV radiation has a wavelength of 260 nm, the wavelength most effectively absorbed by DNA. Major causative effect of ionizing radiation being its distinct ability to the ionization of water, which in turn gives rise to highly reactive hydroxyl radicals. These radicals interact with the cellular organic components, especially the DNA, and thereby kill the cell ultimately.

Sunlight is the major source of radiation on the earth. It includes visible light, ultraviolet radiation, infrared rays and radio waves.

Visible light is immensely beneficial because it is the source of energy for photosynthesis. Yet even visible light when present in sufficient intensity can damages (or) kill microbial cells.

$P \xrightarrow{light} P(\text{activated})$ All micro-organisms possess pigments like chlorophyll, bacterio chlorophyll, cytochromes and flavins which can absorb light energy; become excited (or) activated and act as photosensitizer. The excited photosensitizer (P) transfer its energy to O_2 generating singlet oxygen ($^1O_2$)

$$P(\text{activated}) + O_2 \rightarrow P + {}^1O_2$$

8.2.9 Extreme Cold Environment

Extreme cold micro-organisms in glaciers and permanently frozen lakes

- Micro-organisms that reside in ice has remained frozen for thousands of years.
- Surprisingly, microbes within glaciers are not dormant.
- Life in these ecosystems depends on the photosynthetic activity of microbial psychrophiles.
- Lakes that lie below the glaciers are blocked from solar radiation. These communities are driven by chemosynthesis.
- Geothermal heating, pressure and insulation of the overlying ice keep these lakes in a liquid state.
- Oxygen concentration increases with depth due to increased oxygen solubility in cold waters and at a high pressure.
- The overlying ice also harbors similar micro-organisms at lower population densities.
- To know whether these microbial populations are active or not radioactive substrates were added to samples incubated at an Antarctic laboratory.
- The micro-organisms living in glaciers and frozen lakes involve novel and creative techniques.
- Microbes are protected from shorter wavelengths of UV light because they are absorbed by oxygen.
- Longer wavelengths of UV light are not absorbed by oxygen and so reach the earth surface. They can harm micro-organisms because they induce the breakdown of tryptophan to toxic photo products.
- One form of electromagnetic radiation is ionizing radiation. Although micro-organisms are more resistant to ionizing radiation than larger organisms, they will still be destroyed by a sufficiently large dose.
- Excessive exposure to UV light outstrips the organisms' ability to repair the damage and causes the death.
- Glaciers have traditionally been regarded as areas that do not contribute to global carbon budget.

8.2.10 Effects and Microbial Adaptations to Environmental Conditions

Adaptation to Environmental Conditions

Adaptation

All life is still based on organic molecules dissolved in water, and we all use the same basic cellular machinery. Extremophiles have not fundamentally changed the way and or strategies to look for life, but they have bolstered the optimism with which, liquid water is considered a possible habitat for all forms of life.

Extremophiles are defined as organisms living in extreme environment. Extreme environments are considered "hostile to higher forms of life" and uninhabitable by other organisms. Physico-chemical factors of the extreme environments effect the life of that area which is why there is a limited diversity and some groups of organisms are missing. Victor Shelford (1913) in his "law of tolerance", postulated that organism will usually be limited by abiotic factors. Each particular factor that an organism responds to in an ecological system has what he called limiting effects. The factors function within a range, that is, a maximum value and a minimum value for the factors exist, which Shelford designated "limits of tolerance". For an organism to succeed in a given environment each of a complex set of conditions must remain within the tolerance range of that organism, and if any condition exceeds the minimum or maximum tolerance of that organism, it will fail to thrive.

The environmental factors that affect growth are

- Cell structure and growth

Adaptations to environmental factors

- Cold adaptation in SRB
- Growth above 100 °C
- Temperature
- pH (Fig. 8.6 shows pH of some important materials)

pH and microbial growth

- pH range for growth limited to 2 units
- *Picrophilus oshimae* (pH 0.7-2)
- Sea water in general well buffered around pH 8
- Water availability

Water availability

Water activity, osmosis and halophiles

- All organisms require water
- Water content and substances dissolved in water
- Sea water contains about 3% NaCl
- Halophiles: salt-loving organisms

- Oxygen
- Pressure
- Light and radiation

(Energy & carbon source)

The factors affecting Growth are:

Transport

Biosynthesis

Maintenance of highly organized structure regulation, reproduction, and detoxification.

- Osmophiles: live in environments high in sugars
- Xerophiles: live in very dry environment

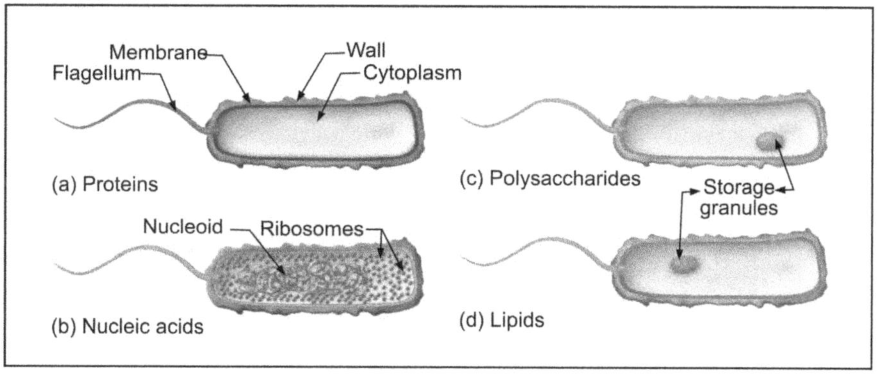

Fig. 8.4 Different biomolecules in bacterial cell

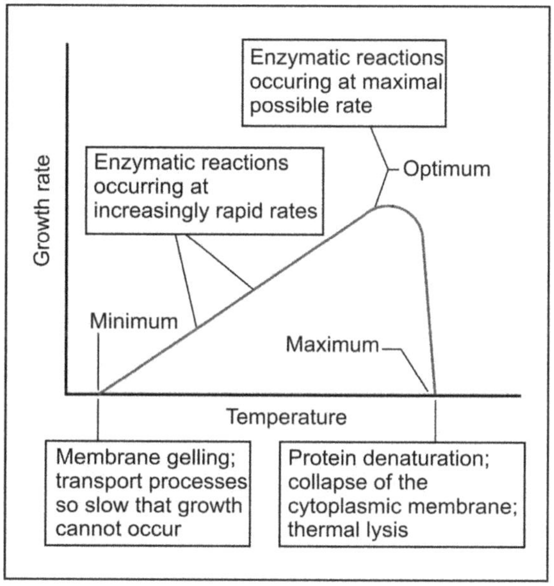

Fig. 8.5 The relation between temperature and growth rate

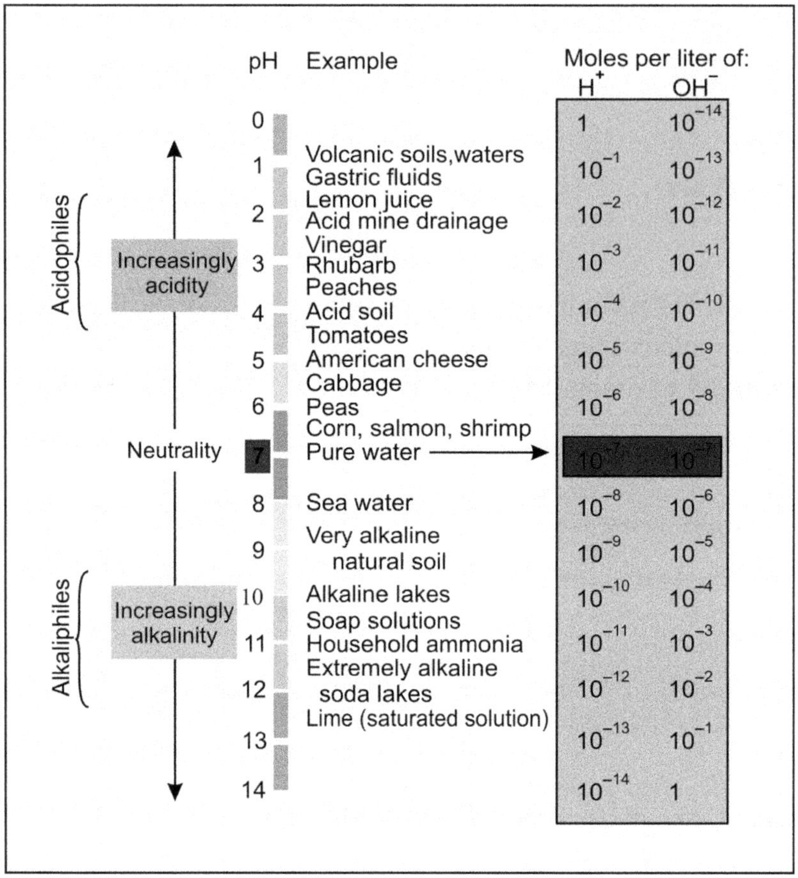

Fig. 8.6 pH of different materials

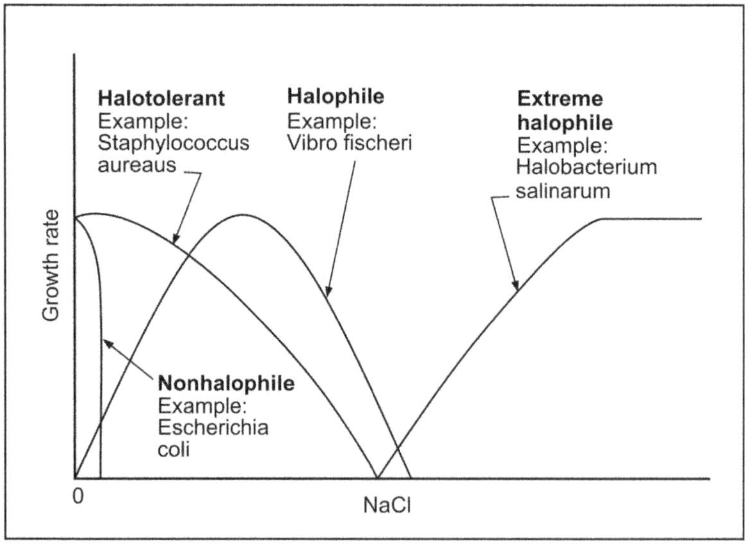

Fig. 8.7 Different groups of microbes basing on salt concentration

Toxic forms of Oxygen

(By-products during O_2 reduction)

$$O_2 + e^- \rightarrow O_2^- \quad \text{Superoxide}$$

$$O_2^- + e^- + 2H^+ \rightarrow H_2O_2 \quad \text{Hydrogen peroxide}$$

$$H_2O_2 + e^- + H^+ \rightarrow H_2O + OH \quad \text{Hydroxyl radical}$$

$$OH + e^- + H^+ \rightarrow H_2O \quad \text{Water}$$

$$\text{Overall: } O_2 + 4e^- + 4H^+ \rightarrow 2H_2O$$

(a) $H_2O_2 + H_2O_2 \rightarrow 2\,H_2O + O_2$

(b) $H_2O_2 + NADH + H^+ \rightarrow 2\,H_2O + NAD^+$

(c) Superoxide dismutase: $O_2^- + O_2^- + 2H^+ \rightarrow H_2O_2 + O_2$

(d) Superoxide dismutase/catalase in combination:

$$4O_2^- + 4H^+ \rightarrow 2\,H_2O + 3O_2$$

(e) Superoxide reductase: $O_2^- + 2H^+ + cyt\ c_{reduced} \rightarrow H_2O_2 + \text{cyt c}_{oxidized}$

8.2.11 Electricity

Wound healing, especially in people with diabetic neuropathies, can be extremely difficult to accomplish.

For example, of people who have diabetic ulcers on their feet, inability of wounds to heal causes an average amputation rate to be about 25%

Many diabetic ulcers and even decubitus ulcers can take months, years, or never heal a tall.

This inability of conventional medical practice to heal wounds has been termed "*a failure of the health care system*".

Even newer therapies such as myocutaneous flaps, water debridement, and other techniques have not increased the healing rate appreciably in the past fifty years or the rate of reoccurrence.

One modality that has been studied is electrical stimulation.

Many papers point to the use of electrical stimulation across wounds to increase wound healing. However, even this technology does not always work.

Some papers show wound healing with DC micro currents while others show only healing with strong AC currents. Some papers report that in the early stages of wound healing the polarity needs to be positive near the wound and negative away from the wound and other papers report the opposite.

In fact, in a summary of different studies on wound healing, Yarkony reported nothing conclusive in setting the intensity of currents, whether it was DC or AC stimulation or the frequency of electrical stimulation in the ability of electrical stimulation to heal wounds.

Recent evidence, however, links this disparity to possibly being linked to room temperature. Vasoconstriction of the circulation during treatment due to a cool or cold examination room blocks the blood flow increase due to electrical stimulation of the wound.

If the room is warmed, blood flow increases and wounds heal well with electrical stimulation.

Numerous mechanisms have been suggested on why electrical stimulation promotes wound healing including increased circulation, increased angiogenesis increased proliferation of epidermal tissue, and a bacteria static effect of electrical stimulation.

The possible bacteria static effect of electrical stimulation was first reported over 30 years ago by Rowley & McKenna. Using high voltage electrical stimulation (300 volts), bacteria (*E. coli*) died after a brief session of electrical stimulation. While a few studies have used similar voltages for clinical electrical stimulation of wounds most studies that report healing use a fraction of these voltages and currents. The stimulation voltages used by Rowley et al. would be extremely painful for the patient.

Further, since DC micro current has been shown, in some studies, to aid in healing of wounds, when the voltages used by Rowley and colleagues are compared to DC micro currents, they are thousands of times higher. Thus, the currents used in these studies were not clinically relevant and, therefore, the application of these studies to real life situations is questionable.

The present investigation was conducted to study the effect of electrical stimulation on bacterial growth (Fig. 8.8) in three common bacteria that are seen in wounds, *Escherichia coli, Pseudomonas aeruginosa,* and *Staphylococcus aureus*. These bacteria were grown in culture and then exposed to either DC microcurrent (100 μamps) or biphasic sine wave stimulation at 5 or 20 ma for 30 minutes. These currents are normal currents used in wound healing. Bacterial growth was then assessed after 24 hours of incubation to see if the normal currents that are used with electrical stimulation clinically to heal wounds can alter bacterial growth.

One of the mechanisms causing wounds to not heal is bacterial invasion. Bacteria rupture cell membranes and maintain chronic inflammation to prevent wound healing Many studies show that either DC microcurrent or low current AC stimulation has the ability to increase wound healing. In earlier studies, Rowley and colleagues published data showing that electrical stimulation has a bacteria static effect on *Escherichia coli* and several other bacteria. Barranco et al. showed inhibition in *Staphylococcus aureus* growth with 400μA DC stimulation. But the electrodes were metal and at 400 μamps, corrosion was noted. Other in vitro studies with 100 μA DC stimulation also showed a bacteria static effect but here silver electrodes were also used.

Other studies showed a bacteria static effect of DC at 1, 5, or 10 ma but not AC stimulation. These studies showed large changes in pH with DC stimulation, probably due to the fact that, unlike clinical situations where stimulation is a 30 minute modality, the current was left on for hours. This pH change was seen also with AC stimulation at 500 volts. But these studies were conducted in vitro with a small separation distance between the electrodes. Thus the current per mm of distance on the bacterial cultures were large. Further, metal ions like silver can kill bacteria in themselves.

In addition, these studies were conducted at very high stimulation voltages (over 300 volts). In wounds, nerve endings are sensitized by the release of cytokines. Even mild electrical stimulation can therefore be painful. In previous studies, the current used to heal wounds was less than 20 ma. Therefore this was the current used in these studies.

In the present investigations, the density of the broth, size of the chamber and size of electrodes were adjusted so that the electrodes were separated by the distance seen in a typical wound treatment. The impedance of the broth matched that of a human wound, about 1200 ohms between the electrodes. This, in itself, is different than previous studies where large current densities were seen due to high voltages being applied to small bacteria cultures. While we used a large chamber for the broth, the current density may have still been somewhat higher than in a limb due to the higher volume in a limb. However, while current density may have been somewhat higher than in a wound here, earlier in vitro studies used a fraction of the volume used here between the electrodes and electrodes were closer together making current density in e.g. Rowley et al much higher than in wounds.

When currents were applied in the present experiments for a 30 minute stimulation period, similar to a standard treatment period for wound healing, DC stimulation had no effect on bacteria growth. AC had some effect on each of the bacteria but the only real effect on growth with electrical stimulation was on pseudomonas. Any effect seen on *Escherichia E.coli and Staphylococcus aureus* was small. For *pseudomonas*, the growth reduction at either AC current was large.

However, bacteria can still be destroyed by electrical stimulation through another mechanism in wounds. Electrical stimulation and, electrical stimulation of wounds causes the release of prostaglandins and other cytokines. These prostaglandins and other cytokines attract macrophages to the area where electrical stimulation is applied. Therefore, although electrical stimulation may not have a direct effect on bacteria in wounds, there is some evidence that white blood cells such as macrophages are attracted as a secondary effect of the electrical stimulation, this may explain why electrical stimulation may be associated with bacterial death.

The present studies still remain in direct contradiction to the studies by Rowley et al showing a direct effect of electrical stimulation on inhibiting growth in *Escherichia coli.*

However, while *Escherichia E.coli* and *Staphylococcus aureus* showed either a statistically insignificant change in growth or an insignificant clinical change in growth with electrical stimulation, this is not to say that electrical current does not alter bacterial behavior.

Bacterial motility and attachment to substrates appears to be impaired by stimulation with electric currents. This is especially true for *pseudomonas* where flagella are needed for mobility. The fact that *pseudomonas* here did have some impaired growth may be due to the fact that there are two flagella proteins involved in its mobility and attachment- if either is impaired, growth is reduced. Here, these flagella, since they use contractile proteins and ion channels for movement, may be impaired with electric current. This makes these bacteria different from the other 2 which do not move by this mechanism.

However, there are conditions where electrical stimulation will inhibit growth in all 3 bacteria. While currents of up to 20ma in themselves with these same bacteria did not reduce bacterial growth, in combination with antibiotics, the reduced ability of the bacteria to attach to substrates made them more susceptible to attack by the antibiotics.

Thus while antibiotics alone or electrical stimulation alone did not kill these bacteria, the combination of the two did. Thus, electrical stimulation with either DC or weak AC currents may have an unseen effect which may kill bacteria in vivo but not under these circumstances in vitro. Further investigation is warranted. Here, for example, current was used for 30 minutes, a standard treatment modality. Perhaps longer exposure to current would have a more dramatic effect *in vivo*.

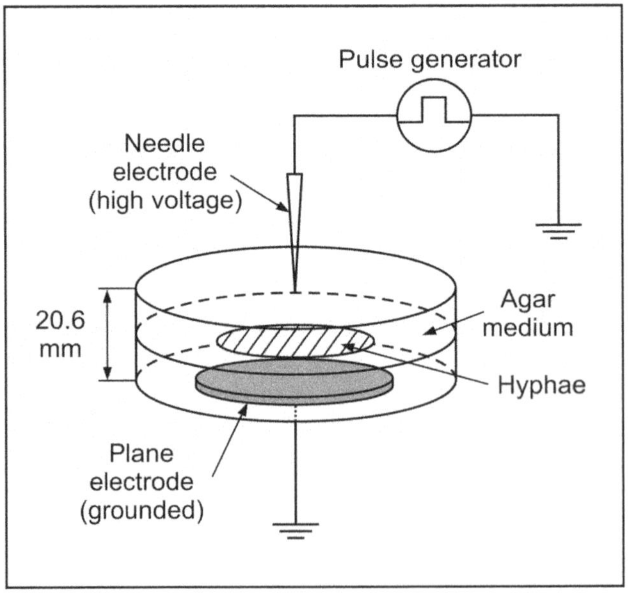

Fig. 8.8 Study of effect of electricity on micro-organisms

8.2.12 Mechanical Impact

Microbial stress due to the impaction of micro-organisms onto an agar collection surface was studied experimentally. The relative recovery rates of aerosolized *Pseudomonas fluorescens* and *Micrococcus luteus* were determined as a function of the impaction velocity by using a moving agar slide impactor operating over a flow rate range from 3.8 to 40 liters/min yielding impaction velocities from 24 to 250 m/s. As a reference, the sixth stage of the Andersen Six-Stage Viable Particle Sizing Sampler was used at its operating flow rate of 28.3 liters/min (24 m/s) (Fig. 8.9). At a collection efficiency of close to 100% for the agar slide impactor, an increase in sampling flow rate and, therefore, in impaction velocity produced a significant decline in the percentage of micro-organisms recovered. Conversely, when the collection efficiency was less than 100%, greater recovery and lower injury rates occurred. The highest relative rate of recovery (approximately 51% for *P. fluorescens* and approximately 62% for *M. luteus*) was obtained on the complete (Trypticase soy agar) medium at 40 and 24 m/s (6.4 and 3.8 liters/min), respectively. *M. luteus* demonstrated less damage than *P. fluorescens*, suggesting the hardy nature of the gram-positive strain versus that of the gram-negative microorganism. Comparison of results from the agar slide and Andersen impactors at the same sampling velocity showed that recovery and injury due to collection depends not only on the magnitude of the impaction velocity but also on the degree to which the micro-organisms may be embedded in the collection medium.

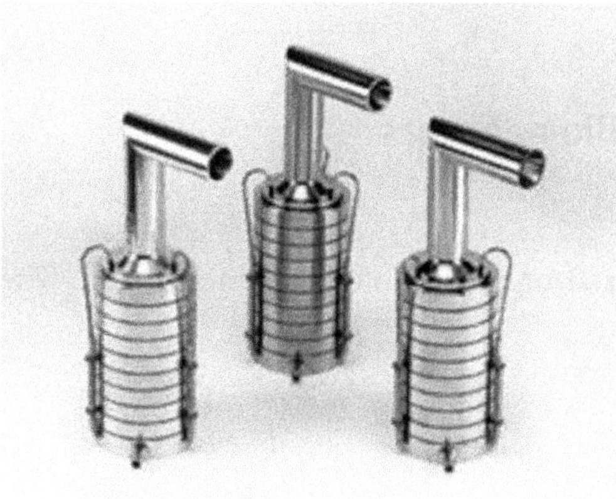

Fig. 8.9 Andersen impactors

Cascade impactors operate on the principle of inertial impaction. Each stage of the impactor comprises a series of nozzles or jets through which the sample laden air is drawn, directing any airborne towards the surface of the collection plate for that particular stage.

Whether a particular particle impacts on that stage is dependent on its aerodynamic diameter. Particles having sufficient inertia will impact on that particular stage collection plate, whilst smaller particles will remain entrained in the air stream and pass to the next stage where the process is repeated.

The stages are normally assembled in a stack or row in order of decreasing particle size. As the jets get smaller, the air velocity increases such that smaller particles are collected. At the end of the test, the particle mass relating to each stage is recovered using a suitable solvent and then analysed usually using HPLC to determine the amount of drug actually present.

8.3 Bioindicators

8.3.1 Introduction

Bioindicators are considered to be more reliable for the assessment of the status of the system over some chemical tests. The micro-organisms which exist in any environment are direct indicators of the conditions of that area. The types of micro-organisms are all a direct results of the nutrient concentration and environmental conditions. The functions of microbes in the environment, nutrient status and direct microscopic examination are used as a bioindication of the system.

In the event of pollution the physical and chemical structure of the system undergoes a change resulting in biota. Some species are sensitive to the changed situations while some are tolerant. The sensitive organisms therefore disappear and their place is taken by the tolerant species. This mode of identification of organisms indicates the degree of pollution.

8.3.2 Pharmaceutical Applications of Bioindicators

Methods

The degree of eco systems imbalance is measured only by biological information. The following criteria:

- Species composition
- Diversity of the species
- Distribution pattern
- The presence or absence of indicator organism.

Biologically each zone offers optimal conditions for certain species or communities or organisms which are known as "Indicator organisms" or "Indicator community".

The saprobic (it is a condition in which living things that are living in or being in an environment rich in organic matter but lacking oxygen) zones are classified as:

- Polysaprobic (gross pollution)
- α-mesosaprobic (heavy pollution)

- β-mesosaprobic (moderate pollution)
- Oligo saprobic less pollution (clean water)

Table 8.1 Indication of Organic Pollution

Genera	Pollution Index	Genera	Pollution Index
		Micractinum	01
Anacystis	01	Phacus	02
Ankistrodesmus	02	Navicula	03
Chlorella	03	Oscillatoria	04
Chlamydomonas	04	Synedra	02
Euglena	05	Nitzschia	03
		Stigeoclonium	02

If an algal sample has the genera *Chlorella, Oscillatoria, Stigeoclonium, Synedra, Nitzschia, Chlamydomonas and Navicula*, the score according to above list is 3 + 5 + 2 + 3 + 4 + 3 = 22. A score of 20 or more for a sample is an indication of organic pollution shown in Table 8.1. This confirms the high organic pollution of this water sample. A score of 15 to 19 is a probable of high organic pollution. Lower figures indicate that the organic pollution is not high.

Analytical Methods

Saprobic index: The Saprobic zones(S) are expressed as:

1. Oligosaprobic - S - 1
2. β -Mesosaprobic - S - 2
3. α -Mesosaprobic - S - 3
4. Polysaprobic - S - 4

The product of frequency (h) and saprobic zones(S) expresses the saprobic value.

- *Biotic Index:* The Biotic indices are developed on the basis of tolerance of the organisms to the various zones of pollution.

  $$B_1 = 2(\text{n class I}) + (\text{n class II})$$

  where n = no. of organisms in each class. In class I the organisms are little tolerant to organic pollution. In class II the organisms are tolerant to organic pollution but not to an aerobic conditions. The index value range between 0 to 10.

Gabriel used as index (I) based on the number of decomposers, B(bacteria), producers (P) algae etc., and consumers, C (ciliates etc.,)

$$I = 2P/(B + C)$$

Biological Index of pollution developed by Morasawa is estimated with the following formula.

$$BIP = [A/(A+B)] \times 100$$

Where A is the number of chlorophyll bearing organisms

B is the number of non chlorophyll bearing organisms

This concept of bioindication has originated from the recognition of fact that each species in the animal and plant community has specific and optimum ecological requirements for its best survival propagation and growth.

The basic interest of pollution is due to its effects on living organisms and hence the essesment of pollution is a biological problem. The physical and chemical data gives quantitative information while biological data only qualitative in nature hence in the establishment of the pollution status the physico-chemical was considered as ideal base for the biological analysis has been tedious and expensive. The degree of ecosystem imbalance is measured by

1. Species composition
2. Diversity of the species
3. Distribution pattern
4. The presense or the absence of indicator organisms.

- Bioindicators are organisms, chemical markers or biological processes whose change point can be observed to altered environmental conditions and can be used to identify and quantify the effects of pollutants on the environment.
- It can also be defined as anthropogenically induced response in biomolecular, biochemical and physiological effects on one or more organisms, population, community or ecosystem level of biological organization.
- Bioindicators can tell us about the cumulative effects of different pollutants in the ecosystem (Fig. 8.10) and about how long a problem may persist.

For example

A. Abundance of large marine organism or darkening of coral pigmentation may indicate that a reef has been exposed to poor quality of water for several weeks or months

B. Reduced photosynthesis in plants or coral may indicate stress due to exposure of herbicides.

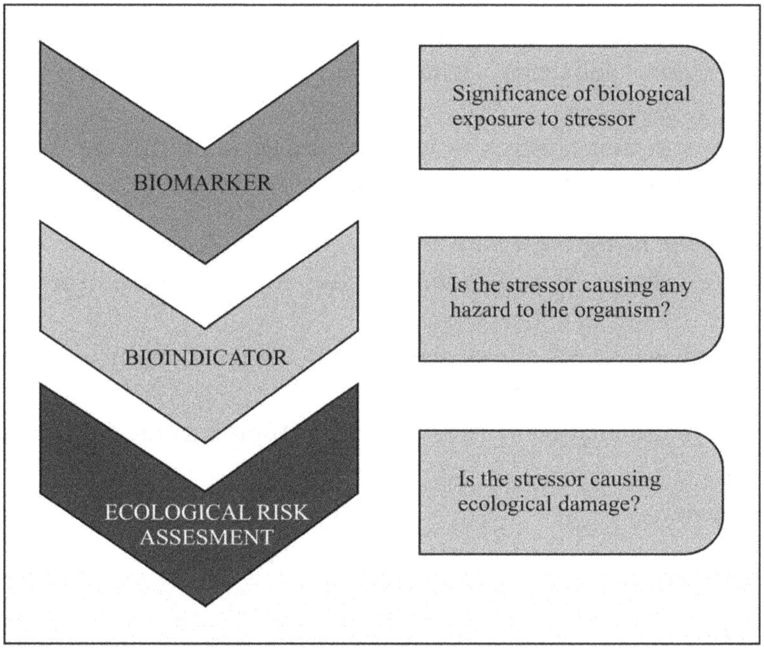

Fig. 8.10 Bioindicators and effect of pollutants on the environment

Criteria for Selecting Bioindicators

- Indicator should have casual relationship to ecological significant end point.
- Indicator should have specific dose responsiveness to specific stressor i.e., should be sensitive and specific
- Indicator should have wide temporal and spatial distribution.
- Indicator should be available all the year and should have low variability to noise in the system.
- Indicator should have results which are transparent and reproducible.
- Indicator should sometime even surrogate the role of other responses.
- Indicator should be easy to collect and should be cost-effective.

Types of Bio Indicators

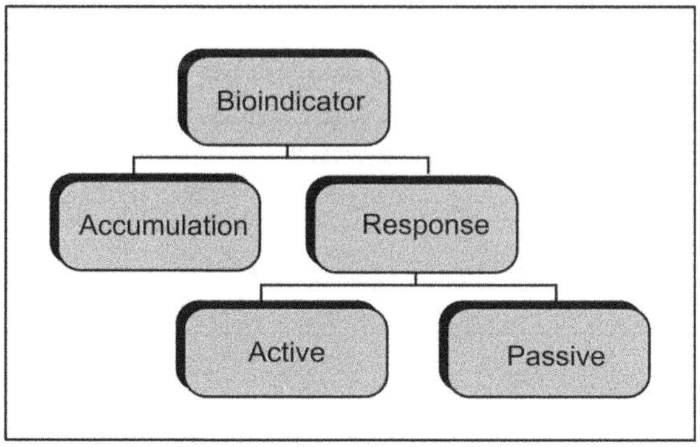

Fig. 8.11 Types of bioindicators

Bio indicators may be of two types

Accumulation bioindicator: Store pollutants without any evident changes in their metabolisms; shown in Fig. 8.11.

Response bioindicator: React with cell changes or visible symptoms of damage when taking up even small quantity of harmful substances.

Types of responses observed while using them may be

Ecological changes: Involving changes in population density, key species and species diversity;

Behavioral changes: Can be changes in feeding activities, bacterial mobility or web spinning;

Physiological changes: Can be accumulation of heavy metal, CO_2 production, BOD and microbial activity.

Micro-organisms as bioindicators

- Micro-organisms are diverse group of organisms found in large quantities and are easier to detect and sample.
- The presence of some micro-organisms is well correlated with particular type of pollution and it serves as standard indicator of pollution.
- Some bacteria produce stress proteins in response to contaminant like cadmium and benzene.

Bacterial characteristics for water analysis

- The indicator bacterium should be present whenever enteric pathogens are present.
- The indicator bacterium should not reproduce in contaminated water and produce inflated values.
- It should survive longer than the hardiest enteric pathogen.
- It should have greater specificity.
- Its detection assay should be easy to perform.
- It should be harmless to humans.
- Its level in water should have some direct relationship with faecal pollution.

Table 8.2 Some bio indicators indicating status of aquatic systems

Micro organism/bacteria	Status of aquatic system
Escherichia coli	Fecal origin
Streptococcus faecalis	do
Klebsiella	do
Clostridium perfringens	do

Table 8.2 *Contd...*

Micro organism/bacteria	Status of aquatic system
C.perfringens	Fecal origin
Spirillium volutants spores	Industrial chemicals and toxic chemical waste
Thiothrix	Effulent from oil refineries containing dehydrapen sulphide
Vogesella indigofera	heavy metal contamination
Vibrio harveyi	Mutagenic pollution

Bioluminescent bacteria as bioindicators

- Bioluminescent bacteria (Fig. 8.12): These are used to test water for environmental toxins
- If there are toxins present in the water, the cellular metabolism of bacteria is inhibited or disrupted
- This affects quality or amount of light emitted by bacteria
- It is very quick method and takes just 30 minutes complete but could not identify the toxin shown in Table 10.8.

Examples of such luminous bacteria include

- *Photobacterium fischeri, P. phosphor reum*

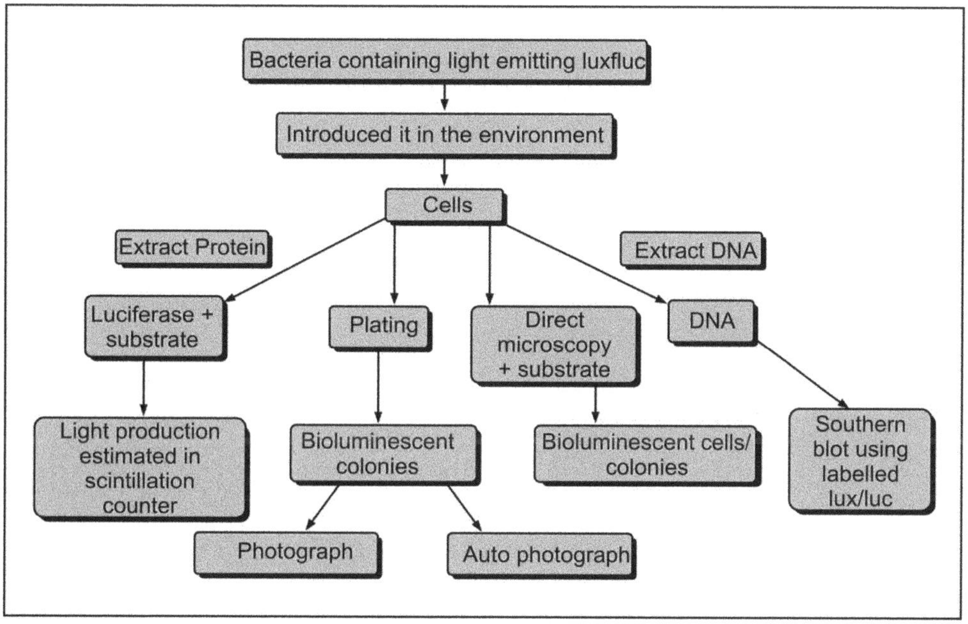

Fig. 8.12 Schematic diagram of assay to check for the presence of toxic contaminant using bioluminescent bacteria

Essay Questions

1. Write a note on the effect of Hydrostatic pressure on micro-organisms
2. Explain the effect of radiation action in the inactivation of micro-organisms
3. Explain the role of osmosis in Preservation of foods from microbial contamination
4. Explain the role of oxygenases in inhibiting the growth of aerobic micro-organisms
5. Write a note on effects of vibration in causing fragmentation and lysis of micro-organisms by agitation.
6. Explain the Ionic effect and its mode of action in inhibiting the growth of micro-organisms
7. Write a note on microbial adaptations to environmental conditions

Multiple Choice Questions

1. Which of the following aerotolerant uses manganese ions instead of superoxide dismutase to destroy superoxide radical
   (a) Lactobacillus
   (b) Enterococcus
   (c) Serratia
   (d) Streptococci
2. Micro-organisms growing at 55 °C to 65 °C are called
   (a) Thermopiles
   (b) Mesophiles
   (c) Psychrophiles
   (d) Facultative psychrophiles

Answers

1. (a) 2. (a)

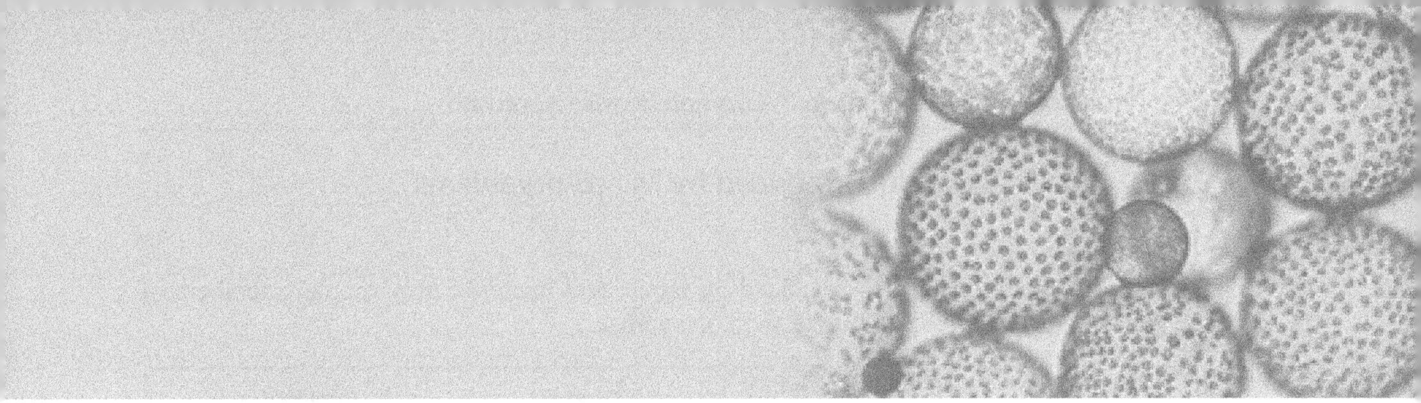

9 APPLICATIONS OF MICROBES IN PHARMACY

LEARNING OBJECTIVES

After studying the chapter the students familiarize themselves with concepts in:

- *Understanding Immunity against fungal infections*
- *Distinguishing pharmaceuticals produced by various micro-organisms*
- *Understanding pharmaceutical significance of bacteria, fungi and algae*

9.1 Introduction

Before recognizing the existence of micro-organisms in the universe, they were being used to produce useful products by human beings. Ancient civilizations had used yeast to make alcohol. Food products and beverages were also being produced by microorganism from ancient times. However, it took several thousands of years to recognize the role of microorganism in these processes. Scientific approaches and inventions in 19th century, paved the way for understanding the microbial role and evolving the branch of microbiology. In the industrial microbiology point of view micro-organisms are considered as mini chemical factories. Micro-organisms have the capacity to convert raw material into intermediate or end product. Since those microbial products are useful for human beings, people started exploiting microorganism for their needs. The major inventions in microbiology are discovery of antibiotics and manipulation of micro-organisms genetically (recombinant DNA technology) to produce new products followed by immunological products. Currently there is a wider contribution of microbiology to the pharmaceutical sciences. Specific pharmaceutical applications of major groups of micro-organisms are briefly introduced.

9.1.1 Pharmaceuticals produced by Micro-organisms

Dextran

Dextrans are polysaccharides produced by lactic acid bacteria, in particular members of the genus *Leuconostoc* following growth on sucrose.

Type of Dextran	Average Molecular Weight in Daltons	Product	Clinical Uses
Dextran 40	40,000	10% w/v in 5% w/v glucose injection or 0.9% w/v NaCl injection	*IV infusion*: improves blood flow and tissue function in burns and conditions associated with local ischaemia
Dextran 70	70,000	6% w/v in 5% w/v glucose injection or 0.9% w/v NaCl injection	*IV*: used to produce an expansion of plasma volume in conditions associated with loss of plasma proteins
Dextran 110	110,000	6% w/v in 5% w/v glucose injection or 0.9% w/v NaCl injection	*IV*: as for dextran 70
Iron dextran	5000-7500 (complex with ferric chloride)	Colloidal solution in 0.9% w/v NaCl injection	*Deep IM*: non-deficiency anaemia IV (slow infusion) = non-deficiency anaemia
Dextran sodium sulphate	–	Powder for preparing solution	Anticoagulant (I.V use of solution)
Chemically cross linked dextrans	–	–	*Water-insoluble*: Chromatographic techniques (fractionation and purification)

9.1.2 Vitamins, Amino Acids and Organic Acids

Pharmaceutical	Organism preferred for production industries	Use
Riboflavin (vitamin B_2)	*Eremothecium ashbyii, Ashbya gossypii*	Treatment of vitamin B_2 deficiency disease
Cyanocobalamin (vitamin B_{12})	*Propionibacterium freundenreichii* *Propionibacterium shermanii* *Pseudomonas denitrificans*	Treatment of pernicious anaemia

Contd...

Pharmaceutical	Organism preferred for production industries	Use
Amino acids e.g., glutamate, lysine	*Corynebacterium glutamicum, Brevi bacterium flavum*	Supplementation of feeds/food, IV infusion fluid constituents
Antibiotics e.g., Benzyl penicillin Gentamicin Nystatin	*Penicillium notatum,* *P. chrysogenum, Micromonospora purpurea, Streptomyces noursei*	Antibacterial drug antibacterial drug antifungal drug
Organic acids e.g., citric acid	*Aspergillus niger*	Effervescent products, sodium citrate used as an anticoagulant, potassium citrate used to treat cystitis
Lactic acid	*Lactobacillus delbrueckii, Rhizopus oryzae*	Calcium lactate is a convenient source of Ca^{+2} for oral administration; constituent of intraperitoneal dialysis solutions
Gluconic acid	*Gluconobacter suboxydans, Aspergillus niger*	Calcium gluconate is a source of Ca^{+2} for oral administration; gluconates used to render bases more soluble e.g., chlorhexidine gluconate

9.1.3 Enzymes

Name of Enzyme	Microbial Source	Uses
Diastase	*Aspergillus oryzae*	Manufacture of glucose, syrup, digestive aid
Acid-resistant amylase	*A. niger*	Digestive aid
Invertase	*S. careviseae*	Candy manufacture
Pectinase	*S. clerotinalibertina*	Clarification of fruit juices
Protease	*A. niger*	Digestive aid
Protease	*B. subtilis*	Detergents, removal of gelatine from photographic films to recover silver
Streptokinase	*Streptococcus* species	Promotes healing of wounds and burns

Contd...

Name of Enzyme	Microbial Source	Uses
Collogenase	*Clostridium histolyticum*	Promotes healing of wounds and burns
Lipase	*Rhizopus* species	Digestive aid
Cellulose	*Trichoderma konigi*	Digestive aid

Micro-organisms	Process	Product
Lactobacillus bulgaricus	Lactic acid fermentation	Buttermilk
L. bulgaricus + *Streptococcus thermophillus*	Lactic acid fermentation	Yogurt
Streptococcus lactis + *L. bulgaricus* + Lactose fermenting yeasts	Alcoholic and lactic acid fermentations	**Kefir** fermented milk drink made with kefir "grains" (ayeast/bacterial fermentation starter)
S. Lactis, S. Cremoris (various thermophilic lactic acid bacteria principally lactobacilli)	Initial lactic acid, fermentation temperature 35 °C	Cheeses
Various lactic acid bacteria within the cheese	Proteolysis and lipolysis	Hard cheeses e,g., cheddar and swiss
Surface growth initially of fungi (*geotrichum, candidum* and *pencillium species*) sometimes followed by *bacterium linens* and *Bacterium erythrogenes*	Proteolysis and lipolysis	Soft cheeses e.g., Camembert, Bric, limburges
Propionibacterium species	Propionic acid fermentation	
Penicillium roqueforti	Lipolysis and production of blue mold pigment	Roquefort (a soft cheese)

Micro-organisms have found wide spread uses in the performance of bioassays for

1. Determining the concentration of certain compounds (e.g., amino acids, vitamins and some antibiotics) in complex chemical mixtures or in body fluids.
2. Diagnosing certain diseases
3. Testing chemicals for potential mutagenicity or carcinogenicity
4. Monitoring purpose involving the use of immobilized enzymes
5. Sterility testing of antibiotics

9.2 Pharmaceutical Significance of Bacteria

Organism	Characteristics	Pharmaceutical relevance
Bacillus subtilis	Gram-positive rod, aerobic, spore former	Used to validate and monitor dry heat and ethylene oxide sterilization
Bacillus pumilis	Gram-positive rod, aerobic, spore former	Used to validate and monitor radiation sterilization process
Bordetella pertussis	Gram-negative rod, aerobe	Vaccine against Whooping cough
Clostridium tetani	Gram-positive, anaerobe, spore former	Vaccine against Tetanus
Corynebacterium diphtheriae	Gram-positive, aerobe	Vaccine against diphtheria
Haemophilus influenza type b	Gram-negative enteric rod, aerobe	Vaccine against H1B functions
Leuconostoc mesenteroides	Gram-positive rod	Dextran production
Nesseria meningitidis	Gram-negative cocci, aerobic	Vaccine against Meningitis C
Pseudomonas aeruginosa	Gram-negative, micro-aerobic	Alginate production Kelsey-Sykes disinfectant capacity test
Salmonella typhi	Gram-negative enteric rod, facultative anaerobe	Chick martin/rideal walker disinfectant coefficient test
Actinomyces species	Gram + ve, filamentous rods	Antibiotic production
Bacillus stearothermophilus	Gram + ve rod, aerobic, spore former	Used to validate and monitor moist heat sterilization processes

9.2.1 Uses of Bacteria

Single-cell protein (SCP) is a sources of mixed protein extracted from pure or mixed cultures of algae, yeasts, fungi or bacteria (grown on agricultural wastes) used as a substitute for protein-rich foods, in human and animal feeds.

Microbes employed to produce SCP include yeasts *Kluyveromyces marxianus* is a species of yeast. It is produced as a nutritional yeast and bonding agent for fodder and pet food, and as a source of ribonucleic acid in pharmaceuticals. Other yeasts including *Saccharomyces cerevisiae*, *Pichia pastoris*, *Candida utilis=Torulopsis* and *Geotrichum candidum =Oidium lactis*.

SCP producing fungi are *Aspergillus oryzae*, *Fusarium venenatum*, *Sclerotium rolfsii*, *Polyporus* and *Trichoderma.*

SCP producing bacteria are *Rhodopseudomonas capsulata, Methylococcus, Methylotrophs.*

SCP producing algae are *Chlorella* and *Spirulina* genera of cyanobacteria are edible, but also because they provide many health benefits.

9.2.2 Idli Fermentation

"Idli" is a traditional cereal/legume-based naturally fermented steamed product with a soft and spongy texture which is highly popular and widely consumed as a snack food item in India. *Candida versatilis, Levconostoc mesentoids, Streptococcus fecalis, Pediococcus.*

9.2.3 Cabbage Fermentation

Sauerkraut means "sour cabbage", is finely cut cabbage that has been fermented by various lactic acid bacteria, including *Leuconostoc mesenteroides*, *Lactobacillus plantarum*, and *Pediococcus*.[1][2] It has a long shelf life and a distinctive sour flavor, both of which result from the lactic acid that forms when the bacteria ferment the sugars in the cabbage. Sauerkraut is also used as a condiment upon various foods, such as meat dishes and hot dogs *Pediococcus* is a genus of Gram-positive lactic acid bacteria.

9.2.4 Swiss Cheese

Propionibacterium freudenreichii ssp *shermanii* is a Gram-positive, non-motile bacterium that plays an important role in the creation of Emmental cheese and to some extent, Jarlsberg cheese, Leerdammer and Maasdam cheese. Its concentration in Swiss-type cheeses is higher than in any other cheese. Propionibacteria are commonly found in milk and dairy products.

9.2.5 Cyanocobalamin (Vitamin B-12)

Bacillus megatherium, Steptomyces griseus, Bacillus megatherium, Streptomyces aureofaciens or Streptomyces griseus Aerobacter aerogenes.

9.2.6 Riboflavin(Vitamin B_2)

Biotechnological processes used for industrial scale riboflavin biosynthesis by using different micro-organisms, including filamentous fungi such as *Ashbya gossypii*, *Candida famata* and *Candida flaveri*, as well as the bacteria *Corynebacterium ammoniagenes* and *Bacillus subtilis*.

9.2.7 β- carotene

β-Carotene is a strongly colored red-orange pigment abundant in plants and fruits. It has been used to treat various disorders such as erythropoietic protoporphyria, to reduce the risk of breast cancer in women before menopause, and the risk of age-related macular degeneration (AMD). β-carotene is synthesized by mated fungal strains of *Blakeslea trispora*. For the large scale production of Carotenods microbes like (green micro algae) *Dunaliella salina* (green micro algae), *Xanthophyllomyces dendrorhous* (yeast), *Haematococcus pluvialis* (green algae).

9.2.8 Food-grade Lactic Acid Bacteria

Food grade lactic acid bacteria have been safely consumed by humans for centuries in fermented foods. *Lactococcus lactis* is widely used in the dairy industry as a starter, *Lactobacillus lactis*:

9.2.9 Yogurt

Lactobacillus delbrueckii subsp. *bulgaricus* is one of several bacteria used for the production of yogurt. *Lactobacillus delbrueckii* subsp. *bulgaricus* is also found in other naturally fermented products.

9.2.10 Nystatin

Nystatin (originally named **Fungicidin**) is a polyene antifungal medication that is derived from a bacterium, *Streptomyces noursei*. It was discovered by Rachel Fuller Brown and Elizabeth Lee Hazen in 1950. Many molds and yeast infections are sensitive to Nystatin, most notably *Candida*.

9.2.11 Bacteriocins (Nisin)

Bacteriocins (Nisin) are antibacterial proteins produced by bacteria that kill or inhibit the growth of other bacteria. Many lactic acid bacteria (LAB) produce a high diversity of different bacteriocins. Though these bacteriocins are produced by LAB found in numerous fermented and non-fermented foods, Nisin is currently the only Bacteriocin widely used as a food preservative.

9.3 Pharmaceutical Significance of Fungi

- **Vitamins**

  Riboflavin is produced commercially in good yields by the moulds. *Eremothecium ashbyii* grows on protein digest medium

- **Organic Acids**

  Citric acid is produced by *Aspergillus niger*. It is used in effervescent products

  Sodium citrate: Anticoagulant

  Potassium citrate: Treating cystitis

- **Iron Chelating Agent**

  Growth of many micro-organisms in iron deficient growth media results in the secretion of low mol. wt iron chelating agents called as siderophores

- **Deferoxamine**

  Deferoxamine (also known as desferrioxamine B, desferoxamine B, DFO-B, DFOA, DFB or desferal) is a bacterial siderophore produced by the *Actinobacteria Streptomyces pilosus*. It has medical applications as a chelating agent used to remove excess iron from the body.[18] The *mesylate salt* of DFO-B is commercially available.

- **Enzymes**

  Glucose oxidase is produced from *Aspergillus niger* which is used in blood glucose analysis.

- **Antibiotics**

  Antibiotics are produced from various moulds such as *streptomyces*.

  Pencillin is produced from *Penicillium notatum* and *P. chrysogenum*.

  Nystatin is produced from *Streptomyces noursei* which acts as antifungal drug.

- **Steroid Biotransformation**

  Conversion of progesterone to 11 α-hydroxy progesterone is mediated by *Rhizopus nigricans*

- **Vitamin Assays**

  Saccharomyces uvarum is used in the assay of inositol.

- **Models of Mammalian Drug Metabolism**

  Microbial systems can be used as *in vitro* models for drug metabolism studies e.g., Imipramine is metabolized to 5 major metabolites 2-hydroxy imipramine, 10-hydroxy imipramine, iminodibenzyl, imipramine N-oxide and desipramine

  Cunnighamella blakesleeana produces the hydroxylated metabolites such as

  2 hydroxy Imipramine and 10- hydroxy Imipramine

  Aspergillus flauipes produces N-oxide derivateand *Fusarium oxysporum* f.sp.*cepae* yield *iminodibenzyl*

  Pharmacologically active metabolite Desipramine which is a Tricyclic Antidepressant is produced by *Mucor griseocyanus*.

- **Genetic Manipulation of Fungi**

  Saccharomyces cerevisiae expression system can be used for producing recombinant proteins

  Yeast has been employed for the production of small hepatitis B surface protein for use in recombinant vaccine

  Antimalarial vaccine component is produced by *S. cerevisiae*

  Protoplasts from fungi are used to generate strains capable of enhanced ethanol production or capable of metabolism of novel carbohydrates

9.4 Pharmaceutical Significance of Protozoa

- Protozoa serves as important link in the food chain of communities in aquatic environment
- Biological sewage treatment involves both anaerobic and aerobic *Protozoans* digestion
- Anaerobic e.g., *Metopus, Saprodinum* and *Epalxis.*
- Aerobic e.g.: *Paramecium*, *Vorticella*
- Inorganic material is removed from water by *Protozoans* for their own synthesis

- Autotrophs are skimmed from the water surface and used as fertilizer
- Protozoans are important research organisms as they are easily cultured and maintained in the laboratory
- *Tetrahymena*, *Euplotes* and *Paramecium* have been used to study cell cycle, Nucleic acid, biosynthesis during cell division

9.5 Pharmaceutical Significance of Algae

- **Algae as a Source of Pharmaceuticals**

  Macro algae derived compounds have a broad range of biological activities such as antibiotic, antiviral, antineoplastic, anti-inflammatory, cytotoxic and antimitotic

  The highest percentage of antimicrobial activity was found in *Phaeophyceae* (84%), *Rhodophyceae* (67%) and *Chlorophyceae* (44%)

  Red and brown macro algae extracts show significant potential as anti-pathogenic agents for use in fish aquaculture

- **Neuro Protective Product**

  Both macro algae and microalgae are neuroprotective agents and promote nerve cell survival

  Spirulina platesis may be useful in the development of novel treatments for neurodegenerative disorders such as Alzheimer or Parkinson disease

- **Human Therapeutic Proteins**

  Microalgae usually find extensive use as therapeutic and diagnostic proteins

  Expression of recombinant proteins in green algal chloroplast holds substantial promise as a platform for algae as a source of pharmaceuticals.

- **Drugs**

  Compounds isolated from blue green algae hold significant promise as anticancer drugs

  Microalgae produce incredibly potent alkaloidal neurotoxins such as Saxitoxin used as anticancer drugs

- **Algae as a Source of Neutraceuticals**

  Physiologically active Neutraceuticals from algae include food supplements, dietary supplements; value added processed foods as well as non-food supplements such as tablets, soft gels, capsules etc.

9.6 Some of the Products Derived from Algae

- Omega 3 polyunsaturated fatty acids: The polyunsaturated omega-3 fatty acids like Eicosa Pentaenoic Acid (EPA, and Docosa Hexaenoic Acid (DHA,) are derived from microalgae e.g. *Isochrysis, Tetraselmis, Chaetoceros, Thalassiosira,Nannochloropsis.*
- *Cyanobacterium spirulina* is rich in γ-Linolenic acid and thus is a good source for the purification of this polyunsaturated fatty acid
- The Red algae, *Porphyridium* contain more than 30% of total fatty acids as Arachidonic acid
- Algae are a rich source of carbohydrates, protein, enzymes and vitamins A, C, B_1, B_2, B_6, iodine, Mg, Ca etc.
- Algae act as biofilters, thus used in the treatment of waste water and in controlling pollution.
- Algae used to produce biodiesel, and is used to yield bioethanol and biobutanol can prove to be effective in regulating global warming
- Algae also produce natural pigment, which can be used as dyes as a substitute for chemical dyes
- Brown algae is a source of Alginic acid used as thickening, stabilizing and emulsifying agent in ice creams, dairy products and in the textile industry
- Genetically engineered algae are used to produce straight vegetable oil
- *Chlorella*, particularly a transgenic strain which carries an extra mercury reductase gene, has been studied as an agent for environmental remediation due to its ability to reduce Hg^{2+} to the less toxic elemental mercury.

Essay Questions

1. Write a note on pharmaceuticals produced by various micro-organisms
2. Explain the pharmaceutical significance of bacteria, fungi and algae

Multiple Choice Questions

1. Which amongst the following microorganism is used for the production of swiss cheese
   (a) Propinionibacterium species
   (b) Streptococcus species
   (c) Lactobacillus species
   (d) Candidum species

2. Which among the following enzyme is used in the manufacturing of glucose, syrup, digestive acid
   (a) Inverstase
   (b) Pectinase
   (c) Diastase
   (d) Acid resistant amylase
3. Which of the following organic acid is used as anticoagulant
   (a) Sodium citrate
   (b) Potassium citrate
   (c) Ammonium carbonate
   (d) Lithium carbonate
4. Which among the following microorganism is used to validate and monitor moist heat sterilization processes
   (a) Actinomyces species
   (b) Bacillus species
   (c) Salmonella
   (d) Nesseria species
5. Conversion of progesterone to 11 alpha hydroxy progesterone is mediated by
   (a) Rhizopus nigricans
   (b) Psuedomonas aeruginosa
   (c) Leuconostoc mesentoids
   (d) Salmonella typhi

Answers

1. (a)	2. (c)	3. (a)
4. (b)	5. (a)	

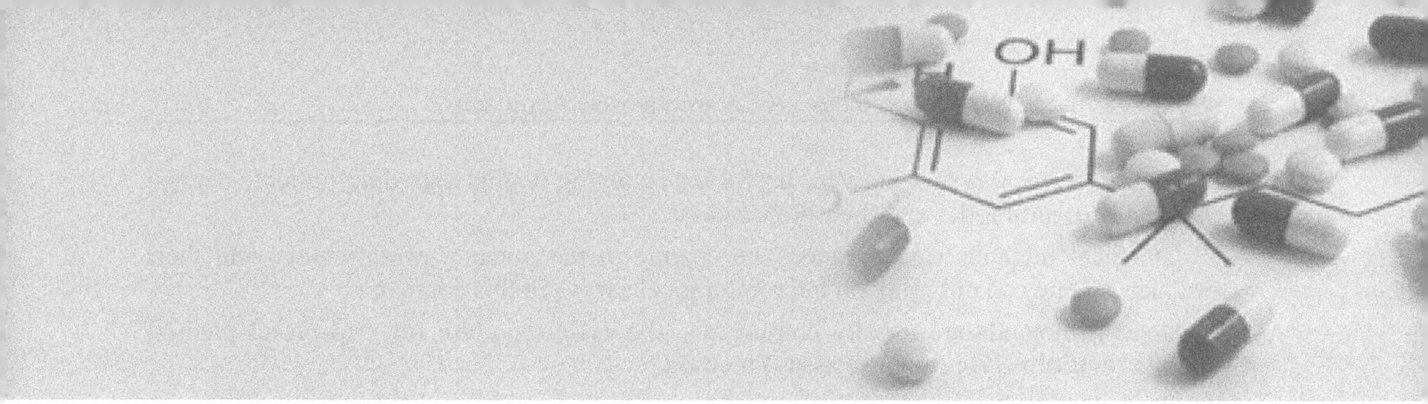

10 MICROBIOLOGICAL ASSAYS

LEARNING OBJECTIVES

After studying the chapter the students familiarize themselves with concepts in:

- *Understanding requirements of Antibiotic assay*
- *Understanding precision of microbiological assays*
- *Understanding various bio indicators and their applications*
- *Understanding biosensors and their applications in pharma industry*
- *Understanding various tests for specified micro-organisms*

10.1 Introduction

The microbiological assay is based upon the comparison of the inhibition of growth of micro-organisms by measured concentrations of the antibiotics to be examined with that produced by known concentrations of a standard preparation of the antibiotic having a known capacity.

Principle: The potency (activity) of an antibiotic product is expressed as the ratio of the dose that inhibits the growth of a suitable susceptible microorganism to the dose of an International Biological Standard, an International Biological Reference Preparation, or an International Chemical Reference Substance of that antibiotic that produces similar inhibition. Properly validated secondary reference materials may also be utilized in the assay. To carry out the assay a comparison is made between the inhibition of the growth of micro-organisms produced by known concentrations of the reference material and that produced by measured dilutions of the test substance. This response can be measured by the diffusion method or in a liquid medium by the turbid metric method.

The inhibition of microbial growth under standardised conditions may be utilized for demonstrating the therapeutic efficacy of antibiotics.

Microbiological assays are very useful for resolving doubts regarding possible change in potency of antibiotics and their preparations.

Chemical methods cannot detect the change in the potency of antibiotics and their products so one can only rely on microbiological assays in this context.

General methods are usually employed – the **cylinder-plate (or cup-plate)** method and the **turbidimetric (or tube assay)** method.

The cylinder-plate method (method A) depends upon diffusion of the antibiotic from a vertical cylinder through a solidified agar layer in a petridish or plate to an extent such that growth of the added microorganism is prevented entirely in a zone around the cylinder containing a solution of antibiotic.

The turbidimetric method (method B) depends upon the inhibition of growth of a microbial culture in a uniform solution of the antibiotic in a fluid medium that is favourable to its rapid growth in the absence of the antibiotic.

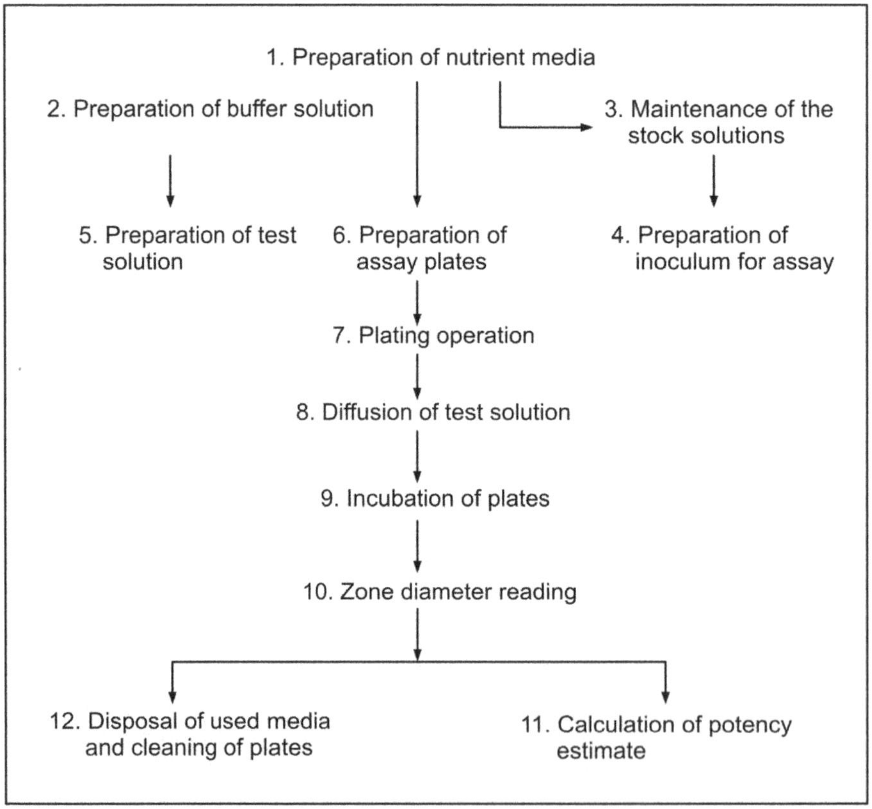

Fig. 10.1 Flowchart showing operations in the microbiological diffusion assay

Note: Due to space constrain Tables 1 to 5 given in Indian Pharmacopoeia(IP) 2014 volume I were not reproduced in this book, so reader need to refer IP2014 Volume I suggested pages to carry out the following microbiological assays.

The assay is designed in such a way that the mathematical model on which potency equation is based can be proved to be valid. If a parallel-line model is chosen, the two log dose-response lines of the preparation being examined and the standard preparation should be parallel; they should be rectilinear over the range of doses used in the calculation.

These conditions should be verified by validity tests for a given probability.

Conventional plate assays require several hours' incubation and consequently the possibility of using rapid microbiological assay methods has been studied.

10.2 Requirements of Antibiotic Assay

(i) ***Standard preparation and units of activity***: A standard preparation is an authentic sample of the appropriate antibiotic for which potency has been precisely determined by reference to the appropriate international standard. The potency of the standard preparation may be expressed in international units or in ug per mL of the pure antibiotic shown in Flowchart.

- The standard preparations for India are maintained at the Central Drugs Laboratory, Calcutta.
- A unit, is the specific activity contained in such an amount of the respective standard preparation as is indicated by the Ministry of Health and Family Welfare, Government of India from time to time.
- A standard preparation may be replaced by a working standard prepared by any laboratory which should be compared at definite intervals with the standard.

(ii) ***Media***: Minor modifications of the individual ingredients may be made, provided the resulting media have equal or better growth-promoting properties and give a similar standard curve response.

Dissolve the ingredients in sufficient water to produce 1000 mL and add sufficient 1M sodium hydroxide or 1M Hydrochloric acid, as required, so that after sterilization the pH is as given in Table 10.1

(iii) ***Buffer solutions***: Buffer solutions are prepared by dissolving the following quantities of dipotassium hydrogen phosphate and potassium dihydrogen phosphate in sufficient water to produce 1000 mL after adjusting the pH with 8M phosphoric acid or 10M potassium hydroxide. The table gives the information regarding buffer number quantity of dipotassium hydrogen phosphate, K_2HPO_4 (g) quantity of potassium dihydrogen phosphate, KH_2 PO_4 (g); pH adjusted after sterilization (Table 10.2).

Preparation of the Standard Solution

To prepare a stock solution, dissolve a quantity of the standard preparation of a given antibiotic, accurately weighed and previously dried as indicated in the solvent specified in the table, and then dilute to the required concentration as indicated. Store in a refrigerator and use within the period indicated on the day of assay, prepare from the stock solution five or more test dilutions, the successive solutions increasing stepwise in concentration, usually in the ratio 1: 1.25 for method A or smaller for method B. Use the final diluent specified and a sequence such that the middle or median has the concentration specified in Table 10.3.

Preparation of the sample solution: From the information available for the substance being examined (the "un known") assign to it an assumed potency per unit weight or volume and on this assumption prepare on the day of the assay a stock solution and test dilution as specified for each antibiotic in but with the same final diluent as used for the standard preparation. The assay with 5 levels of the standard requires only one level of the unknown at a concentration assumed equal to the median level of the standard.

Test organisms: The test organism for each antibiotic is listed in Table 10.4, together with its identification number in the American Type Culture Collection (ATCC) and the Nation Collection of Type Cultures (NCTC) or the National Collection of Industrial Bacteria (NCIB).

Preparation of inoculums: The method of preparation of the microbial suspensions for preparing the inoculum for the assay is given in Table 10.5. If the suspensions are prepared by these methods, growth characteristics are sufficiently uniform so that the inoculum can be adequately determined by the following trials.

For Method A: After the suspension is prepared, as given under table 5, add different volumes of it to each of several different flasks containing 100 mL of the medium specified in Table 10.3. Using these inocula, prepare inoculated plates as described for the specific antibiotic assay.

While conducting cylinder-plate assays, double layer plates may be prepared by pouring a seed layer (inoculated with the desired microorganism) over a solidified uninoculated base layer. For each Petridish, 21 mL of the base layer and 4 mL of the seed layer may be generally suitable. Fill each cylinder with the median concentration of the antibiotic and then incubate the plates. After incubation, examine and measure the zones of inhibition. The volume of suspension that produces the optimum zones of inhibition with respect to both clarity and diameter determines the inoculum to be used for the assay.

For Method B: Proceed as described for method A and using the several inocula, carry out the procedure as described for the specific antibiotic assay running only the high and low concentrations of the standard response curve. After incubation, read the absorbances of appropriate tubes. Determine which inoculum produces the best response between the low and high antibiotic concentrations and use these inoculums for the assay.

Apparatus: All equipment is to be thoroughly cleaned before and after each use glass ware should be sterilised by dry heat or by steam.

Temperature control: Thermostatic control is required in several stages of a microbial assay, when culturing a microorganism and preparing its inoculum and during incubation in a plate assay.

Spectrophotometer: Measuring transmittance within a fairly narrow frequency band requires a suitable spectrophotometer in which the wavelength of the light source can be varied or restricted by the use of a 580 nm filter. For preparing inocula of the required density, or with a 530 nm filter for reading the absorbance in a tube assay.

Cylinder-plate assay receptacles (containers): Use rectangular glass trays or glass or plastic Petri dishes (approximately 20 × 100 mm) having covers of suitable material and assay cylinders made of glass, porcelain, aluminium or stainless steel with outside diameter 8 mm ± 0.1 mm, inside diameter 6 mm ± 0.1 mm and length 10 mm ± 0.1 mm.

Carefully clean the cylinders to remove all residues. An occasional acid-bath eg: with about 2M nitric acid or with chromic acid solution is needed.

Turbidimetric assay receptacles (containers): For assay tubes, use glass or plastic test tubes e.g., 16 mm × 125 mm or 18 mm × 150 mm that are relatively uniform in length, diameter and thickness and substantially free from surface blemishes and scratches.

Assay designs: Microbial assays gain markedly in precision by the segregation of relatively large sources of potential error through suitable experimental designs.

- In a cylinder-plate assay, the essential comparisons are restricted to relationships between zone diameter measurements within plates, exclusive of the variation between plates in their preparation and subsequent handling.
- For a turbidimetric assay the difference in observed turbidity will reflect the differences in the antibiotic concentration.
- Within these restrictions, two alternative designs are recommended; i.e., a 3-level (or 2-level) factorial assay, or a 1-level assay with a standard curve.
- For a factorial assay, prepare solutions of 2 or 3 corresponding test dilutions for both the standard and the unknowns on the day of the assay, as described under preparation of the standard and preparation of the sample.
- For a one-level assay with a standard curve, prepare instead solutions of five test dilutions of the standard and a solution of a single median test level of the unknown as described in the same sections.
- Consider an assay as preliminary if it's computed potency with either design is less than 60% or more than 150% of that assumed in preparing the stock solution of the unknown. In such a case, adjust its assumed potency accordingly and repeat the assay.
- Microbial determinations of potency are subject to inter-assay variables as well as intra-assay variables, so that two or more independent assays are required for a reliable estimate of the potency of a given assay preparation or unknown.

- Starting with separately prepared stock solutions and test dilutions of both the standard and the unknown, repeat the assay of a given unknown on a different day. If the estimated potency of the second assay differs significantly, as indicated by the calculated standard error, from that of the first, conduct one or more additional assays.

10.2.1 Methods

The microbiological assay of antibiotics may be carried out by method-A or method-B

Cylindrical-plate or cup-plate method: Inoculate a previously liquefied medium appropriate to the assay (Table 10.1 and 10.3) with the requisite quantity of suspension of the microorganism, add the suspension to the medium at a temperature between 40° and 50° and immediately pour the inoculated medium into petridishes or large rectangular plates to give a depth of 3 to 4 mm. Ensure that the layers of medium are uniform in thickness, by placing the dishes or plates on a level surface.

The prepared dishes or plates must be stored in a manner so as to ensure that no significant growth or death of the test organism occurs before the dishes or plates are used and that the surface of the agar layer is dry at the time of use.

Using the appropriate buffer solutions indicated in Table 10.2 and 10.3 prepare solutions of known concentration of the standard preparation and solutions of the corresponding assumed concentrations of the antibiotic to be examined. After preparing the solution with the help of directions given in the individual monograph, these should be further diluted as indicated in Table 10.3. Apply the solutions to the surface of the solid medium in sterile cylinders or in cavities prepared in the agar. The volume of solution added to each cylinder or cavity must be uniform and sufficient almost to fill the holes when these are used.

When paper discs are used these should be sterilized by exposure of both sides under a sterilizing lamp and then impregnated with the standard solutions or the test solutions and placed on the surface of the medium.

When petridishes are used, arrange the solutions of the standard preparation and the antibiotic to be examined on each dish so that they alternate around the dish and so that the highest concentrations of standard and test preparations are not adjacent.

When plates are used, place the solutions in a Latin square design, if the plate is a square, or if it is not, in a randomised block design. The same random design should not be used repeatedly.

Leave the dishes or plates standing for 1 to 4 hours at room temperature or at 4°C, as appropriate, as a period of pre-incubation diffusion to minimize the effects of variation in time between the applications of the different solutions. Incubate them for about 18 hours at a temperature indicated in Table 10.3. Accurately measure the diameters or areas of the circular inhibition zones and calculate the results.

10.2.2 One-level Assay with Standard Curve

Standard solution: Dissolve an accurately weighed quantity of the standard preparation of the antibiotic, previously dried where necessary, in the solvent specified in table 10.3 and then dilute to the required concentration, as indicated, to give the stock solution. Store in a refrigerator and use within the period indicated on the day of the assay, prepare from the stock solutions, 5 dilutions (solutions S_1 to S_5) representing five test levels of the standard and increasing step-wise in the ratio of 4:5. Use the diluents specified in table 10.3 and a sequence such that the middle or median has the concentration given in the table.

Sample solution: From the information available for the antibiotic preparation which is being examined (the "unknown") assign to it an assumed potency per unit weight or volume and on this assumption prepare on the day of the assay a stock solution with the same solvent as used for the standard. Prepare from this stock solution a dilution to a concentration equal to the median level of the standard to give the sample solution.

Method: For preparing the standard curve, use a total of 12 petridishes or plates to accommodate 72 cylinders or cavities. A set of three plates (18 cylinders or cavities) is used for each dilution on each of the three plates of a set fill alternate cylinders or cavities with solution S_3 and each of the remaining 9 cylinders or cavities with one of the other 4 dilutions of the standard solution. Repeat the process for the other 3 dilutions of the standard solution.

For each unknown preparation use a set of three plates (18 cylinders or cavities) and fill alternate cylinders or cavities with the sample solution and each of the remaining 9 cylinders of cavities with solution S_3.

Incubate the plates for about 18 hours at the specified temperature and measure the diameters or the zones of inhibition.

Estimation of potency: Average the readings of solution S_3 and the readings of the concentration tested on each set of three plates, and average also all 36 readings of solution S_3. The average of the 36 readings of solution S_3 is the correction point for the curve. Correct the average value obtained for each concentration (Fig. 10.2) (S_1, S_2, S_4 and S_5). Thus, in correcting the value obtained with any concentration, say S_1, if the average of 36 readings of S_3 is, for example, 18.0 mm and the average of the S_3 concentration on one set of three plates is 17.8 mm, the correction is + 0.2 mm. If the average reading of S_1 is 16.0 mm, the corrected reading of S_1 is 16.2 mm. Plot these corrected values including the average of the 36 readings for solutions S_3 on two-cycle semi-log paper, using the concentrations in units or µg per ml (as the ordinate logarithmic scale) and the diameter of zones of inhibition as the abscissa. Draw the straight response line either through these points by inspection or through the points plotted for the highest and lowest zone diameters obtained by means of the following expressions.

$$L = \frac{3a + 2b + c - e}{5}$$

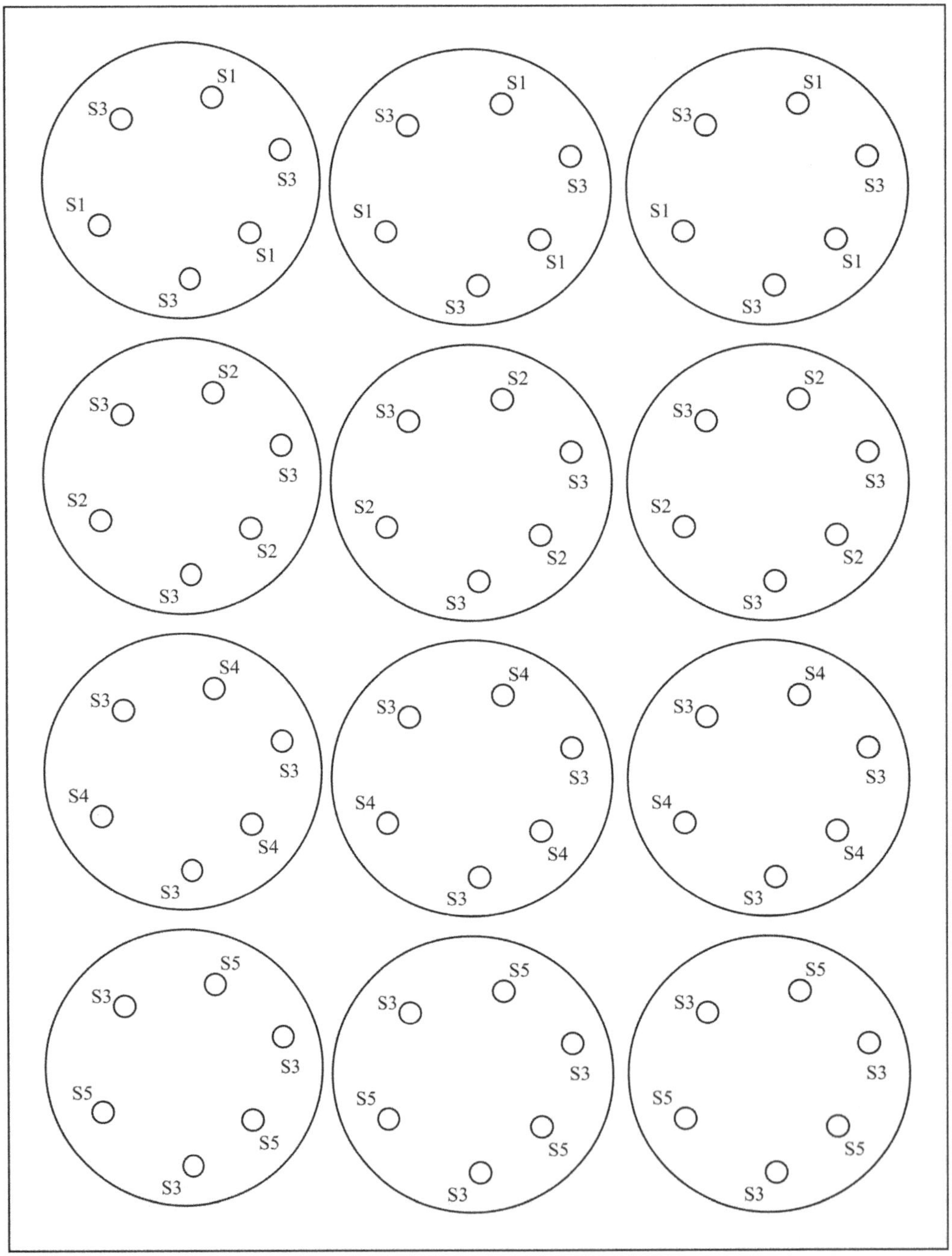

Fig. 10.2 One- level assay plates for preparing the standard curve S3 the median concentration of the standard solution; S1, S2, S4, S5 are dilutions of standard solutions. A set of 3 plates for each standard solution like S1, S2, S4, and S5 are used

$$H = \frac{3e + 2d + c - a}{5}$$

where

L = the calculated zone diameter for the lowest concentration of the standard curve response line.

H = the calculate zone diameter for the highest concentration of the standard curve response line.

c = average zone diameter of 36 readings of the reference point standard solution.

a, b, d, e = corrected average values for the other standard solutions, lowest to highest concentrations, respectively.

Average the zone diameters for the sample solution and for solution S_3 on the plates used for the sample solution. If the sample gives a large average zone size than the average of standard (solution S3), add the difference between them from the zone size of solution S_3 of the standard response line. From the response line read the concentration corresponding to these corrected values of zone sizes. From the dilution factors, the potency of the sample may be calculated.

Average the zone diameter of unknown on the plates used for unknown sample

Average the zone diameter of S3 on the plates used for unknown sample given in Fig. 10.3.

If sample unknown gives large average zone diameter (i.e., for example 20 mm) than average zone diameter of standard (S3) (i.e., for example 18 mm)

The difference between the two average zone diameters is 20-18 = 2

Add" 2" to the zones of S3 of standard response line

If sample unknown gives smaller average zone diameter (i.e. for example 18 mm) than average zone diameter of standard (S3) (i.e., for example 20 mm)

The difference between the two average zone diameters is 20-18 = 2

Subtract the difference" 2" from the zones of S3 of the standard response line shown in Fig. 10.4.

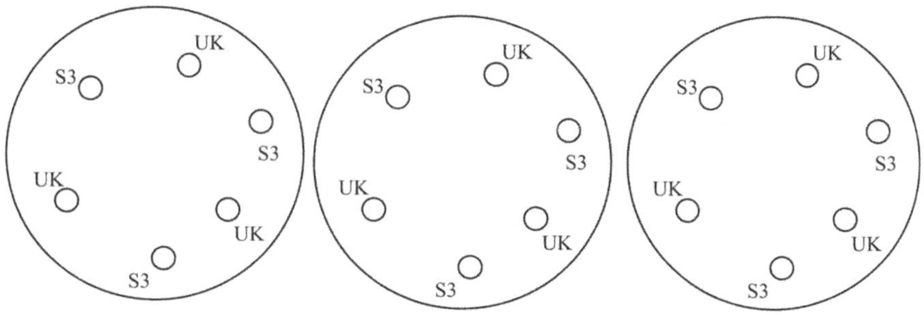

Fig.10.3 A set of 3 Plates containing standard solution S3 and unknown solution (UK) samples in one-level assay

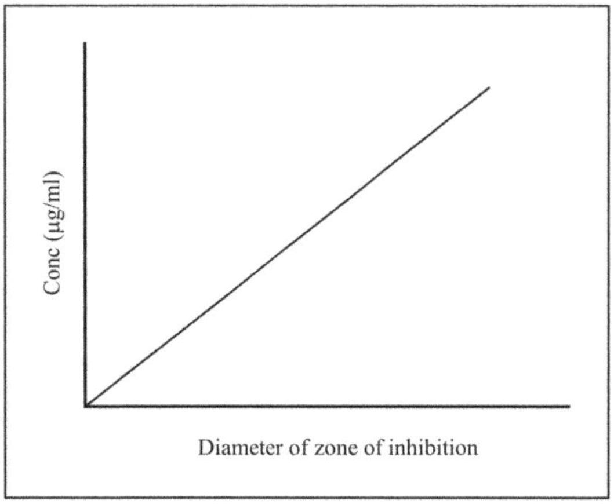

Fig. 10.4 Standard response line to measure the unknown concentration of the drug with the corresponding inhibition zone

10.2.3 Two-Level Factorial Assay (Fig. 10.5)

Prepare parallel dilutions containing 2 levels of both the standard (S_1 and S_2) and the unknown (U_1 and U_2). On each of four or more plates, fill each of its four cylinders or cavities with a different test dilution, alternating standard and unknown. Keep the plates at room temperature and measure the diameters of the zone of inhibition shown in Fig. 10.4.

Estimation of potency: Sum the diameters of the zones of each dilution and calculate the percentage potency of the sample (in terms of the standard) from the following equation

$$\% \text{ potency} = \text{Antilog } (2.0 + a \log I)$$

a may have a positive or negative value and should be used algebraically and

$$a = \frac{(U_1 + U_2) - (S_1 + S_2)}{(U_1 + U_2) + (S_1 - S_2)}$$

where U_1 and U_2 are the sums of the zone diameters with solutions of the unknown of high and low levels.

S_1 and S_2 are the sums of the zone diameters with solutions of the standard of high and low levels.

$$I = \text{ratio of dilutions}$$

If the potency of the sample is lower than 60% or greater than 150% of the standard, the assay is invalid and should be repeated using higher or lower dilutions of the same solution.

The potency of the sample may be calculated from the expression

$$\frac{\% \text{ potency} \times \text{assumed potency of the sample}}{100}$$

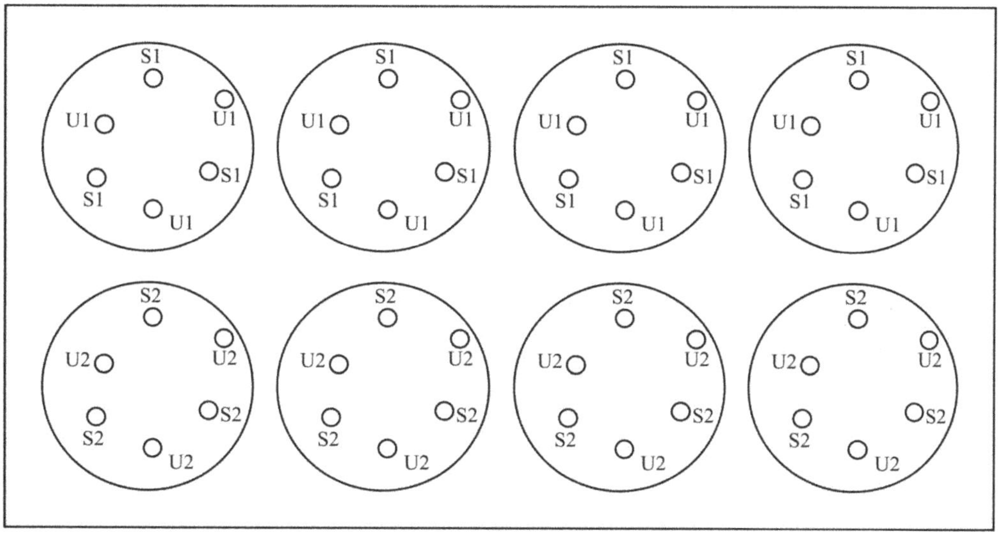

Fig. 10.5 Two- level factorial assay plates

Other designs

1. Factorial assay containing parallel dilution of three test levels of standard and the unknown.
2. Factorial assay using two test levels of standard and two test levels of two different unknowns.

10.2.4 Turbidimetric or Tube Assay Method (Fig. 10.6)

This method has the advantages of shorter incubation period for the growth of the test organism (usually 3 to 4 hours) but the presence of solvent residues or other inhibitory substances affects this assay more than the cylindrical-plate assay and care should be taken to ensure freedom from such substances in the final test solutions. This method is not recommended for cloudy or turbid preparations.\

Prepare five different concentrations of the standard solution for preparing the standard curve by diluting the stock solution of the standard preparation of the antibiotic (Table 10.3) and increasing stepwise in the ratio 4:5. Select the median concentration (Table 10.3) and dilute the solution of the substance being examined (unknown) to obtain approximately this concentration. Place 1 mL of each concentration of the standard solution and of the sample solution in each of the tubes in duplicate. To each tube add 9 mL of nutrient medium previously seeded with the appropriate test organism (Table 10.3).

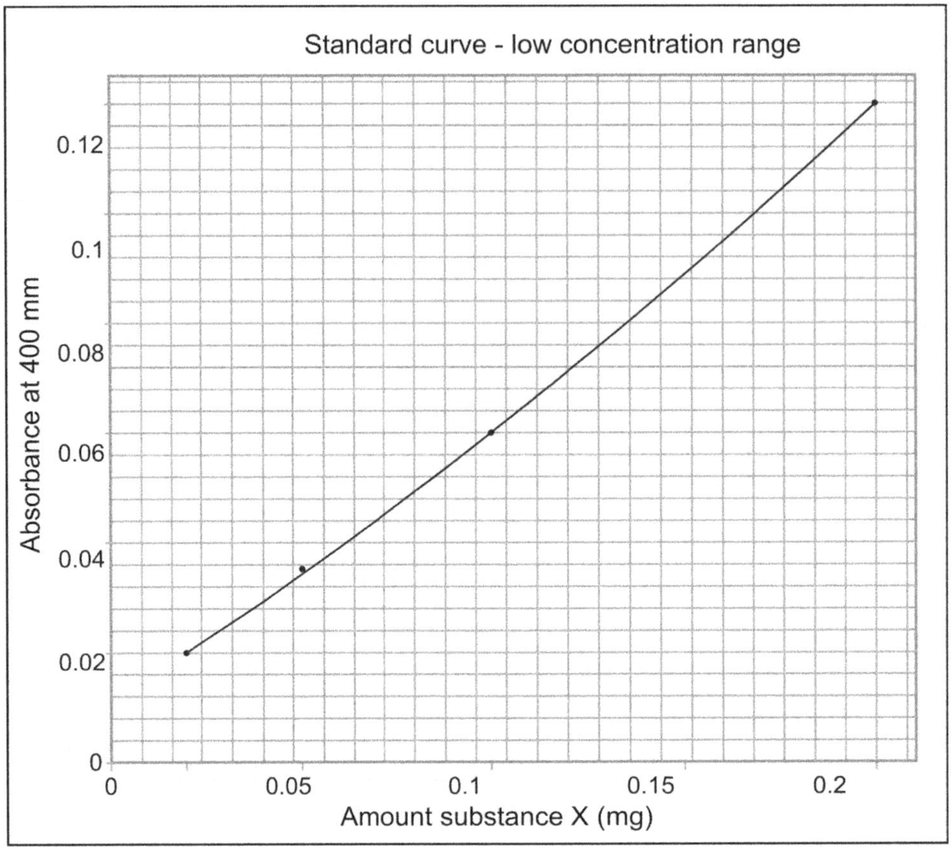

Fig. 10.6 Response line of tube assay

At the same time prepare three control tubes, one containing the inoculated culture medium (culture control), and another identical with it but treated immediately with 0.5 mL of dilute formaldehyde solution (blank) and a third containing uninoculated culture medium.

Place all the tubes, randomly distributed or in a randomized block arrangement, in an incubator or a water-bath and maintain them at the specified temperature (Table 10.3) for 3 to 4 hours. After incubation add 0.5 mL of dilute formaldehyde solution to each tube. Measure the growth of the test organism by determining the absorbance at about 530 nm of each of the solutions in the tubes against the blank.

Estimation of Potency: Plot the average absorbances for each concentration of the standard on semi-logarithmic paper with the absorbances on the arithmetic scale and concentrations on the logarithmic scale. Construct the best straight response line through the points either by inspection or by means of the following expressions.

$$L = \frac{3a + 2b + c - e}{5}$$

$$H = \frac{3e + 2d + c - a}{5}$$

where

L = the calculated absorbance for the lowest concentration of the standard response line.

H = the calculated absorbance for the highest concentration of the standard response line

a, b, c, d, e = average absorbance values for each concentration of the standard response line lowest to highest respectively.

Plot the values obtained for L and H and connect the points. Average the absorbances for the sample and read the antibiotic concentration from the standard response line. Multiply the concentration by the appropriate dilution factors to obtain the antibiotic content of the sample shown in Fig. 10.7.

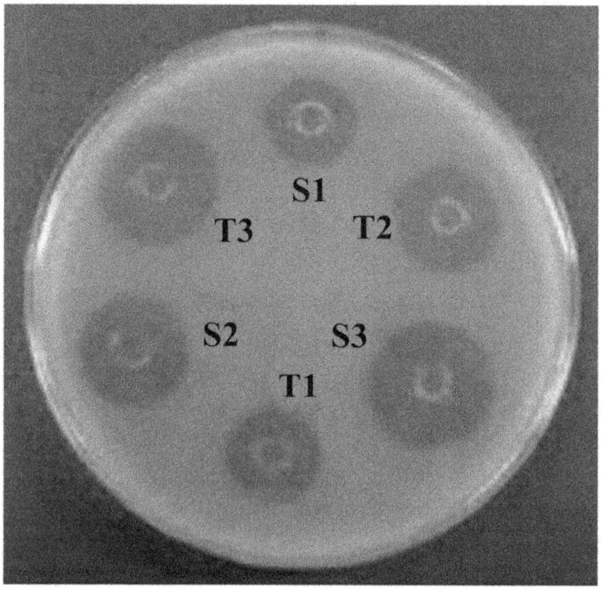

Fig. 10.7 Plate showing the inhibition zones due to addition of antibiotic

10.2.5 Precision of Microbiological Assays

The limits of error of the estimated potency should be not less than 95% and not more than 105% of the estimated potency unless otherwise stated in the individual monograph.

This degree of precision is the minimum acceptable for determining that the final product complies with the official requirements and may be inadequate for those deciding, for example, the potency which should be stated on the label or used as the basis for calculating the quantity of an antibiotic to be incorporated in a preparation. In such circumstances, assay of greater precision may be desirable with, for instance, fiducial limits of error of the order of 98% to 120%. By using this limit, instead of the estimated potency, to assign a potency to the antibiotic either for labeling or for calculating the quantity to be included in a preparation, there is less likelihood of the final preparation subsequently failing to comply with the official requirements for potency.

10.2.6 Microbiological Assay of Streptomycin

In the microbiological assay of streptomycin, the test organism employed is *Bacillus subtilis* (or) *Klebsiella pneumoniae* and the assay method employed is both method A and method B, the prior drying is required in both method A and method B. The initial solvent used is water. The final stock concentration per ml required is 1 mg. It should be used before 30 days after preparation. The final diluent used is water. The median dose µg or units per mL in case of method A is 1.0 µg and method B is 30 µg. The incubation temperature for method A is 32-35 °C and for method B 35-37 °C.

Urease assay: The inhibition of urease property of aminoglycoside antibiotics can be utilized to measure the potency of aminoglycoside antibiotics. When *Proteus mirabilis* grows in a urea containing medium it hydrolyses the urea to ammonia and consequently raises the pH of the medium.

A simple method is described for the rapid assay of aminoglycoside antibiotics in serum.

The method is based on the inhibition by these antibiotics of the urease activity of *Proteus spp*., and is devised to reduce errors attributable to the varying pH values and buffering capacities of the serum of individual patients. The method is as accurate as plate-assay and tube-dilution techniques, gives results within 3 hours of the specimen being taken, is not influenced by concurrently administered penicillin or cephalosporin antibiotics, uses routine laboratory materials, offers no technical difficulties, and has the advantage, over previously described methods based on pH change, of assaying aminoglycoside activity over an alkaline range of pH.

***Luciferase assay*:** In this technique, firely luciferase enzyme is used to measure small amounts of ATP in a bacterial culture, ATP levels being reduced by the inhibitory action of aminoglycoside antibiotics.

10.3 Microbiological Assay of Vitamin-B_{12}

Requirement: A fundamental requirement in a microbial assay for the activity of a vitamin or amino acid (factor) is the inability of the test organism to synthesize the factor being assayed. Furthermore, the test organism must require the factor being assayed for normal growth and should be sensitive to very small amounts of the required factor. For these types of microbial assays, special media are prepared that are nutritionally complete in all respects except for the factor under study. Control tubes containing the suitable media inoculated with the test species exhibit no, or only minimal, growth. If the basic requirements specified above are satisfied, the growth response of the test organism is, within limits, proportional to the amount of factor added to the medium.

- The extent of the growth response may be determined by turbidity or spectrometric measurement, or by titration of the acid produced as metabolic waste.
- The turbidity of the culture is proportional to the amount of microbial growth; the development of acidity also reflects quantitatively the growth response.

Assay preparation: Place a suitable quantity of material to be assayed, previously reduced to a fine powder if necessary and accurately measured or weighed, in an appropriate vessel containing, for each g or mL of material taken, 25 mL of an aqueous extracting solution prepared just prior to use to contain, in each 100 mL, 1.29 g of disodium phosphate, 1.1 g of anhydrous citric acid, and 1.0 g of sodium metabisulfite.

Autoclave the mixture at 121 °C for 10 minutes. Allow any undissolved particles of the extract to settle, and filter or centrifuge if necessary.

Dilute an aliquot of the clear solution with water so that the final test solution contains vitamin B_{12} activity approximately equal to that of the standard cyanocobalamin solution which is added to the assay tubes.

Standard cyanocobalamin stock solution: To a suitable quantity of USP cyanocobalamin RS, accurately weighed, add sufficient 25% alcohol to make a solution having a known concentration of 1.0 μg of cyanocobalamin per ml. Store in a refrigerator.

Standard cyanocobalamin solution: Dilute a suitable volume of standard cyanocobalamin stock solution with water to a measured volume such that after the incubation period, the difference in transmittance between the inoculated blank and the 5.0 mL level of the standard cyanocobalamin solution is not less than that which corresponds to a difference of 1.25 mg in dried cell weight. This concentration usually falls between 0.01 mg and 0.04 mg per mL of standard cyanocobalamin solution. Prepare a fresh standard solution for each assay.

Basal Medium Stock Solution

L - Cystine	-	0.1 gm
L - Tryptophane	-	0.05 gm
1N HCl	-	10 mL

Adenine-Guanine-Uracil solution	-	5 mL
Xanthine solution	-	5 mL
Vitamin solution I	-	10 mL
Vitamin soltuion II	-	10 mL
Salt solution A	-	5 mL
Salt solution B	-	5 mL
Asparagine solution	-	5 mL
Acid-hydrolyzed casein solution	-	25 mL
Dextrose, anhydrous	-	10 g
Sodium Acetate, Anhydrous	-	5 gm
Ascorbic acid	-	1 g
Polysorbate 80 solution	-	5 mL

Acid-hydrolyzed casein solution: Mix 100 gm of vitamin-free casein with 500 mL of 6N HCl, and reflux the mixture for 8 to 12 hours. Remove the HCl from the mixture by distillation under reduced pressure until a thick paste remains. Redissolve the resulting paste in water, adjust the solution with 1N NaOH to a pH of 3.5 ± 0.1 and add water to make 1000 mL. Add 20 gm of activated charcoal, stir for 1 hour and filter. Repeat the treatment with activated charcoal. Store under toluene in a refrigerator at a temperature not blow 10°. Filter the solution if a precipitate forms during storage.

Adenine-guanine-uracil solution: Dissolve 200 mg each of adenine sulfate, guanine hydrochloride, and uracil, with the aid of heat, in 10 mL of 4N hydrochloric acid, cool and add water to make 200 mL. Store under toluene in a refrigerator.

Asparagine solution: Dissolve 2.0 mL of L-asparagine in water to make 200 mL. Store under toulene in a refrigerator.

Xanthine solution: Suspend 0.20 g of xanthine in 30 ml to 40 mL of water, heat to about 70°, add 6.0 mL of 6N ammonium hydroxide, and stir until the solid is dissolved. Cool, and add water to make 200 mL. Store under toulene in a refrigerator.

Salt solution A: Dissolve 10 gm of monobasic potassium phosphate and 10 gm of dibasic potassium phosphate in water to make 200 ml. Add 2 drops of HCl, and store under toulene.

Salt solution B: Dissolve 4.0 gm of Mg SO_4, 0.20 gm of NaCl, 0.20 gm of $FeSO_4$ and 0.20 gm of manganese sufate in water to make 200 ml. Add 2 drops of HCl, and store under toluene.

Polysorbate 80 solution: Dissolve 20 gm of polysorbate 80 in alcohol to make 200 mL. Store in a refrigerator.

Vitamin solution I: Dissolve 10 mg of riboflavin, 10 mg of thiamine hydrochloride, 100 µg of biotin, and 20 mg of niacin in 0.02N glacial acetic acid to make 400 mL. Store, protected from light, under toluene in a refrigerator.

Vitamin solution II: Dissolve 20 mg of paraaminobenzoic acid, 10 mg of calcium pantothenate, 40 mg of pyridoxine hydrochloride, 40 mg of pyridoxal hydrochloride, 8 mg of pyridoxamine dihydrochloride, 2 mg of folic acid in dilute neutralized alcohol (1 in 4) to make 400 mL. Store, protected from light in a refrigerator.

Tomato juice preparation: Centrifuge commercially canned tomato juice so that most of the pulp is removed. Suspend about 5 gm per L of analytical filter-aid in the supernatant, and filter with the aid of reduced pressure, through a layer of the filter aid. Repeat if necessary, until a clear, straw-coloured filtrate is obtained. Store under toluene in a refrigerator.

Culture medium: Dissolve 0.75 gm of water soluble yeast extract, 0.75 gm of dried peptone, 1.0 gm of anhydrous dextrose, 0.20 gm of potassium biphosphate in 60 ml to 70 mL of water. Add 10 mL of tomato juice preparation and 1 mL of polysorbate 80 solution. Adjust the solution with 1N NaOH to a pH of 6.8, and add water to make 100 mL. Place 10 mL portions of the solution in test tubes and plug with cotton. Sterilize the tubes and contents in an autoclave at 121 °C for 15 min. cool as rapidly as possible to avoid color formation resulting from overheating the medium.

Suspension medium: Dilute a measured volume of basal medium stock solution with an equal volume of water. Place 10 mL portions of the diluted medium in test tubes sterilize and cool as directed for the culture medium.

Stock culture of Lactobacillus leichmannii: To 100 mL of culture medium add 1.0 gm to 1.5 g of agar and heat the mixture, with stirring on a steam bath, until the agar dissolves. Place approximately 10 mL portions of the hot solution in test tubes, cover the tubes suitably, sterilize at 121 °C for 15 minutes in an autoclave and allow the tubes to cool in an upright position. Inoculate three or more of the tubes, by stab transfer of the pure culture of *Lactobacillus leichmannii*. (Before first using a fresh culture in this assay, make no fewer than 10 successive transfers of the culture in a 2-week period).

Incubate 16 to 24 hours at any selected temperature between 30° and 40° but held constant to within ±0.5°, and finally store in a refrigerator.

Prepare fresh stab cultures at least three times each week and do not use them for preparing the inoculums if more than 4 days old.

The activity of the microorganism can be increased by daily or twice-daily transfer of the stab culture, to the point where definite turbidity in the liquid inoculums can be observed 2 to 4 hours after inoculation.

A slow-growing culture seldom gives a suitable response curve and may lead to erratic results.

Inoculum: Make a transfer of cells from the stock culture of *Lactobacillus leichmannii* to 2 sterile tubes containing 10 mL of the culture medium each.

Incubate these cultures for 16 to 24 hours at any selected temperature between 30° and 40° but held constant to within ±0.5°.

Under aseptic conditions, centrifuge the cultures, and decant the supernatant.

Suspend the cells from the culture in 5 mL of sterile suspension medium and combine. Using sterile suspension medium, adjust the volume so that a 1 in 20 dilution in saline TS produces 70% transmittance when read on a suitable spectrophotometer which should be set at a wavelength of 530 nm, equipped with a 10 mm cell and read against saline TS set at 100% transmittance.

Prepare a 1 in 400 dilution of the adjusted suspension using basal medium stock solution, and use it for the test inoculums.

Calibration of spectrophotometer: Check the wavelength of spectrophotometer periodically, using a standard wavelength cell or other suitable device.

Before reading any tests, calibrate the spectrophotometer for 0% and 100% transmittance, using water and with the wavelength set at 530 nm.

Procedure

Cleanse meticulously by suitable means, followed preferably by heating at 250 °C for 2 hours, hard-glass test tubes, about 20 mm × 150 mm in size, and other necessary glassware because of the high sensitivity of the test organism to minute amounts of vitamin B_{12} activity.

- To the test tubes add, in duplicate, 1.0 mL, 1.5 mL, 2.0 mL, 3.0 mL, 4.0 mL and 5.0 mL respectively, of the standard cyanocobalamin solution. To each of these tubes and to four similar empty tubes add 5.0 mL of Basal medium stock solution and water to make 10 mL.
- To similar test tubes add, in duplicate, respectively, 1.0 mL, 1.5 mL, 2.0 mL, 3.0 mL and 4.0 mL of the assay preparation. To each tube add 5.0 mL of Basal medium stock solution and water to make 10 mL. Place one complete set of standard and assay tubes together in one tube rack and the duplicate set in a second rack or section of a rack, preferably in random order.
- Cover the tubes suitably to prevent bacterial contamination, and sterilize the tubes and contents in an autoclave at 121 °C for 5 minutes, arranging to reach this temperature in not more than 10 minutes by preheating the autoclave, if necessary. Cool as rapidly as practicable to avoid colour formation resulting from overheating the medium.
- Take precautions to maintain uniformity of sterilizing and cooling conditions throughout the assay, since packing tubes too closely in the autoclave, or overloading it, may cause variation in the heating rate.
- Aseptically add 0.5 mL of inoculums to each tube so prepared, except two of the four containing no standard cyanocobalamin solution (the uninoculated blanks). Incubate the tubes at a temperature between 30° and 40° held constant to within ±0.5°, for 16 to 24 hours.
- Terminate the growth by heating to a temperature not lower than 80 °C for 5 minutes. Cool to room temperature. After agitating its contents, place the container in a spectrophotometer that has been set at a wavelength of 530 nm and read the

transmittance when a steady state is reached. This steady state is observed a few seconds after agitation when the reading remains constant for 30 seconds or more. Allow approximately the same time interval for the reading on each tube.

- With the transmittance set at 100% for the uninoculated blank, read the transmittance of the inoculated blank. If the difference is greater than 5% or if there is evidence of contamination with a foreign microorganism, disregard the results of the assay.
- With the transmittance set at 100% for the uninoculated blank, read the transmittance of each of the remaining tubes. Disregard the results of the assay if the slope of the standard curve indicates a problem with sensitivity.

Calculation: Prepare a standard concentration-response curve by the following procedure. Test for and replace any aberrant individual transmittances. For each level of the standard, calculate the response from the sum of the duplicate values of the transmittances as the difference,

$$Y = 2.00 - \text{transmittance}$$

Plot this response on the ordinate of cross section paper against the logarithm of the ml of standard cyanocobalamin solution per tube on the abscissa, using for the ordinate either an arithmetic or a logarithmic scale, whichever gives the better approximation to a straight line. Draw the straight line or smooth curve that best fits the plotted points.

- Calculate the response, y, adding together the two transmittances for each level of the assay preparation. Read from the standard curve the logarithm of the volume of the standard preparation corresponding to each of those values of y that falls within the range of the lowest and highest points plotted for the standard.
- Subtract from each logarithm so obtained the logarithm of the volume, in ml, of the assay preparation to obtain the difference, x for each dosage level.
- Average the values of x for each of three or more dosage levels to obtain
- $\bar{x} = M$; The log-relative potency of the assay preparation
- Determine the quantity, in µg, of USP cyanocobalamin RS corresponding to the cyanocobalamin in the portion of material taken for assay by the equation

  $$M = \text{antilog}\left(M' + 10g\ R\right)$$

  R = number of µg of cyanocobalamin that was assumed to be present in each mg (or capsule or tablet) of the material taken for assay.

Replication: Repeat the entire determination at least once, using separately prepared assay preparations.

- If the Difference between the two 10 g potencies M is not greater than 0.08, their mean, $\overline{M}$, is the assayed 10 g potency of the test material.

- If the two determinations differ by more than 0.08, conduct one or more additional determinations.
- From the mean of two or more values of M that do not differ by more than 0.15, compute the mean potency of the preparation under assay.

10.4 Microbial Assay of Niacin (Vitamin B_3)

Niacin, also known as vitamin B_3 and nicotinic acid, is an organic compound with the formula $C_6H_5NO_2$ and, depending on the definition used, one of the 20 to 80 essential human nutrients. Pharmaceutical and supplemental niacin are primarily used to treat hypercholesterolemia (high cholesterol) and pellagra (niacin dediciency). Insufficient niacin in the diet can cause nausea, skin and mouth lesions, anemia, headaches, and tiredness. The lack of niacin may also be observed in pandemic deficiency disease, which is caused by a lack of five crucial vitamins (niacin, vitamin C, thiamin, vitamin D, and vitamin A) and is usually found in areas of widespread poverty and malnutrition. Niacin has not been found to be useful in decreasing the risk of cardiovascular disease in those already on a statin (lipid lowering drugs) but appears to be effective in those not taking a statin.

Principle of Microbial Assay

Numerous bacteria have been found to require niacin for their metabolic processes. This has permitted the development of microbiological methods for assay of niacin. These methods are quite sensitive and usually measure niacin-active compounds more specifically then chemical methods.

Micro-organism for Assay

The selection criteria of the organism for this assay depends on its ability to utilize only the forms of niacin that are available to the host in which they normally grow and are unable to synthesize it for themselves. The requirements are satisfied by Latcobacillus plantarum, a non-pathogenic, acid forming organism. This organism is easy to culture and affected only to a lesser extent by stimulatory or inhibitory substances normally found in pharmaceutical preparation containing niacin. It is grown on a simple slab culture medium containing gelatin, yeast extract, and glucose. For assay it is cultured in the assay tubes by transferring to the liquid medium consisting of the basic medium containing and optimum amount of added niacin. The range of niacin added to the series of standard tubes is 0.50 µg/tube. Thus the niacin content of extremely small amounts of biological materials may be measured readily.

Test Solution Preparation

The first step in assay procedure is the preparation of test solution of material to be assayed. If the sample is a dry or semi-solid material, the niacin is extracted by heating the sample in a measured volume of dilute H_2SO_4 in an autoclave for 30 min, liquid preparations re autoclaved 30 minutes after addition of H_2SO_4 to give a concentration of 1 N H_2SO_4 preparation of test solution is completed by neutralizing with strong NaOH solution, then diluting to a volume that contains 0.1g of niacin per ml.

Standard Niacin Stock Solution I

50 mg of U.S.P Niacin RS is dissolved in 500 ml of alcohol. Each ml of this contains 100 µg/ml of U.S.P. Niacin RS.

Standard Niacin Stock Solution II

100 ml of standard niacin stock solution I is diluted with 1000 ml of water. Each ml of this solution contains 10µg/ml of U.S.P Niacin RS.

Standard Niacin Solution

Standard niacin stock solution II is suitably diluted with water to obtain concentration beween 10 ng and 40 ng of niacin per ml.

Basal Medium Stock Solution

Ingredients	Quantity
Acid-hydrolysed casein solution	25 ml
Cystine-tryptophane solution	25 ml
Dextrose, anhydrous	10 g
Sodium acetate, anhydrous	5 g
Adenine-guanine-uracil solution	5 ml
Ribofavin-thiaminehydrochloride-biotin solution	5 ml
Aminobenzoic acid-calcium pantothenate-pyridoxine hydrochloride solution	5 ml
Salt solution A	5 ml
Salt solution B	5 ml

The medium preparation is done by dissolving anhydrous dextrose and sodium acetate in the previously mixed solutions, adjusting the ph to 6.8 with 1n sodium hydroxide, and finally, making up the volume to 250 ml with water.

Culture medium: To each of a series of test tubes containing 5 ml of the basal medium stock solution 5 ml of water containing 1 µg of niacin are added. Plug these tubes with cotton and sterilize in an autoclave at 121 °C for 15 minutes.

Inoculum: Make a transfer of cells from the stock culture of *Lactobacillus Plantarum* to a sterile tube containing 10 ml of culture medium. Incubate this culture for 16 to 245 hours at 30 to 37 °C. The cell suspension so obtained is the inoculums.

Niacin Assay Procedure

First Step: To prepare a standard curve of the Niacin standard transmittance

1. Preparation of Standard Niacin Tubes (in duplicate)

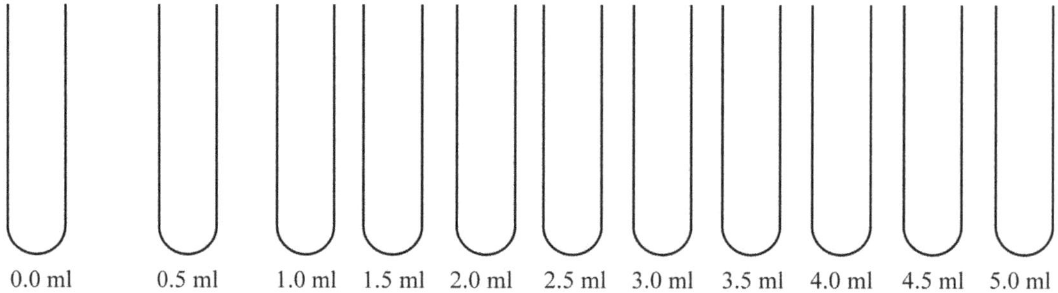

2. Add Basal Medium Stock Solution 5 ml each
3. Add water to make up volume to 10 ml

Second Step: Preparation of Tubes of material to be assayed

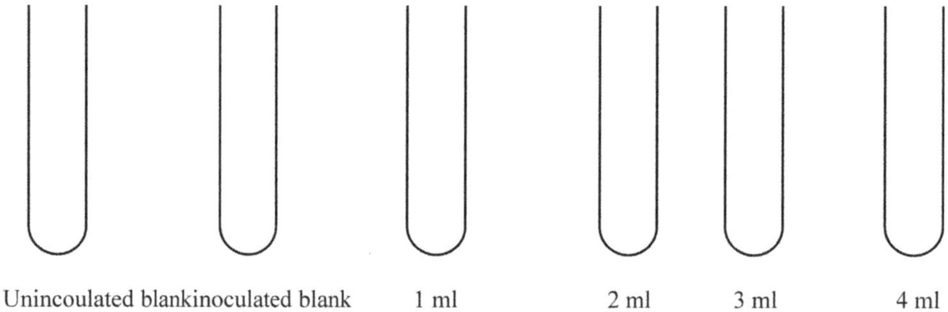

4. To each tube add 5 ml of Basal Medium Stock Solution
5. Add water to make up the volume to 10 ml
6. Mix the contents of each tube
7. Plug the tubes with cotton
8. Sterilize in an autoclave at 121° to 123 °C
9. Cool the tubes
10. Aseptically inoculate each tube with 1(one) drop of inoculum.
11. Incubate for 16 to 24 hours as selected temperature between 30° and 37 °C.
12. Mix the contents of each tube
13. Add 1(one) drop of antifoaming agent
14. Transfer it to optical container (cuvette)

15. Agitate the contents
16. Place the cuvette in spectrophotometer at the wavelength between 540 nm and 660 nm.
17. Read the transmittance
18. Set the transmittance at 1.0 for un-inoculated blank
19. Record the transmittance of the inoculated blank
20. The transmittance set at 1.00 for the inoculated blank
21. Read the transmittance for each of the remaining tubes
22. Prepare a standard curve (Fig. No) of the niacin standard transmittances for each level of Standard Niacin Solution plotted against µg of niacin contained in the respective tubes
23. From the standard curve (Fig. No.), by interpolation the niacin content of the test solution is determined in each tube.
24. The niacin content of the test material is calculated from the average values obtained from not less than six tubes that do not vary by more than $\pm$ 10 percent from the average.
25. Multiply the values obtained by 0.992 if the results are to be expressed as Niacinamide.

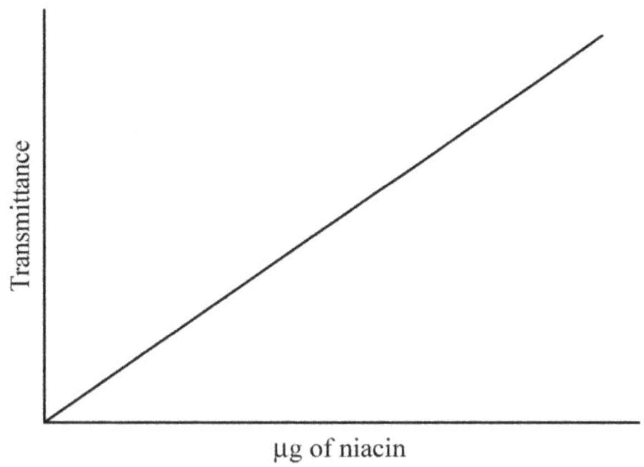

Fig. 10.8 Standard curve of the niacin standard transmittance

Limitations

Un-inoculated Blank

- The transmittance in un-inoculated blank reading corresponds to a dried cell weight greater than 600 microgram per tube, disregard the results of assay.

- Or if there is evidence of contamination with a foreign microorganism, disregard the results of the assay.

Inoculated Blank

- In the transmittance of inoculated blank if the difference between the transmittance observed at the highest level of the standard and that of the inoculated blank is less than the difference corresponding to a dried cell weight of 1.25 mg per tube, disregard the results of the assay.
- Transmittance values of inoculated blank exceeding readings corresponding to dried cell weights of more than 600 µg per tube indicate the presence of an excessive amount of niacin in the Basal Medium Stock Solution and invalidate the assay.

Standard Niacin Solution

Disregard transmittance values equivalent to less than 0.5 mL or more than 4.5 mL

Niacin in the Test Material

If the transmittance values of less than six tubes containing the test solution are within the range of the 0.5 to 4.5 mL levels of the niacin standard tubes, the data are insufficient to permit calculation of the test material.

10.5 Microbial Assay of Amino Acids

The described method for the assay of the ten essential aminoacids, namely histidine, arginine, lysine, leucine, isolucine, valine, methionine, threonine, tryptophane and phenylalanine applies to *Pediococcus acidilactici* ATCC™ 8042 as the test organism.

Procedure

Assay medium

Amino acid assay media are prepared for using in the microbiological assay of amino acids. Three types of media are used for this purpose:

1. Maintenance Media: For carrying the stock culture to preserve the viability and sensitivity of the test organism for its intended purpose;
2. Inoculum Media: To condition the test culture for immediate use;
3. Assay Media: To permit quantitation of the amino acid under test. They contain all the factors necessary for optimal growth of the test organism except the single essential amino acid to be determined.

The Amino Acid Assay Media used in the microbiological assay of amino acids using *Pediococcus acidilactici* ATCC™ 8042 as the test organism is Lysine Assay Medium or Cystine Assay Medium

Principles of the Procedure

Lysine Assay Medium and Cystine Assay Medium contain all the factors essential for the growth of *Pediococcus acidilactici* ATCC 8042, except the amino acid under assay. The addition of the amino acid in specified increasing concentrations gives a growth response by the test organism.

All amino acid assay media contain the following formula.

Approximate Formula	Per Liter
Dextrose	50.0 g
Sodium Acetate	40.0 g
Ammonium Chloride	6.0 g
Monopotassium Phosphate	1.2 g
Dipotassium Phosphate	1.2 g
Magnesium Sulfate	0.4 g
Ferrous Sulfate	20.0 mg
Manganese Sulfate	40.0 mg
Sodium Chloride	20.0 mg
Adenine Sulfate	20.0 mg
Guanine Hydrochloride	20.0 mg
Uracil	20.0 mg
Xanthine	20.0 mg
Thiamine Hydrochloride	1.0 mg
Pyrodoxine Hydrochloride	2.0 mg
Pyridoxamine Hydrochloride	600.0 mg
Pyridoxal Hydrochloride	600.0 mg
Calcium Pantothenate	1.0 mg
Riboflavin	1.0 mg
Nicotinic Acid	2.0 mg
p-Aminobenzoic Acid	200.0 µg
Biotin	2.0 µg

Folic Acid	20.0 μg
Glycine	0.2 g
DL-Alanine	0.4 g
Asparagine	0.8 g
L-Aspartic Acid	0.2 g
L-Proline	0.2 g
DL-Serine	0.1 g
DL-Tryptophan	80.0 mg
L-Glutamic Acid	0.6 g
L-Histidine Hydrochloride	124.0 mg
DL-Phenylalanine	0.2 g
DL-Threonine	0.4 g
L-Tyrosine	0.2 g
DL-Valine	0.5 g
DL-Isoleucine	0.5 g
DL-Leucine	0.5 g
L-Arginine Hydrochloride	484.0 mg
DL-Methionine	0.2 g
L-Cystine	0.1 g
L-Lysine Hydrochloride	0.5 g

**Adjusted and/or supplemented as required to meet performance criteria.*

Assay Medium Preparation

Suspend the ingredients required for the basal media preparation, as directed in the above formula. Heat with frequent agitation and boil for 2-3 minutes to completely dissolve the powder and dispense in 5 mL amounts into tubes, evenly dispersing the precipitate. Finally add standard or test samples adjusting tube volume to 10 mL with purified water and autoclave the media at 121°C for 10 minutes.

Cultural Response

Lysine Assay Medium or Cystine Assay Medium

Prepare the medium as per the label directions. These media support the growth of *Pediococcus acidilactici* ATCC™ 8042 when prepared in single strength and supplemented with the appropriate amino acid. Lysine Assay Medium should produce a standard curve when tested with L-Lysine at 0.0 to 300 µg per 10 ml. Cystine Assay Medium should produce a standard curve when tested with L-Cystine at 0 to 50 µg per 10 ml. Incubate tubes with caps loosened at 35-37°C for 16-20 hours. Read the percent transmittance at 660 nm.

Preparation of Stock Culture and Inoculum

Stock cultures of *Pediococcus acidilactici* ATCC 8042 are prepared by stab inoculation into tubes of Lactobacilli Agar AOAC or Micro Assay Culture Agar. Incubate cultures at 35-37°C for 24 hours. The stock cultures are stored at 2-8°C. Make transfers at monthly intervals in triplicate.

The inoculum for assay is prepared by subculturing the test organism into 10 mL Lactobacilli Broth AOAC or Micro Inoculum Broth. Incubate at 35-37°C for 16-24 hours. After incubation, centrifuge the cells under aseptic conditions and decant the liquid supernatant. Wash the cells 3 times with 10 mL sterile 0.85% NaCl solution. After the third wash, resuspend the cells in 10 mL sterile 0.85% NaCl solution. Dilute the 10 mL cell suspension with the appropriate amount of sterile 0.85% NaCl solution. One drop of the diluted inoculums suspension is used to inoculate each of the assay tubes.

Amino Acid Solution

Stock solutions of each amino acid are prepared. Increasing amounts of the standard or the unknown and sufficient purified water to give a total volume of 10 ml per tube are added to the test tubes containing 5 mL of the assay medium. Measure the growth response turbidimetrically or titrimetrically. Turbidimetric readings are made after incubation at 35-37°C for 16-20 hours. Titrimetric readings are made after incubation at 35-37°C for 72 hours.

It is essential that a standard curve be constructed each time an assay is run. Conditions of autoclaving and temperature of incubation that influence the standard curve readings cannot always be duplicated.

Results

1. Prepare a standard concentration response curve by plotting the response readings against the amount of standard in each tube, disk or cup.
2. Determine the amount of amino acid at each level of assay solution by interpolation from the standard curve.
3. Calculate the concentration of amino acid in the sample from the average of these values. Use only those values that do not vary more than ±10% from the average. Use the results only if two-thirds of the values do not vary more than ±10%.

Limitations of the Procedure

1. The test organism used for inoculating an assay medium must be cultured and maintained on media recommended for this purpose.

2. Aseptic technique should be used throughout the assay procedure.
3. The use of altered or deficient media may cause mutants having different nutritional requirements that will not give a satisfactory response.
4. For successful results of these procedures, all conditions of the assay must be followed precisely.

Table 10.1 Media: Quantities in g of ingredients per 1000 ml

Ingredient	Medium									
	A	B	C	D	E	F	G	H	I	J
Peptone	6.0	6.0	5.0	6.0	6.0	6.0	9.4	-	10.0	-
Pancreatic digest of casein	4.0	-	-	4.0	-	-	-	17.0	-	15.0
Yeast extract	3.0	3.0	1.5	3.0	3.0	3.0	4.7	-	-	-
Beef extract	1.5	1.5	1.5	1.5	1.5	1.5	2.4	-	10.0	-
Dextrose	1.0	-	1.0	1.0	-	-	10.0	2.5	-	-
Papaic digest of soyabean	-	-	-	-	-	-	-	3.0	-	5.0
Glycerin	-	-	-	-	-	-	-	-	10.0	-
Polysorbate 80	-	-	-	-	-	-	-	10.0*	-	-
Sodium chloride	-	-	3.5	-	-	-	10.0	5.0	3.0	5.0
Di-potassium hydrogen phosphate	-	-	3.68	-	-	-	-	2.5	-	-
Potassium dihydrogen phosphate	-	-	1.32	-	-	-	-	-	-	-
Final pH (after sterilisation)	6.5-6.6	6.5-6.6	6.95-7.05	7.8-8.0	7.8-8.0	5.8-6.0	6.0-6.2	7.1-7.3	6.9-7.1	7.2-7.4

*Quality in ml, to be added after boiling the media to dissolve the agar.

Table 10.2 Buffer Solutions

Buffer No.	Dipotassium hydrogen phosphate, K_2HPO_4 (g)	Potassium dihydrogen phosphate, KH_2PO_4 (g)	pH adjusted after sterilization to
1.	2.0	8.0	6.0 ± 0.1
2.	16.73	0.523	8.0 ± 0.1
3.	-	13.61	4.5 ± 0.1
4.	2.0.	80.00	6.0 ± 0.1
5.	35.0	-	10.5 ± 0.1*
6.	13.6	4.0	7.0 ± 0.2

*After addition of 2 ml of 10M potassium hydroxide

Table 10.3 Stock Solutions and Test Dilutions of Standard Preparation

Standard stock solution						Test Dilution		
Antibiotic	Assay method	Prior Drying	Initial solvent, (further diluents, if different)	Final stock concentration per ml	Use before (number of days)	Final diluents	Final median dose µg or Units per ml	Incubation temp. (°)
Amikacin	B	No	Water	1 mg	14	Water	10 µg	32-35
Amphotericin B	A	Yes	DMSO[11]	1 mg	Same day	B5	1.0 µg	29-31
Bacitracin	A	Yes	0.01M HCl	100 units	Same day	B1	1.0 Unit	32-35
Bleomycin	A	Yes	B6[8]	2 units	14	B6	0.04 Unit	32-35
Capreomycin	B	Yes	Water	1 mg	7	Water	100 µg	35-37
Carbenixillin	A	No	B1	1 mg	14	B6	20 µg	36-37.5
Chlortetracycline	A[1]	No	0.1 M HCl	1 mg	4	Water	2.5 µg	37-39
	B[10]	No	0.1 M HCl	1 mg	4	Water	0.24 µg	35-37
Colistimethate sodium	A	Yes	Water	1 mg	Same day	B4	1.0 Unit	35-39
	B	Yes	Water	1 mg	Same day	B6	1.0 Unit	35-37
Colistin sulphate	A	No	Water	1 mg	14	B6	1.0 µg	35-37
Erythromycin	A	Yes	Methanol (10 mg/ml)[8]B2	1 mg	14	B2	1.0 µg	35-37
Framycetin	A	Yes	B2	1 mg	14	B2	1.0 µg	30-35
Gentamicin	A	Yes	B2	1 mg	30	B2	0.1 µg	36-37.5
Gramicidin	B	Yes	Methanol	1 mg	30	B6[12]	0.1 Unit	35-37
Kanamycin sulphate	A[1]	NO	B2	800 units	30	B2	0.8 Unit	37-39
	B[2]	No	Water	1000 units	30	Water	10 Units	32-35
Netilmicin sulphate	A	Yes	Water	1 mg	7	B2	1.0 Unit	32-35

Table 10.3 ***Contd...***

	Standard Tock solution					Test Dilution		
Antibiotic	Assay method	Prior Drying	Initial solvent, (further diluents, if different)	Final stock concentration per ml	Use before (number of days)	Final diluents	Final median dose μg or Units per ml	Incubation temp. (°)
Novobiocin	A	Yes	Ethanol (10 mg/ml)[9], (B2) DMF[7]	1 mg	5	B4	0.5 μg	32-35
Nystatin	A	Yes	DMF[7]	1000 Units	Same day	B4	20 Units	29-31
Oxytetracycline	A[3]	No	0.1 M HCl	1 mg	4	B3	2.5 μg	32-35
	B[2]	No	0.1 M HCl	1 mg	4	Water	0.24 μg	35-37
Polymyxin B	A	Yes	Water, (B4)	10,000 Units	14	B4	10 Units	35-39
Sisomicin	A	Yes	B2	1 mg	14	B2	0.1 μg	32-35
Spiramycin	A[4]	No	Methanol	1 mg	1	B2	12-50 Units	30-32
Streptomycin	A[4]	Yes	Water	1 mg	30	Water	1.0 μg	32-35
	B[5]	Yes	Water	1 mg	30	Water	30 μg	35-37
Teicoplanin	A	Yes	B4	1 mg	Same day	B4	1.0 Unit	32-35
Tetracycline	A[3]	No	0.1M HCl	1 mg	1	Water	2.5 μg	32.5
	B[6]	No	0.1M HCl	1 mg	4	Water	0.24 μg	35-37
Tobramycin	B	Yes	Water	1 mg	14	Water	2.5 μg	32-35
Tylosin	B[10]	No	*	1 mg	Same day	*	0.05-0.25 Unit	36-38
Tyrothricin	B	Yes	Ethanol	1 mg	Same day	Ethanol	1.0 Unit	36-38
Vancomycin	A	No	Water	1 mg	7	B3	10 μg	32-35

1. With *Bacillus pumilus* ATCC 14884 as test organism; 2. With *Staphylococcus aureus* ATCC 29737 as test Organism; 3. With Bacikkus cereus var mycoides ATCC 11778 as test organism; 4. With *Bacillus subtilis* ATCC 6633 as test organism; 5. With *Klebsiella pneumonia* ATCC 10031 as test organism; 6. With *Staphylococcus aureus* ATCC 29737 as test organism; 7. DMF = Dimethylformamide 8. In columns 4 & 7, b denotes buffer solution and the number following refers to the buffer.

Table 10.4 Test Organism for Microbial assay of Antibiotics

Antibiotic	Test Organism	ATCC[1] No.
Amikacin	*Staphylococcus aureus*	29737
Amphotericin B	*Saccharomyces cerevisiae*	9763
Bacitracin	*Micricocus luteus*	10240
Bleomycin	*Mycobacterium smegmatis*	607
Capreomycin	*Klebsiella pneumoniae*	10031
Carbenixillin	*Pseudomonas aeruginosa*	25619
Chlortetracycline	*Bacillus pumilus*	14884
Colistimethate sodium	*Bordetella bronchiseptica*	4617
	Escherichia coli	10536
	Escherichia coli	9637
Colistin sulphate	*Bordetella bronchiseptica*	4617
	Escheichia coli	10536
Erythromycin	*Kocuria rhizophila*	9341
Framycetin	*Bacillus pumilus*	14884
Gentamicin	*Bacillus subtilis*	6633
Gramicidin	*Entrococcus hirae*	10541
	Staphylococcus aureus	6538
Kanamycin sulphate	*Bacillus pumulus*	14884
	Staphyococcus aureus	29737
Neomycin	*Staphyococcus epidermidis*	12228
Netilmicin sulphate	*Staphyococcus aureus*	6538
Novobiocin	*Staphyococcus epidermidis*	12228
Nystatin	*Saccharomyces cerevisiae*	2601
Oxytetracycline	*Bacillus cereus var, mycoides*	11778
	Staphylococcus aureus	29737
Polymyxin B	*Bordetella bronchiseptica*	4617
Sisomicin	*Staphylococcus epidermidis*	12228
Spiramycin	*Bacillus subtilis*	6633
Streptomycin	*Bacillus subtilis*	6633
	Klebsiella pneumoniae	10031
Teicoplanin	*Bacillus subtilis*	6633
Tetracycline	*Bacillus cereus*	11778
	Staphylococcus aureus	29737
Tobramycin	*Staphylococcus aureus*	29737
Tylosin	*Staphylococcus aureus*	9144
Tyrothricin	*Staphylococcus aureus*	10541
Vancomycin	*Bacillus subtilis*	6633

American type culture collection, 21301 Park Lawn Drive, Rockville, MD20852, USA

Table 10.5 Preparation of •noculum

Test Organism	Incubation condition			Suggested dilution factor	Suggested inoculum composition		
	Medium/ Method of Preparation	Temp. (°)	Time		Medium	Amount (ml per 100 ml)	Antibiotics assayed
Bacillus cereus var. mycoides (11778)	$A^1/2$	32-35	5 days	-	F	As required	Oxytetracycline Tetracycline
Bacillus pumilus (14884)	$A^1/2$	32-35	5 days	-	D	As required	Chlortetracycline Framycetin Kanamycin sulphate
Bacillus subtilis (6633)	$A^1/2$	32-35	5 days	-	E	As required	Framycetin
					E	As required	Kanamycin B
					B	As required	Spiramycin
					A	As required	Streptomycin
					E	As required	Teicoplanin
					A	As required	Vancomycin
Bordetella bronchiseptica (4617)	A/1	32-35	24 hr	1:20	H	0.1	Colistimethate sodium
					H	0.1	Colistin sulphate
					H	0.1	Polymyxin B
Escherichia coli (10536)	A///1	35-39	24 hr	1:20	H	0.1	Colustimethate sodium
Escherichia coli (9637)	A/1	35-37	24 hr	-	C	0.1	Colistimethate sodium
Entrococcus hirae (10541)	A/1	36-37	24 hr	-	C	1.0	Gramicindin

Table 10.5 ***Contd...***

Test Organism	Incubation condition			Suggested dilution factor	Suggested inoculum composition		
	Medium/ Method of Preparation	Temp. (°)	Time		Medium	Amount (ml per 100 ml)	Antibiotics assayed
					C	1.0	Tyrothricin
Klebsiella pneumonia (10031)	A/1	36-38	16-18 hr	-	C	1.0	Capremycin
							Streptomycin
Kocuria rhizophila (9341)	A/1	32-35	24 hr	1:40	D	15	Erythromycin
MIcrococus luteus (10240)	A/1	32-35	24 hr	1:35	A	0.3	Bacitracin
Mycobacterium smegmatis (607)	J/4	36-37.5	48 hr	As determined	I	1.0	Bleomycin
Pseudinibas aeruginosa (25619)[2]	A/1	36-37.5	24 hr	1:25	H	0.5	Carbenicillin
Saccharomyces cerevisiae (9763)	G/3	29-31	48 hr	As determined	G	1.0	Amphotericin B
Saccharomyces cerevisiae (2601)	G/3	29-31	48 hr	As determined	G	1.0	Nystatin
Saccharomyces aureus (6538)	A/1	32-35	16-18 hr	-	C	1.0	Gramicidin
			24 hr	-	A	1.0	Netilmicin sulphate
Staphyococcus aureus (29737)	A/1	32-35	24 hr	1:20	C	0.1	Amikacin
							Doxycycline
							Oxytetracycline
							Tetracycline
							Tobramycin

Table 10.5 *Contd...*

Test Organism	Incubation condition			Suggested dilution factor	Suggested inoculum composition		
	Medium/ Method of Preparation	Temp. (°)	Time		Medium	Amount (ml per 100 ml)	Antibiotics assayed
					C	0.2	Kanamycin sulphate
Staphylovovvus epidermidis (12228)	A/1	32-35	24 hr	1:40	D	0.03	Gentamicin
					D	0.4	Neomycin
					A	4.0	Novobiocin
					D	0.03	Sisomicin

Use medium a containing 300 mg of manganese sulphate per litre

10.6 Biosensors

A biosensor is an analytical device which converts a biological response into an electrical signal (Fig. 10.9). The term 'biosensor' is often used to cover sensor devices used in order to determine the concentration of substances and other parameters of biological interest even where they do not utilise a biological system directly.

Biosensors represent a rapidly expanding field, at the present time, with an estimated 60% annual growth rate; the major impetus coming from the health-care industry (e.g. 6% of the western world are diabetic and would benefit from the availability of a rapid, accurate and simple biosensor for glucose) but with some pressure from other areas, such as food quality appraisal and environmental monitoring. Research and development in this field is wide and multidisciplinary, spanning biochemistry, bioreactor science, physical chemistry, electrochemistry, electronics and software engineering. Most of this current approach concerns potentiometric and amperometric biosensors and colorimetric paper enzyme strips. A successful biosensor must possess at least some of the following beneficial features:

1. The biocatalyst must be highly specific for the purpose of the analyses, be stable under normal storage conditions and, show good stability over a large number of assays (i.e. much greater than 100).
2. The reaction should be as independent of such physical parameters as stirring, pH and temperature as is manageable.
3. The response should be accurate, precise, reproducible and linear over the useful analytical range, without dilution or concentration. It should also be free from electrical noise.
4. If the biosensor is to be used for invasive monitoring in clinical situations, the probe must be tiny and biocompatible, having no toxic or antigenic effects. If it is to be used in fermenters it should be sterilisable. This is preferably performed by autoclaving but no biosensor enzymes can presently withstand such drastic wet-heat treatment. In either case, the biosensor should not be prone to fouling or proteolysis.
5. The complete biosensor should be cheap, small, portable and capable of being used by semi-skilled operators.
6. There should be a market for the biosensor

The biological response of the biosensor is determined by the biocatalytic membrane which accomplishes the conversion of reactant to product. Immobilised enzymes possess a number of advantageous features which makes them particularly applicable for use in such systems. They may be re-used, which ensures that the same catalytic activity is present for a series of analyses. This is an important factor in securing reproducible results and avoids the pitfalls associated with the replicate pipetting of free enzyme proportionality constant, k_L, in equation. Even if total dependence on the external diffusional rate is not achieved (or achievable), any increase in the dependence of the reaction rate on external or internal diffusion will cause a reduction in the dependence on the pH, ionic strength, temperature and inhibitor concentrations.

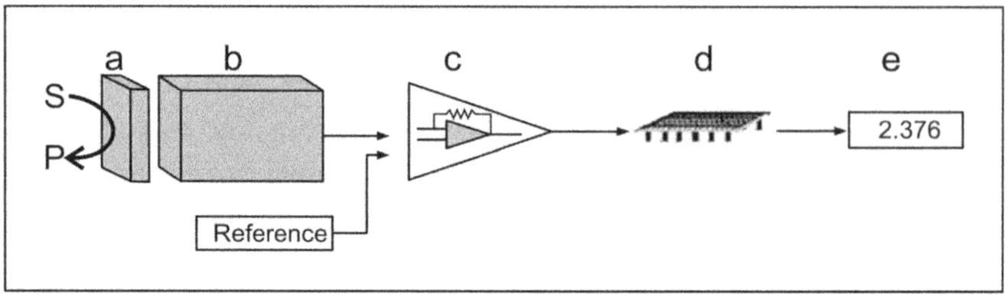

Fig. 10.9 Schematic diagram showing the main components of a biosensor. The biocatalyst **(a)** converts the substrate to product. This reaction is determined by the transducer **(b)** which converts it to an electrical signal. The output from the transducer is amplified **(c)** processed **(d)** and displayed **(e)**.

The key part of a biosensor is the transducer (shown as the 'black box' in Figure 10.8) which makes use of a physical change accompanying the reaction. This may be

1. The heat output (or absorbed) by the reaction (calorimetric biosensors),
2. Changes in the distribution of charges causing an electrical potential to be produced (potentiometric biosensors),
3. Movement of electrons produced in a redox reaction (amperometric biosensors),
4. Light output during the reaction or a light absorbance difference between the reactants and products (optical biosensors), or
5. Effects due to the mass of the reactants or products (piezo-electric biosensors).

There are three so-called 'generations' of biosensors;

First generation biosensors where the normal product of the reaction diffuses to the transducer and causes the electrical response, second generation biosensors which involve specific 'mediators' between the reaction and the transducer in order to generate improved response, and third generation biosensors where the reaction itself causes the response and no product or mediator diffusion is directly involved.

The electrical signal from the transducer is often low and superimposed upon a relatively high and noisy (i.e. containing a high frequency signal component of an apparently random nature, due to electrical interference or generated within the electronic components of the transducer) baseline.

The signal processing normally involves subtracting a 'reference' baseline signal, derived from a similar transducer without any biocatalytic membrane, from the sample signal, amplifying the resultant signal difference and electronically filtering (smoothing) out the unwanted signal noise. The relatively slow nature of the biosensor response considerably eases the problem of electrical noise filtration. The analogue signal produced at this stage may be output directly but is usually converted to a digital signal and passed to a microprocessor stage where the data is processed, converted to concentration units and output to a display device or data store.

10.6.1 Calorimetric Biosensors

Many enzyme catalyzed reactions are exothermic, generating heat (Table 10.6) which may be used as a basis for measuring the rate of reaction and, hence, the analyte concentration. This represents the most generally applicable type of biosensor. The temperature changes are usually determined by means of thermistors at the entrance and exit of small packed bed columns containing immobilized enzymes within a constant temperature environment (Figure 10.10). Under such closely controlled conditions, up to 80% of the heat generated in the reaction may be registered as a temperature change in the sample stream. This may be simply calculated from the enthalpy change and the amount reacted. If a 1 mM reactant is completely converted to product in a reaction generating 100 kJ $mole^{-1}$ then each ml of solution generates 0.1 J of heat. At 80% efficiency, this will cause a change in temperature of the solution amounting to approximately 0.02 C. This is about the temperature change commonly encountered and necessitates a temperature resolution of 0.0001 C for the biosensor to be generally useful.

Table 10.6 Heat output (molar enthalpies) of enzyme catalyzed reactions.

Reactant	Enzyme	Heat output -DH (kJ $mole^{-1}$)
Cholesterol	Cholesterol oxidase	53
Esters	Chymotrypsin	4 - 16
Glucose	Glucose oxidase	80
Hydrogen peroxide	Catalase	100
Penicillin G	Penicillinase	67
Peptides	Trypsin	10 - 30
Starch	Amylase	8
Sucrose	Invertase	20
Urea	Urease	61
Uric acid	Uricase	49

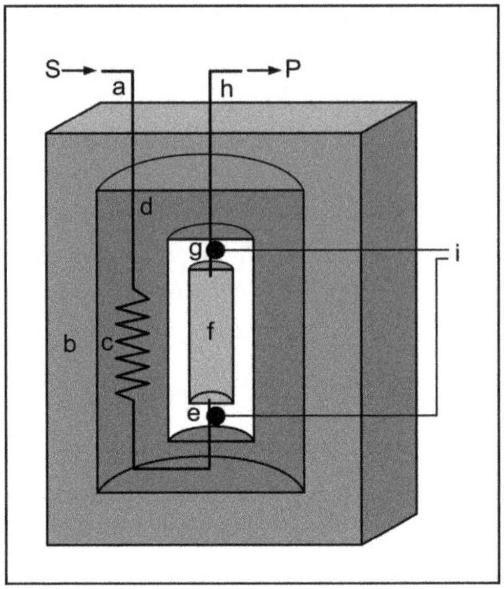

Fig. 10.10 Schematic diagram of a calorimetric biosensor. The sample stream **(a)** passes through the outer insulated box **(b)** to the heat exchanger **(c)** within an aluminium block **(d)**. From there, it flows past the reference thermistor **(e)** and into the packed bed bioreactor **(f)** 1ml volume), containing the biocatalyst, where the reaction occurs. The change in temperature is determined by the thermistor **(g)** and the solution passed to waste **(h)**. External electronics **(I)** determines the difference in the resistance, and hence temperature, between the thermistors.

10.6.2 Potentiometric Biosensors

Potentiometric biosensors make use of ion-selective electrodes in order to transduce the biological reaction into an electrical signal. In the simplest terms this consists of an immobilised enzyme membrane surrounding the probe from a pH-meter (Figure 10.11), where the catalysed reaction generates or absorbs hydrogen ions (Table 10.3). The reaction occurring next to the thin sensing glass membrane causes a change in pH which may be read directly from the pH-meter's display. Typical of the use of such electrodes is that the electrical potential is determined at very high impedance allowing effectively zero current flow and causing no interference with the reaction.

There are three types of ion-selective electrodes which are of use in biosensors:

1. Glass electrodes for cations (e.g. normal pH electrodes) in which the sensing element is a very thin hydrated glass membrane which generates a transverse electrical potential due to the concentration-dependent competition between the cations for

specific binding sites. The selectivity of this membrane is determined by the composition of the glass. The sensitivity to H^+ is greater than that achievable for NH_4^+,

2. Glass pH electrodes coated with a gas-permeable membrane selective for CO_2, NH_3 or H_2S. The diffusion of the gas through this membrane causes a change in pH of a sensing solution between the membrane and the electrode which is then determined.
3. Solid-state electrodes where the glass membrane is replaced by a thin membrane of a specific ion conductor made from a mixture of silver sulphide and a silver halide. The iodide electrode is useful for the determination of I^- in the peroxidase reaction (Table 10.3) and also responds to cyanide ions.

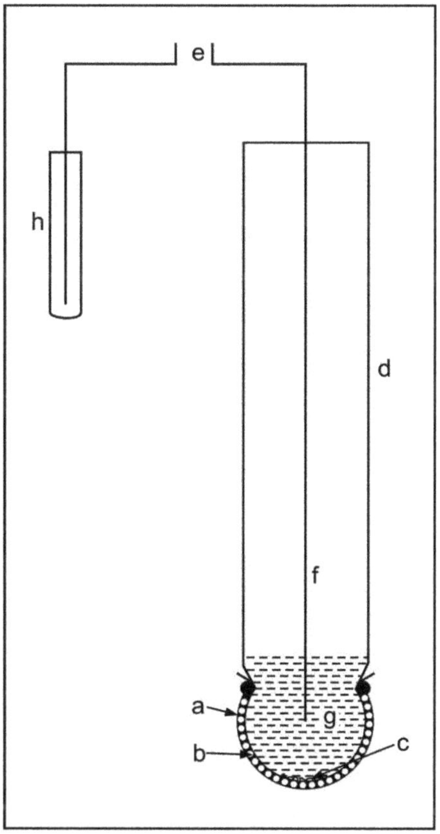

Fig. 10.11 A simple potentiometric biosensor. A semi-permeable membrane **(a)** surrounds the biocatalyst **(b)** entrapped next to the active glass membrane **(c)** of a pH probe **(d)**. The electrical potential **(e)** is generated between the internal Ag/AgCl electrode **(f)** bathed in dilute HCl **(g)** and an external reference electrode **(h)**.

Table 10.7 Reactions involving the Release or Absorption of Ions that may be utilized by Potentiometric Biosensors.

(a)	H^+ cation,
	glucose oxidase H_2O
	D-glucose + O_2 $\rightarrow$ D-glucono-1,5-lactone + H_2O_2 $\rightarrow$ D-gluconate + H^+
	penicillinase
	penicillin $\rightarrow$ penicilloic acid + H^+
	urease (pH 6.0)[a]
	$H_2NCONH_2 + H_2O + 2H^+ \rightarrow 2NH_4^+ + CO_2$
	urease (pH 9.5)[b]
	$H_2NCONH_2 + 2H_2O \rightarrow 2NH_3 + HCO_3^- + H^+$
	lipase
	neutral lipids + H_2O $\rightarrow$ glycerol + fatty acids + H^+
(b)	NH_4^+ cation,
	L-amino acid oxidase
	L-amino acid + O_2 + H_2O $\rightarrow$ keto acid + NH_4^+ + H_2O_2
	asparaginase
	L-asparagine + H_2O $\rightarrow$ L-aspartate + NH_4^+
	urease (pH 7.5)
	$H_2NCONH_2 + 2H_2O + H^+ \rightarrow 2NH_4^+ + HCO_3^-$
(c)	I^- anion,
	peroxidase
	$H_2O_2 + 2H^+ + 2I^- \rightarrow I_2 + 2H_2O$
(d)	CN^- anion,
	b-glucosidase
	amygdalin + $2H_2O$ $\rightarrow$ 2glucose + benzaldehyde + H^+ + CN^-
	[a] Can also be used in NH_4^+ and CO_2 (gas) potentiometric biosensors.
	[b] Can also be used in an NH_3 (gas) potentiometric biosensor.es80ll66bp

A recent development from ion-selective electrodes is the production of ion-selective field effect transistors (ISFETs) and their biosensor use as enzyme-linked field effect transistors (**ENFET**s, Fig. 10.14). Enzyme membranes are coated on the ion-selective gates of these electronic devices, the biosensor responding to the electrical potential change via the current output. Thus, these are potentiometric devices although they directly produce changes in the electric current. The main advantage of such devices is their extremely small size (<< 0.1 mm^2) which allows cheap mass-produced fabrication using integrated circuit technology. As an example, a urea-sensitive FET (ENFET containing bound urease with a reference electrode containing bound glycine) has been shown to show only a 15% variation in response to urea (0.05 - 10.0 mg ml^{-1}) during its active lifetime of a month. Several analytes may be determined by miniaturised biosensors containing arrays of ISFETs and ENFETs. The sensitivity of FETs, however, may be affected by the composition, ionic strength and concentrations of the solutions analysed.

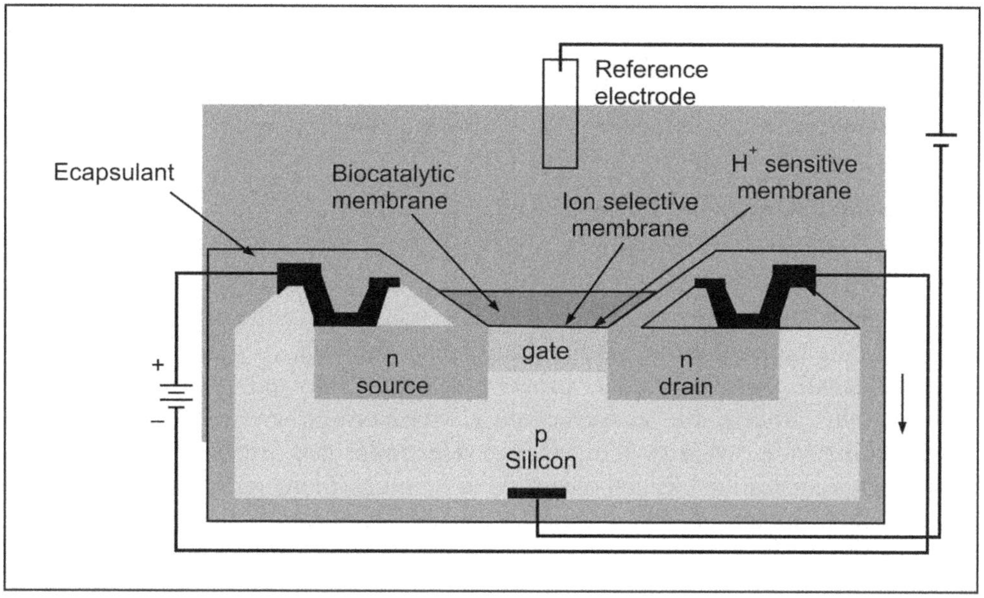

Fig. 10.12 Schematic diagram of the section across the width of an ENFET

The actual dimensions of the active area are about 500 mm long by 50 mm wide by 300 mm thick. The main body of the biosensor is a p-type silicon chip with two n-type silicon areas; the negative source and the positive drain. The chip is insulated by a thin layer (0.1 mm thick) of silica (SiO_2) which forms the gate of the FET. Above this gate is an equally thin layer of H^+-sensitive material (e.g. tantalum oxide), a protective ion selective membrane, the biocatalyst and the analyte solution, which is separated from sensitive parts of the FET by an inert encapsulating polyimide photopolymer. When a potential is applied between the electrodes, a current flows through the FET dependent upon the positive potential detected at the ion-selective gate and its consequent attraction of electrons into the depletion layer. This current (I) is compared with that from a similar, but non-catalytic ISFET immersed in the same solution. (Note that the electric current is, by convention, in the opposite direction to the flow of electrons).

10.6.3 Amperometric Biosensors

Amperometric biosensors function by the production of a current when a potential is applied between two electrodes. They generally have response times, dynamic ranges and sensitivities similar to the potentiometric biosensors. The simplest amperometric biosensors in common usage involve the Clark oxygen electrode (Figure 10.13). This consists of a platinum cathode at which oxygen is reduced and a silver/silver chloride reference electrode. When a potential of -0.6 V, relative to the Ag/AgCl electrode is applied to the platinum cathode, a current proportional to the oxygen concentration is produced. Normally both electrodes are bathed in a solution of saturated potassium chloride and separated from the bulk solution by an oxygen-permeable plastic membrane (e.g. Teflon, polytetrafluoroethylene). The following reactions occur:

$$\text{Ag anode } 4Ag^0 + 4Cl^- \rightarrow 4AgCl + 4e^-$$

$$\text{Pt cathode } O_2 + 4H^+ + 4e^- \rightarrow 2H_2O$$

The efficient reduction of oxygen at the surface of the cathode causes the oxygen concentration there to be effectively zero. The rate of this electrochemical reduction therefore depends on the rate of diffusion of the oxygen from the bulk solution, which is dependent on the concentration gradient and hence the bulk oxygen concentration. It is clear that a small, but significant, proportion of the oxygen present in the bulk is consumed by this process; the oxygen electrode measuring the rate of a process which is far from equilibrium, whereas ion-selective electrodes are used close to equilibrium conditions. This causes the oxygen electrode to be much more sensitive to changes in the temperature than potentiometric sensors. A typical application for this simple type of biosensor is the determination of glucose concentrations by the use of an immobilized glucose oxidase membrane.

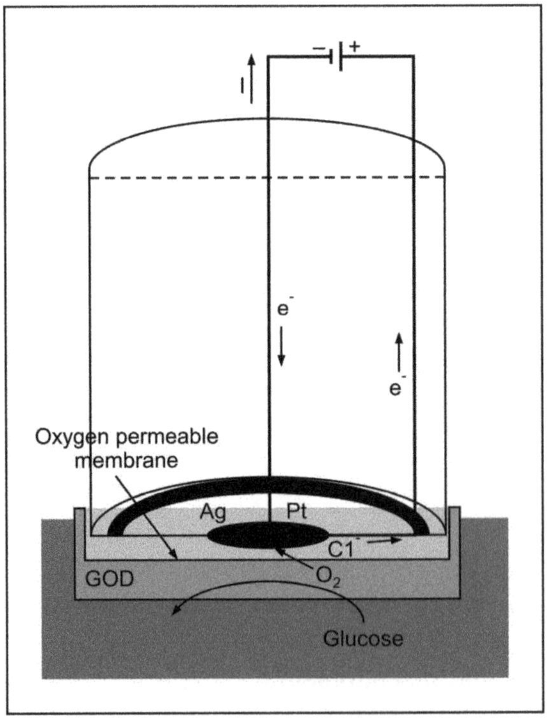

Fig. 10.13 Schematic diagram of a simple amperometric biosensor

A potential is applied between the central platinum cathode and the annular silver anode. This generates a current (I) which is carried between the electrodes by means of a saturated solution of KCl. This electrode compartment is separated from the biocatalyst (here shown glucose oxidase, GOD) by a thin plastic membrane, permeable only to oxygen. The analyte solution is separated from the biocatalyst by another membrane, permeable to the substrate(s) and product(s). This biosensor is normally about 1 cm in diameter but has been scaled down to 0.25 mm diameter using a Pt wire cathode within a silver plated steel needle anode and utilizing dip-coated membranes.

An alternative method for determining the rate of this reaction is to measure the production of hydrogen peroxide directly by applying a potential of +0.68 V to the platinum electrode, relative to the Ag/AgCl electrode, and causing the reactions:

Pt anode $H_2O_2 \rightarrow O_2 + 2H^+ + 2e^-$

Ag cathode $2AgCl + 2e^- \rightarrow 2Ag^0 + 2Cl$

10.6.4 Optical Biosensors

There are two main areas of development in optical biosensors.

These involve determining changes in light absorption between the reactants and products of a reaction, or measuring the light output by a luminescent process. The former usually involve the widely established, if rather low technology, use of colorimetric test strips. These are disposable single-use cellulose pads impregnated with enzyme and reagents. The most common use of this technology is for whole-blood monitoring in diabetes control. In this case, the strips include glucose oxidase, horseradish peroxidase (EC 1.11.1.7) and a chromogen (e.g. *o*-toluidine or 3,3',5,5'-tetramethylbenzidine). The hydrogen peroxide, produced by the aerobic oxidation of glucose), oxidising the weakly colored chromogen to a highly coloured dye.

10.6.4.1 Peroxidase

$$\text{Chromogen(2H)} + H_2O_2 \rightarrow \text{dye} + 2H_2O$$

The evaluation of the dyed strips is best achieved by the use of portable reflectance meters, although direct visual comparison with a colored chart is often used. A wide variety of test strips involving other enzymes are commercially available at the present time. A most promising biosensor involving luminescence uses firefly luciferase (*Photinus*-luciferin 4-monooxygenase (ATP-hydrolysing), EC 1.13.12.7) to detect the presence of bacteria in food or clinical samples. Bacteria are specifically lysed and the ATP released (roughly proportional to the number of bacteria present) reacted with D-luciferin and oxygen in a reaction which produces yellow light in high quantum yield.

10.6.4.2 Luciferase

ATP + D-luciferin + O_2 → oxyluciferin + AMP + pyrophosphate + CO_2 + light (562 nm)

The light produced may be detected photometrically by use of high-voltage, and expensive, photomultiplier tubes or low-voltage cheap photodiode systems. The sensitivity of the photomultiplier-containing systems is, at present, somewhat greater (< 10^4 cells ml^{-1}, < 10^{-12} M ATP) than the simpler photon detectors which use photodiodes. Firefly luciferase is a very expensive enzyme, only obtainable from the tails of wild fireflies. Use of immobilized luciferase greatly reduces the cost of these analyses.

10.6.5 Piezo-Electric Biosensors

Piezo-electric crystals (e.g. quartz) vibrate under the influence of an electric field. The frequency of this oscillation (f) depends on their thickness and cut, each crystal having a characteristic resonant frequency. This resonant frequency changes as molecules adsorb or desorb from the surface of the crystal, obeying the relationships

$$\Delta f = \frac{kf^2 \Delta m}{A}$$

Where **Δf** is the change in resonant frequency (Hz), **Δm** is the change in mass of adsorbed material (g), **K** is a constant for the particular crystal dependent on such factors as its density and cut, and **A** is the adsorbing surface area (cm^2). f = frequency of piezoelectric quartz crystal in MHz, for any piezo-electric crystal, the change in frequency is proportional to the mass of absorbed material, up to about a 2% change. This frequency change is easily detected by relatively unsophisticated electronic circuits. A simple use of such a transducer is a formaldehyde biosensor, utilizing a formaldehyde dehydrogenase coating immobilized to a quartz crystal and sensitive to gaseous formaldehyde.

The major drawbacks: These devices are the interference from atmospheric humidity and the difficulty in using them for the determination of material in solution.

Advantages: They are, however, inexpensive, small and robust, and capable of giving a rapid response.

10.6.6 Immunosensors

Biosensors may be used in conjunction with enzyme-linked immunosorbent assays (**ELISA**). The principles behind the ELISA technique are shown in 10.13. ELISA is used to detect and amplify an antigen-antibody reaction; the amount of enzyme-linked antigen bound to the immobilized antibody being determined by the relative concentration of the free and conjugated antigen and quantified by the rate of enzymic reaction. Enzymes with high turnover numbers are used in order to achieve rapid response. The sensitivity of such assays may be further enhanced by utilizing enzyme-catalyzed reactions which give intrinsically greater response; for instance, those giving rise to highly colored, fluorescent or bioluminescent products. Assay kits using this technique are now available for a vast range of analyses.

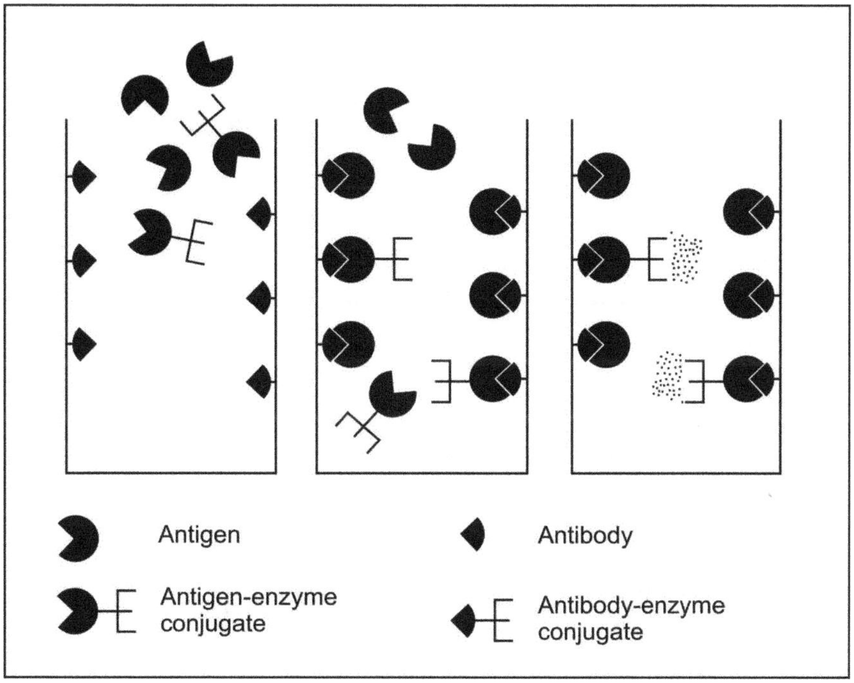

Fig. 10.14 Principles of a direct competitive ELISA. **(i)** Antibody, specific for the antigen of interest is immobilized on the surface of a tube. A mixture of a known amount of antigen-enzyme conjugate plus unknown concentration of sample antigen is placed in the tube and allowed to equilibrate. **(ii)** After a suitable period the antigen and antigen-enzyme conjugate will be distributed between the bound and free states dependent upon their relative concentrations. **(iii)** Unbound material is washed off and discarded. The amount of antigen-enzyme conjugate that is bound may be determined by the rate of the subsequent enzymic reaction.

Recently ELISA techniques have been combined with biosensors, to form **immunosensors**, in order to increase their range, speed and sensitivity. A simple immunosensor configuration is shown in Figure 10.1f (a), where the biosensor merely replaces the traditional colorimetric detection system. However more advanced immunosensors are being developed (Figure 10.15 (b)) which rely on the direct detection of antigen bound to the antibody-coated surface of the biosensor. Piezoelectric and FET-based biosensors are particularly suited to such applications.

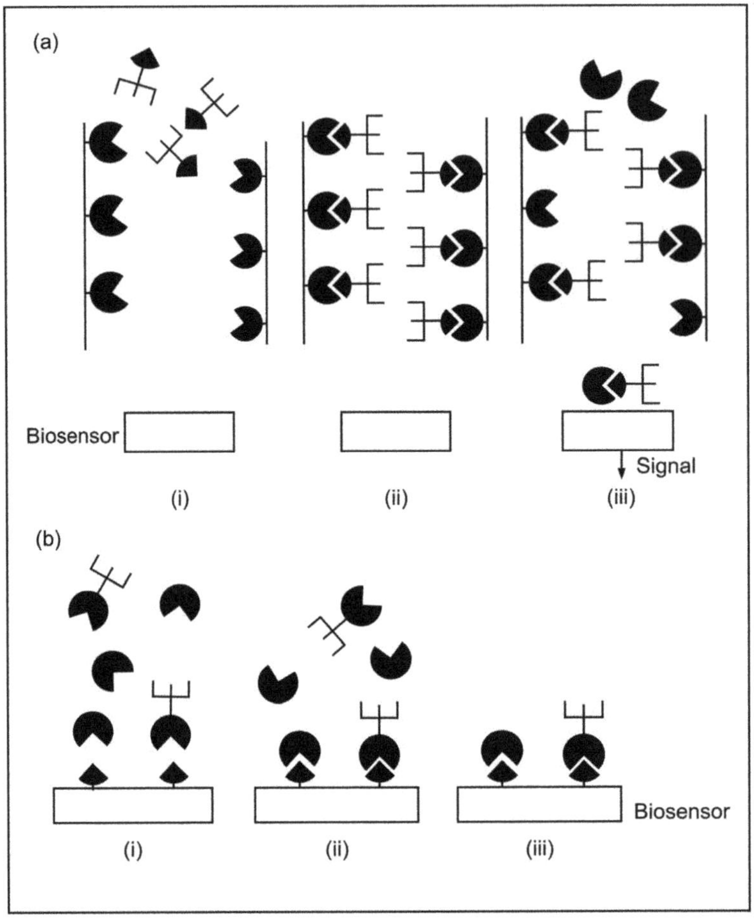

Fig. 10.15 Principles of immunosensors. **(a)(i)** A tube is coated with (immobilized) antigen. An excess of specific antibody-enzyme conjugate is placed in the tube and allowed to bind. **(a)(ii)** After a suitable period any unbound material is washed off. **(a)(iii)** The analyte antigen solution is passed into the tube, binding and releasing some of the antibody-enzyme conjugate dependent upon the antigen's concentration. The amount of antibody-enzyme conjugate released is determined by the response from the biosensor. **(b)(i)** A transducer is coated with (immobilized) antibody, specific for the antigen of interest. The transducer is immersed in a solution containing a mixture of a known amount of antigen-enzyme conjugate plus unknown concentration of sample antigen. **(b)(ii)** After a suitable period the antigen and antigen-enzyme conjugate will be distributed between the bound and free states dependent upon their relative concentrations. **(b)(iii)** Unbound material is washed off and discarded. The amount of antigen-enzyme conjugate bound is determined directly from the transduced signal.

10.6.7 Microbial Biosensors

- A biosensor is a device that detects, transmits and records information regarding a physiological or biochemical change.
- Technically, it is a probe that integrates a biological component with an electronic transducer thereby converting a biochemical signal into a quantifiable electrical response.
- Biosensors make use of a variety of transducers such as electrochemical, optical, acoustic and electronic.
- The function of a biosensor depends on the biochemical specificity of the biologically active material.
- The choice of the biological material will depend on a number of factors viz the specificity.
- storage, operational and environmental stability.
- Selection also depends on the analyte to be detected such as chemical compounds antigens, microbes, hormones, nucleic acids or any subjective parameters like smell and taste.
- Enzymes, antibodies, DNA, receptors, organelles and micro-organisms as well as animal and plant cells or tissues have been used as biological sensing elements.
- Some of the major attributes of a good biosensing system are its specificity, sensitivity, reliability, portability, (in most cases) ability to function even in optically opaque solutions, real-time analysis and simplicity of operation.

10.6.7.1 Use of microbial cells as Biosensing Elements

- Advantages of microbes as biological sensing materials in the fabrication of biosensors
- Present ubiquitously
- Able to metabolise a wide range of chemical compounds
- Great capacity to adapt to adverse conditions
- Develop the ability to degrade new molecules with time
- Microbes are also amenable for genetic modifications through mutation or through recombinant DNA technology
- Serve as an economical source of intracellular enzymes
- In the construction of biosensors purified enzymes have been most commonly used due to their high specific activities as well as High analytical specificity
- Limitation
- Expensive
- Unstable

- Over 90% of the enzymes known to date are intracellular
- In this respect, the utilization of whole cells as a source of intracellular enzymes has been shown to be a better alternative to purified enzymes in various industrial processes (Bickerstaff, 1997; D'Souza, 1999).

10.6.7.2 Reasons for using microbes as biosensor

- It avoids the lengthy and expensive operations of enzyme purification
- Preserves the enzyme in its natural environment
- Protects it from inactivation by external toxicants such as heavy metals
- Whole cells also provide a multipurpose catalyst especially when the process requires the participation of a number of enzymes in sequence
- Whole cells ~ usage ~viable or non-viable form
- Viable cells are gaining considerable importance in the fabrication of biosensors (Burlage and Kuo, 1994; Riedel, 1998; Arikawa et al.,1998;Simonian et al., 1998).
- Viable microbes metabolise various organic compounds either an aerobically or aerobically resulting in various end products like ammonia, carbon dioxide, acids etc., that can be monitored using a variety of transducers.
- Viable cells are mainly used when the overall substrate assimilation capacity of micro-organisms is taken as an index of respiratory metabolic activity, as in the case of estimation of biological oxygen demand (BOD) or utilization of other growth or metabolically related nutrients like vitamins, sugars, organic acids and nitrogenous compounds (Riedel, 1998). Another mechanism used for the viable microbial biosensor involves the inhibition of microbial respiration by the analyte of interest, like environmental pollutants (Arikawa et al., 1998).

10.6.7.3 Limitation

- Diffusion of substrate and products through the cellwall resulting in a slow response as compared to enzyme- based sensors (Rainina et. al., 1996).
- One of the ways to obviate this problem is to use permeabilised cells.
- Permeablisation can be achieved via Physical (freezing and thawing),
- Chemical (organic solvents/detergents) and
- Enzymatic (lysozyme, papain) approaches
- The most common technique uses organic solvents such as toluene, chloroform, ethanol and butanol or detergents like

  N-cetyl-N, N, N-trim ethyl ammonium bromide (CTAB), Na-deoxycholate and digitonin (Patil and D'Souza, 1997).
- Such chemical treatment creates minute pores by removing some of the lipids from the cell membranes, thereby allowing for the free diffusion of small

molecular weight substrates/products across the cell membrane while retaining most of the macromolecular compounds like the enzymes inside the cell.

- The Permeablisation process, however, renders the cell non-viable but can serve as an economical source of intracellular enzymes.
- In the case of periplasmic enzymes such as invertase and catalase in yeast (D'Souza and Nadkarni, 1980; Svitel et al., 1998) and uniease and phosphatases in bacteria (Kamath and D'Souza, 1992; Macaskie et al.,1992) whole cells can be used without Permeablisation
- One of the recent advances is to engineer the cell to transport the intra cellular enzyme and anchor it into the peri-plasmic space.
- Such an approach has been applied to obtain recombinant *Escherichia coli* cells with surface expressed oragno phosphorous hydrolase (OPH), an enzyme useful in the fabrication of biosensors for the detection of organophosphate compounds (Mulchandani et al., 1998a,b).
- These cells could degrade the organophosphates more efficiently (Mulchandani et. al., 1998a,b) without the diffusional limitations otherwise observed in engineered cells expressing OPH intra-cellular (Rainina et al., 1996).
- The above approach is an important development in the field of microbial-biosensors as it provides a cell system with no membrane transport problems and at the same time will not affect the cellular structure and activity.
- This is in contrast to chemically permeabilised cells which result in loss of cell viability
- These types of genetic approaches may have major significance in the future, especially for sensors like BOD wherein polymers such as protein, starch, lipid etc., have to be broken down to monomers before they can be metabolised.
- Another limitation in using whole cells is the low specificity as compared to biosensors containing pure enzymes.
- This is mainly due to the unwanted side reactions catalyzed by other enzymes in a cell.
- Several approaches are being investigated to minimize such non-specific reactions.
- Permeabilisation of the cell empties it of most of the small molecular weight cofactors etc., thus minimizing the unwanted side reactions (D'Souza, 1989a).
- Thus a whole cell of yeast containing intracellular –galactosidase converts lactose to ethanol and CO_2 whereas the same cell on permeabilisation converts lactose only to glucose and galactose due to the loss of cofactors from the cell (Rao et al., 1988; Joshi et al.,1989).
- Side reactions, which can occur due to the presence of other enzymes in a cell, can also be minimised by inactivating such enzymes either by physical (heat) or

chemical means when non-viable cells are used (Godboleet al., 1983; Di Paolantonio and Rechnitz,1983; D'Souza, 1989a; Riedel, 1998).

- Another approach that is of significance in viable cell-based biosensors is the blockage of unwanted metabolic pathways or transport systems.
- Thus, for the determination of glutamic acid in the presence of glucose by Bacillus subtilis, the glucose up take carrier system of the cell was blocked using a thiol inhibitor like chloromercuri benzoate and also the glycolysis was reversibly inhibited by NaF (Riedel and Scheller, 1987). .
- Microbial biosensors based on light emission from luminescent bacteria are being applied as a sensitive, rapid and non-invasive assay in several biological systems (Burlage and Kuo, 1994; Matrubutham and Sayler, 1998).
- Bioluminescent bacteria are found in nature, their habitat ranging from marine (Vibrio fischeri) to terrestrial (Photorhabdus luminescens) environments.
- Bioluminescent whole cell biosensors have also been developed using genetically engineered micro-organisms (GEM) for the monitoring of organic, pesticide and heavy metal contamination.
- The micro-organisms used in these biosensors are typically produced with a constructed plasmid in which genes that code for luciferase are placed under the control of a promoter that recognizes the analyte of interest.
- When such microbes metabolise the organic pollutants, the genetic control mechanism also turns on the synthesis of luciferase, which produces light that can be detected by luminometers.
- One approach to environmental monitoring is to detect changes in gene expression patterns induced by adverse conditions.
- Bacterial strains that increase light production in the presence of specific chemicals have been constructed using bioluminescence genes (lux) as reporters of transcriptional responses.
- A typical example is the *Pseudomonas fluorescens* HK44, a lux -based bioluminescent bio-reporter that is capable of emitting light upon exposure to naphthalene, salicylate and other substitute danalogues.

10.6.7.4 Immobilization of Bio Materials

- The basic requirement of a biosensor is that the biological material should bring the physico-chemical changes in close proximity of a transducer.
- Immobilisation not only helps in forming the required close proximity between the biomaterial and the transducer, but also helps in stabilising it for reuse.
- The biological material has been immobilised directly on the transducer or in most cases, in membranes, which can subsequently be mounted on the transducer.

- Biomaterials can be immobilised either through adsorption, entrapment, covalent binding, cross-linking or a combination of all these techniques (D'Souza, 1989a, 1999; Bickerstaff, 1997).
- *e.g.*, Covalent binding, commonly used technique for the immobilisation of enzymes and antibodies.

10.6.7.5 Microbial Biosensors for Environmental Applications

Table 10.8 Microbial Biosensors for Environmental Applications

Analysis	Microorganism	Transducer/immobilization	Detection limit	Reference
BOD	*Trichosperum cutaneum*	Miniature oxygen electrode (UV cross-linking resin (ENT – 3400)	0.2 – 18 mg/*l*	Yang et.al (1996)
BOD	*T. cuteneum*	Miniature oxygen electrode array (photo cross-linkable resin)	<32 mg/*l*	Yang et.al (1997)
BOD	*T.cutaneum*	Oxygen electrode (entrapment)	10-70 mg/*l*	Marty et. al (1997)
BOD	*P.putidex*	Oxygen electrode (adsorption on porous nitro cellulose membrane)	> 0.5 mg/*l*	Chee et. al (1999)
BOD	Activated sludge (mixed microbial consortium)	Oxygen electrode/flow injection system (entrapped in dialysis membrane)	> 3.5 mg/*l*	Lin et. al (2000)
BOD	Salt tolerant mycelia yeast A. adeinvarans 1.53	Oxygen electrode (PVA)	2.61-524 mg/*l*	Tag et. al (2000)
Bioavailable organic carbon in oxic sediments	Yeast cells	Oxygen electrode (PVA)	Microscale	Neudoerfer and Meyer (1997)
Aniomic surfactants (linear alky benzene sulfonates (LAS)	LAS degrading bacteria isolated from activated sludge	Oxygen electrode, (reactor type sensor, ca-alginate)	< 6 mg/*l*	Nomura et. al (1994)
Acrylamide acrylic acid	*Broxibacterium.* sp	Oxygen electrode (free celis)	0.01-0.075 and 0.01-0.1 g/*l*	Ignatov et. al. (1997)
Phenotic compounds	*Ps. parido*	Oxygen electrode (reactor with cells adsorbed on PEI glass)	100 uM	Nandakumar and Mattiason (1999 a)

Table 10.8 *Contd...*

Analysis	Microorganism	Transducer/immobilization	Detection limit	Reference
Nitrite	*Nurobacter vulgaris* DSM 10236 *S.cerevisine*	Oxygen electrode (adsorption on Whatman paper)	> 10 □m	Reshetilov et. al (2000)
Cyanide	*S.cerevisiae*	Oxygen electrode (PVA)	0.15-15 nM	Tkebukaro et. al (1996)
Chlorophenols	*Rhodococcus sp., Trichosporon beigelli Ps. Putida*	Oxygen electrode (PVA)	0.004-0.04 and 0.002-0.04 mM	Riedel et. al (1993, 1995)
3-Chloro-benzoate	*Ps. putida*	Oxygen electrode (PVA)	40-200 µN	Riedel et. al (1991)
Chlorinated and brominated hydrocarbons (l-chlorobutane and ethylenebromide)	*Rhodococcus sp.* DSM 6344	Ion selective electrodes (alginate)	0.22 and 0.04 mg/*l*	Peter et. al (1996)
Polycyclic aromatic hydrocarbons (Naphthalene)	*Sphingomonus yanolkuvate* B1 or *Ps. Fluorescens* WW 4	Oxygen electrode	0.01-3.0 mg/*l*	Keenig et al. (1996, 1997a)
Organophosphate nerve agents (paraxon, methyl parathion, diazinon)	GEM[b] *E.coli* (organophosphorous hydrolase)	Potentiometric (adsorption on electrode surface)	0.055-1.8, 0.06-0.91 and 0.46-8.5 mM	Mulchandani et. al. (1998a)
Organophosphate nerve agents (paraxon, parathion, coumaphos)	GEM[b] *E.coli* (organophosphorous hydrolase)	Fiber-optic (agarose)	0.0-0.6, 0.0-0.03 and 0.0-0.075 mM	Mulchandani et.al. (1998b)
Pollutants such as diuron and mercuric chloride	*Synechacaccus sp.* PCC 7942	Photoelectro chemical (photo cross linkable PVA bearing styrylpyridium group)	0.2 and 0.06 µM	Rouillon et al (1999)
Herbicides (diuron and atrazine)	Chloroplast/thylakoid membranes	Pt-electrode in microelectrochemical cell (photo cross linkable PVA bearing styrylpyridium group	2×10^{-5} and 2×10^{-4} mM	Rouition et al (1995)
Mono and polyphenols (atrazine)	Potato (S. tuberosum) slices (polyphenol oxidase inhibition)	Oxygen electrode (tissue slice sandwitched between membranes)	20-130 µM	Mazzel et. al (1993)

Table 10.9 Applications of Bioluminescence-based Biosensors

Application	Microorganism	Reference
Monitoring toxicity of compounds to eukaryoles	*S. cerevislae* was genetically modified to express firefly luciferase	Hollis et. al. (2000)
On-line monitoring of microbial growth	*E.coli* engineered for constitutive bioluminescence	Marincs (2000)
Toxicity of Zn, Cu and Cd, alone or in combination	*E.coli* HB101 and Ps. Fluorescens 10586 genetically modified with luxCDABE	Presion et. al (2000)
Polycyclic aromatic hydrocarbons	Ps. Fluorescens HK44 genetically modified with luxCDABE	Webb et.al. (1997), Sayler et al. (1999), Ripp et. al. (2000)
Exotoxicity assessment of organotins and their initial breakdown products (tributyltin, dibutyltin, triphenyltin and diphenyltin)	Microtox and hexCDABE modified *Ps. Fluorescens*	Bundy et. al. (1997)
Ethanol as a model toxicant	*E.coli TV* 1061, *harboring* the plasmid pGrpELux5	Gu et. al. (1996), Rupani et al. (1996)
Monitoring of biocides	Bioluminescent strain of E.coli produced by recombinant DNA technology.	Fabricant et. al. (1995)
Metals, solvents, crop protection chemicals etc	*E.coli* heat shock promoters, dnak and grpE were fused with lux genes of V,fischeri	Van Dyk et. al (1994)
Identifying constraints to bioremediation of BTEX contaminated sites	luxCDABE modified Ps. Fluorescens	Sousa et. al. (1998)
Assessment of the toxicity of metals in soils amended with sewage sludge	luxCDABE modified Ps. Fluorescens	McGrath et. al. (1999)

10.6.8 Summary

There is a vast potential market for biosensors which is only beginning to be exploited.

(a) Biosensors generally are easy to operate, analyze over a wide range of useful analyte concentrations and give reproducible results.

(b) The diffusional limitation of substrate(s) may be an asset to be encouraged in biosensor design due to the consequent reduction in the effects of analyte pH, temperature and inhibitors on biosensor response.

The following are the polymers and their functions(table 10.6)

Table 10.10 Polymers and their Functions

Polymer	Function
Polyacetylene	Redox polymer
Polyacrylamide	Polymer gel
Polyaniline	Redox polymer
Polyethylene	Membrane
Poly ethyleneimine	Membrane
Poly Ethylene Phthalate	Enzyme membrane
Poly methacrylate	Enzyme membrane
Poly pyrrole	Redox polymer
Poly styrene	Optical fiber
Poly thiophene	Redox polymer
Poly urethane	Enzyme membrane
Poly vinyl alcohol	Polymer matrix
Poly vinyl chloride	Polymer matrix

Applications

Transducers and their applications are:

Table 10.11 Different Transducers and their Applications

Transducer	Applications
Ion selective electrodes	Ion in biological Media, Enzyme electrodes
Thermistors	Enzyme organelle, gases, antibiotic, pollutants
Fibre optic and optoelectronic devices	pH, enzyme substrates, Immuno logical systems
Piezoelectric Crystals	Volatile gases

Advantages

- Very low concentration of biological substance measured
- Wide range of sensitivity for analysis
- Rapid response and low cost
- Continuous real time assay
- Disposable, reagent-less nature
- Computer compatibility

Current and Future Challenges of Biosensors

1. Novel techniques for the mass production of biosensors
2. Molecular engineering of the biosensor

3. Direct transduction of biorecognition events
4. Micro fabricated biosensors

Function

To interact specifically with a target compound i.e., the compound to be detected, it must be capable of detecting the presence of a target compound in the test solution.

The ability of a bio-element to interact specifically with target compound (specificity) is the basis for biosensor.

Response of a bio element

- Heat absorbed (or liberated) during the interaction.
- Movement of electrons produced in a radox reaction.
- Light absorbed (or liberated) during the interaction.
- Effect due to mass of reactants or products

Types of bio sensors

- Electrochemical biosensor
- Optical biosensor
- Thermal biosensor
- Resonant biosensor
- Ion-sensitive biosensor

10.7 Assessment Methods of New Antibiotics

1. ***Dilution method*:** The Broth dilution method involves subjecting the isolate to a series of concentrations of antimicrobial agents in a broth environment. Microdilution testing uses about 0.05 to 0.1 ml total broth volume and can be conveniently performed in a microtiter format. Macrodilution testing uses broth volumes at about 1.0 ml in standard test tubes. For both of these broth dilution methods, the lowest concentration at which the isolate is completely inhibited (as evidenced by the absence of visible bacterial growth) is recorded as the minimal inhibitory concentration or MIC. The MIC is thus the minimum concentration of the antibiotic that will inhibit this particular isolate. The test is only valid if the positive control shows growth and the negative control shows no growth.

   A procedure similar to broth dilution is agar dilution. Agar dilution method follows the principle of establishing the lowest concentration of the serially diluted antibiotic concentration at which bacterial growth is still inhibited.

2. ***Disk diffusion method***: Because of convenience, efficiency and cost, the disk diffusion method is probably the most widely used method for determining anti-microbial resistance in private veterinary clinics.

   A growth medium, usually Mueller-Hinton agar, is first evenly seeded throughout the plate with the isolate of interest that has been diluted at a standard concentration (approximately 1 to 2 x 10^8 colony forming units per ml). Commercially prepared disks, each of which are pre-impregnated with a standard concentration of a particular antibiotic, are then evenly dispensed and lightly pressed onto the agar surface

   The test antibiotic immediately begins to diffuse outward from the disks, creating a gradient of antibiotic concentration in the agar such that the highest concentration is found close to the disk with decreasing concentrations further away from the disk. After an overnight incubation, the bacterial growth around each disc is observed. If the test isolate is susceptible to a particular antibiotic, a clear area of "no growth" will be observed around that particular disk.

   The zone around an antibiotic disk that has no growth is referred to as the zone of inhibition since this approximates the minimum antibiotic concentration sufficient to prevent growth of the test isolate. This zone is then measured in mm and compared to a standard interpretation chart used to categorize the isolate as susceptible, intermediately susceptible or resistant. MIC measurement cannot be determined from this qualitative test, which simply classifies the isolate as susceptible, intermediate or resistant.

3. ***E-test***: E-test (AB Biodisk, Solna, Sweden) is a commercially available test that utilizes a plastic test strip impregnated with a gradually decreasing concentration of a particular antibiotic. The strip also displays a numerical scale that corresponds to the antibiotic concentration contained therein. This method provides for a convenient quantitative test of antibiotic resistance of a clinical isolate. However, a separate strip is needed for each antibiotic, and therefore the cost of this method can be high.

4. ***Automated antimicrobial susceptibility testing systems***: Several commercial systems have been developed that provide conveniently prepared and formatted microdilution panels as well as instrumentation and automated reading of plates. These methods are intended to reduce technical errors and lengthy preparation times.

   Most automated antimicrobial susceptibility testing systems provide automated inoculation, reading and interpretation. These systems have the advantage of being rapid (some results can be generated within hours) and convenient, but one major limitation for most laboratories is the cost entailed in initial purchase, operation and maintenance of the machinery. Some examples of these include: Vitek System (bioMerieux, France), Walk-Away System (Dade International, Sacramento,

Calif.), Sensititre ARIS (Trek Diagnostic Systems, East Grinstead, UK), Avantage Test System (Abbott Laboratories, Irving, Texas), Micronaut (Merlin, Bornheim-Hesel, Germany), Phoenix (BD Biosciences, Maryland) and many more.

5. ***Mechanism-specific tests*:** Resistance may also be established through tests that directly detect the presence of a particular resistance mechanism. For example, beta lactamase detection can be accomplished using an assay such as the chromogenic cephalosporinase test (Cefinase disk by BD Microbiology Systems, Cockeysville, MD and BBL DrySlide Nitrocefin, Becton Dickinson, Sparks, MD) and detection for chloramphenicol modifying enzyme chloramphenicol acetyltransferase (CAT) may utilize commercial colorimetric assays such as a CAT reagent kit (Remel, Lenexa, Kansas).

6. ***Genotypic methods*:** Since resistance traits are genetically encoded, we can sometimes test for the specific genes that confer antibiotic resistance. However, although nucleic acid-based detections systems are generally rapid and sensitive, it is important to remember that the presence of a resistance gene does not necessarily equate to treatment failure, because resistance is also dependent on the mode and level of expression of these genes. Some of the most common molecular techniques utilized for antimicrobial resistance detection are:

   Polymerase chain reaction (PCR) is one of the most commonly used molecular techniques for detecting certain DNA sequences of interest. This involves several cycles of denaturation of sample DNA, annealing of specific primers to the target sequence (if present), and the extension of this sequence as facilitated by a thermostable polymerase leading to replication of a duplicate DNA sequence, in an exponential manner, to a point which will be visibly detectable by gel electrophoresis with the aid of a DNA-intercalating chemical which fluoresces under UV light.

***DNA hybridization*:** This is based on the fact that the DNA pyrimidines (cytosine and thymidine) specifically pair up with purines (guanine and adenine; or uracil for RNA). Therefore, a labeled probe with a known specific sequence can pair up with opened or denatured DNA from the test sample, as long as their sequences complement each other. If this "hybridization" occurs, the probe labels this with a detectable radioactive isotope, antigenic substrate, enzyme or chemiluminescent compound.

***Modifications of PCR and DNA hybridization*:** With these basic principles, several modifications have been introduced which further improve the sensitivity and specificity of these standard procedures. Examples of such development were the use of 5'-fluorescence-labeled oligonucleotides, the development of molecular beacons, development of DNA arrays and DNA chips, among many others.

10.8 Microbial Limit Tests

The following tests (Fig. 10.18) are designed for the estimation of number of viable aerobic micro organ present and for detecting the presence of designated species in pharmaceutical substances.

The term 'growth' is used to designate the presence and presumed proliferation of viable micro-organisms.

10.8.1 Preliminary Testing

- The methods given herein are invalid unless it is demonstrated that the test specimens to which they are applied do not, of themselves, inhibit the multiplication under the test conditions of micro-organisms that can be present.
- Therefore prior to doing the tests, inoculate diluted specimens of the substances being examined with separate viable cultures of "*Escherichia coli*", *Salmonella* species, *Pseudomonas aeruginosa* and *Staphylococcus aureus*.

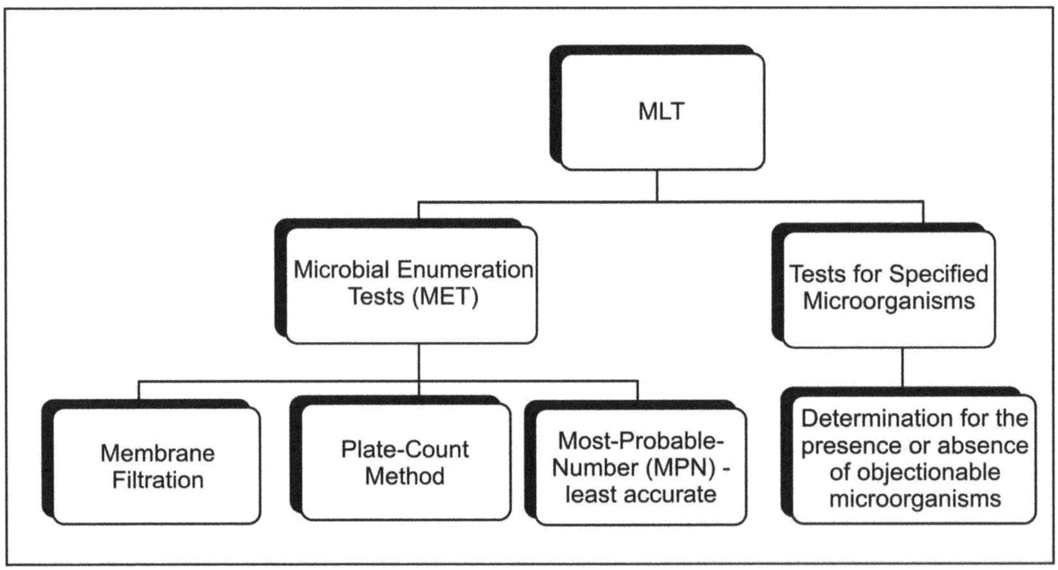

Fig.10.16 Schematic diagram of microbial limit test methods

- This can be done by adding 1 mL of not less that 10-3 dilutions of a 24 hr broth culture of the micro-organisms to first dilution (in buffer solution pH 7.2 fluid Soyabean – casein digest medium or fluid lactose medium) of the test material and following the test procedure.

- If the organisms fail to grow in the relevant medium the procedure should be modified by
  - (a) Increasing the volume of diluent with the quantity of test material remaining same
  - (b) Incorporating a sufficient quantity of suitable inactivating agent in the diluents.
  - (c) Combining the aforementioned modifications so as to permit growth of organisms in media.

If inhibitory substances are present in the sample, 0.5% of soya lecithin and 4% polysorbate 20 may be added to the culture.

Alternatively, repeat the test as described using fluid casein-digest-soya-lecithin-polysorbate 20 medium to demonstrate neutralization of preservatives or other antimicrobial agents in test-material. Apply membrane filtration method.

Limitations: Though suitable inactivating agents incorporated and volume of the diluents is increased, recovering of the viable cultures was not possible and the article is not suitable for applying the membrane filtration method.

The failure to isolate the inoculated organism may be due to the bactericidal activity of the product.

This may indicate that the article is not likely to be contaminated with the given species of micro-organisms.

However, monitoring should be continued to establish **the spectrum of inhibition** and **bactericidal activity** of the article.

Sampling: Use 10 mL or 10 g specimens for each of the tests specified in the individual monograph

Precautions

- The microbial limit tests should be carried out under conditions designated to avoid accidental contamination during the test.
- The precautions taken to avoid contamination must be such that they do not adversely affect any micro-organisms that should be revealed in the test.

10.8.2 Methods

Total Aerobic Microbial Count

Pretreat the sample of the product being examined as described below:

10.8.2.1 Water soluble products

Dissolve 10 g or dilute 10 mL of preparation being examined unless otherwise specified in buffered sodium chloride peptone solution pH 7.0 or any other suitable medium shown to have no antimicrobial activity under the conditions of the test and adjust the volume to 100 ml with the same medium. If necessary adjust pH to about 7.

10.8.2.2 Products Insoluble in Water (Non fatty)

Suspend 10 g or 10 mL of the preparation being examined unless otherwise specified, in buffered sodium chloride – peptone solution pH 7.0 or any other suitable medium shown to have no anti microbial activity under the conditions of the test and adjust the volume to 100 mL with the same medium

- A suitable surfactant such as 0.1% w/v polysorbate 80 may be added to assist the suspension of poorly wettable substances. If necessary adjust the pH of suspension to 7.

10.8.2.3 Fatty Products

Homogenise 10 g or 10 mL of the preparation being examined unless otherwise specified with 5 g of polysorbate 20 or polysorbate 80. If necessary heat to not more than 40 °C. Mix carefully while maintaining the temperature in water bath or in oven. Add 85 mL of buffered sodium chloride – peptone solution pH – 7.0 or any other suitable medium shown to have no antimicrobial activity under the conditions of the test heated to not more than 40 °C if necessary maintain this temperature for the shortest time necessary for formation of an emulsion and in any case for not more than 30 min. If necessary adjust the pH to 7.

10.8.2.4 Examining Methods

Determine the total aerobic microbial count in the substance being examined by any of the following.

Membrane Filtration

- Use membrane filters 50 mm in diameter and having a nominal pore size of not greater than 0.45 μm the effectiveness of which is retaining bacteria has been established for the type of preparation being examined
- Sterilise and assemble the filtration apparatus described under tests for sterility
- Transfer 10 mL or a quantity of each dilution containing 1 g of the preparation being examined to each of two membrane filters and filter immediately.
- If necessary dilute the predicated preparation so that a colony count of 10-100 may be expected.
- Wash each membrane by filtering through it three or more successive quantities each of about 100 mL of a suitable liquid such as buffered sodium-chloride peptone solution pH 7.
- For fatty substances add to the liquid *poly sorbate* 20 or *polysorbate* 80.

- Transfer one of the membrane filters, intended for the enumeration of bacteria, to the surface of a plate of *Casein soyabean digest agar* and other intended for enumeration of fungi to the surface of a plate of *Sabouraud dextrose agar with antibiotics.*
- Incubate the plates for 5 days, unless a more reliable count is obtained in shorter time, at 30 °C-35 °C in the test for bacteria and 20 °C to 25 °C in test for fungi.
- Count the number of colonies that are formed.
- Calculate number of micro-organisms per 'g' or per 'ml' of preparation being examined.
- If necessary count bacteria and fungi separately.

10.8.2.5 Plate count

***For bacteria*:** using Petri dishes 9-10 cm in diameter, add to each dish a mixture of 1 ml of the pretreated preparation and about 15 ml of the liquefied *Casein soyabean digest agar* at not more than 45 °C

- Alternatively, spread the pretreated preparation on the surface of the solidified medium in a Petri dish of the same diameter
- If necessary dilute the pretreated preparation as described above so that a colony count of not more than 300 may be expected
- Prepare at least two such Petri dishes using the same dilution and incubate 30 °C-35 °C for 4 days unless a more reliable count is obtained in a shorter time
- Count the number colonies that are formed
- Calculate the results using plates with the greatest number of colonies but taking 300 colonies per plate as the maximum consistent with good evaluation.

For fungi: Proceed the method similar to bacteria but use Sabourand dextrose agar with antibiotics in place of Casein soyabean digest agar and incubate the plates at 20 °C-25 °C for 5 days, unless a more reliable count is obtained in a shorter time. Calculate the results using plates with not more than 100 colonies.

10.8.2.6 Multiple – Tube or Serial Dilution Method

- In each of fourteen test-tubes of similar size, place 9.0 mL of sterile fluid soyabean casein digest medium.
- Arrange 12 of the tubes in four sets of three tubes each.
- Put aside one set of three tubes to serve as controls.
- Into each of three tubes of one set ("100") and into fourth tube (A) pipette 1 ml of the solution of the suspension of the test specimen and mix.
- From tube (A) pipette 1 mL of its contents into the one remaining tube (B) not included in the set and mix shown in Table. 10.10.

- These two tubes contain 100 mg (or 100 μl) and 10 mg (or 10 μl) of specimen respectively.
- Into each of the second set ("10") of the three tubes pipette 1 ml from tube A, and into each tube of third set ("1") pipette 1 mL from tube B.
- Discard the unused contents of tube A and B.
- Close well and incubate all of the tubes.
- After incubation period examine the tube for growth
- The three control tubes remain clear.

Observations in the tubes containing the test specimen, when interpreted by reference to the Table 10.12, indicate the most probable number of micro-organisms per 'g' or per 'mL' of test specimen.

Table 10.12 Most Probable Total Count by Multiple Tube or Serial Dilution Method

Observed combination of number of tube showing growth in each set			Most probable number of micro-organisms per 'g' or per 'mL'
No. of mg (or mL) of specimen per tube			
100 (100 μl)	10 (10 μl)	1 (1 μl)	
3	3	3	> 1100
3	3	2	1100
3	3	1	500
3	3	0	200
3	2	3	290
3	2	2	210
3	2	1	150
3	2	0	90
3	1	3	160
3	1	2	120
3	1	1	70
3	1	0	40
3	0	3	95
3	0	2	60
3	0	1	40
3	0	0	23

10.8.2.7 Tests for Specified Microorganism

Pretreatment of samples being examined

The procedure for pretreatment is proceeded as test for **total aerobic microbial count** but using *lactose broth* or any other medium that have no antimicrobial activity under the conditions of test in place of *buffered* sodium chloride-peptone solution pH-7.

Test Species *Escherichia coli*

Place the prescribed quantity in a sterile screw-capped container add 50 ml of nutrient broth shake, allow to stand for 1 hour and shake again. Loosen the cap and incubate at 37°C for 18-24 hr.

10.8.2.7.1 Primary Test

- Add 1 mL of the enrichment culture to a tube containing 5 mL of Mac Conkey Broth.
- Incubate in a water bath at 36 °C-38 °C for 48 hours
- If the contents of the tube show acid and gas carryout the secondary test.

10.7.2.7.2 Secondary Test

- Add 1 mL of the contents of the tubes containing
- 5 ml of *Mac Conkey broth*
- 5 ml of *Peptone water*
- Incubate in water bath at 43.5° to 44.5° for 24 hr and examine tube (a) for acid and gas and tube (b) for indole
- To test for indole add 0.5 ml of Kovac's reagent, shake well and allow to stand for 1 min.

Observation: If a red colour is produced in the reagent layer Indole is present. Also the presence of acid and gas and of indole in the secondary test indicates the presence of *"Escherichia coli"*.

Carryout a control test by repeating the primary and secondary tests adding 1.0 mL of the enrichment culture and a volume of broth containing 10-50 *Escherichia coli* (NCTC 9002) organisms, prepared from a 24-hour culture in nutrient broth to 5 mL of *Mac Conkey broth*.

- The test is not valid unless the results indicate that the control contains *Escherichia coli*.

10.8.2.7.3 Alternative Method

With inoculating loop, streak a portion from the enrichment culture on the surface of Mac Conkey agar medium present in the Petri dish.

- Cover and invert the dishes and incubate
- Upon examination, if none of the colonies are brick-red in colour and have a surrounding zone of precipitated bile, the sample meets the requirements of the test for the absence of *Escherichia coli.*
- If the colonies described above are found, transfer the suspect colonies individually to the surface of Levine eosin - methylene blue agar medium plated on Petri dishes.
- Cover and invert the plates and incubate
- Upon examination if none of the colonies exhibit both a characteristic metallic sheen under reflected light and a blue - black appearance under transmitted light, the sample meets the requirements of the test for the absence of *Escherchia coli*
- The presence of *E. coli* may be further confirmed by further suitable cultural and biochemical tests.

10.8.2.8 Salmonella

Transfer a quantity of pretreated preparation being examined containing 1g or 1ml of product to 100ml of Nutrient broth in sterile screw capped jar, shake & incubate at 35 to 37 for 24hr.

Preliminary test; Add 1.0 ml of enrichment culture to each of two tubes containing (A) 10ml of Selenite F broth & (B)Tetrathionet -bile- brilliant green broth &incubate at 36 to38° for 48 hr. From each of this two cultures subculture on following four agar medium & incubate at 36 to 38°for24 hr• if none of colonies conform to description given in table 10.15, sample meet requirement for absence of *salmonella.*

Table 10.13 Results of Microbial Limit Test for *Salmonella*

Selective Medium	Characteristic Colonial Morphology
Brilliant Green Agar Medium	Small, transparent, colorless or pink to white opaque (frequently surrounded by pink to red zone)
Xylose-Lysine Desoxycholate Agar Medium	Red, with or without black centers
Bismuth sulfite Agar Medium	Black or green

Secondary test: subculture any colonies showing characteristics given in table in triple sugar-iron agar by first inoculating the surface of slope & at the same time inoculate a tube of urea broth &incubate both at 36 to 38 for 18 to 24 hr. The absence of acidity from the surface growth in triple sugar iron agar & together with absence of red colour in urea broth, indicates the presence of *salmonella.*

For Control: Repeat the primary & secondary test using 1.0 ml of enrichment culture & volume of broth containing 10 to 50 *salmonella* organism, prepare from 24hr broth culture in nutrient broth, for inoculation of tubes (a) & (b). The result is not valid unless the result indicate that the control contains salmonella.

10.8.2.9 Pseudomonas aeroginosa

Inoculate 100 ml of fluid soya bean casein digest medium with quantity of solution, suspension or emulsion thus obtained containing 1 g or 1 ml of preparation being examined & incubates at 35 to 37 for 24 to 48 hr

If upon examination none of colonies having characteristics listed in table for media used, sample meet requirement for absence of micro- organisms.

- If colony conform to description in table, carry out oxidase & pigment test.
- Oxidase & Pigment Test Streak representative suspect colony from cetrimide agar medium on surface of *pseudomonas* agar medium for detection of florescein & pseudomonas agar medium for detection of pyocyanin contained in Petri dish & incubate at 33 to 37 °for NLT 3 days.
- Examine the streak surface under u.v light.
- Examine plate to determine whether colonies conforming to description in table are present. If, growth of suspect colonies occur, place 2 or 3 drops freshly prepared 1%w/v solution of N, N- tetramethyl-4-phenylenediamine dihydrochloride on filter paper & smear with colony.
- If there is no development of pink colour changing to purple, the sample meet requirements of test for absence of *Pseudomonas aeruginosa.*

Table 10.14 Results of Microbial Limit Test for *Pseudomonas Aeroginosa*

Selective Medium	Characteristic Colonial Morphology	Flourescence in UV Light	Oxidase Test	Gram Stain
Centrimide Agar Medium	Generally Greenish	Greenish	Positive	Negative rods
Pseudomonas Agar Medium for Detection of Fluorescin	Generally colorless to yellowish	Yellowish	Positive	Negative rods
Pseudomonas Agar Medium for Detection of Pyocyanin	Generally Greenish	Blue	Positive	Negative rods

10.8.2.10 *Staphylococcus aures*

Proceed as described under the test for *Psudomonas aerugino.* If upon examination of incubated plate, none of them contain colony having characteristics listed in the table, the sample meets requirement for the absence of *S.aureus*. If, growth occurs, carry out

COAGULASE test. Transfer representative suspect colony from agar surface to individual tubes, each containing 0.5ml of mammalian, preferably horse or rabbit plasma with or without additive. Incubate in water bath at 37 °C and examine tubes at 3hour & subsequently at suitable intervals up to 24 hours. If no coagulation is observed sample meets the requirement of test for absence of *S.aureus*

Table 10.15 Results of Microbial Limit Test for *Staphylococcus Aures*

Selective Medium	Characteristic Colonical Morphology	Gram Stain
Vogel-Johnson Agar Medium	Black Surrounded by yellow zone	Positive cocci (in clusters)
Mannital-Salt Agar Medium	Yellow colonies with yellow zones	Positive cocci (in clussters)
Baird-Parker Agar Medium	Black, shiny, surrounded by clear zones 2 to 5 mm	Positve coccid (in clusters)

10.9 Some of the Media used in the Microbial Limit Tests

Culture media may be prepared according to the medium composition formula (or) dehydrated culture medium may be used provided when reconstituted as directed by manufacturer, these should be similar to the formulae given for each medium.

- To the formula agar is specified in a formula use agar that has a moister content of > 15% where water called purified water is used.

Different types of media are

1. Baird-parker Agar Medium

Pancreatic digest of casein	10.0 g
Beef extract	5.0 g
Yeast extract	1.0 g
Lithium chloride	5.0 g
Agar	20.0 g
Glycine	12.0 g
Sodium pyruvate	10.0 g
Water up to	1000 ml

Method: Heat with frequent agitation and boil for 1 minute. Sterilize cool to between 45 to 50 °C and add 10 mL of 1% w/v solution of sterile *potassium tellurite* and add 50 ml of egg yolk emulsion. Mix intimately but gently and pour into plates. (Prepare the egg-yolk emulsion by disinfecting the surface of whole shell eggs aseptically cracking the eggs and separating out intact yolks into a sterile graduated cylinder. Add to a sterile saline solution, get a 3 to 7 ratio of egg-yolk to saline. Add to sterile blender cup and mix at high speed for 5 secs). Adjust pH after sterilization to 6.0 ± 0.2.

2. Bismuth sulphite agar medium

Formula

Solution (1)

Beef extract	6.0 g
Peptone	10.0 g
Agar	24.0 g
Ferric citrate	0.4 g
Brilliant green	10 mg
Water to	1000 mL

Method: Dissolve with aid of heat and sterilise by maintaining at 115 °C for 30 min

Solution (2)

Ammonium Bismuth citrate	3.0 g
Sodium sulphate	10.0 g
Anhydrous Disodium hydrogen phosphate	5.0 g
Dextrose monohydrate	5.0 g
Water	1000 mL

Method: Mix, heat to boiling, cool to room temperature add 1 volume of solution (2) to 10 volumes of solution (1) previously melted and cooled to a temperature of 55 °C and pour.

Storage: Bismuth sulphite agar medium should be stored at 2-8 °C for 5 days before use.

3. Brilliant green agar medium

Peptone	10.0 g
Yeast extract	3.0 g
Lactose	10.0 g
Sucrose	10.0 g
NaCl	5.0 g
Phenol red	80.0 g
Brilliant green	12.5 g
Agar	12.0 g
Water	1000 ml

Method: Mix allow to stand for 15 min. Sterilise by maintaining at 115 °C for 30 min and mix before pouring.

4. Buffered Sodium chloride – peptone solution (pH – 7)

Potassium hydrogen

phosphate	3.56 g
Disodium hydrogen phosphate	7.23 g
Sodium chloride	4.3 g
Peptone (Meat/casein)	1.0 g
Water	1000 mL

Method: 1% w/v polysorbate 20 or polysorbate 80 may be added. Sterilise by heating in an autoclave at 121 °C for 15 min.

5. Casein soyabean digest agar medium

Formula	Quantity
Paninealic digest of casein	15.0 g
Papaic digest of soyabean meal	5.0 g
Sodium chloride	5.0 g
Agar	15.0 g
Water	1000 mL

Method: Adjust pH after sterilization to 7.3 ± 0.2

6. Cetrimide agar medium

Panereatic digest of gelatin	20.0 g
Magnesium chloride	1.4 g
Potassium sulphate	10.0 g
Cetrimide	0.3 g
Agar	13.6 g
Glycerine	10.0 g
Water	1000 mL

Method: Heat to boiling 1 minute with shaking. Adjust the pH so that after sterilization it is 7.0-7.4 sterilize at 121 °C for 15 min.

7. Deoxy cholate – citrate agar medium

Beef extract	5.0 g
Peptone	5.0 g
Lactose	10.0 g
Tri sodium citrate	8.5 g
Sodium thio sulfate	5.4 g
Ferric citrate	1.0 g
Sodium desovy cholate	5.0 g

Neutral red	0.2 g
Agar	12 g
Water	1000 mL

Method: Mix and allow to stand for 15 min with continuous stirring, bring gently to boil and at boiling point until solution is complete. Cool it rapidly.

Note: Desoxy cholate agar should not be over heated. It should not be remelted and the surface of the plates should be dried before use.

8. Mac Conkey agar medium

Pancreatic digest of gelatin	17.0 g
Peptone	
(meat and casein in equal parts)	3.0 g
Lactose	10.0 g
Sodium chloride	5.0 g
Bile salts	1.5 g
Agar	13.5 g
Neutral red	30 mg
Crystal violet	1 mg
Water	1000 mL

Method: Boil the mixture of solids and water for 1 min to effect solution. Adjust pH after sterilization to 7.1 ± 0.2

9. Pseudomonas agar medium for detection of fluorescein

Panereatic digest of casein	10.0 g
Peptic digest of animal tissue	10.0 g
Anhydrous dibasic	
potassium phosphate	1.5 g
Magnesium sulphate	1.5 g
Glycerine	10 ml
Agar	15 g
Water	1000 mL

Dissolve the solid components in water before adding glycerine. Heat with frequent agitation and boil 1 min to effect solution. Adjust the pH after sterilization to 7.2 ± 0.2.

Essay Questions

Essay Questions

1. Write a note on various bio indicators and their applications
2. Write a note on biosensors and their applications in pharma industry

Multiple Choice Questions

1. Which of the following saprophobic zones are classified as heavy pollution zones
   (a) Polysaprobic zones
   (b) oligo saprobic
   (c) alpha saprobic
   (d) beta saprobic zones
2. Poly vinyl alcohol is used as
   (a) Redox polymer
   (b) Polymer gel
   (c) Polymer matrix
   (d) Enzyme polymer
3. Piezoelectric crystals are used as
   (a) Enzyme substrates
   (b) Ions in biological media
   (c) Volatile gases
   (d) Enzyme electrodes
4. Polyacyrlamaide is used as
   (a) Polymer gel
   (b) Enzyme membrane
   (c) Optical fiber
   (d) Dox polymer
5. Which among the following genera has the highest pollution index
   (a) Anacystis
   (b) Ankistrodesmus
   (c) Chlorella
   (d) Euglena

Answers

1. (c)	2. (c)	3. (c)
4. (a)	5. (d)	

11

MICROBIAL SPOILAGE AND PRESERVATION OF PHARMACEUTICAL PRODUCTS

LEARNING OBJECTIVES

After studying the chapter the students familiarize themselves with concepts in:

- *Understanding Physico-chemical deterioration of pharmaceuticals*
- *Understanding various factors affecting spoilage of pharmaceutical products*
- *Understanding protection of micro-organisms within pharmaceutical products*
- *Understanding standards for non-sterile pharmaceutical products*
- *Understanding mechanisms of various microbes and their manifestations*
- *Developing an insight into the preservation of pharmaceutical products*
- *Understanding fast and high thorough put preservative efficacy testing*
- *Understanding potable water standards*

11.1 Microbial Spoilage Introduction

Pharmaceutical products used in prevention, treatment and diagnosis of disease contain a wide variety of ingredients, present is complex physico-chemical status. Such products should meet current pharmaceutical Good Manufacturing Practice (GMP) requirements for quality, safety and efficiency and sufficiently elegant to be acceptable to patients.

Microbial spoilage is a phenomenon where the pharmaceutical product undergo chemical and physico-chemical deterioration in their formulation resulting unfit for use and are therapeutically inactive.

- Microbial spoilage can be caused by bacteria, yeasts or fungi which are extremely versatile in their metabolic activities.
- Inadvertent use of contaminated products may present a potential health hazard to patients, resulting in outbreaks of medicament-related infections and therefore contributing to the spread of disease.

The consequences of contamination of few organisms in pharmaceutical products are:

1. Heavy contamination of product with opportunist pathogens like Pseudomonas species has resulted in the spread of "nosocomial" (hospital-acquired) infections.
2. Low levels of contamination with pathogen such as salmonella have attracted considerable attention due to contamination of products with toxic metabolites.

11.2 Spoilage - Chemical and Physicochemical Deterioration of Pharmaceuticals

Micro organisms form a major part of natural recycling process for biological matter in the environment also possess a wide variety of degradative capabilities, which are able to exert under mild physico chemical conditions.

Mixed natural communities are more effective co-operative biodeteriogens than individual species and sequences of attack of complex substrates occur where intial attack by one group of micro-organisms renders then susceptible to further deterioration by secondary and subsequent micro-organisms.

Under suitable environment selection pressures, Novel degradative pathways may emerge with the capability to attack newly introduced synthetic chemical. But the rates of degradation of materials released into the environment can vary greatly, from half-lives of hours (phenol) to months (hard detergents) to years (halogenated pesticides).

The overall rate of deterioration of a chemical will depend upon:

(a) Molecular structure

(b) Physico chemical properties of particular environment

(c) The type and quantity of microbes present.

(d) Whether the metabolites produced can serve as source of ustable energy and precursors for the biosynthesis of cellular components.

11.2.1 Pharmaceutical Ingredients Susceptible to Microbial Attack

Pharmaceutical products are dosage forms that are formulated by suitable ingredients. The ingredients include therapeutic agents and other additions. The pharmaceutical ingredients susceptible to microbial attack are

1. Therapeutic agents
2. Surface active agents
3. Organic polymers

4. Humectants
5. Fats and oils
6. Sweetening, flavoring and coloring agents.
7. Preservatives and Disinfectants.

Therapeutic Agents

- Spoilage of therapeutic agents (or) Active ingredients results in drug metabolism making it less potent or chemically inactive forms.

Under laboratory conditions a variety of micro organisms metabolize a wide assortment of drugs resulting in loss of activity.

Therapeutic agents like

I. Alkaloids
   (a) Morphine
   (b) Strychnine
   (c) atropine
II. Analgesics
   (a) Aspirin
   (b) Paracetamol
III. Barbiturates
IV. Thalidomide
V. Steroid Esters
VI. Mandelic acid

Can be metabolized and can serve as substrates for growth.

Advantage

The use of micro-organisms to carry out subtle transformations on steroid molecules forms the basis of the commercial production of potent therapeutic steroidal agents.

Examples

(a) Metabolism of Atropine in eye drops by contaminating fungi.
(b) Inactivation of penicillin injections by β- lactamase producing bacteria.
(c) Steroid metabolism in damp tablets and creams by fungi.
(d) Microbial hydrolysis of aspirin in a suspension by esterase producing bacteria.
(e) Chloramphenicol deactivation in an oral medicine by a chloramphenicol acetylase-producing contaminant.

Surface Active Agents

Various types of surface active agents used in the formulation of pharmaceutical dosage form are

(i) Anionic surfactants
(ii) Non-ionic surfactants
(iii) Ampholytic surfactants
(iv) Cationic surfactants

Anionic Surfactants

- Anionic surfactants such as the alkali metal and amine soaps of fatty acids are stable due to slightly alkaline pH of the formulations.

Mechanism of degradation in chemical structure of anionic surfactants due to spoilage

- Alkyl and alkyl benzene sulphonates and sulphate esters are metabolized by co-oxidation of their terminal methyl groups followed by sequential β-oxidation of the alkyl chains and fission of the aromatic rings.
- The presence of chain branching involves additional α-oxidative processes.

Effect of chain length in ease of degradation: Ease of degradation decreases with increase in chain length and complexity of branching of alkyl chain.

Non-Ionic Surfactants

- Non-ionic surfactants such as "alkyl polyoxy ethylene alcohol" emulsifiers are readily metabolized by a wide variety of micro-organisms.

Mechanism of degradation in chemical structure of Non-ionic Surfactant due to spoilage

- "Alkyl phenol polyoxyethylene alcohols" are attacked by microbes but are significantly resistant
- "Fatty acids of sorbitan esters," "Polysorbates" and "sucrose esters" undergo Lipolytic clearage followed by degradation of cyclic nucleus, producing numerous small molecules readily utilizable for microbial growth.

Ampholytic Surfactants

Based on "Phosphatides", "betaines" and "alkylamino substituted aminoacids" are important group of surfactant those are reasonably biodegradable.

Cationic Surfactants

These surfactants are used as antiseptics and preservatives in pharmaceutical application undergo slow degradation at high dilution.

e.g., *Pseudomonas* species are found to be growing readily in quaternary ammonium Antiseptic solutions.

Organic Polymers

Organic polymers are added to the pharmaceutical preparations to increase their stability, uniform distribution of drug in given system etc.

Many "thickening agents" and "suspending agents" used in pharmaceutical formulations are subjected to microbial depolymerization by specific classes of extracellular enzymes (Table 11.1) yielding nutritive fragments and monomers.

Table 11.1 Organic Polymers and their Depolymerizing Enzymes

Substrates	Enzymes
1. Starches	Amylases
2. Pectine	Pectinases
3. Carboxy methy cellulose (exception with alkyle cellulose)	Cellulases
4. Polyuronides (Tragacanth, Acacia)	Veronidases
5. Dextrans	Dextranases
6. Proteins	Proteases

Some other organic polymer and their significance

- Agar an inert polymer which is used as a solidifying agent in microbiological culture media.
- Synthetic packaging polymers such as nylon, poly styrene and polyester are extremely resistant to attack.
- Modified cellulose called cellophane is also susceptible to spoilage under humid conditions

Humectants

Humectants are low molecular weight materials like glycerol and sorbitol, which are included in some formulation to reduce water loss.

- Since they are metabolized easily they should be present in higher concentrations.

Fats and Oils

- In an emulsion hydrophobic materials are attacked extensively due to their dispersion. Aided by high solubility of O_2 in many oils, sometimes it is called Rancidity of oils
- Fungal attack can be seen in condensed moisture films on the surface of oils in bulk, or where water droplets have contaminated bulk oil phase.
- But microbial metabolism of pharmaceutical hydrocarbon oils are rarely seen.
- Problem occurs when water droplets have accumulated in oil storage tanks and subsequent fungal colonization catalyses causes serious corrosion.

Mechanism of degradation: Lipolytic recapturing of triglycerides liberates glycerol and fatty acids and followed by β-oxidation of alkyl chains of fatty acid and produces odoriferous Ketones.

Sweetening, Flavoring and Coloring Agents

- Many of sugars and other artificial sweetening agents used in pharmacy are ready substrates for microbial growth.

But some are used in very high concentrations to reduce water activity in aqueous products and inhibit microbial attack.

- At one time, a variety of coloring agents like tartrazine and Amaranth and flavoring agents like peppermint water were kept stock solutions for extemporaneous dispensing purposes but they supported the growth of *pseuodomonas species* including "*Pseudomonas aeruginosa*".

Such solution should be preserved at proper conditions (or) freshly made when required. Alcoholic solutions are much less susceptible to microbial attack.

Preservatives and Disinfectants

- Many preservatives and disinfectants are metabolized by a wide variety of Gram-negative bacteria at concentrations below their effective 'use' levels.
- Growth of *Pseudomonas* in stock solutions of quaternary ammonium antiseptics and chlorhexidine has resulted in infection of patients.
- *Pseudomonas* species have metabolized 4-hydroxybenzoate ester preservatives contained in eye-drops thus resulting in serious eye infections.
- They also metabolize oral suspensions and solutions.

So selection of suitable preservative for formulation of pharmaceutical products to avoid contamination can be done by studying the properties of various preservatives and their susceptibility to microbial contamination.

11.2.2 Manifestations and Mechanism of Action

Toxic Effects

Microbial Toxins

- Endotoxin produced by gram negative bacteria such as *Escherichia E.coli.*
- Toxins of this type are poorly absorbed by the oral route but are important in connection with injectable products, particularly perfusion fluids

- Exotoxins are highly lethal produced by Clostridium botulinum
- *Staphylococcus aureus* produce a toxin, characterized as a specific polysaccharide
- *Aspergillus* commonly infects peanuts, cotton seed and grain which are all components of animal food.

Metabolic Products

- In addition to microbial toxins there are metabolic products and are simpler catabolic products such as organic acids and Amines are toxic to man
- Compounds of less toxic relatively high concentrations should be attained before a spoiled product causes illness.

Irritancy

Contaminants provide a source of foreign protein evoking an allergic contact dermatitis reaction or that high level of a microbial metabolite will cause a primary irritant reaction.

Change of Activity

- Destruction of penicillium by pencillinase enzymes produced by a broad range of micro-organisms. Microbial enzymes which inactivate chloramphenicol are also known and destruction of preservatives and disinfectants.
- Loss of Atropine of up to 20% in eye drops could be caused by *corynebacterium* and *Pseudomonas* spp. isolated from the eye drops
- *Corynebacterium hoffnaii* metabolised the analgesics aspirin, phenacetin and pacacetmol.
- *Acinetobacter toffi*, obtained from distilled water utilized aspirin as a sole carbon source in a mineral salt solution.

Visibility Effects

(i) Visible Growth

- In liquid formulation contaminants may be seen as sediment, turbidity, colonies, coloured of bacteria, yeasts or moulds may form.

(ii) Colour Changes

- Members of pseudomonas germs produced soluble pigments ranging in colour from blue-green to brown.

(iii) Gas Production

- Products containing carbohydrates or other fermentable substrates are particularly susceptible to this type of spoilage.

(iv) Taste

- The products taste peen liar indicates spoiled

(v) Texture

- Creams can become lumpy or gritty and changes in viscosity of liquid preparations.
- Humidifiers, incubators, ventilators, resuscitators and other apparatus require proper maintenance and decontamination after use.

11.2.3 Observable Effects of Microbial attacks on Pharmaceutical Products

- Microbial contaminants create an environment for biosynthesis and energy products before they replicate by attacking formulation ingredients and results in "Spoilage".

Example: 10^6 microbes have an overall degradative effect around 10^6 times faster than one cell. But growth and attack may well be localized in surface moisture films or very un-evenly distributed within the bulk of viscous formulations like creams.

- Early indications of spoilage are organoleptic with the release of unpleasant smelling, tasting metabolites such as 'sour' fatty acids, 'Fishy' amines bad eggs', bitter, earthy or sickly tastes and smells.
- Products may become un-appealingly discolored by microbial pigments of various shades.
- Thickening and suspending agents such as Tragacanth, acacia, carboxy methyl cellulose can be depolymerized resulting in loss of viscosity.
- Microbial polymerization of sugars and surfactant molecules can produce slimy, viscous masses in syrups, shampoos and creams and also fungal growth in creams produces gritty textures.
- Change in pH takes place due to release of acidic or basic metabolites.
- Gaseous metabolites may be seen as trapped bubbles within viscous formulations.
- Lipolytic release of fatty acids from oils will lower pH and encourage coalescence of oil globules and cracking of the emulsion.
- Fatty acids and their ketonic oxidation products will provide a sour taste and unpleasant smell. While the bubbles of gaseous metabolites may be visible trapped in product and pigment may discolor it.

11.2.4 Factors Affecting Microbial Spoilage of Pharmaceutical Products

By understanding the influence of environmental parameters on micro-organisms it may be possible to manipulate the environmental conditions as unfavorable as possible for growth and spoilage within the limits of patients' acceptability and therapeutic efficacy.

The final pharmaceutical product characteristics will indicate its susceptibility to attack by various classes of micro-organisms.

Factors that affect the formulation are:

1. Types and size of contaminant inoculums
2. Nutritional factors
3. Moisture content: water Activity (A_w)
4. Redox potential
5. Storage temperature
6. pH
7. Packaging design
8. Protection of micro-organisms within pharmaceutical products.

Types of Size of Contaminant Inoculum

Formulation of a dosage form successfully against microbial attack depends up on the pharmacist prediction also understanding the challenges faced in life enables him to build-in as much protection as possible against microbial attack.

Knowledge of microbial ecology and careful identification of contaminants can be useful in tracking down the defective steps in the production process.

Low levels of contaminants may not cause appreciable spoilage, if unable to replicate in products. Inoculum size alone is not always a reliable indicator of likely spoilage potential.

e.g., Low levels of aggressive *Pseudomonas* in a weakly preserved solution suggest greater risk than tablets containing fairly high numbers of fungal and bacterial spores.

Various chances of contaminants are:

- Raw materials were unusually contaminated.
- There was a lapse in plant-cleaning protocol.
- A biofilm detached itself within supplying pipe work.
- May be product is grossly misused during administration.

Process of contamination and further growth

- When an aggressive microorganism contaminates a medicine, there may be an appreciable lag period before significant spoilage begins, the duration of which decreases disproportionately with increasing contaminant loading.
- As there is usually a considerable delay between manufacture and administration of factory-made medicines, growth and attack could happen during this period unless additional steps were taken to prevent it.

Nutritional Factors

- The simple nutritional requirements and metabolic adaptability of many common spoilage micro-organisms, enable them to utilize many formulation components as substrates for biosynthesis and growth.
- The use of crude vegetable or animal products in a formulation provides an additionally nutritious environment.
- Demineralized water prepared by good ion-exchange methods will normally contain sufficient nutrients to allow significantly growth of many water-brone Gram-negative bacteria such as *Pseudomonas* species.
- Acute pathogens require specific growth factors normally associated with the tissues they infect but which are often absent in pharmaceutical formulations. So they do not multiply although they may remain viable and infective for an appreciable time.

Moisture Content: Water Activity (A_w)

- Micro-organisms require readily accessible water in appreciable quantities for growth to occur.
- By measuring a product's Water Activity (A_w), it is possible to obtain an estimate of the proportion of uncomplexed water that is available in the formulation to support microbial growth using a formula.

$$A_W = \frac{\text{vapor pressure of formulation}}{\text{vapor pressure of water}}$$

- The greater the solute concentration, the lower is the water activity, with exception of halophilic bacteria most micro-organisms grow best in dilute solutions (high A_w) and as solute concentration rises (lowering A_w) growth rates decline until a minimal growth-inhibitory A_w is reached.

Table 11.2 Water Activity of Microbes

Bacteria	**A_w**
1. *Gram negative rods*	0.95
2. *Staphylococci*	0.90
3. *Micrococci*	0.90
4. *Lactobacilli*	0.90
5. *yeasts*	0.88

Table 11.3 Water Activity of Fungi

Fungi	**A_w**
1. *Aspergillus glaucus*	0.61

- The A_w of aqueous formulations can be lowered to increase resistance to microbial attack by the addition of high concentrations of sugars (or) polyethylene glycols.
- A_w can also be reduced by drying, although the dry often hygroscopic medicines will require suitable packing to prevent resorption of water and consequent microbial growth.
- Tablet film coatings are available which reduce water vapour uptake during storage and allows ready dissolution in bulk water.
- Condensed water films can accumulate on the surface of 'dry' products such as tablet or bulk oils following storage in damp atmospheres with fluctuating temperature resulting in sufficiently high localized A_w to initiate fungal growth.

Redox Potential

- The ability of microbes to grow in an environment is influenced by its oxidation-Reduction balance (redox potential) as they will require compatible terminal electron acceptors to permit their respiratory pathways to function.
- The redox potential even in viscous emulsions may be quite high due to appreciable solubility of oxygen in most fats and oils.

Storage Temperature

- The particular storage temperature may selectively determine the types of micro-organisms involved in spoilage.
- A deep freeze at –20°C or lower is used for long-term storage of some pharmaceutical raw materials and short-term storage of dispensed total parenteral nutrition (TPN) feeds prepared in Hospitals.
- Reconstituted syrups and multi-dose eye-drop packs are dispensed with instruction to "Store in cool place" such as a domestic fridge (8° – 12°C), partly to reduce the risk of growth of contaminants.
- Conversely water for injection (EP) should be held at 80°C after distillation and before packing and sterilization to prevent possible regrowth of Gram-negative bacteria and the release of endotoxins.

pH

Extremes of pH prevent microbial attack.

Various bacterial species are reported to grow in neutral pH.

e.g., (i) Gram-negative bacteria growing in Antacid mixtures

(ii) some grow in flavored mouthwashes and demineralised water

- above pH 8 spoilage is rare
- in products with low pH levels like fruit juice-flavored syrup with a pH 3-4 mould or yeast can be possible. Yeasts metabolize organic acids and raise the pH to levels where secondary bacterial growth can occur.
- Although use of low pH adjustment to preserve food stuffs is well established, it is not practicable to make deliberate use of this for medicines.

Packaging Design

Packaging can have a major influence on microbial stability of few formulations in controlling the entry of contaminants during both storage and use.

- The idea of designing the container for parenteral administration got significance as we can avoid the contamination that results in high risk of infections.
- Self-sealing rubber wads must be used to prevent microbial entry into multiple-dose injection containers following withdrawals with a hypodermic needle.
- Wide mouthed cream jars are replaced by narrow nozzles and flexible screw capped tubes, thereby removing the operator-induced contamination during use of product.
- Where medicines rely on their A_w to prevent spoilage, packaging such as strip foils must be of water vapour-proof materials with fully efficient seals.
- Cardboard outer packaging and labels themselves can become substrates for microbial attack under humid conditions and preservatives are often included to reduce the risk of damage.

Protection of Micro-organisms within Pharmaceutical Products

- The survival of microorganism in particular environment is influenced by the presence of relatively inert materials.
- Thus, microbes can be more resistant to heat or desiccation in the presence of polymers like starch acacia, gelatin etc
- Adsorption onto naturally occurring particulate material may aid establishment and survival.
- It was believed that presence of some surfactants suspending agents and proteins can increase the resistance of micro-organisms to preservatives.

Table 11.4 Contaminants Found in Pharmaceuticals

Year	Product	Contaminant
1907	Plague Vaccine	*Clostridium tetani*
1943	Fluorescein eye drops	*Pseudomonas aeruginosa*
1946	Talcum powder	*Clostridium tetani*
1948	Serum vaccine	*Staphylococcus aureus*
1955	Chloroxylenol Disinfectant	*Pseudomonas aeruginosa*
1966	Thyroid tablets	*Salmonella muenchen*
1966	Antibiotic eye ointment	*Pseudomonas aeruginoxa*
1966	Saline solution	*Serratia Marce scens*
1967	Carmine powder	*Salmonella cubana*
1967	Hand cream	*Klebsiella pneumonia*
1969	Peppermint water	*Pseudomonas aeruginosa*
1970	Chlorhexidine –cetrimide antiseptic solution	*Pseudomonas cepacia*
1972	Intravenous fluids	*Pseudomonas, Erwinia Enterobacter spp.*
1972	Pancreatin powder	*Salmonella agona*
1977	Contact lens solution	*Serratia and enterobacter.*
1981	Surgical dressings	*Clostridium spp.*
1982	Iodophor solution	*Pseudomonas aeruginosa*
1983	Aqueous soap	*Pseudomonas stutzeri*
1984	Thymol mouth wash	*Pseudomonas aeruginosa*
1986	Antiseptic mouth wash	*Coliforms*

11.3 Sources and Control of Contamination

In Manufacture

Regardless of whether manufacture takes place in industry or on small scale in the hospital pharmacy, the microbial/microbiological quality of finished product will be determined by:

1. Formulation components used
2. Environment in which they are manufactured
3. Manufacturing process itself.

Quality must be maintained at all stages like:

(a) Raw materials particularly water and those of natural origin must be of high microbiological standard.

(b) All processing equipment should be subject to planned preventive maintenance and should be properly cleaned after use to prevent cross-contamination between batches.

(c) Cleaning equipment should be appropriately cleaned and properly maintained.
(d) Manufacture should take place in suitable premises supplied with filtered air.
(e) The end product requires suitable packaging which will protect it from contamination during its shelf life.

Hospital Manufacture

Manufacture in hospital premises raises certain additional problems with regard to contamination control

Water

Mains water in hospitals is frequently stored in large roof tanks which may be relatively inaccessible and poorly maintained.

- Water for pharmaceutical manufacture require the further treatments like:
  (a) Distillation
  (b) Reverse osmosis
  (c) Deionization
  (d) A combination of these

Depending on intended use of water.

- Such a process need careful monitoring and maintaining the microbiological standards after treatment
- May be Gram-negative opportunistic pathogens can survive on traces of organic matter in treated water and will readily multiply to high numbers at room temperature.
- Water should be stored at a temperature in excess of 80°C and circulated in the distribution system at a flow rate of 1-2 m/s to prevent the buid up of bacterial bio films in the piping.

Environment

- The microbial flora of the hospital pharmacy environment is a reflection of the general hospital environment and the activities undertaken there.
- Free living opportunist pathogens such as *Pseudomonas aeruginosa* are normally found in web sites like drain, sinks and taps, buckets and scrubbing machines are responsible for distributing these around pharmacy.

Steps to avoid contamination

Contamination levels in the production environment may be minimized by observing:

- Good manufacturing practices

- By installing heating traps is sink-u-bends results in destruction of reservoir of contaminants
- Proper maintenance and storage of equipment.

Packaging

- Materials like sacking, cardboard, card liners, works and paper are unsuitable for packing pharmaceuticals as they are heavily contaminated.
- In olden-days packaging in hospitals has been frequently reused for economic reasons for this purpose large number of containers may be returned to pharmacy bringing with them microbial contaminants introduced during use in the wards.
- Re-usable containers must be thoroughly washed and dried and never use directly.
- Another common practice in hospitals is repackaging of products purchased in bulk into small containers.
- Increased handling of product inevitably increases the risk of contamination.

In use

We can know the sources of contamination during the usage of pharmaceutical products. Abuse of the product and cross-contamination in the hospitals, especially multidose products are vulnerable to contamination during use. Contaminations in use are reduced by improvement in packaging and changes in nursing practices.

Human Sources

During normal usage, patients may contaminate their medicine with their own microbial flora.

Topical products are considered to be most at risk; as the product will probably be applied by hands thus introducing contaminants from resident skin flora of staphylococci, micrococcus species.

The opportunities for contamination may be reduced by using disposable applicators for topical products or by giving oral products by disposable spoon.

- Multi-dose products once contaminated can be served as a vehicle of cross-contamination or cross-infection between patients.

Environmental Sources

Small numbers of air borne contaminants may settle in products left open to the atmosphere; in this some die during storage and some remain static level of about $10^2 - 10^3$ colony forming unit (CFU) per 'g' or per 'mL'.

Large numbers of water borne contaminants are accidently introduced into topical products by wet hands or by 'splash-back mechanism' survive by utilizing nutritional requirements multiply subsequently and may exceed 10^6 CFU per 'g' or per 'mL'.

Equipment sources

- Patients and nursing staff may use a range of applicators (pads, sponges, brushes and spatulas) during medicament administration like topical products. When reused results in contamination between fresh stocks of product.

11.4 Microbial Standards for Non-Sterile Pharmaceutical Products

Few raw materials used in making pharmaceutical products are sterile as received and special treatment may be required to render them microbiologically acceptable for use. Strict adherence to effective environmental control and sanitation, equipment cleaning practices and good personal hygiene practices in pharmaceutical manufacture is vital in minimizing both the type and number of micro-organisms.

The significance of micro-organisms in non-sterile pharmaceutical products should be evaluated in terms of:

(a) use of product

(b) the nature of product

(c) potential hazard to the user

(d) also processing of product in relation to an acceptable quality for pharmaceutical purposes

- Certain categories of products should be tested routinely for total microbial count and for specified indicator microbial contaminants

  e.g., Natural plant, animal and mineral products for *salmonella species*

  (i) Oral solutions and suspensions for *E.coli*

  (ii) Articles applied topically for *Pseudomonas aeruginosa and Staphylococcus aureus*.

- Articles intended for rectal, urethral vaginal administration for yeasts and molds.
- Definitivemicrobial limits are incorporated into specific monographs on the basis of a major criterion like:

(a) Potential of the stipulated micro-organisms counts etc.

- Relevant tests for determining the total count of viable aerobic micro-organisms and total combined molds and yeast count, and for identification and detection of designated species are given under "Microbial Limit Test".

- The presence of certain micro-organisms in non-sterile preparations may have the potential to reduce or ever inactivate therapeutic activity of the product and has a potential to adversely affect the health of the patient.

Microbial examination of non sterile products is perfumed according to the methods given in the texts on "Microbiological Examination of Non Sterile Products", "Microbial Enumeration Test", "Tests for Specified Organisms".

Acceptance criteria are based on individual results or the average replicate counts when replicates counts are performed.

When an acceptance criterion for microbiological quality is prescribed

10^1 cfu: maximum acceptable count = 20

10^2 cfu: maximum acceptable count = 200

10^3 cfu: maximum acceptable count = 2000

Acceptance is based on total aerobic microbial count (TAMC) and total combined yeasts and molds count (TYMC).

Table 11.5 Acceptance Criteria for Microbiological Quality of Non-Sterile Substances for Pharmaceutical use

	Total aerobic Microbial count (cfu/g (or) cfu/ml)	Total combined yeasts/Molds count (cfu/g (or) cfu/ml)
Substances for pharmaceutical use	10^3	10^2

Table 11.6 Acceptance Criteria for Microbiological (Quality) of Non Sterile Dosage Forms

Route of administration	Total Aerobic Microbial count (cfu/g or cfu/mL)	Total combined yeasts/molds count (cfu/g (or) cfu/mL)	Specified Micro-organisms
Non aqueous preparations for oral use	10^3	10^2	Absence of *Escherichia* (1 g or 1 mL)
Aqueous preparations for oral use	10^2	10^1	Absence of *Escherichia* (1 g or 1 mL)
Rectal use	10^3	10^2	
Oro mucosal use	10^2	10^1	Absence of *Staphylococcus aureus*
Gingival use	-	-	-
Coetaneous use	-	-	-
Nasal use	-	-	Absence of *pseudomonas aeruginosa(P)*
Auricular use	-	-	-

Table 11.6 ***contd....***

Route of administration	Total Aerobic Microbial count (cfu/g or cfu/mL)	Total combined yeasts/molds count (cfu/g (or) cfu/mL)	Specified Micro-organisms
Vaginal	10^2	10^1	Absence of *Pseudomonas aeruginosa*
Transdermal patches (limits for one patch including adhesive layer and backing)	10^2	10^1	Absence of *Staphylococcus aureus* Absence of *Candida albicans* Absence of *Staphycoccus aureus* Absence of *Pseudomonas aeruginosa*
Inhalation use (special requirements apply to liquid preparations for nebulization)	10^2	10^1	Absence of *Staphylococcus aureus* Absence of *Pseudomonas aeruginosa* Absence of bile-tolerant gram negative bacteria

In addition to the micro-organisms; the significance of other micro-organisms recovered should be evaluated in terms of the following:

The use of the product: hazard varies according to the route of administration (eye, nose, respiratory tract).

- The nature of product
- The method of application
- The intended recipient: risk may differ for neonates, infants the debilitated
- Use of immunosuppressive agents, corticosteroids
- The presence of disease, wounds, organ damage

Table 11.7 Standard Saturated Salt Solutions used to Caliberate Water Activity Determination Instruments

Saturated salt solution	ERH%	a_w
1. Potassium sulfate ($K_2 SO_4$)	97.3	0.97
2. Berium chloride ($Ba Cl_2$)	90.2	0.902
3. Sodium chloride (NaCl)	75.3	0.753
4. Magnesium Nitrate ($Mg (NO_3)_2$)	52.9	0.529
5. Magnesium chloride ($Mg Cl_2$)	32.8	0.328

Table 11.8 Water Activities (a_w) required to support the Growth of Representative Micro-Organisms

Bacteria	Water Activity (a_w)	Molds and yeast	Water Activity (a_w)
Pseudomonas aeruginosa	0.97	*Rhyzopus nigricans*	0.93
Bacillus cereus	0.95	*Mucor plumbeus*	0.92
Clostridium botulinum TYPE A	0.95	*Rhodotonela Mucilaginosa*	0.92
Escherichia coli	0.95	*Sacchoromyces cerevisiae*	0.90
Clostridium perfrigens	0.95	*Paecilomyces variotti*	0.84
Lacto bacillus viridescens	0.95	*Pencillium chrysogenum*	0.83
Salmonella s_{pp}	0.95	*Aspergillus fumigates*	0.82
Enterobacter aerogenes	0.94	*Pencicillium globrum*	0.81
Micrococcus lysodekticus	0.93	*Aspergillus niger*	0.77
Bacicuss subticis	0.90	*Aspergillus flavus*	0.78
Staphylococeus aureus	0.86	*Zygosachnaromyces rouxii (osmophilic yeast)*	0.62
Halobacterium halobium (halophilic baceterium)	0.75	*Xeromyces bisporus (xero philic fungi)*	0.61

Table 11.9 Microbial Limit Testing Strategy for Representative Pharmaceutical and OTC Drug Products based on Water Activity

S. no.	Products	Water Activity	Greatest Potential Contaminants	Tests Recommended
1.	Nasal inhalant	0.99	Gram-negative bacteria	TAMC, TCYMC absence of S. *aureus* and P. *aeruginosa*
2.	Hair shampoo	0.99	Gram-negative bacteria	TAMC, TCYMC absence of S. *aureus* and P. *aeruginosa*
3.	Antacid	0.99	Gram-negative bacteria	TAMC, TCYMC absence of E. *coli* and *salmonella spp*
4.	Topical cream	0.77	Gram-positive bacteria	TAMC, TCYMC absence of S. *Aureus* and P. *Aeruginosa*
5.	Oral liquid	0.90	Gram-positive bacteria and fungi	TAMC and TCYMC
6.	Oral suspension	0.87	Fungi	TAMC and TCYMC
7.	Topical ointment	0.55	None	Reduced testing
8.	Lip balm	0.36	None	Reduced testing
9.	Vaginal and rectal suppositories	0.30	None	Reduced testing
10.	Compressed tablets	0.36	None	Reduced testing
11.	Liquid-filled capsule	0.30	None	Reduced testing

11.5 Preservation of Pharmaceutical Products

An antimicrobial 'Preservative' may be included in a formulation to minimize the risk of spoilage and to kill low levels of contaminants introduced during storage.

Properties of an ideal preservative

- A broad spectrum of activity and a rapid rate of killing
- Selectivity in reacting with the contaminants and not the formulation ingredients
- Non-irritant and non-toxic to patients
- Stable and effective throughout the life.
- Preservatives are antimicrobial agents that can be found in nearly all consumer products including foods. Without preservatives many consumer products we take for granted soaps, shampoos, cosmetics, cleaners, would literally spoil on the store shelf and supports the growth of pathogenic micro-organisms
- Not all products must be preserved with chemical preservatives. One of the most common ways to prevent the growth of micro-organisms in consumer products is to adjust the pH of the product to the point where it should not support the growth of microbes.
- If we use the products those are contaminated with microbes then it would be nothing but self inoculation with pathogens.

Antimicrobial test laboratories specializes the testing of the consumer called preservative efficacy challenge test; the efficacy of a preservative is measured in the laboratory setting using a preservative challenge test. Preservative challenge test consist of the following basic steps.

1. The product is evaluated for the presence of pathogens after manufacturing
2. The product is separated out into separate container
3. Each container is inoculated with a different microorganism at a fairly high concentration and the initial challenge concentration is found.
4. The product is incubated approximately room temperature for an extended period of time.
5. The product is re-evaluated for the presence of the micro-organisms that were inoculated into it.
6. The product is incubated further, sometimes analyzed at 14, 21 and 28 days.
7. The product is re-inoculated with even more micro-organisms and allowed to incubate further.

The typical micro-organisms used for preservative challenge studies are:

1. *Pseudomonas aeruginosa*: Gram-negative, hard bacterium
2. *Escherichia coli*: Gram-negative bacterium, similar to many pathogens

3. *Staphylococcus aureus*: Gram-positive bacterium opportunistic pathogen
4. *Candida albicans*: Fungus (yeast), opportunistic pathogen
5. *Asperigillur niger*: Fungus (mold), opportunistic pathogen.

11.6 Useful method for Fast and High thorough put Preservative Efficacy Testing

Introduction

Microbial contamination of cosmetic products is of great importance for the suppliers and the consumers

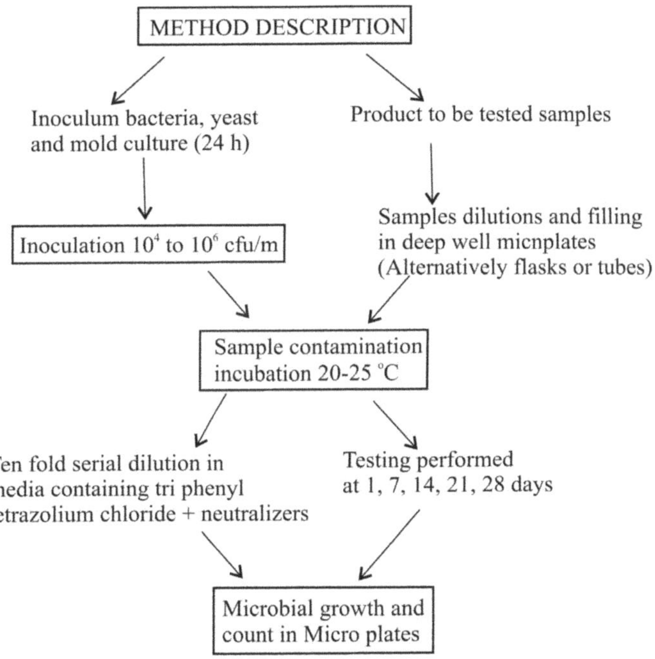

- The microbial growth is at the origin of organoleptic and formulation alterations (viscosity, color).
- To prevent microbial contamination, addition of system preservatives are needed
- according to microbial sensibility of the cosmetic product and its use by consumers
- Identification of potential new preservatives for products need large screening of samples.
- Preservatives must be used at concentration as low as possible in order to avoid any toxic effects (except against the microbial strains)

- The new preservative system must be compatible with the formulation and the practices of use of the end product.

Based on the reports, the challenge test that allows the screening of hundred of sample simultaneously are developed.

- Samples were contaminated in deep well micro plate format allowing the study 90 samples per micro plate per microbial strain
- Micro-organisms used include all the strains recommended in the current regulatory method for cosmetic preservative efficacy testing
- Counting was performed at each time (1, 7, 14, 21, 28) with triphenyl tetrazolium assay in 96 wells micro plates for the yeast and bacteria and with the conventional agar plating method for the mold *Aspergillus niger*.
- The culture media containing tripheny tetrazolium was designed in order to naturalize the preservative properties (neutralization products included). This adaptation eliminates the need of neutralization step at each sampling
- The counting of microbial population and the interpretation of the results are fast and easy. Results can be read on micro plate reader (data traceability, automatization).
- Validation conducted on samples of raw materials or end products shows a good accuracy with regulatory challenge test.

Conclusion

The micro-challenge test is cost effective and method of choice for research projects and need for the discovery of new preservatives or control of anti microbial efficacy where the regulatory method is not required.

11.7 Microbial Assessment

Microbial assessments are guidelines to provide an approach of engineers without borders (EWB) to assess the impact of potable water system

- The guidelines will outline a systematic and scientific process for EWB members to conduct a microbial assessment of a water treatment system
- This will also function as a tool that describes how to train local community members to continually assess and monitor the system to build capacity and demonstrate sustainability
- Guidelines for the microbial evaluation of a potable water system will provide EWB project managers and team members a tool to evaluate the effectiveness of the system that is intended to reduce microbial contaminants and therefore burden of disease causing pathogens

Potable Water Standards

Depending on the country, standards for potable water quality will vary. According to 'WHO'

"Water quality targets are usually set by national authorities who should decide on the tolerable risk level and derive the water quality targets that result in compliance with this risk level".

- It is important to identify the standards for *Thermo tolerant coli* form, pH, turbidity and chlorine level used by the country of interest

Table 11.10 Frame Work

Time Frame	Activity	Major Goals	Outcome
I. Pre intial site assessment	1. Choose assessment team leader	Designate leader to co-ordinate the activities and direct decisions and follow up data analysis	Effective operational management
	2. Prepare for Data collection	If there is no in-country laboratory, obtain kits and prepare material for data collection (sheets, binders)	All materials needed for site visit
II. Onsite, pre-intial site assessment	3. Prepare for data collection	♦ Identify laboratory for processing of samples ♦ . Identify possible catchment sources of water supply	Set up of source of samples and manner in which they will be processed
During intial site assessment	4. Collect data	♦ . Obtain samples of water from catchment to be used for system in take ♦ . Deliver to lab in a timely fashion	Raw data output from laboratory analysis
	5. Analyze data	Record data from laboratory as base line data	Source of data for comparison with future sampling

Table 11.11 Post Implementation Assessment

Time Frame	Activity	Major Goals	Outcome
After system has been designated and set-up	1. Prepare for data collection	Use same kits and methods used for intial assessment	All materials needed for assessment ready for use
	2. Collect data	♦ Obtain samples from out –take of system ♦ Obtain samples from randomly selected distribution sites	Raw data output from laboratory analysis
After water samples have been processed	3. Analyses data	♦ Have values to directly compare to base line ♦ Assess for the reduction of microbial indicators	Quantitative analysis of samples
After data analyses	4. Distribute data	Disseminate data to EWB	Follow-up to results of assessment

Community Member training			
Time frame	1. Prepare materials	Translate data collection sheets into appropriate language ♦ Identify translater ♦ Identify community members willing to be trained ♦ Set up a notification system for community collected data to be disseminated to project managers	All the materials needed for training ready for use
After post system assessment	2. Training	♦ Train community member in how to collect samples, where to collect samples and how to deliver samples to lab ♦ Train community members on how to record data, and how to disseminated it to EWB project managers	Trained community members capable of assessing the system appropriately post implementation of the system

Essay Questions

1. Explain the various Physico chemical deterioration of pharmaceuticals
2. Write a note on various factors affecting spoilage of pharmaceutical products
3. Write a note on protection of micro-organisms within pharmaceutical products
4. Explain the standards for non-sterile pharmaceutical products
5. Write a note on mechanisms of various microbes and their manifestations

Multiple Choice Questions

1. The contaminant present in talcum powder is
   (a) Pseudomonas aeruginosa
   (b) Clostridium tetani
   (c) Salmonella cubana
   (d) Staphylococcus aureus
2. Storage temperature for reconstituted syrups is
   (a) 8-12 °C (b) 2-4 °C
   (c) 4-6 °C (d) 6-8 °C
3. The enzyme acting on polyuronides is
   (a) Protease
   (b) Veronidase
   (c) Detranase
   (d) Cellulose

Answers

1. (b) 2. (a) 3. (b)

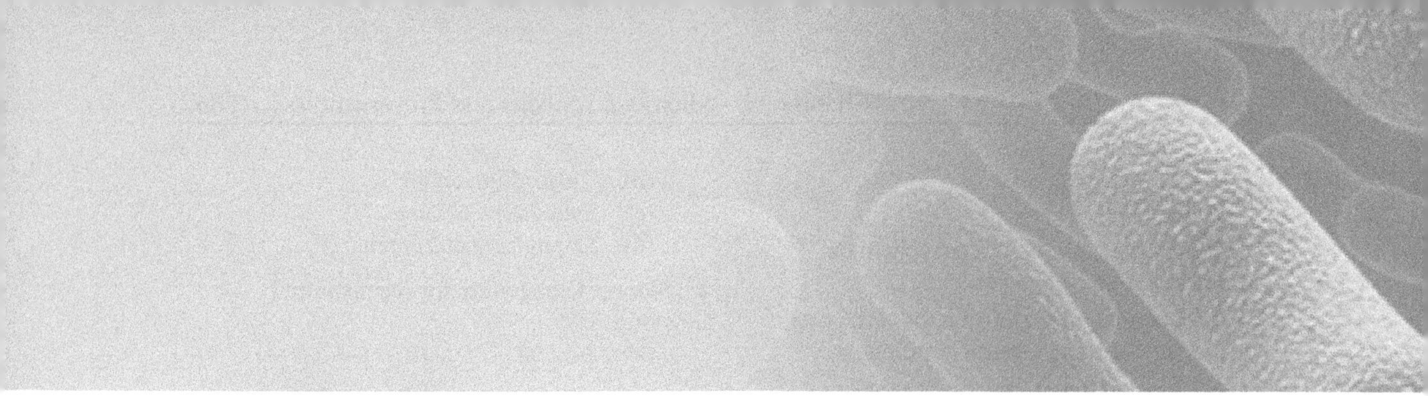

12 MISCELLANEOUS TOPICS

LEARNING OBJECTIVES

After studying the chapter the students familiarize themselves with concepts in:

- *Developing an insight on soil microbiology*
- *Understanding details of food microbiology*
- *Understanding Industrial microbiology with various fermentative methods*
- *Understanding modes of actions of antibiotics such as peniciliins, tetracyclines*
- *Understanding aero microbiology*
- *Understanding microbiology of water*
- *Understanding microbiology of milk*
- *Understanding microbiology of cheese*

12.1 Soil Microbiology

Soil is the outer region of earth-crust consisting of loose material formed by gradual weathering of rock and gives to plant both mechanical and nutritional support. Soil can be defined as the space-time continum forming the upper part of the earth crust.

Soil as a Habitat for Micro-organisms

Soil is a unique habitat which harbours a variety of microflora and fauna and gives mechanical and nutritional support to higher plants on which human civilization is based. Structural components of soil and its major constituents determine soil quality.

1. *Soil quality*: Soil quality can be defined as the capacity of a soil to function within the boundaries of ecosystem to sustain biological productivity, maintain environmental quality and promote plant and animal health.

   Soil quality encompasses its capacity for (i) rop productivity (ii) food safety (iii) health of animals and humans.

2. *Physico-chemical properties of soil*: Physico-chemical properties of soil include soil texture, water, air, inorganic chemical and organic matter.

- Mechanical composition (texture) of soil is determined on the basis of size of soil particles i.e., sand, silt and clay particles.
- The sources of inorganic material in soil are the parent raises which get changed by the physical and chemical processes of weathering.

3. *Is 'Habitat' a Better Term for Micro-organism*: It is rather better to use the term 'niche' than 'habitat', as the habitat is the place where an organism lives, whereas niche speaks the habitat as well as role of the organism in that habitat with respect to other organisms and the environment. Odum (1971) has used the two analogies, 'address' for habitat and 'profession' for niche of the organisms.
4. *Microbial balance*: Soil is a complex ecosystem in a state of dynamic equilibrium, bounded by physico-chemical parameters. The relative stability of this system depends upon the relative stability of its biological composition and regulating parameters. The equilibrium is possible only when, during coexistence action and interaction between different micro-organisms of varied potential go on.

12.1.1 Rhizosphere and Rhizoplane Micro-organisms

Rhizosphere is defined as an area of intense microbiological activity that extends several millimeter from the root system of the growing plants. The term rhizoplane refers to the root surface.

Micro-organisms growing under the influence of roots are often qualitatively and quantitatively different from those inhabiting remote from this influence in the soil environment.

Rhizosphere is a unique subterranean habitat for micro-organisms. The rhizosphere microflora of one plant differ from the rhizosphere microflora of the other plant. Thus, rhizosphere micro-organisms differ plant to plant both qualitatively and quantitatively.

1. *Reasons of Increased Microbial activity in Rhizosphere*: The outer epidermal walls of living root hairs and all plant roots are covered with mucilage and cuticle organic and inorganic compounds accumulated in cytoplasm of root cells are diffused out. The phenomenon of loss of organic and inorganic compounds from root surface is known as root exudation.

   All these root tissues and organic and inorganic compounds constitute a food base (for micro-organisms) which are generally lacking in non-rhizosphere soil. The micro-organisms colonize the rhizosphere to utilize them as food and in turn release exudates from their own cells. Thus, they are regarded as selective sieves.
2. *Composition of Root exudates*:

   (a) Root exudates contain carbohydrates, organic acids, nucleotides, flavanones, enzymes etc.

(b) Atleast ten sugars such as glucose, fructose, sucrose, xylose, maltose, rhamnose, arabinose and a few oligosaccharides have been identified in the exudates

(c) Aminoacids

(d) Vitamins

3. *Factors affecting exudation*:
   - Temperature
   - Light
   - Secondary metabolites

   All the three factors increase the exudation process

4. *Rhizosphere micro-organisms*: The rhizosphere region is highly favourable habitat for the proliferation and metabolisms of numerous types of micro-organisms on screening the rhizosphere and non-rhizosphere microfungi of soyabean both qualitatively and quantitatively it was found that the rhizosphere microfungi was higher than non-rhizosphere fungi.

   The dominant fungi of rhizosphere were *Aspergillus Flavus, Atomigatus, A.niger* etc.
   - Bacteria reported from the rhizosphere and rhizoplane regions irrespective of their dominance are *Arthrobacter, Pseudomonas, Bacillus brevis, B.polymyxa* etc.
   - Actinomycetes are also important constituents of rhizoplane rhizosphere.

5. *The rhizosphere effect*: Rhizosphere effect is defined as the stimulation that can be measured an quantitative basis by the use of rhizosphere: Soil (R:S) ratio, obtained by dividing the number of micro-organism in the rhizosphere soil by the number of micro-organisms in the non-rhizosphere soil.

6. *Effect of Micro flora on Host plant*: The rhizosphere micro-organisms have either beneficial or harmful effects on the development of plant.

   Micro-organisms in the rhizosphere zone change the availability or toxicity of sulphur to plants.

   The micro-organisms catalyze the reactions in the rhizosphere and produce CO_2 and form organic acids that in turn solubilize the inorganic nutrients of plants.

Factors affecting microbial community in soil:

- Soil moisture
- Organic and inorganic chemicals
- Soil organic matter
- Types of vegetation and its growth stages
- Different seasons

12.1.2 Organic Matter Decomposition

Decomposition and photosynthesis are the two important process of an ecosystem. Litter (the organic remains of biological origin) is an organic chemical-carrier of nutrients present in different ecosystems. The structural components of litter governs the rate of decomposition.

1. ***Composition of litter:***
   - Cellulose
   - Hemicellulose
   - Lignin
   - Water-soluble components
   - Ether and Alcohol-soluble components
   - Proteins
2. ***Carbon Assimilation and Immobilization*:** The process of conversion of substrate to protoplasmic carbon is known as assimilation. About 20-40% substrate is assimilated and the rest is released as CO_2 or accumulates as waste.
   - Accumulation of inorganic substance by the micro-organisms and making the plants nutrient-deficient is known as immobilization. The magnitude of immobilization is proportional to net quantity of microbial cells formed.
3. ***Organic matter dynamics in soil*:** When organic matter is present in soil it is gradually rendered into a uniform, dark coloured amorphous mass by micro-organisms which is designated as humus. Humus serves as a source of energy for the development of various groups of micro-organisms and as a result of decomposition CO_2, NH_3 and other products are given off. During the course of decomposition, the water-soluble components are metabolised first. Thereafter, cellulose and hemicellulose disappear gradually. The lignins disappear in the last stage of decomposition because they are resistant to decomposition.
4. ***Micro-organisms Associated with organic matter decomposition*:**

   (a) Cellulose decomposers

   Fungi: *Aspergillus, penicillium, fusarium*

   Bacteria: *Bacillus, cellulomonas, corynebacterium*

   (b) Hemicellulose decomposers

   Fungi: *Aspergillus, Fusarium, penicillium*

   Bacteria: Bacillus, pseudomonas

   Streptomycetes: Streptomyces

   (c) Lignin decomposers

   Fungi: *Agaricus, polyporus, poria*

   Bacteria: Arthrobacter, pseudomonas, micrococcus

5. ***Factors affecting organic matter decomposition:***
   - Litter quality
   - Temperature
   - Soil pH
   - Inorganic chemicals
   - Moisture
6. ***Microbial biomass as an index of soil fertility*:** Microbial biomass, irrespective of soil types, is a part of soil organic matter which includes the living microbial components i.e., *bacteria, actinomycetes, fungi, algae, protozoa.* Cultivation leads to considerable loss of soil organic matter and therefore microbial biomass also changes. The turn over time of microbial biomass is estimated at 1-3 years. Since microbial biomass is the most active fraction of soil organic matter, therefore, any change in organic matter may be supposed that microbial biomass too has changed.
7. ***Soil fertility*:** Soil fertility is the sustainable capacity of a soil to produce good yields of high quality on the basis of chemical, physical and biological factors shown in Fig.12.1.

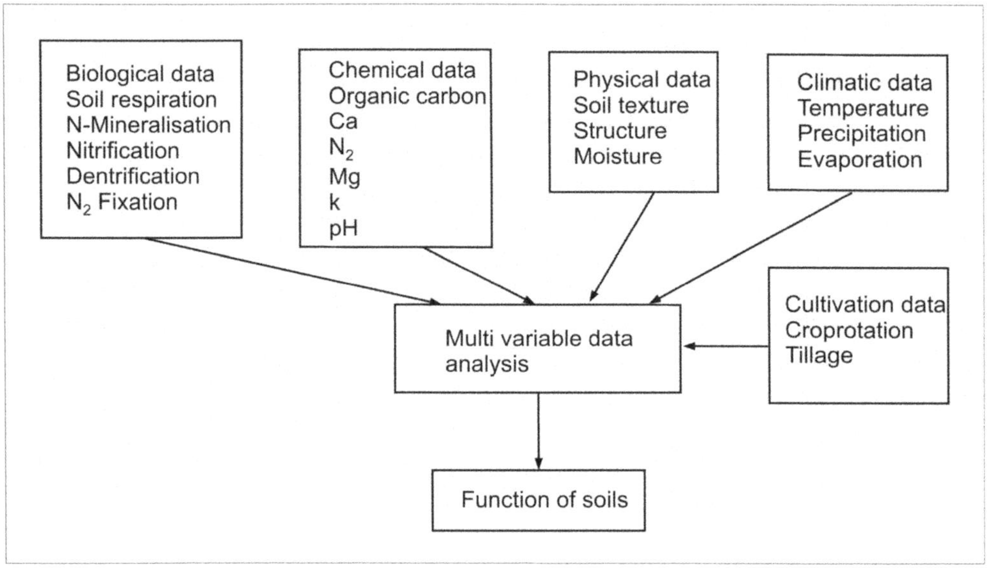

Fig. 12.1 Factors effecting soil fertility

Soil function

- Primary production by creating a rooting substrate
- To support above ground
- To decompose organic material

12.2 Biogeochemical Cycling

The major plant nutrients derived from soil are nitrogen, phosphorus and potassium out of these three nutrients nitrogen stands out as most susceptible to microbial transformations as it builds up protein. Phosphorus is second to nitrogen which is required by both plants and micro-organisms. Potassium is the major cation that plants obtain from soil.

THE CARBON CYCLE

The carbon cycle is one of the major biogeochemical cycles describing the exchange of carbon exchanged among the biosphere, pedosphere, geosphere, hydrosphere, and atmosphere of the Earth. It is required for the building of all organic compounds and involves the participation of many of the earth's key forces.

In Terrestrial Ecosystems: The atmospheric carbon dioxide is virtually the only source of carbon which is the basic constituent of all the organic compounds. A major source of atmospheric CO_2 is the process of photosynthesis, respiration, degassing from volcanic activity and the decomposition of organic material. Carbon dioxide is captured by plants throughout their lives and heterotrophic organisms in turn obtain a part of this carbon. The element is transferred from organism to organism when plants are eaten by herbivores which are in turn eaten by carnivores along the food chain. All these organisms go through respiration, excrete organic waste, and eventually die and decompose which releases carbon into the soil either as carbonates or fossil fuels. Through time and pressure, the organic material buried in soil and sediments may eventually become fossil fuels such as coal and oil, which then become additional sources of carbon. When these are burned, they emit tremendous amounts of carbon back into the atmosphere. The burning of fossil fuels, however, is occurring at much higher rates than is their production.

In Marine Ecosystems: The absorption of carbon dioxide into the world's oceans is influenced by the presence of widespread viruses within ocean water that infect many species of bacteria. The resulting bacterial deaths spawn a sequence of events that lead to greatly enlarged respiration of carbon dioxide, enhancing the role of the oceans as a carbon sink.

The carbon dioxide drawn into marine ecosystems is eventually released through oceanic respiration. In the oceans, dissolved carbonate can combine with dissolved calcium to precipitate solid calcium carbonate, $CaCO_3$, mostly as the shells of microscopic organisms. When these organisms die, their shells sink and accumulate on the ocean floor. Over time these carbonate sediments form limestone which is the largest reservoir of carbon in the carbon cycle.

Effects of Carbon Cycle on Global Climate

At present, there is a fear of the greenhouse effect increasing global warming. The excess carbon dioxide from the burning of fossil fuels is responsible for the gradual yet constant rise in temperature over the past few decades. Certain wave lengths coming from the sun, mainly infrared radiation, are trapped by greenhouse gases and kept in the earth's atmosphere. These gases block the re-radiation of infrared waves back out into space, causing the global temperature to increase.

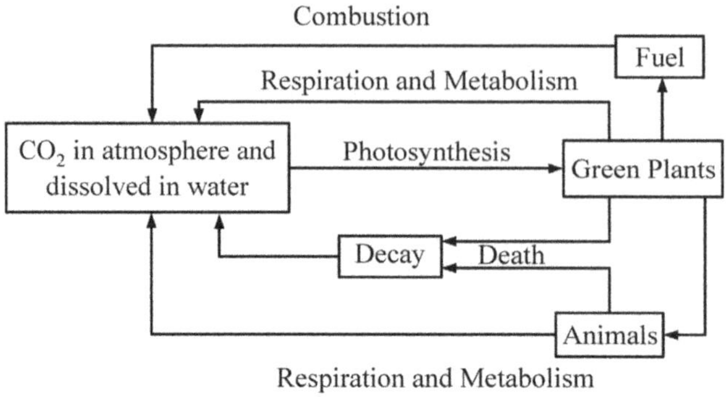

Fig. 12.2 Basic carbon cycle flow diagram

THE NITROGEN CYCLE

The nitrogen cycle is a biogeochemical cycle where nitrogen undergoes chemical reactions, changes form, and moves through different reservoirs on earth, including living organisms.

The majority of the earth's atmosphere (about 78%) is composed of atmospheric nitrogen, but it is not in a form that is usable to living things. Complex species interactions allow organisms to convert nitrogen to usable forms and exchange it between themselves. Nitrogen is required by organisms in the synthesis of proteins, nucleic acids, and other nitrogenous compounds.

Nitrogen Cycle Process

The nitrogen cycle composes of the following stages:

(i) Ammonification
(ii) Nitrification
(iii) Nitrogen uptake
(iv) Nitrogen fixation
(v) Denitrification

Ammonification

Ammonification is a process of converting the organic nitrogen of plants and animals after their death to ammonium ions (NH_4) by the action of saprotrophic fungi and bacteria. The saprotrophs use the ammonia (NH_3) to synthesize their own proteins and other nitrogen-containing organic compounds.

Nitrification

Nitrification is a process of oxidizing ammonium ions added to the soil by ammonification. It occurs in two stages. In the first stage, ammonium (NH_4^+) is converted to nitrite (NO^{2-}). Bacteria of the genus Nitrosomonas oxidize NH_3 to nitrites (NO_2^-). The second stage of nitrification involves the oxidation of nitrite (NO_2) to nitrate (NO_3. Bacteria of the genus Nitrobacter oxidize the nitrites to nitrates (NO_3^-).

Nitrification occurs only in oxygen-rich environments like circulating or flowing waters and the very surface layers of soils and sediments. Ammonium ions are positively charged and therefore stick (are sorbed) to negatively charged clay particles and soil organic matter. The positive charge prevents ammonium nitrogen from being washed out of the soil (or leached) by rainfall. In contrast, the negatively charged nitrate ion is not held by soil particles and so can be washed down the soil profile, leading to decreased soil fertility and nitrate enrichment of downstream surface and groundwater's.

Nitrogen Uptake

Nitrate (NO_3^-) formed by the process of nitrification is used by plants as a mineral metabolite and may be converted by them into amino groups and other nitrogen-containing compounds. Nitrates are also added to the soil through rock dissolution and combination of atmospheric nitrogen with oxygen. However, many plants also absorb ammonium from the soil.

Nitrogen Fixation

The reduction of atmospheric nitrogen (N_2) to the ammonium ion (NH^+_4) is called nitrogen fixation. Three processes are responsible for most of the nitrogen fixation in the biosphere:

- Atmospheric fixation by lightning
- Biological fixation by certain microbes alone or in a symbiotic relationship with some plants and animals
- Industrial fixation

Atmospheric Fixation

The enormous energy of lightning breaks nitrogen molecules and enables their atoms to combine with oxygen in the air forming nitrogen oxides. These dissolve in rain, forming nitrates that are carried to the earth. Atmospheric nitrogen fixation probably contributes some 5-8% of the total nitrogen fixed.

Industrial Fixation

Under great pressure, at a temperature of 600°C, and with the use of a catalyst, atmospheric nitrogen and hydrogen (usually derived from natural gas or petroleum) can be combined to form ammonia (NH_3). Ammonia can be used directly as fertilizer, but most of it is further processed to urea and ammonium nitrate (NH_4NO_3).

Biological Fixation

Nitrogen fixing bacteria often form symbiotic relationships with host plants. This symbiosis is well-known to occur in the legume family of plants (e.g. beans, peas, and clover). In this relationship, nitrogen fixing bacteria inhabit legume root nodules and receive carbohydrates and a favorable environment from their host plant in exchange for some of the nitrogen they fix. There is also nitrogen fixing bacteria that exist without plant hosts, known as free-living nitrogen fixers. In aquatic environments, blue-green algae are an important free-living nitrogen fixer.

Denitrification

Through de-nitrification, oxidized forms of nitrogen such as nitrate and nitrite (NO_2) are converted to di-nitrogen (N_2) and, to a lesser extent, nitrous oxide gas. De-nitrification is an anaerobic process that is carried out by denitrifying bacteria, which convert nitrate to nitrogen in the following sequence:

$$NO_3^- \text{->} NO_2^- \text{->} NO \text{->} N_2O \text{->} N_2$$

Nitric oxide and nitrous oxide are both environmentally important gases. Nitric oxide (NO) contributes to smog, and nitrous oxide (N_2O) is an important greenhouse gas, thereby contributing to global climate change.

Human Impact on Nitrogen Cycle

Humans affect the nitrogen cycle through activities that increase the amount of nitrogen that is biologically available in an ecosystem. The major culprits are fossil fuel combustion and the application of nitrogen-based fertilizer. Fossil fuel combustion releases nitric oxides and combines with other elements in the air to form smog and acid rain, thus enhancing green house effect.

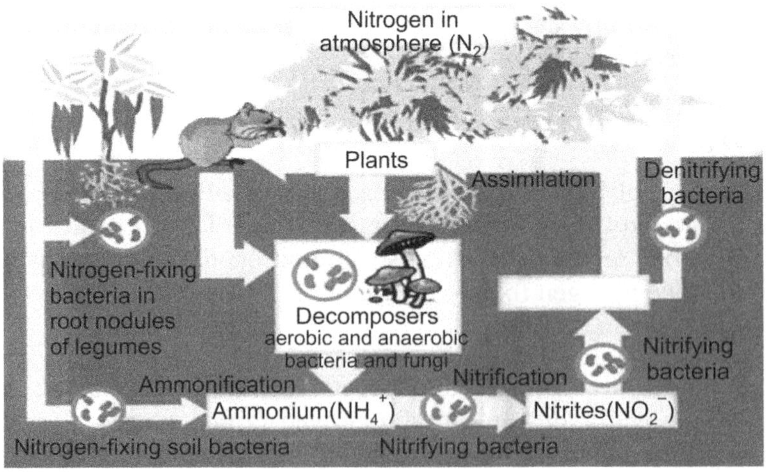

Fig. 12.3 Nitrogen cycle

THE PHOSPHORUS CYCLE

The **Phosphorus cycle** is defined as the biogeochemical cycle which describes the movement of phosphorus through the spheres of the ecosystem. Phosphorus is an essential nutrient for animals and plants. It plays a critical role in cell development and is a key component of molecules that store energy, such as ATP, DNA and lipids.

Phosphorus Cycle Process

The largest reservoir of phosphorus is in sedimentary rock. When it rains, phosphates are removed from the rocks (via weatherings) and are distributed in soils and water. Plants take up the inorganic phosphate from the soil. The plants may then be consumed by animals. Once in the plant or animal, the phosphate is incorporated into organic molecules such as DNA. When the plant or animal dies, it decays, and the organic phosphate is returned to the soil. Within the soil, organic forms of phosphate can be made available to plants by bacteria that break down organic matter to inorganic forms of phosphorus. This process is known as mineralization. Phosphorus in soil can end up in waterways and eventually oceans and sediments over time.

The same process occurs within the aquatic ecosystem. Phosphorus is not highly soluble, binding tightly to molecules in soil; therefore it mostly reaches waters by traveling with runoff soil particles. These phosphates tend to settle on ocean floors and lake bottoms. As sediments are stirred up, phosphates may reenter the phosphorus cycle, but they are more commonly made available to aquatic organisms by being exposed through erosion. Water plants take up the waterborne phosphate which then travels up through successive stages of the aquatic food chain.

Human Impact on Phosphorus Cycle

The phosphorous cycle is affected by human activities. Artificial phosphorous can cause over growth of algae and plants in aquatic ecosystems. When the excess plant material is broken down, the decomposing bacteria can use up all the oxygen in the water causing dead zones. Most bodies of water gradually become more productive over time through the slow, natural accumulation of nutrients in a process called eutrophication. However, overgrowth of algae due to phosphorous fertilizer is called "cultural eutrophication" or "hypertrophication," and is generally negative for ecosystems.

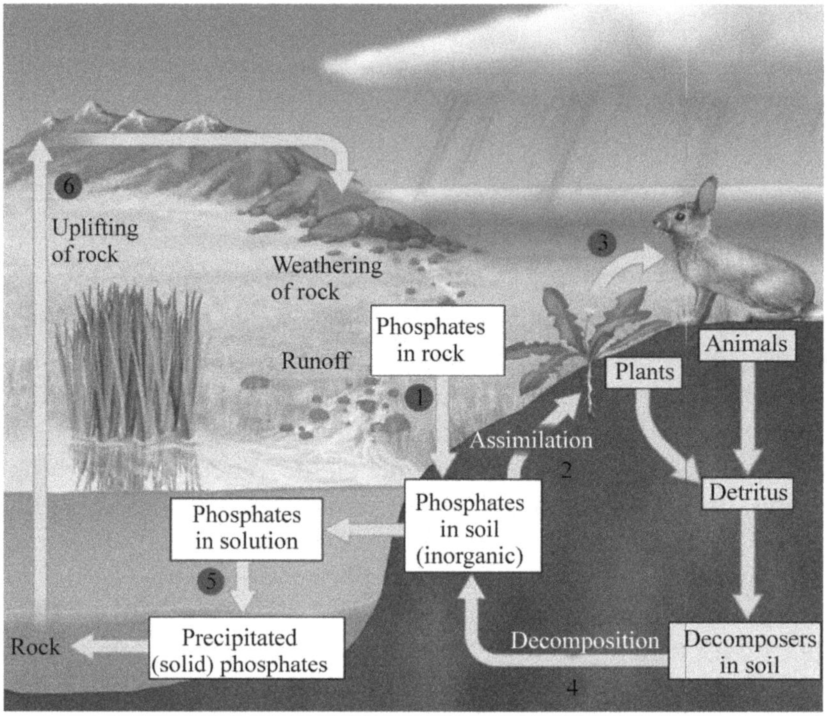

Fig. 12.4 The phosphorous cycle

THE SULPHUR CYCLE

The **sulfur cycle** is a biogeochemical cycle by which sulfur is exchanged between minerals (including the waterways) and living systems. Sulphur is the most abundant and widely distributed element in the nature and found both in free as well as combined states

The sulfur cycle contains both atmospheric and terrestrial processes. Within the terrestrial portion, the cycle begins with the weathering of rocks, releasing the stored sulfur. The sulfur then comes into contact with air where it is converted into sulfate (SO_4). The sulfate is taken up by plants and microorganisms and is converted into organic forms; animals then consume these organic forms through foods they eat, thereby moving the sulfur through the food chain. As organisms die and decompose, some of the sulfur is again released as a sulfate and some enters the tissues of microorganisms. There are also a variety of natural sources that emit sulfur directly into the atmosphere, including volcanic eruptions, the breakdown of organic matter in swamps and tidal flats, and the evaporation of water.

Sulfur eventually settles back into the Earth or comes down within rainfall. A continuous loss of sulfur from terrestrial ecosystem runoff occurs through drainage into lakes and streams, and eventually oceans. Sulfur also enters the ocean through fallout from the Earth's atmosphere. Within the ocean, some sulfur cycles through marine communities, moving through the food chain. A portion of this sulfur is emitted back into the atmosphere from sea spray. The remaining sulfur is lost to the ocean depths, combining with iron to form ferrous sulfide which is responsible for the black color of most marine sediments.

Sulphur Cycle Process

The essential steps of the sulfur cycle are:

- Mineralization of organic sulfur to the inorganic form, hydrogen sulfide: (H_2S).
- Oxidation of sulfide and elemental sulfur (S) and related compounds to sulfate, (SO_4^{2-}).
- Reduction of sulfate to sulfide.
- Microbial immobilization of the sulfur compounds and subsequent incorporation into the organic form of sulfur

These are often termed as follows:

Assimilative sulfate reduction, in which sulfate (SO_4^{2-}) is reduced to organic sulfhydryl groups (R-SH) by plants, fungi, and various prokaryotes. The oxidation states of sulfur are +6 in sulfate and -2 in R-SH

Desulfuration, in which organic molecules containing sulfur can be desulfurated, producing hydrogen sulfide gas (H_2S), oxidation state = -2.

Oxidation of hydrogen sulfide, produces elemental sulfur (S^o), oxidation state = 0. This reaction is done by the photosynthetic green and purple sulfur bacteria and some chemolithotrophs (organisms using inorganic compounds for ATP production).

Further *oxidation of elemental sulfur* by sulfur oxidizers produces sulfate.

Dissimilative sulfur reduction, in which elemental sulfur can be reduced to hydrogen sulfide

Dissimilative sulfate reduction, in which sulfate reducers generate hydrogen sulfide from sulfate

Human Impact on Sulphur Cycle

Human impact on the sulfur cycle is primarily in the production of sulfur dioxide (SO_2) from industry (such as burning coal) and the internal combustion engine. Sulfur dioxide can precipitate onto surfaces where it can be oxidized to sulfate in the soil (it is also toxic to some plants), reduced to sulfide in the atmosphere, or oxidized to sulfate in the atmosphere as sulfuric acid, a principal component of acid rain.

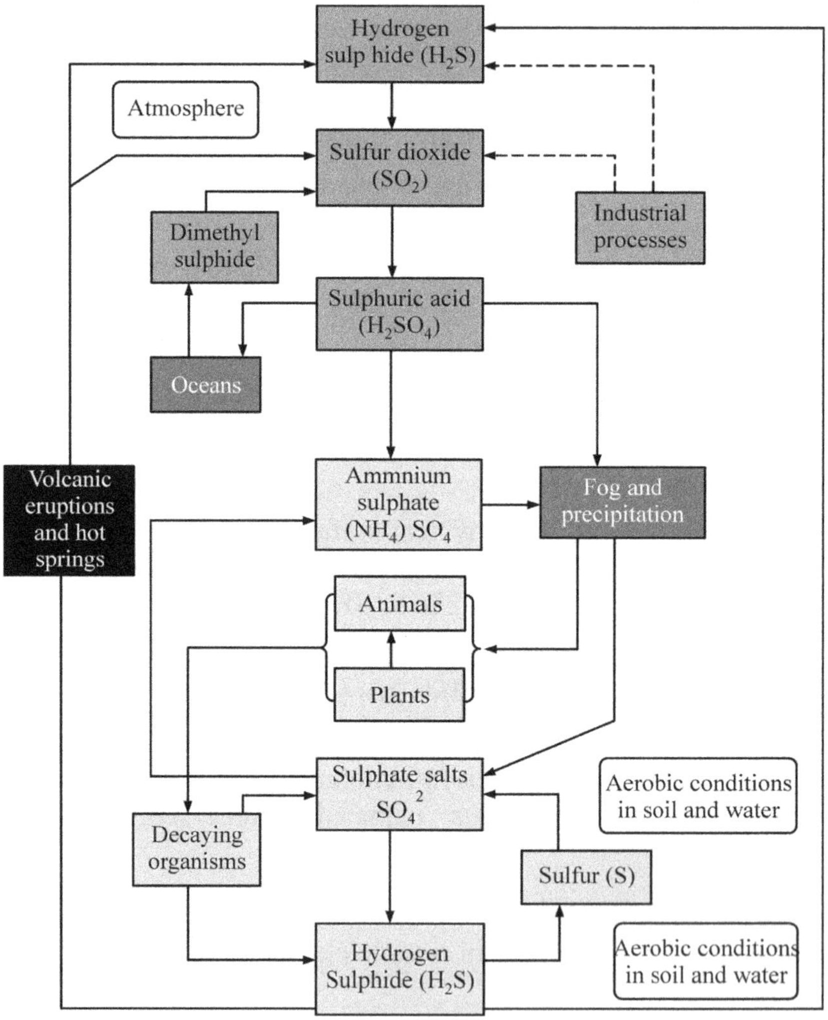

Fig. 12.5 Sulphur cycle

12.3 Food Microbiology

Micro-organisms influence the quality, availability and quantity of our food. Food can serve as a medium for the growth of micro-organisms and this growth may cause the food to undergo decomposition and spoilage.

1. ***Microbial flora of fresh foods***: The inner tissues of healthy plants and animals are free of micro-organisms (sterile). However the surface of raw vegetables and meats are contaminated with a variety of micro-organisms. It is desirable to maintain very low microbial level of contamination on raw foods.

   Meats: Fresh meat cut from the chilled carcass has its surface contaminated with micro-organisms characteristic of the environment and the implements used to cut the meat. Among the more common species of bacteria occurring on fresh meats are *pseudomonas, staphylococci, micrococci* etc.

   Poultry: Freshly dressed poultry have a bacterial flora on their surface that originates from the bacteria normally present on the live birds and from the manipulations during killing, defeathering and evisceration. *Pseudomonas* constitute the major contaminants on the skin of freshly dressed poultry.

   Eggs: Micro-organisms, particularly bacteria and molds, may enter the egg through cracks in the shells or penetrate the shells when the bloom (thin protein coat) covering the shell deteriorates.

   Fruits and Vegetables: Fruits and vegetables are normally susceptible to infection by *bacteria, fungi* and *viruses.* Microbial contamination of fruits and vegetables pertains to their post-harvest handling.

   Shellfish and Finfish: The microbial flora of freshly caught oysters, clams, fish and other aquatic specimens is very largely a reflection of the microbial quality of the waters where they are harvested. The marine bacterium *Vibrio parachaemolyticus* has been responsible for a number of gastroenteritis epidemics in the united states due to consumption of raw or inadequately cooked seafood.

2. ***Microbial spoilage of foods***: The type of food substance and the method by which it is processed and preserved may favor contamination by certain groups of micro-organisms. When micro-organisms are given a chance to grow, the organisms will produce changes in appearance, flavor, odor and other qualities of foods. These degradation processes are as follows shown in Table 12.1.

Putrefaction

Protein foods + proteolytic micro-organisms → Aminoacids + amines + Ammonia + Hydrogen sulfide

Fermentation

Carbohydrate foods '+' carbohydrate-fermenting micro-organisms → acids + gases + alcohols

Rancidity:

Fattyfoods + lipolytic micro-organisms → fattyacids + glycerol

Fresh foods:

Table 12.1 Microbial Spoilage of Foods

Food	Type of spoilage	Micro-organisms Involved
Bread	Moldy	*Rhizopus nigricans, penicillium, Aspergillus niger*
Fish	Discoloration Putrefaction	*Pseudomonas, Alcaligenes*
Poultry	Slime, odor	*Pseudomonas, Alcaligenes*
Fresh meat	Putrefaction	*Alcaligenes, clostridium*
Pickles, saverkraut	Film yeasts, pink yeasts	*Rhodotorula*

Canned foods: Spore formers like clostridium and bacillus constitute the most important group of micro-organisms in the canning industry because of their heat resistance. The following are the most important types of microbiological spoilage of commercially canned foods are:

1. Flat sour spoilage
2. Thermophilic anaerobe spoilage
3. Putrefaction

12.3.1 Food Preservation Methods

(i) Physical preservation method

(a) *Asepsis*: Asepsis is the process of prevention of growth of micro-organisms and their contaminants or both. The covering or wrapping, prevents primarily contamination during handling.

(b) *High temperature*: The killing of micro-organisms at high temperature is supposed to be caused by the denaturation of the proteins and especially by inactivation of enzymes required for metabolism

- The heat treatment also kills micro-organisms or their spores.
- The heat resistance of micro-organisms usually expressed in terms of their thermal death time, which is defined as the time it takes at a certain temperature to kill a stated number of cells or spores under specific conditions.
- Pasteurization is another method in which micro-organisms are killed by heat treatment usually involves the application of temperature below 100 °C.

(c) *Canning*: Canning is defined as the preservation of foods in sealed containers and usually implies heat treatment as the major factor. Nicholas Appert, who has been called the "father of canning", performed heating of foods in sealed containers

- The temperature used for canning foods ranges from 100 °C for high-acid foods to 121 °C for low-acid foods.
- The most important organism to be eliminated in canned foods is the spore forming an aerobe *Clostridium botulinum*, which is capable of producing a very potent lethal toxin.

(ii) Chemical preservation methods

Food additives are specially added to prevent the deterioration or decomposition of food, has been referred to as chemical preservatives. The food deterioration may be due to micro-organisms, by food enzymes or by purely chemical reactions.

- Lactic acid, acetic acid, propionic and citric acids or their salts are used as preservatives.
- Citric acid used in syrup, drinks, jams and jellies as a substitute for fruit flavours and for preservation.
- Lactic and acetic acids are added to drinks of various kinds, green olives etc
- Propionic acid affects the cell membrane permeability
- Nitrates and nitrites used in curing meats, primarily for the preservation of colour.

Radiation: Ultraviolet light of sufficient intensity and time of exposure is microbicidal to exposed micro-organisms. Ultraviolet radiation is limited to the control of micro-organisms because of its very limited penetration.

- Ionizing radiations are lethal to micro-organisms. They are microbicidal at room temperature and have the ability to penetrate
- Gamma rays and electron beams have been experimented with extensively for use in the food industry.
- Canned and packaged foods can be sterilized by an appropriate radiation dosage. Cold sterilization produces a rise in temperature of the product of only a few degrees

- Radiation pasteurization is a term describing the killing of over 98% but not 100% of the organisms by intermediate doses of ionizing radiation.

(iii) Wood smoke

Wood smoke contains a large number of volatile compounds that may have bacteriostatic or bactericidal effect. Smoking of foods usually adds desired flavours and acts as preservatives besides, improvement in the colour of the inside of meat formaldehyde is considered as most effective. Other compounds in smoke are aliphatic acids, alcohols, ketones etc. Wood smoke is more effective against vegetative cell than against spores.

12.3.2 Micro-organisms as Food – Single – Cell Protein

The term single cell protein first given by Wilson. Single – cell protein defined as micro-organism or microbial biomass utilized as food. Bacteria, yeast, algae produced in massive quantities, are attractive sources of food for animals as well as humans.

- Yeast – cell crops harvested from the vats used to produce alcoholic beverages have been used as a food supplement for generations.

The attractiveness of single – cell protein as a food substitute or supplement is apparent from the following characteristics.

1. Micro-organisms grow very rapidly and produce a high yield. It has been calculated that 1000 lb of yeast would produce several tons of protein in one day. Algae grown in ponds can produce 20 tons of protein per acre per year
2. Protein content of the microbial cells is very high. Dried cells of pseudomonas species grown on petroleum products have 69% protein
3. The protein of selected micro-organisms contains all the essential aminoacids.
4. Some micro-organisms, particularly yeast, have a high vitamin content.

Oriental foods: Traditionally, oriental foods are used in many countries including India.

1. Mycoprotein: Product such as Tempeh and Koji contain a significant amount of mould biomass (mycelium) which is a source of food. Mycoproteins, marketed in some foreign countries under the name quorn, is essentially the mycelium of *Fusarium graminerarum* grown in continuous culture in a medium containing glucose, ammonium salts and a few growth factors.

   (i) *Tempeh*: This is the fermented food of Indonesians. The most popular type is produced from soyabeans and also called as tempeh kedele.

   (ii) *Soy sauce*

(iii) *Miso*: Molds are involved in the preparation of most of the oriental foods. Miso is prepared by the starter termed koji (by japaness) and chou (Chinese), molds serve the source of enzymes.

(iv) *Idli*

(v) *Natto*: It is a soya bean product

(vi) *Minchin*: In this case starch free but gluten rice wheat is used

(vii) *Poi*: The bulbs and the corns of the taro plant are steamed for 2-3 hours, cooled, trimmed, scrapped and finally ground.

12.4 Microbiology of Air (Aeromicrobiology)

The term aerobiology was used to denote air-borne spores (e.g., Fungi and other micro-organisms) and pollen grains shown in Table 12.2.

- Aeromicrobiology deals with the study of air-borne micro-organisms and viruses along with important particulate matter of air, especially smoke, dust, radionuclides and pesticides.
- The important gases that affect the micro-organisms are H_2S, SO_2, CO, Cl, HF, O_3 etc.

Table 12.2 Some Common Aeroallergens

Aeroallergens	Sources
Pollen grains	Wind-pollinated plants eg: grasses, weeds, trees
Moulds	Saprophytic fungi multiply on dead organic substrate
Danders	Feathers of chickens, ducks, hairs of cat, dogs, sheep, cattle
House dust	A composite of all dust containing specific components related to mites, algae
Cosmetics	Talcs, perfume, hair tonics, lotions
Insecticides	Insecticides containing pyrethrum as a common Ingredient
Paint and vanishes	Linseed oil, organic solvents act as irritant

A. Significance of Air

- Air plays dual role i.e., creating the health and diseased condition.
- The cool mild breeze coming through a garden brings fragrance and solace to humans in such a condition of experiences comfort. Moreover, such conditions are better for control of exhalation and inhalation of air i.e., *"pranayam"*.

- In addition, the stormy air (wind) becomes dangerous sometimes causing a great damage to both the natural/man-made structures on the earth.
- Air containing foul smelling and pathogenic micro-organisms is not fit for human health. Such air causes many human diseases including allergy.
- The allergy causing air-borne agents are called aeroallergens that include biotic and abiotic factors.

B. Vedic technology for air purification

- The seers were aware of making their surroundings pure by vedic technology one of which is the *agnihotra* i.e., the smallest form of Vedic Home.
- *Agnihotra* was the daily duty of offerings to fire, twice in a day (at morning and evening) for air purification in their houses and surroundings
- Gases are produced after burning of various substances of fire oblations (e.g., ghee, cereals, medicinal herbs, forest herbs) and diffused in surroundings. These gases kill/inhibit various kinds of micro-organisms present in air.
- The action of gases is potentiated by increased temperature that causes decline in relative humidity of the atmosphere
- These gases act as antimicrobial and insect repellant.

C. Works on Aeromicrobiology in India

1. *Fungi*: The first systematic work was carried out by *Cunningham* which he published in the form of a book, microscopic examination of air
   - Later on prof. K. C. Mehta of Agra college, Agra extensively investigated the air for the presence of wheat rust spores.
   - He discovered that rust spores survive on wheat and barley. The wind currents carry the inoculum to the hills when climatic conditions of plains are unfavourable. When these are favourable, spores are brought back to plains to start reinfection on fresh wheat plants.

(i) **Occurrence and epidemiology:** Brown and black rust of wheat are disseminated from the hills of south India to central India by "hop jump" in which a storm depression formed in Bay of Bengal/Arabian sea reaches central India.

- Satellite television cloud photography is a possible tool for forecasting the spread of several plant pathogens such as *Alternaria, Cercospora, Helminthosporium, Puccinia* etc.

(ii) **Aflatoxins by Aerofungi:** Aflatoxins are the 2° metabolites of some saprophytic fungi injurious for human health.

- The species of fungi secreting aflatoxins are *Aspergillus flavus*, *A. Parasiticus* others etc.
- *A. Flavus* is known to cause cancer

- Rati and Ramalingam surveyed *A. flavus* in air samples in outdoor air and air of poultry shed. They found that 72% of these were toxigenic, and the incidence of toxigenic strain was found to be greater in winter months.
- Organs other than liver are also affected by aflatoxins such as kidney, adrenal glands, lungs skin
- Aflatoxin B_1 is known to cause mutagenicity through chromosomal aberrations and DNA breakage in plant and animal cells.

2. *Algae*:
   - The most common algae found in air are the species of *Chlorella, Chlorococcum, Chlamydomonas, Aulosira, Nostoc* and *Phormidium*

D. Indoor Aero-Microbiology

Indoor aero microbiology deals with micro-organisms present in air inside the houses. There are many micro-organisms which are responsible for biodeterioration of storage materials, equipment, library materials and archives

1. *Aeromicrospora of pharmacy*: Sharma and Navneet reported aero fungi from the fermentation unit of Gurukul Kangri Pharmacy, Haridwar.
2. *Aeromicroflora of hospitals*: Hospital is an important indoor environment responsible for spread of air-borne pathogens.
   - It acts as reservoir of pathogens which later on is transmitted to the other individuals like patients, hospital workers, visitor etc.
   - The hospital transmitted pathogens are *Mycobacterium tuberculosis, S.aeureus, Influenza virus, A.flavus, A.fumigatus*

   Even house dust has been investigated for the presence of allergenic constituents.
3. *Aeromicroflora of storage materials*:
   (i) *Library*: The major constituent of paper is the cellulose. Therefore, cellulose degrading micro-organisms colonise and degrade the papers. The common cellulose degrading fungi are the species of *Alternia, Aspergillus, Curvularia, Bispora, Rhizopus, Fusarium.*
   (ii) *Wall paintings*: The world fame wall paintings at Ajanta and Ellora caves have shown the sign of biodeterioration probably aerofungi have deteriorated the wall paintings. Growth of aerofungi is supported by the excreta of bats which probably serve as a substrate.

E. Aeroallergens and Aero allergy: The allergy causing agents present in air are called aeroallergens, and the allergy caused by them is called aero allergy shown in Table 12.3.

Table 12.3 Examples of Aeroallergens

Aeroallergens	Examples
Algae	*Aulosira, Chlamydomonas, Nostoc, diatoms, Chlorella*
Fungi	*Alternaria, Aspergillus, Candida, Curvularia, Fusarium*
Lichens	*Cladonia, Heterodermia, Parmelia*
Pollen grains	*Amaranthus species, Azadirachta indica, carica papaya, cocos nucifera, Datura metel, catharanthus roseus, ocimum sanctum etc*
Others	*Dust, mites, viruses, bacteria, protozoa, moss spores*

1. *House dust allergens*: House dust is a mixture of hairs, moulds, bacteria, decomposed parts of cloths or furniture, small insects, mites etc
   - These are inhaled by individuals who later on suffers from allergy
   - The most common fungal spores isolated from the allergic individuals are the species of *Aspergillus, Rhizopus, Curvularia, Helminthosporium, Fusarium, Cephalosporium* etc
   - *D. pteronyssinus* is commonly known as house dust mite
2. *Pollen grains*: In India aeroallergenic pollen grains are contributed mainly from the plants belonging to the family *Poaceae, Chenopodiaceae, Amaranthaceae* and *Asteraceae.*
   - After attaining maturity, the pollen grains get disseminated and dispersed through vectors like wind, water and insects.
3. *Cosmetics*: Cosmetics are the articles that someone applies to, sprinkles on or rubs into their body to cleanse, beautify or promote attractiveness or alter their appearance
   - The examples of cosmetics of daily use are creams, gels, powders, lotions, oils, dyes etc
   - These cosmetics show dermatological problems
   - The causes of allergies are

   (a) the quality products of cosmetics

   (b) spoilage of cosmetics by micro-organisms like *E.coli, Aerobacter aerogenes, Subtilis, Aspergillus*

   (c) secretion of toxins by micro-organisms

   (d) chemical ingredients of cosmetics

   (f) phylloplane microflora

   - Phyllosphere describe the leaf surface as the habitat of micro-organisms
   - The leaf surface acts as the landing stage for the microbial propagules. These are deposited by impaction, by boundary layer exchange, by sedimentation under the influence of gravity and in rain and splash droplets

- The spores present on leaf surface get nutrients defused from leaf and also from pollengrains present on leaf surface
- Micro-organisms colonise the leaves when it remain in infolding stage
- Some common phylloplane microflora are bacteria (*Beijernickiasp pseudomonas trifoli* etc), yeasts (*Candida albicans, Cryptococcus diffluens, S.cerevisiae*) and fungi (*A.niger, cephalosporium, Alternia*) shown in Table 12.4.

1. *Phylloplane pathogens*: The micro-organisms living on phylloplane are of several types i.e., saprophytes, symbionts and pathogens

Table 12.4 Some Phylloplane Pathogens

Pathogens	Disease
Albugo candida	White rust of crucifers
Alternaria	Leaf spot of crucifers
Helminthosporium oryzae	Brown spot of paddy
A. Solani	Early blight of potato

2. *Microflora of floral parts*
   - Flowers produce pollengrains, nector and several chemicals that attract micro-organisms. Therefore, a variety of micro-organisms fall on petals, sepals, ovary etc
   - Among those, both beneficial and pathogenic micro-organisms are present
   - One of the pathogenic group of fungi is the smuts of *graminaceous* plants
   - Fruit infection occurs sometimes by the micro-organisms of floral parts for example *Pestalotia psidii* causing fruit rot of guava.
   - In addition to pathogenic micro-organisms, floral parts also harbour beneficial micro-organisms,

For example: Dhataki flowers (*Woodfordia fructicosa*) are used in Ayurvedic pharmacy in the production of "Amritarishta" one of the widely used medicine in the treatment of fever.

Characteristics of Phylloplane Microflora

Phylloplane term is used in ecology which means the surface of a leaf considered as a habitat, especially for micro-organisms It is also called as phyllosphere

(i) *Morphological characteristics*: The phylloplane inhabitants possess morphological characteristics for their survival. These include the development of pigment in their mycelia, spores, pycnidia, apothecia for protection against strong light and desiccation. The dark pigments act as light screen. These pigments are often referred to as melanin.

(ii) *Physiological Characteristics*:

(a) *Nutrition*: Phylloplane microfungi have ability to decompose cellulose by producing cellulases

- In addition, pectinases, cutinases, proteases have also been estimated in many fungi e.g., *Alternaria alternata, Cladosporium herbarum*

(b) *Radiations*: High intensity light inhibits mycelial growth

- Light of normal intensity is not harmful to phylloplane fungi
- Fungi containing melanin pigment are resistant to UV exposure
- Hyaline spores of *Aureobasidium* and *Sporobolomyces* are killed by exposure of UV for 5 minutes, whereas dark spores of *Alternia* and *Epicoccum* survive even after exposure for 35 minutes

(c) *Relative humidity*: During rain and dew formation, high relative humidity on leaf surface is found. But when there is wind the micro environment is reduced.

- Phylloplane fungi get advantages at low levels of relative humidity.
- Generally, a faster growth rate of the germ tube and mycelium of some fungi occurs at 100% relative humidity.

(d) *Temperature*: The phylloplane fungi are mesophilic growing at temperature 20-25 °C. Even some fungi (*e.g., Alternaria alternata, Cladosporium herbarum*) can grow below 0 °C.

Microbial Interaction on Leaf Surface

- Many kinds of interactions occur on phylloplane region between the pathogens and saprophytes
- The most significant effect was observed when the spores of leaf surface fungi or their metabolites were sprayed on leaves prior to inoculation of the pathogens.

12.5 Microbiology of Water

- Water is the elixir of life. It is an essential part of protoplasm and creates a state for metabolic activities to occur smoothly.
- There are thousands of micro-organisms which live in water and are transported through it.
- Water receives micro-organisms from air, soil, sewage, organic wastes, dead plant and animals etc

A. Types of water: Natural water is commonly grouped into four well-marked classes: (a) atmospheric water (b) surface water (c) stored water (d) ground water

1. *Atmospheric water*:
   - Rain and snow are included under the atmospheric water
   - Micro-organisms in the form of cells/dormant propagules and dust particles remain suspended in water and snow.
   - Considerable number of bacteria can be isolated from rain water
   - After heavy rain or snow fall, the dust particles and bacteria are washed from the atmosphere
2. *Surface water*: The water present on earth surface is known as surface water
   - As soon as raindrops or snow touches the earth, it becomes contaminated by the micro-organisms present in soil.
   - Total microbial content in water depends on microbial population of soil, types of soil, types of organic materials present in soil and also on types of micro-organisms and their activities
3. *Stored water*: The stagnant land water present in ponds, lakes etc are called stored water.
   - During storage, in general, the number of micro-organisms gets reduced; thus it establishes the purity and stability to some extent.
   - However, in stored water the micro-organisms are affected by several factors such as sedimentation, UV light, temperature, osmotic effects, food supply, and activities of other micro-organisms.
4. *Ground water*: Soil consists of particles of varying size, therefore, soil pore size varies. The large pores allow a free percolation of water due to gravitational force. This is known as gravitational water. The gravitational water moves down and accumulates in the form of ground water.
   - A huge amount of fresh water is present in the form of ground water.

B. Water micro-organisms: A large number of micro-organisms both saprophytes and pathogens are found in water which fall under the groups bacteria, fungi, algae, protozoa and nematodes

- The majority of bacteria found in water belongs to groups: fluorescent bacteria (*e.g., Pseudomonas, Algimonas* etc)

Chromogenic rods (*Xanthomonas*)

Coliform group (*E.coli, Aerobacter*)

Proteus group, non-chromogenic and non-spore forming rods spore formers of the genus Bacillus

Pigmented and non pigmented cocci

Some of Aquatic Fungi in Different Water Bodies

Aquatic fungi	Sources
Achlya americana	Tap water, fish parasite
A. androcomposita	Tank water
A. debaryana	Water, fish pathogen
Blastocladia simplex	Gujar lake
Rhizophydium species	Gujar lake

Some of the water-borne pathogenic microbes

Micro-organisms Bacteria	Reservoir	Other features
Mycobacterium tuberculosis	Free-living, infected person	Tuberculosis
Vibrio cholerae	Free-living	Diarrhoea
Pseudomonas aeruginosa	Free-living	Swimer's ear
Protozoa		
Giardia lamblia	Sheep, dogs, cats	Diarrhoea
Entamoeba histolytica	Water	Amoebiasis

1. Marine Microbiology

- Marine microbiology deals with micro-organisms living in sea.
- Pressure in the marine environment increases by about 1 atm/10 meters in depth.
- The bacteria growing in vertically differentiated marine environment can be categorized in three groups:
  - (a) barotolerant (bacteria growing optimally between 0 and 400 atm but best at normal atmospheric pressure)
  - (b) moderate barophiles (bacteria growing optimally at 400 atm, but still grow at 1 atm) and
  - (c) extreme barophiles (bacteria growing only at higher pressure i.e., 6000 to 11,000 meter depth)
- In the marine system, the major source of organic matter is phytoplanktons i.e., free floating plants
- A common planktonic alga is synecoccus which can reach to a density of 10^4 to 10^5 cells/ml at the ocean surface
- Picocyano bacteria may represent 20 to 80% of total phytoplankton biomass
- Recently, a very interesting group of bacteria (Archaeobacteria) has been discovered from the marine system.

2. Fresh water microbiology

- Lakes and rivers provide the major fresh water bodies which are used for portable water.
- The nutrient poor lakes are known as oligotrophic lakes, whereas the nutrient rich lakes are called eutrophic lakes
- The nutrient rich lakes contain high amount of bottom sediments containing organic matter.
- Eutrophication (enrichment of lake due to high concentration of nutrients) of lakes occur by multifarious ways where anthropogenic activities are of much importance.
- The eutrophic lakes support luxuriant growth of bacteria and algae.
- Some of the fast growing algae at optimum condition bloom well showing their maximum population. This phenomenon is known as water blooming, and micro-organisms associated with it are called water blooms.
- The two most important lakes of India which are fully eutrophicated are Dal lake and Naina lake which are the only source of potable water.

The micro-organisms growing in lakes are the genera:

- *Anabaena*
- *Microcystis*
- *Nostoc*
- *Oscillatoria*
- *Spirulina*
- *Diatoms*
- *Protozoa*

C. Microbiological Analysis of water purity

- The natural water bodies such as lakes, streams, rivers contain sufficient amount of nutrients that support the growth of micro-organisms.
- People suffering from communicable diseases also discharge pathogenic microbes in water through their excreta, for example amoebic dysentery, typhoid fever, bacillary dysentery, poliomyelitis etc
- Bacteria multiply in water at 35 °C and at 20 °C.

The Fecal coli forms: On the basis of microbiological examination of water, its portability may be ascertained.

- Intestinal bacteria present in water generally do not survive in aquatic environment due to physiological stress but if entered human system in the mean while, they cause serious problems
- The characteristic group of intestinal bacteria are the coliforms

- Coliforms are defined as facultatively anaerobic, gram-ve, non-sporing rod shaped bacteria that ferment lactose with gas formation within 48 hours at 35 °C
- The coliform groups are present in water due to faecal contamination i.e., discharge of faeces by human and other animals in water.
- Coliforms are the members of the family enterobacteriaceae which includes *E.coli*, *Enterobacter aerogenes*, salmonella and *Klebsiella pneumoniae.*
- If such bacteria are not detectable in water in 100 ml, the water can be said as portable water

1. ***Sanitary tests for coli forms***: The original test for the presence of coliform in water is done by standard multiple tube fermentation technique. This method involves the three routine standard tests:
   (a) the presumptive test
   (b) the confirmed test
   (c) the complete test
   (i) *Presumptive test*: A series of fermentation tubes each containing lactose broth or lauryl tryptose broth of known concentration are inoculated with known amount of water.
      - These tubes are incubated for 24-48 hours at 35 °C
      - Inoculate 15 tubes (5 tubes with 10 ml, 5 with 1 ml and 5 with 0.1 ml water)
      - At the end of 24 hours of incubation, the tubes indicate that the coliforms are absent
      - These tubes are incubated for an additional 24 hour to be sure for the absence of coliforms (i.e., gas production)

   (ii) *Confirmed test*:
      - If a positive test of gas production is obtained, it does not mean that coliforms are present
      - The other organisms too also give false positive presumptive test because they are also capable of fermenting lactose with formation of acid and gas.
      - The positive presumptive test is resulted due to synergism i.e., joint action of two micro-organisms on a carbohydrate with the production of gas which is not formed if both are grown separately.
      - In addition, if yeasts, species of clostridium and some other micro-organisms are present, gas is also produced. Therefore, a confirmed test is performed for the presence of coliforms.
      - All fermentation tubes showing gas within 48 hours at 35 °C are used for confirmed test. It is of two types

      The positive presumptive fermentation tube is gently shaken. A drop of its culture is transferred to brilliant green lactose bile broth fermentation tube. The tubes are incubated for 48 hours at 35 °C. The appearance of gas within this period indicates for positive confirmed test. The dye (brilliant green) inhibits the gram positive bacteria and synergistic reactions of gram positive and gram negative bacteria for a common food base.

- The second confirmed test is done by *Eosine methylene blue (EMB) agar* or *Endo agar* method.
- In *Eosine methylene blue agar* method, a definite amount of two stains (eosin and methylene blue) is added to a melted lactose agar.
- The medium is poured into Petri dishes. Over the surface of EMB agar medium, a loopful culture from each positive fermentation tube is streaked
- Plates are incubated at 35 °C for 24 hours keeping them in inverted position.
- There develops three types of colonies:
  (a) typical colonies (nucleated)
  (b) a typical colonies (non nucleated, pink)
  (c) negative colonies (all other types)
- The development of typical colonies shows that the confirmed test is positive.

(iii) Completed test: Completed test is performed to ascertain about the presence of coliforms in water.

- The purpose of the completed test is to determine whether
  (a) the colonies growing on EMB or endo agar are again capable of fermenting lactose and forming acid and gas, and
  (b) the organisms transferred to agar slants show the morphological appearance of coliform group.
- Each colonies form positive confirmed test is transferred to lactose fermentation tube and to nutrient agar slants
- The tubes are incubated at 35 °C for 48 hours.
- Production of gas in fermentation tubes and, demonstration of gram-negative, non spore forming rods on the agar slants constitute a positive completed test for coliforms.
- The absence of gas and the rod production confirms for negative test of coliforms.

2. *The most probable number of (MPN) of coli forms:*

- MPN is used to evaluate coli-aerogenes test by fermentation tube method.
- A statistical range of the coliform numbers is determined by observing the number of broth tubes producing gas.

(i) The membrane filter technique:

- Goetz and Tsuneishi described a new method for enumeration of coliform micro-organisms in water to which they named as Millipore filter technique

- This technique has been accepted as the standard method for the microbiological examination of sewage water etc.
- The filtering apparatus consists of a glass or stainless steel funnel, and a flask
- The funnel of stainless steel is clamped to a base containing a molecular filter
- The stem of base is inserted into a filter flask through a rubber stopper. A sterile membrane filter (0.45 μm) disk is placed in the sterilized holding apparatus
- A volume of water is passed through filter disk. Bacteria present in water sample are retained on filter disk. The sides of funnel and membrane are rinsed with sterile distilled water. Thereafter, the membrane filter disc is aseptically removed by a sterile forceps and placed on absorbent disk saturated with culture medium and contained in Petri dish.
- The medium passes through the pores of membrane and nourishes the bacteria present on it. After proper incubation at 35 °C for 24 hours each bacterium multiplies to form a visible colony on membrane
- The colonies are easily counted.

Advantages to Membrane Filter Technique

- This method is very useful in emergency
- It allows the direct counting of micro-organisms instead of counting most probable number
- It permits the small numbers of bacteria from large quantities of water
- It is time saving method.

Disadvantages

- In turbid waters containing algal growth and other materials the pores of membrane filter are clogged.
- Metals and phenols can be absorbed to membrane filter and therefore, inhibit growth of bacteria retained on membrane filter.

3. *The defined substrate test:*

- The defined substrate test is used for both coliforms and *E.coli* in a single 100 mL water sample
- A specialised medium containing O-Nitrophenyl-β-D-Galactopyranoside (ONPG) and 4-Methylumbelliferyl-β-D-Glucuronide (MUG) as the only nutrients are added with a water sample of 100 ml.
- The incubation bottles containing water plus both nutrients along with control are incubated at 35 °C for 24 hours.
- If coliforms are present the medium will turn yellow within 24 hours due to break down of ONPG.
- When *E.coli* is present, the MUG is changed to yield a fluorescent product

- The fluorescence is observed under long-wavelength UV light for the presence of *E.coli*.
- If the color does not develop and give negative report for the presence of coli form, the water is suitable for drinking.

4. ***IMVic tests***:
   - *E.coli* and *Aerobacter aerogenes* are the most important bacteria of coliform group, the former is commonly known as fecal contaminant and the later as non-fecal contaminant.
   - Morphologically both are similar and cannot be distinguished. Therefore, biochemical tests are being used to differentiate each of them.
   - The tests differentiating them are collectively known as IMVic tests (or reactions).
   - The abbreviation IMVic is prepared by using first letter of four different tests: indole, methyl red, voges-proskauer, and citrate tests shown in Table 12.5.

Table 12.5 IMVic Tests Results of Coliform Bacteria

Tests	*E.coli*	*A.aerogenes*
Indole	Indole is produced from tryptophan +	Indole is not produced, (–)
Methyl red	*E.coli* produces acids that drop pH below 4.5. Hence methyl red is turned red	Methyl red remains yellow due to production of less acid, (–)
Voges-proskauer	*E.coli* does not produce acetyl methyl carbinol in glucose-peptone medium, (–)	Acetyl methyl carbinol is produced by this bacterium (+)
Citrate	Citrate as the sole carbon source does not support the growth of *E.coli*, (–)	Citrate supports the growth of this bacterium (+)

D. Purification of water: There are several methods for purification of water the use of which depends on amount and quantity of water. There are three chief methods which are used for the purification of drinking water in municipal supplies, i.e., sedimentation, filtration and disinfection.

1. ***Sedimentation:*** Sedimentation is done when water consists of large sized organic materials such as leaves, and gravels which have run off from the soil.
   - Suspended particles settle down depending on their size and weight and conditions of the stored water.
   - Sedimentation is done in large reservoirs or in restricted area of settling tank.

- The rate of sedimentation is enhanced by adding alum, iron, salts, colloid silicates which act as coagulants
- The suspended materials and micro-organisms are entrapped by coagulants and settle down rapidly. This procedure is called coagulation or flocculation.
- The micro-organisms remain viable for some time. Thus, sedimentation provides partial reduction of micro-organisms in water due to their settling down on bottom but does not sterilize the polluted water.

2. ***Filtration:*** It is second step of purification
   - After sedimentation the water is further purified by passing to filtration unit.
   - It is the effective means of removing micro-organisms and the other suspended material from the water.
   - There are two types of sand filters which are used in water purification such as slow sand filter and rapid sand filter.

   (i) *Slow sand filter*: In slow sand filtration plants the rate of filtration of water is slow, hence the plant requires a considerable area.
   - This plant consists of a concrete floor containing drainage tiles (for collection of filtered water).
   - The tile is covered with first coarse sand and finally 2 to 1 feet of fine sand at the top of plant.
   - Water is passed through this plant. Water passes slowly through the filter and collected by tile drain pipes at the bottom which later on is pumped into a reservoir.
   - Sand grains have positive charges and bacterial cell walls have negative charge. Therefore, bacteria are adsorbed on the surface of sand.

   (ii) *Rapid sand filter*: This plant consists of layers of sand, gravel and rock.
   - Before filtration, water is treated with alum or ferrous sulphate in a settling tank where precipitates settle down. Then water is allowed to pass through rapid sand filter plant.
   - This plant depends on physical trapping of fine particles and flocks or coagulants.
   - The pores of the plants are soon clogged. It is cleaned by forcing cleaned water backward i.e., back washing through the beds of gravels and sands without disturbing the fine sand.
   - About 99% of bacteria are removed by this plant shown in Fig. 12.4.

3. ***Disinfection***
   - Disinfection is the final step of water purification.
   - Solutions of sodium hypochlorite are treated in small towns but in recent years, chlorination of public water supply has become popular.

- Chlorination involves the release of chlorine gas in water which gets readily mixed up with water
- The amount of chlorine required depends on organic matter and number of micro-organisms present in water, and duration of time to act upon.
- High concentration of chlorine quickly acts upon micro-organisms. Therefore, the amount of chlorine required for disinfection is called chlorine demand
- Water is chlorinated to contain about 0.1 to 0.2 ppm of residual chlorine which reaches to this concentration after 20 minutes of its addition.
- After reacting with water, chlorine is converted into Hypochlorous acid which in turn quickly releases nascent oxygen.
- The nascent oxygen soon oxidases the cellular components of micro-organisms as well as organic matter.

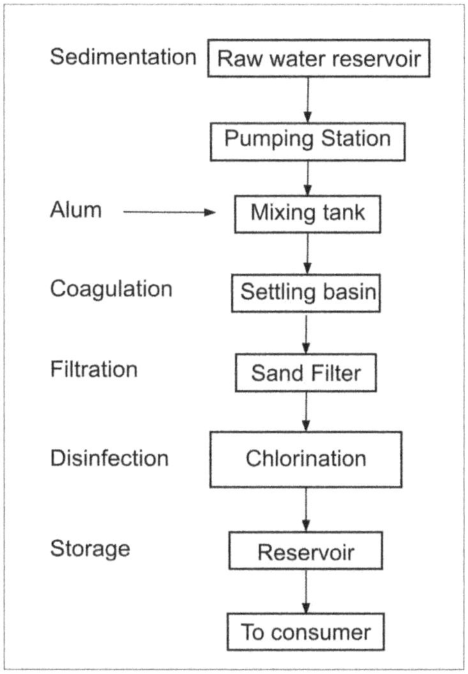

Fig. 12.6 Flow diagram of usual procedure in municipal Water purification

12.6 Microbiology of Milk

- Milk is secreted by mammals for the nourishment of their young ones. It is in liquid form without having any colostrums. The milk contains water, fat, protein and lactose. About 80-85% of the proteins is casein protein.

- Due to moderate pH (6.4 - 6.6), good quantity of nutrients, high water content etc make milk an excellent nutrient for the microbial growth.
- It is mainly the udder interior, teats surrounding environment and manual milking process, make the source of contamination.
- These organisms mainly are *Micrococci, Streptococci* and *Diphtheroid Coryne bacterium boris*
- An inflammatory disease of mammary tissues called mastitis is due to many micro-organisms such as *S.aureus, E.coli, Streptococcus agalactiae, S.uberis, P.aeruginosa and Corynebacterium pyogenes.*
- *Clostridium butyricum* can get into milk from silage fed to cows. This causes the problem called late blowing in some cheese.

Measures to minimize the Contamination

- The dairy industry needs enough cleaning, preventing muddy area wherever possible not to allow to leave urine and feces, shaving udders and trimming tails.
- There should be a regular washing of teats with warm water containing some disinfectants such precautions are to be taken to minimize milk contamination so as to improve the microbiological quality of milk.
- In raw milk, Gram negative rods of the genera pseudomonas, Acinetobacter, flavobacterium, Aerobacter species and Gram positive Bacillus species are dominant micro-organisms shown in Table 12.6.
- The presence of psychotrophs is a traditional test for the microbiological quality of milk based on the reduction of a redox dye such as methylene blue

Table 12.6 Heat Treatment of Milk

Condition	Temperature and holding time
Sterilized	> 100 °C for 20-40 min
High temperature short time	71.7 °C for 15 seconds
Low temperature holding	62.8 °C for 30 min

- A simple phosphatase test is recommended to determine whether milk has been properly pasteurized or not.
- Milk has the alkaline phosphatase inactivated by the time/temperature combinations applied during pasteurization
- Sometimes, raw milk may also contain a number of organisms called thermodurics that can survive mild pasteurization treatments. These are generally Gram-positive bacteria namely *microbacterium, micrococcus, enterococcus* and *Lactobacillus,* but Gram negative, *Alcaligenes tolerans* may also survive
- The thermoduric *Bacillus cereus* causes a flavour defect in the milk by showing appearance of bitty cream phenomenon produced by the lecithinase activity.

Milk Products

(i) *Yoghurt*: Yoghurt is derived from turkish word "Jugurt" which is the most popular fermented milk in the world now-a-days

- It is made from milk, skimmed milk or flavoured milk
- For the preparation of yoghurt, the milk should be free from contamination
- The solid content should be between 11-15% which can be obtained by adding skim or whole milk powder in fresh milk that normally contains 8% solids
- The product can be further improved by adding small amount of modified gums which bind water and impart thickening to the product
- At this stage the size of the fat particles in the milk should be around 2 μm because this improve the milk's viscosity, product's stability and milk appear form
- The milk is then heated 80-90 °C for 30 min, starter culture is added to it
- Heating improves the milk by inactivating immunoglobulins, remove excessive oxygen which supports the growth of starter culture. The milk is now cooled to 40 - 43 °C so as to allow fermentation using starter organisms
- The starter organisms such as *S. salivarius sub Sp. thermophilus and Lb. delbruckii sub Sp. bulgaricus* together at a level of 2% by volume.
- The flavor in yoghurt is due to acetaldehyde shown in Fig. 12.5.
- Microbial pathogens or contaminants generally do not occur in yoghurt due to high acidity and low pH
- A good yoghurt should contain no more than 10 yeast g^{-1} with almost complete absence of coliform and molds

(ii) *Kefir*: Kefir is intact, fermented milk, produced by a mixed lactic acid bacteria and alcoholic yeast

- The microflora responsible is not spread uniformly throughout the milk but is supplemented as discrete kefir 'grains'.
- The kefiran i.e., large layers of polysaccharide material folds upon to produce a cauliflower like florets to produce kefir.
- The outer smooth layer contains lactobacilli while the (inner) rough side contains yeast and lactic acid bacteria

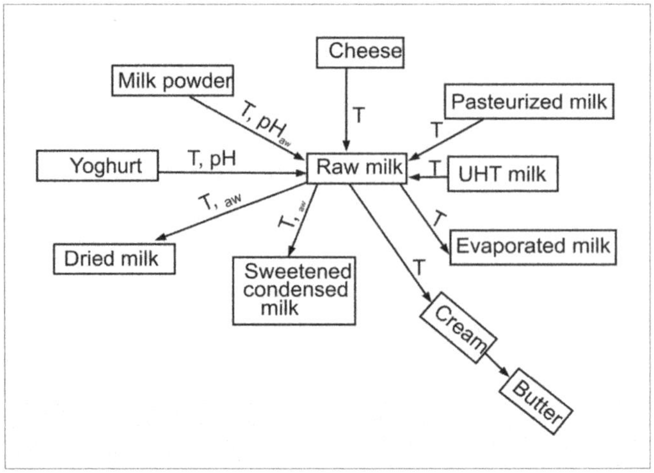

T, elevated temperature pH, reduced pH

aw, reduced water pressure

Fig. 12.7 Milk and milk products

- The capsular homo fermentative *Lactobacillus kefiranflaciens* produces kefiran
- *Lactobacillus kefir* contributes the required effervescence in the product
- For commercial production of kefir, milk is homogenized and heated at 85-95 °C for 3-10 minutes. It is then cooled to 22 °C before addition of kefir grains at a size of 5%.
- The fermentation should be carried out for 8-12 hr.
- The product contains 0.8% acidity, 0.01% to 1.0% ethanol, CO_2, acetaldehyde and diacetyl.

(iii) *Koumiss*: Koumiss is produced from mare's milk which is grayish white drink, produced mostly in east European countries

- It has *L.delbruckii* sub *SP.bulgaricus* and a number of lactose fermenting yeast responsible to produce koumiss.

(iv) *Butter milk*: It is a liquid substance which is separated from cream during churning process

- A mixture of starting cultures such as *Lactobacillus lactis* sub sp.*diacetylactis* and *Leuconostoc mesenteroides* sub sp.*cremoris* produce butter milk
- Since citrate metabolism can provide the pyruvate, lead to the accumulation of diacetyl, hence fresh milk should contain citrate for the production of butter milk.
- For the production, milk is pasteurized, homogenized and fermented at 22 °C for 12-16 hr.

- The final product contains 0.7-0.9% lactic acid

(v) *Butter*: Lactic acid producing bacteria are responsible for subsequent separation of butter fat in the churning process. These organisms (*Leuconostoc citrovorum, Streptococcus cremoris* or *S.lactis*) produce a small amount of acetoin which is spontaneously oxidized to diacetyl. This substance gives butter and similar products with their buttery flavor and aroma.

(vi) *Cheese*: There are about 2000 varieties of cheese made from mammalian milk.

- The cheese name is derived from latin word caseus
- There are two groups of cheese: fresh cheese and ripened cheese.
- The fresh cheese are made up of milk coagulated by acid or high heat eg: cottage cheese
- The ripened cheese are made through lactic acid bacterial fermentation and coagulated by an enzyme preparation.
- There are mainly three categories of cheeses:
  - (a) Soft cheese
  - (b) Hard cheese
  - (c) Semisoft cheese
- The soft cheeses are ripened by the enzymes from yeast and other fungi that grow on the surface.
- Hard cheese ripened by lactic acid bacteria which grows throughout the cheese, die, autolyze and release hydrolytic enzymes
- The semisoft cheeses are ripened by proteolytic and lipolytic organisms which soften the curd and give it flavor.

Microbiology of Cheese

The process of cheese making, involves nine steps:

(a) Preparing the milk
(b) Forming a curd
(c) Cutting
(d) Cooking
(e) Separating the whey
(f) Salting the residue
(g) Applying microbes
(h) Pressing the curd and
(i) Ripening the young cheese shown in Tables 12.7, 12.8

Table 12.7 Some common Cheeses in International Market

Type	Cheese	Method of ripening
Hard cheese	cheddar	Cured at 36-50 °F for eight weeks to 12 months
	Emmentaler (swiss)	Formation of eyes in 3-4 weeks at 72 °F and 80-85% RH. Ripened at 40 °F and higher temperature for 2-10 months
Semisoft cheese	Roque fort	Mold-ripened by *P.roqueforti* cured for 3 months at 48 °F and 95% RH wrapped in foil and stored in a cool room for 2-3 months
Soft	Carrembert	Ripened by *P.candidum* on frames or shelves at 55 °F and about 95% RH for 12 days.

(vii) *Rennin* (*milk-coagulating enzymes*):

- The milk coagulation enzyme, rennet, has its importance in cheese production.
- Rennet is an extract from the fourth stomach of 3-4 week old calves which have been fed on milk. The enzyme so purified, called rennin, chymase or chymosin.
- There are several genera of fungi reported to produce rennin. These are species of *Aspergillus, Candida, Coriolus, Rhizopus, Mucor, Penicillium* etc.

Table 12.8 Examples of Fermented Milk Products

Category	Typical examples
1. Lactic fermentations	
Mesophilic	Butter milk, cultured butter milk, Langofil, Tetmjolk, Ymer
Thermophilic	Yoghurt, laban, Zabadi, labneh, skyr Bulgarian buttermilk
Probiotic	Biograde, Bifighurt Acidophilus milk, Yakult
2. Yeast-lactic fermentations	Kefir, koumiss, acidophilus-yeast milk
3. Mold-lactic fermentations	Viili (a yogurt like mesophilic fermented milk)

12.7 Industrial Microbiology

Industrial microbiology has experienced two dramatic explosions during the last few decades. In the 1940s the discovery of antibiotics, led by penicillin, initiated a major new industry built upon the products of micro-organisms. More recently recombinant DNA technology came into existence.

Micro-organisms and Industry: Micro-organisms, under natural conditions, produce an extremely large number, as well as large variety of chemical substances. Some of these substances are very useful for the treatment of diseases and disorders of people and other animals and hence are attractive to the pharmaceutical industry.

The overall reaction characterizing the industrial application of micro-organisms can be given as follows:

Substrate (raw material) + micro-organisms' → new products

Prerequisites to practical Industrial Microbiological processes: If a micro-organism converts cheap raw materials into a useful product, it may be feasible to perform this reaction on a large industrial scale

1. *The organism*: The organism to be used must be able to produce appreciable amounts of the product.
2. *The medium*: The medium, including the substrate from which the organism produces the new product, must be cheap and readily available in large quantities.
3. *The product*: The method of recovery and purification should be carried out in such a way that the desired end product must be developed.

Micro-organisms used in Industrial processes: Industrial microbiological processes have been developed using specific strains of algae, fungi, bacteria, protozoa and viruses. Microbial species which have potential for industrial application are continually being sought. The attractiveness of a micro-organism may reside in its ability to produce a new product e.g., an antibiotic.

12.7.1 Fermenters and Fermentative Microbes

12.7.1.1 History and Design of Fermenters

What is Fermentation? Fermentation is the chemical transformation of organic substances into simpler compounds by the action of enzymes, complex organic catalysts, which are produced by micro-organisms such as molds, yeasts, or bacteria. Enzymes act by hydrolysis, a process of breaking down or predigesting complex organic molecules to form smaller (and in the case of foods, more easily digestible) compounds and nutrients. The word "fermentation" is derived from the Latin meaning "to boil," since the bubbling and foaming of early fermenting beverages seemed closely akin to boiling. This concept is also known as zymosis.

For the first time, large scale aerobic fermenters were used in central Europe in the year 1930's for the production of compressed yeast.

- The fermenter consisted of a large cylindrical tank with air introduced at the base via network of perforated pipes

- Mechanical impellers were used to increase the rate of mixing and to break up and disperse the air bubbles
- Baffles on the walls of the vessels prevented a vortex forming in the liquid

Basic functions of fermenters: The main function of a fermenter is to provide a controlled environment for growth of a micro-organism;

- The vessel should be capable of being operated aseptically for a number of days and should be reliable for long term operation.
- Adequate aeration and agitation should be provided
- The power consumption should be low

Types of Fermenter

(i) Fluidized bioreactor
(ii) Loop or Air lift bioreactor
(iii) Membrane bioreactor
(iv) Pulsed column bioreactor
(v) Bubble column bioreactor
(vi) Photo bioreactor
(vii) Packed tower bioreactor

Construction of Fermenters: The materials used for the construction of a fermenter should be

1. The materials that have no effect of sterilization
2. Its smooth internal finish. There are two types of such materials

(i) stainless steel
(ii) glass

- Control of temperature is essential
- Aeration and Agitation required to meet the metabolic requirements of the microbes
- The agitator (impeller) is required
- Stirrer gland and bearing
- Baffles to prevent vortex formation
- Sparger to supply sterile oxygen

Design and operation: These are designed to provide support to the best possible growth and biosynthesis for industrially important cultures. These vessels must be strong enough to resist the pressure of large volume of agitating medium.

The achievement and maintenance of Aseptic conditions: The following operations may have to be performed to achieve and maintain aseptic conditions during fermentation:

(i) sterilization of the fermenter
(ii) sterilization of the air supply
(iii) aeration and agitation
(iv) the addition of inoculum, nutrients and other supplements
(v) sampling
(vi) foam control
(vii) monitoring and control of various parameters

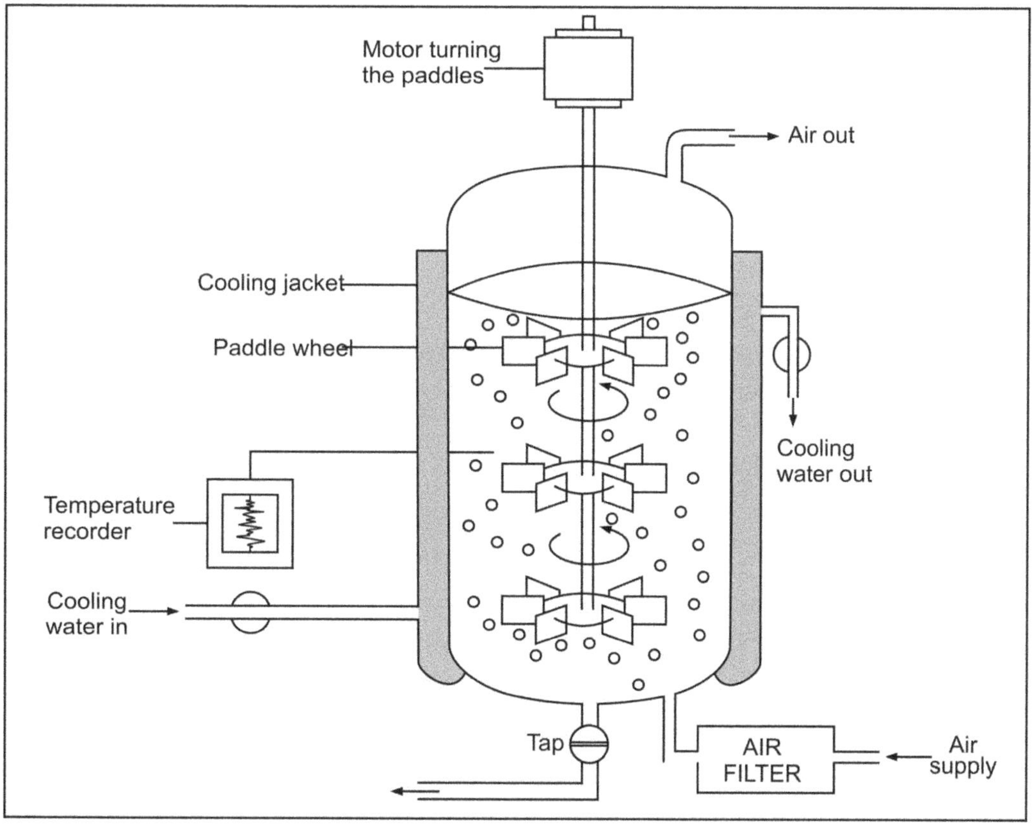

Fig. 12.8 Fermenter

Batch fermentation: Batch fermentation is a process in which a large volume of nutrient medium is inoculated to proceed for the harvest and recovery of the product. This ends the batch fermentation as the vessel is cleansed and desterilized for subsequent batches.

Fed-batch fermentation: In fed-batch fermentation, substrate is added in increments as the fermentation progresses

Continuous fermentation: During continuous fermentation, some parts of the components (media and inoculums) of upstream process are withdrawn intermittently and replacement or withdrawn substances are made by adding the fresh medium or nutrients.

Scale-up fermentations: The determination of the proper incubation conditions to be employed with large scale production tanks as based on information obtained with various sized smaller tanks is called "scale up". This process allows to carryout laboratory procedure at industrial scale.

Culture preservation

1. *Methods of preservations*
   - (a) Agar slant culture
   - (b) Agar slant culture covered with oil
   - (c) Saline suspension
   - (d) Preservation at very low temperature
   - (e) Preservation by drying in vacuum
   - (f) Lyophilization or freeze drying
2. *Stock culture collection centers*
   - (a) American type culture collection, Rockville, Maryland, USA
   - (b) Indian collection of industrial micro-organisms, National chemical laboratory, Pune
   - (c) Institute of Pasteur, Paris (France)
   - (d) Institute of microbial technology, Chandigarh

Criteria used for the Selection of Micro-organisms for Fermentation

The microbes should have following attributes:

- (i) The strain must be genetically stable
- (ii) The strain should be readily maintained for reasonably long period of time
- (iii) The strain must readily produce many vegetative cells, spores or other structures
- (iv) The strains should be able to protect themselves from contamination

1. *Methods of culture maintenance*: There are three methods for culture maintenance:
   - (a) drying organisms on soil or some other solid
   - (b) storing organisms on agar slants and
   - (c) removing the water from the cells or spores by lyophilization and storage of dried product.

12.7.2 Penicillin Fermentation (fed-batch) Method

The process flow begins from the basic raw materials to the downstream processes resulting in the final product. This description is a typical bioprocess flow of any penicillin production facility, it is important to note that in reality, companies generally have their own specific set of standards and hence modification of the process flow is necessary to meet their demands also to optimise quality and quantity.

The actual General Process flow diagram (Fig. 12.9) use in the production of penicillin.

In bioprocess facility, there will be an upstream and downstream process, the upstream processes in this case are referring to processes before input to the fermenter, while the downstream processes refers to the processes that are done to purify the output of the fermenter until it reaches to the desired product.

Medium for *Penicillium*

Medium preparation is necessary in bioprocesses which as it generally involves the use of micro-organism to achieve their products. In the case of the *Penicillium* fungus, the medium usually contain its carbon source which is found in corn steep liquor (a byproduct of starch manufacture) and glucose. Medium also consist of salts such as Magnesium sulphate, Potassium phosphate and Sodium nitrates. They provide the essential ions required for the fungus metabolic activity.

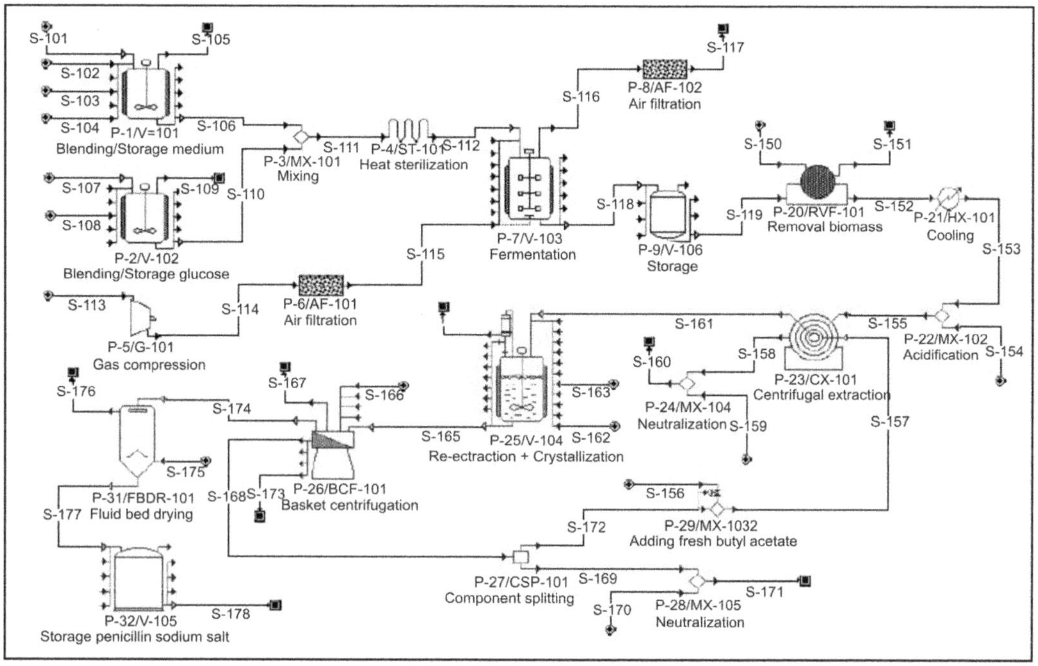

Fig. 12.9 General process flow diagram of penicillin production

Heat Sterilization

Medium is sterilzed at high heat and high pressure usually through a holding tube or sterilsed together with the fermenter. The pressurized steam is used usually and the medium is heated to 121 °C at 30 psi or twice of atmospheric pressure. High temperature short time conditions are used to minimize degradation of certain components of the media.

Fermentation

Fermentation for penicillin is usually done in the fed-batch mode as glucose must not be added in high amounts at the beginning of growth which will result in low yield of penicillin production as excessive glucose inhibit penicillin production. In addition to that, penicillin is a secondary metabolite of the fungus; therefore, the fed-batch mode is ideal for such products as it allows the high production of penicillin. The typical fermentation conditions for the *Penicllium* mold, usually requires temperatures at 20-24 °C while pH conditions are kept in between 6.0 to 6.5. The pressure in the bioreactor is usually much higher than the atmospheric pressure (1.02 atm) this is to prevent contamination from occurring as it prevents external contaminants from entering. Sparging of air bubbles is necessary to provide sufficient oxygen for the viability of the fungus. Depending on the volume of medium, for 2 cubic metres of culture, the sparging rate should be about 2.5 cubic metres per minute. The impeller is necessary to mix the culture evenly throughout the culture medium, fungal cells are much hardy and they are able to handle rotation speed of around 200 rpm shown in Fig. 12.13.

Seed Culture

The seed culture is developed first in the laboratory by the addition of *Penicillium* spores into a liquid medium. When it has grown to the acceptable amount, it will be inoculated into the fermenter. In some cases, the spores are directly inoculated into the fermenter. After 40 hours penicillin begins to be secreted by fungus.

Removal of Biomass

Filtration is necessary at this point of the bioprocess flow, as bio separation is required to remove the biomass from the culture such as the fungus and other impurities away from the medium which contains the penicillin product. There are many types of filtration methods available today, however, the Rotary vacuum filter is commonly employed as it able to run in continuous mode in any large scale operations. Add this point non-oxidizing acid such as phosphoric acid is introduced as pH will be as high as 8.5. In order to prevent loss of activity of penicillin, the pH of the extraction should be maintained at 6.0-6.5.

Adding of Solvent

In order to dissolve the penicillin present in the filtrate, organic solvents such as Amyl acetate or butyl acetate are used as they dissolve penicillin much better than water at physiological pH. At this point, penicillin is present in the solution and any other solids will be considered as waste.

Centrifugal Extraction

Centrifugation is done to separate the solid waste from the liquid component which contains the penicillin. Usually a tubular bowl or chamber bowl centrifuge is use at this point. The supernatant will then be transferred further in the downstream process to continue with extraction.

Extraction

Penicillin dissolve in the solvent will now undergo a series of extraction process to obtain better purity of the penicillin product. The acetate solution is first mixed with a Phosphate buffer, followed by a Chloroform solution and mixed again with a Phosphate buffer and finally in an Ether solution. Penicillin is present in high concentration in the Ether solution and it will be mixed with a solution of Sodium bicarbonate /potassium bicarbonate to obtain the penicillin-sodium salt/penicillin-potassium salt, which allows penicillin to be stored in a stable powder form at room temperature. The penicillin-sodium salt/ penicillin-potassium salt is obtained from the liquid material by basket centrifugation, in which solids are easily removed.

Fluid Bed Drying

Drying is necessary to remove any remaining moisture present in the powdered penicillin salt. In fluid bed drying, hot gas is pumped in from the base of the chamber containing the powdered salt inside a vacuum chamber. Moisture is then removed in this manner and this result in a much drier form of penicillin.

Storage

Penicillin salt is stored in containers and kept in a dried environment. It will then be polished and package into various types of products such as liquid penicillin or penicillin in pills. Dosage of the particular penicillin is determined by clinical trials that are done on this drug.

Industrial uses of bacteria: Lactic acid production, Vinegar production, Amino acid production, L-Lysine production, L-Glutamic acid production

Industrial uses of yeasts: Alcohol production, Baker's yeast, Food yeast

Industrial uses of molds: Penicillin production, Citric acid production, Enzyme production.

12.7.3 Immobilized Enzyme Technology

Enzyme therapy seems to be promising in the treatment of cardiovascular, oncological, intestinal, viral and hereditary diseases. At the same time there exist many limitations for the everyday clinical use of native enzymes. Enzymes are unstable, have a short lifetime in the circulation, cause toxic and immune reactions and are costly, etc. These drawbacks can be at least partially eliminated by enzyme immobilization onto different carriers. Such immobilization can make enzymes more stable, less antigenic and impart a longer circulation lifetime in the organism. Immobilized enzymes can be used as drugs for either local or systemic application (including soluble and insoluble immobilized enzymes for thrombolytic therapy and for the treatment of both malignant diseases and some in-born enzyme deficiencies). Immobilized enzymes can be also used for preparation of artificial cells (based on semi permeable microcapsules, liposomes, cells and cell ghosts). Special attention should be paid to the problem of using the immobilization principles for the construction of drug targeting systems vector protein and antibody immobilization, enzyme-polymer-vector conjugates, etc.

12.7.4 Hybridomas and Monoclonal Antibodies

Antibodies are proteins synthesized in blood against specific antigens just to combat and give immunity in blood. They can be collected from the blood serum of an animal. Such antibodies are heterogeneous and contain a mixture of antibodies (i.e., polyclonal antibodies). Therefore, they do not have characteristics of specificity. If a specific lymphocyte, after the isolation and culture *in vitro*, they become capable of producing a single type of antibody which bears specificity against specific antigen. It is known as 'monoclonal antibodies'. Due to the presence of desired immunity, monoclonal antibodies are used in the diagnosis of diseases.

Genetic research with mico-organisms, particularly at the molecular level, has provided techniques which have been applied to studies with mammalian cells. One of the important outcomes of this research has been the fusion of myeloma cells (cancer cells) with antibody-producing white blood cells (B-Lymphocytes). The resulting hybrid cell is called a hybridoma. Hybridoma cells can be selected and grown to produce a single, specific antibody, an antibody is called a monoclonal antibody.

Uses of Monoclonal Antibodies:

- The human sera have been replaced by monoclonal antibodies produced by hybridomas, for the identification of ABO blood groups
- Diagnosis (including ELISA test for detection of viruses and imaging)
- Immunopurification
- Therapy.

12.7.5 Industrial Aspects of Microorganisms

Biologics for Immunization: Control of infectious diseases through immunization requires the manufacture of immunization preparations on a commercial scale, for a variety of microbiological antigens. Development of effective immunological preparations with the stringent test requirements to ensure their safe use is the major program in many of the major pharmaceutical houses. This topic is thoroughly covered under immunology.

Petrol formation: Mico-organisms are associated with petroleum in its formation, its recovery by drilling, its decomposition and its utilization.

Microbiology and mining: Micro-organisms play a role in the recovery of minerals from ores

Deterioration of materials by micro-organisms: The term materials in this sense, refers to all products other than food stuffs. They are paper, textiles, wood, rubber and metals. Micro-organisms are responsible for a significant amount of this destruction.

Paper: The manufacture of paper involves two major operations. The first consists of physical or chemical treatment of cellulosic material (e.g., wood, cotton) for the purpose of separating and purifying the cellulose fibbers. The second consists of the fabrication of the resulting fibrous pulp. Microbial deterioration in the form of paper-pulp slime may be encountered in the pulp, and other defects may appear on the finished product.

Textiles: Textiles made from natural fibers - cotton, wool, linen and silk - are susceptible to deterioration by micro-organisms. Molds are the principal micro-organisms responsible for this damage.

Painted Surfaces: Painted surfaces are not always resistant to microbial disfiguration. Unless the paint film contains an effective fungicidal ingredient, it may under certain environmental conditions exhibit evidence of mold spotting or discoloration. This deterioration is due to the products of microbial metabolism of organic constituents of the paint.

Packing Material: Prevention of deterioration is accomplished through application of the principles for controlling microbial populations i.e., incorporation of microbicidal agents into the material packaging that protects material from contamination and storage under conditions that inhibit microbial growth (e.g., dehumidification).

12.8 Cell Culture

Cell culture is the multifaceted process through which cells are isolated from animal or plant and then grown under controlled artificial conditions, generally outside their natural environment. In this procedure cells are directly isolated from body or disaggregated by enzymatic or mechanical procedure or they may be derived from cell lines or cell strains. The historical development and methods of cell culture are closely interrelated to those of tissue culture and organ culture. The in vitro propagation of cells has become a common practice in many laboratories for a huge numbers of applications.

Historical events in cell culture development

- 1878: Claude Bernard proposed that physiological systems of an organism can be maintained in a living system after the death of an organism.
- 1885: Roux maintained embryonic chick cells in a saline culture.
- 1897: Loeb demonstrated the survival of cells isolated from blood and connective tissue in serum and plasma.
- 1903: Jolly observed cell division of salamander leucocytes *in vitro.*
- 1907: Harrison cultivated frog nerve cells in a lymph clot held by the 'hanging drop' method and observed the growth of nerve fibers *in vitro* for several weeks. He was considered by some as the father of cell culture.
- 1910: Burrows succeeded in long term cultivation of chicken embryo cell in plasma clots. He made detailed observation of mitosis.
- 1911: Lewis and Lewis made the first liquid media consisted of sea water, serum, embryo extract, salts and peptones. They observed limited monolayer growth.
- 1913: Carrel introduced strict aseptic techniques so that cells could be cultured for long periods.
- 1916: Rous and Jones introduced proteolytic enzyme trypsin for the subculture of adherent cells.
- 1923: Carrel and Baker developed 'Carrel' or T-flask as the first specifically designed cell culture vessel. They employed microscopic evaluation of cells in culture.
- 1927: Carrel and Rivera produced the first viral vaccine - Vaccinia.
- 1933: Gey developed the roller tube technique
- 1940s: The use of the antibiotics penicillin and streptomycin in culture medium decreased the problem of contamination in cell culture.
- 1948: Earle isolated mouse L fibroblasts which formed clones from single cells. Fischer developed a chemically defined medium, CMRL 1066.
- 1952: Gey established a continuous cell line from a human cervical carcinoma known as HeLa (Helen Lane) cells. Dulbecco developed plaque assay for animal viruses using confluent monolayers of cultured cells.
- 1954: Abercrombie observed contact inhibition: motility of diploid cells in monolayer culture ceases when contact is made with adjacent cells.
- 1955: Eagle studied the nutrient requirements of selected cells in culture and established the first widely used chemically defined medium.

- 1961: Hayflick and Moorhead isolated human fibroblasts (WI-38) and showed that they have a finite lifespan in culture.
- 1964: Littlefield introduced the HAT medium for cell selection.
- 1965: Ham introduced the first serum-free medium which was able to support the growth of some cells.
- 1965: Harris and Watkins were able to fuse human and mouse cells by the use of a virus.
- 1975: Kohler and Milstein produced the first hybridoma capable of secreting a monoclonal antibody.
- 1978: Sato established the basis for the development of serum-free media from cocktails of hormones and growth factors.
- 1982: Human insulin became the first recombinant protein to be licensed as a therapeutic agent.
- 1985: Human growth hormone produced from recombinant bacteria was accepted for therapeutic use.
- 1986: Lymphoblastoid γIFN licensed.
- 1987: Tissue-type plasminogen activator (tPA) from recombinant animal cells became commercially available.
- 1989: Recombinant erythropoietin in trial.
- 1990: Recombinant products in clinical trial (HBsAG, factor VIII, HIVgp120, CD4, GM-CSF, EGF, mAbs, IL-2).

Types of Cell Cultures

(i) **Primary cell culture:** This is the maintenance of growth of cells dissociated from the parental tissue (such as kidney or liver) using mechanical or enzymatic methods, in culture medium using suitable glass or plastic containers. The primary cell culture could be of two types depending upon the kind of cells in culture.

Adherent cells - Cells shown to require attachment for growth are said to be anchorage dependent cells. The adherent cells are usually derived from tissues of organs such as kidney where they are immobile and embedded in connective tissue.

Suspension cells - Cells which do not require attachment for growth or do not attach to the surface of the culture vessels are anchorage independent cells/suspension cells. All suspension cultures are derived from cells of the blood system because these cells are also suspended in plasma in vitro e.g. lymphocytes.

(ii) **Secondary cell cultures:** When a primary culture is sub-cultured, it becomes known as secondary culture or cell line. Subculture (or passage) refers to the transfer of cells from one culture vessel to another culture vessel. This is periodically required to provide fresh nutrients and growing space for continuously growing cell lines. The process involves removing the growth media and disassociating the adhered cells (usually enzymatically). Such cultures may be called secondary cultures.

(iii) Established Cell Line: A cell line or cell strain may be finite or continuous depending upon whether it has limited culture life span or it is immortal in culture. On the basis of the life span of culture, the cell lines are categorized into two types:

Finite cell lines - The cell lines which have a limited life span and go through a limited number of cell generations (usually 20-80 population doublings) are known as finite cell lines. These cell lines exhibit the property of contact inhibition, density limitation and anchorage dependence. The growth rate is slow and doubling time is around 24-96 hours.

Continuous cell lines - Cell lines transformed under laboratory conditions or in vitro culture conditions give rise to continuous cell lines. These cell lines show the property of ploidy (aneupliody or heteroploidy), absence of contact inhibition and anchorage dependence. They grow either in a monolayer or in suspension (see below). The growth rate is rapid and doubling time can be 12-24 hours.

Monolayer cultures - When the bottom of the culture vessel is covered with a continuous layer of cells, usually one cell in thickness, they are referred to as monolayer cultures.

Suspension cultures - Majority of continuous cell lines grow as monolayers. Some of the cells which are non-adhesive e.g. cells of leukemia or certain cells which can be mechanically kept in suspension, can be propagated in suspension.

(iv) Transformed cells: Sometimes eukaryotic cells exhibit unusual and alternative growth characteristics both in culture and in vivo. Such cells are usually referred to as transformed or neoplastic cells.

The transformation of some cells may be induced using viruses.

For example, when cultures of mammalian cells are exposed to Polyoma virus or Simian virus 40 (SV 40), some of the cells in the culture are transformed into a cell line that manifests a number of unusual characteristics, including:

1. The cells continue to grow and divide even after confluence is attained (with the result that they grow on top of one another instead of maintaining a monolayer),
2. The cells are no longer anchorage-dependent (thereby permitting growth in multilayers),
3. The cells grow to an indefinite population size,
4. Growth continues for many more generations than in the corresponding un-transformed cells (i.e., the cells appear to ignore or to have lost the built-in counting mechanism keeping track of the number of cell doublings), and

5. The cells grow irregularly in size and in shape and often reveal an abnormal chromosome content.

One of the most famous (and useful) examples is the "HeLa" line of transformed cells originally derived in 1951 from a cancerous cervical tumor and that has been continuously sub-cultured since that time. (HeLa is an acronym for Henrietta Lacks, the woman from whose uterus the cervical cells were removed.)

The relationship that exists between cellular transformation and cancer should be apparent; indeed, when transformed cells are injected into laboratory animals, the cells form tumors or neoplasms, whereas normal cells do not.

In tissue culture, transformed cells do not form conventional junctional complexes with neighboring cells. Hence, it is easy to understand why, when cellular transformation occurs in vivo, the transformed cells metastasize, that is, spread to other body tissues where they form new tumors, growing and crowding out the tissue's normal cells.

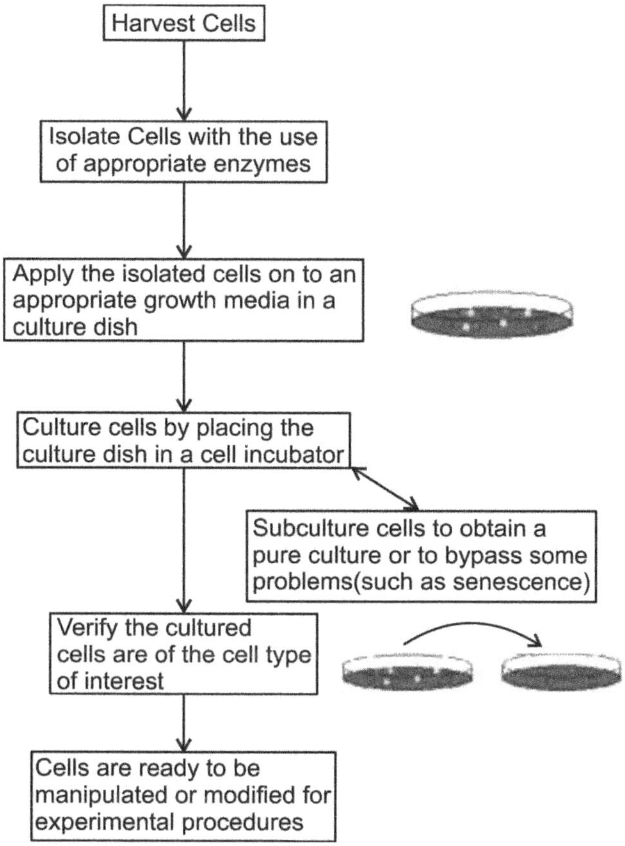

Fig. 12.10 General cell culture procedure

Requirements for Animal Cell Culture

(a) *Sterile Work Area*: Primary animal tissue and micro-organisms must not be cultured in or near the cell culture laboratory and the laboratory must be specifically designated for clean cell culture work.

(b) *Incubation Facilities*: In addition to an airflow cabinet and benching which can be easily cleaned, the cell culture laboratory will need to be furnished with an incubator or hot room to maintain the cells at 30-40°C. The incubation temperature will depend on the type of cells being cultivated. Insect cells will grow best at around 30°C while mammalian cells require a temperature of 37°C.

(c) *Refrigerators and Freezer*: Both items are very important for storage of liquid media at 4°C and for enzymes (e.g., trypsin) and some media components (e.g., glutamine and serum) at -20°C. A refrigerator or cold room is required to store medium and buffers.

A freezer will be needed for keeping pre aliquot stocks of serum, nutrients and antibiotics. Reagents may be stored at a temperature of -20°C but if cells are to be preserved it may be necessary to provide liquid nitrogen or a -70°C freezer.

(d) *Microscopes*: A simple inverted microscope is essential so that cultures can be examined in flasks and dishes. It is vital to be able to recognize morphological changes in cultures since these may be the first indication of deterioration of a culture.

(e) *Tissue Culture Ware*: A variety of tissue culture plastic-ware is available, the most common being specially treated polystyrene. Cells can be maintained in Petri dishes or flasks (25 cm^2 or 75 cm^2) which have the added advantage that the flasks can be gassed and then sealed so that a CO_2 incubator need not be used.

(f) *Washing Up and Sterilizing Facilities*: Pipettes are often plugged with non-absorbent cotton wool before putting into containers for sterilizing. Glassware, such as pipettes, conical flasks, beakers (covered with aluminum foil) is sterilized in a hot air oven at 160°C for one hour.

All other equipment, such as automatic pipette tips and bottles (lids loosely attached) are autoclaved at 121°C for 20 min. Sterilizing indicators such as sterile test strip are necessary for each sterilizing batch to ensure that the machine is operating effectively. Autoclave bags are available for loose items. Aluminum foil also makes good packaging material.

(g) *Liquid Nitrogen Deep Freezer*: The procedure for freezing cells is general for all cells in culture. They should be frozen in exponential phase of growth with a suitable preservative, usually dimethylsulfoxide (DMSO). The cells are frozen slowly at 1°C/min to -50°C and then kept either at -196°C immersed in liquid N_2 (in sealed glass ampoules) or above the liquid surface in the gas phase (screw top ampoules). Deterioration of frozen cells has been observed at -70°C, therefore, -196°C (liquid N_2) seems to be necessary.

(h) *Water Still or Reverse Osmosis Apparatus*: A double distilled or reverse osmosis water supply is essential for preparation of media, and rinsing glassware. Water is sterilized by autoclaving at 121°C for 20 min. The distilled water must be glass distilled and stored in glass if it is to be used for the preparation of media. Storage in plastic may result in leaching of toxic substances from the plastic into the water.

(i) *Filter Sterilization*: Media that cannot be autoclaved must be sterilized through a 0.22 mm pore size membrane filter. These are obtainable in various designs to allow a wide range of volumes to be filtered (e.g., Millipore, Gelman).

(j) *Other Requirements*:

Culture Media

The culture media is prepared in such a way that it provides

(a) The optimum conditions of factors like pH, osmotic pressure, etc.

(b) It should contain chemical constituents which the cells or tissues are incapable of synthesizing.

***There are two types of media used for culture of animal cells*:**

(a) Natural Media: The natural media are the natural sources of nutrient sufficient for growth and proliferation of animal cells and tissues.

The natural media used to promote cell growth fall in three categories:

1. Coagulant, such as plasma clots.
2. Biological fluids such as serum.

   Serum is obtained from human adult blood, placental, cord blood, horse blood, calf blood. The other forms of biological fluids used are coconut water, amniotic fluid, pleural fluid, insect haemolymph serum, culture filtrate, aqueous humour, from eyes etc.
3. Tissue extracts for example Embryo extracts

(b) Synthetic Media: Synthetic media are prepared artificially by adding several organic and inorganic nutrients, vitamins, salts, serum proteins, carbohydrates, cofactors, etc. Different types of synthetic media can be prepared for a variety of cells and tissues to be cultured.

***Synthetic Media are of Two Types*:**

1. Serum containing media (media containing serum)
2. Serum- free media (media without serum).

   Examples of some media are: minimal essential medium (MEM), RPMI 1640 medium, CMRL 1066, F12, etc.

(c) **pH:** Most media maintain the pH between 7 and 7.4. A pH below 6.8 inhibits cell growth. The optimum pH is essential to maintain the proper ion balance, optimal functioning of cellular enzymes and binding of hormones and growth factors to cell surface receptors in the cell cultures.

(d) **Osmolality:** A change in osmolality can affect cell growth and function. Salt, Glucose and Amino acids in the growth media determine the osmolality of the medium. All commercial media are formulated in such a way that their final osmolality is around 300 mOsm.

(e) **Buffering:** Carbon dioxide in the medium is in a developed state and the concentration depends on the atmospheric carbon dioxide tension and temperature. The CO_2 exists in the medium in the form of carbonic acid and protons.

$$CO_2 + H_2O \rightarrow H_2CO_3 \leftarrow H^+ + HCO_3^-$$

It must be noted that there is a direct relationship between the concentration of carbon dioxide, bicarbonate ions and pH of the media. By increasing the atmospheric CO_2, the pH will be reduced making the medium acidic.

(f) **Growth Factors:** In addition to buffering the medium, there are other growth requirements including amino acids, the requirement for which may vary with cell culture type. Commonly the necessary amino acids include cysteine and tyrosine, but some non-essential amino acids may be needed.

(g) **Antibiotics and Antimycotics:** Unless good sterile conditions can be maintained (e.g., using laminar flow hoods) it is necessary to incorporate antibiotics and antimycotics into the media. A wide range of suitable preparations are available from relatively specific antibiotics, e.g., penicillin/streptomycin solutions, to broader spectrum antibacterial/antimycotic agents such as kanamycin or amphotericin B.

The antibiotics chosen should clearly not to be toxic to the cells in culture and may depend on the type of contamination experienced in the individual laboratory.

Animal Culture Procedure

(i) ***Primary Culture*:** When cells are surgically removed from an organism and placed into a suitable culture environment, they will attach, divide and grow. This is called a Primary Culture. There are two basic methods for doing this.

First, for Explant Cultures, small pieces of tissue are attached to a glass or treated in a plastic culture vessel and bathed in culture medium. After a few days, individual cells will move from the tissue explant onto the culture vessel surface or substrate where they will begin to divide and grow.

The second, more widely used method speeds up this process by adding digesting (proteolytic) enzymes, such as trypsin or collagenase, to the tissue fragments to dissolve the cement holding the cells together. This creates a suspension of single cells that are then placed into culture vessels containing culture medium and allowed to grow and divide. This method is called Enzymatic Dissociation.

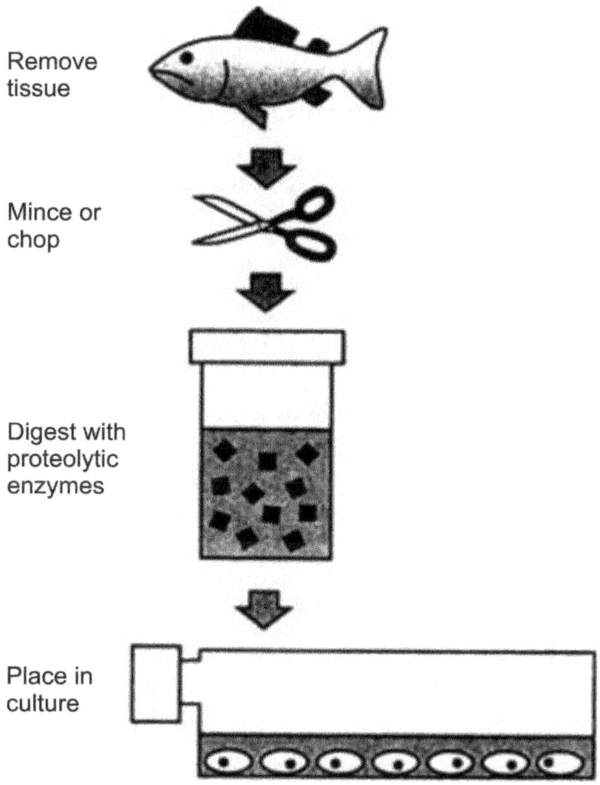

Fig. 12.11 The basic steps of primary cell culture

Advantages of Primary Cell Culture

The major advantages of primary cultures are the retention of:

1. **The Capacity for Biotransformation:** In many cases, the metabolism of a primary cell culture has greater similarity to in vivo than that seen with sub-cellular fractions used as an exogenous source for biotransformation.
2. **The Tissue-Specific Functions:** The second advantage of primary cultures is the retention of tissue specific functions. For example, primary cultures of rat myocardial cells consisting of synchronously beating cells can be prepared. When these cultures were exposed to tricyclic antidepressants that are cardio toxic, beating were observed.

Limitations of Primary Cell Cultures: One limitation of primary cultures is the necessity to isolate cells for each experiment. Procedures to isolate cells require the disruption of the tissue, often with proteolytic enzymes. This may result in the loss or damage of specific membrane receptors, damage to the integrity of the membrane, and loss of cellular products.

(ii) ***Sub-Culturing*****:** When the cells in the primary culture vessel have grown and filled up all of the available culture substrate, they must be Sub-cultured to give them room for continued growth. This is usually done by removing them as gently as possible from the substrate with enzymes. These are similar to the enzymes used in obtaining the primary culture and are used to break the protein bonds attaching the cells to the substrate.

Some cell lines can be harvested by gently scraping the cells off the bottom of the culture vessel. Once released, the cell suspension can then be subdivided and placed into new culture vessels.

Once a surplus of cells is available, they can be treated with suitable cryoprotective agents, such as dimethylsulfoxide (DMSO) or glycerol, carefully frozen and then stored at cryogenic temperatures (below -130°C) until they are needed. The theory and techniques for cryopreserving cells are covered in the Corning Technical Bulletin: General Guide for Cryogenically Storing Animal Cell Cultures.

Advantages of Animal Cell Culture:

- Controlled physiochemical environment (pH, temperature, osmotic pressure, O_2, etc)
- Controlled and defined physiological conditions
- Homogeneity of cell types (achieved through serial passages)
- Economical, since smaller quantities of reagents are needed than in vivo.
- Legal, moral and ethical questions of animal experimentation are avoided

Disadvantages of Animal Cell Culture:

- Expertise is needed, so that behaviour of cells in culture can be interpreted and regulated.
- Ten times more expensive for same quantity of animal tissue; therefore, reasons for its use should be compelling.

Applications of Cell Culture

Cell culture is one of the major tools used in cellular and molecular biology, providing excellent model systems for studying the normal physiology and biochemistry of cells (e.g., metabolic studies, aging), the effects of drugs and toxic compounds on the cells and mutagenesis and carcinogenesis. It is also used in drug screening and development and large scale manufacturing of biological compounds (e.g., vaccines, therapeutic proteins). The major advantage of using cell culture for any of these applications is the consistency and reproducibility of results that can be obtained from using a batch of clonal cells.

I. **Model System:** Cell culture are used as model system to study basic cell biology and biochemistry, to study the interaction between cell and disease causing agents like bacteria, virus, to study the effect of drugs, to study the process of aging and also it is used to study triggers for ageing.

II. **Cancer Research:** The basic difference between normal cell and cancer cell can be studied using animal cell culture technique, as both cells can be cultured in laboratory. Normal cells can be converted into cancer cells by using radiation, chemicals and viruses. Thus, the mechanism and cause of cancer can be studied. Cell culture can be used to determine the effective drugs for selectively destroy only cancer cells.

III. **Virology:** Animal cell cultures are used to replicate the viruses instead of animals for the production of vaccine. Cell culture can also be used to detect and isolate viruses, and also to study growth and development cycle of viruses. It is also used to study the mode of infection.

IV. **Toxicity Testing:** Animal cell culture is used to study the effects of new drugs, cosmetics and chemicals on survival and growth of a number of types of cells. Especially liver and kidney cells. Cultured animal cells are also used to determine the maximum permissible dosage of new drugs.

V. **Vaccine Production:** Cultured animal cells are used in the production of viruses and these viruses are used to produce vaccines. For example vaccines for deadly diseases like polio, rabies, chicken pox, measles and hepatitis B are produced using animal cell culture.

VI. **Genetically Engineered Protein:** Animal cell cultures are used to produce commercially important genetically engineered proteins such as monoclonal antibodies, insulin, hormones, and much more.

VII. **Replacement Tissue or Organ:** Animal cell culture can be used as replacement tissue or organs. For example artificial skin can be produced using this technique to treat patients with burns and ulcers. However research is going on artificial organ culture such as liver, kidney and pancreas. Organ culture techniques and research are being conducted on both embryonic and adult stem cell culture. These cells have the capacity to differentiate into many different types of cells and organs. It is belived that by learning to control the development and differentiation of these cells may be used to treat variety of medical conditions.

VIII. **Genetic Counseling:** Fetal cell culture extracted from pregnant women can be used to study or examine the abnormalities of chromosomes, genes using karyotyping, and these findings can be used in early detection of fetal disorders.

IX. **Genetic Engineering:** Cultured animal cells can be used to introduce new genetic material like DNA or RNA into the cell. These can be used to study the expression of new genes and its effect on the health of the cell. Insect cells are used to produce commercially important proteins by infecting them with genetically altered baculoviruses.

X. **Gene Therapy:** Cultured animal cells can be genetically altered and can be used in gene therapy technique. First cells are removed from the patient lacking a functional gene or missing a functional gene. These genes are replaced by functional genes and altered cells are culture and grown in laboratory condition. Then these altered cells are introduced into the patient. Another method is by using viral vector, functional gene is inserted into the genome of viral vector and then they are allowed to infect the patient, in the hope that the missing gene will be expressed with the help of the viral vector.

XI. **Drug Screening and Development:** Animal cell cultures are used to study the cytotoxicity of new drug. This is also used to find out the effective and safe dosage of new drugs. Now these tests are being conducted in 384 and 1536 well plates. Cell-based assay plays an important role in pharmaceutical industry.

12.9 Industrial Micro-organisms and their Products

12.9.1 *Escherichia E.coli*

(E. coli) are one among the other micro-organisms constituting the micro flora of the gut of the warm blooded animals including humans. These are called as beneficial micro-organisms which are harmless. But the infection caused by a particular strain of E. coli (O157:H7) masks the beneficial effect of the normal E. coli bacteria and it is always seen as an organism of threat by many shown in Fig. 12.11.

The Distinguishing features of E. coli: The simple genome of the E. coli bacteria, the rate of growth, easy to handle, complete gene sequence, the competency as a host, simple cultivation procedure and its ability to grow under both aerobic and anaerobic condition distinguishes these bacteria from others in selection procedure for an experiment. The genome of the E. coli bacteria is very crisp and simple with only 4400 genes, easy to study and understand. The ability of the bacteria to multiply drastically producing a generation in 1200 seconds under suitable growth condition dragged the attention of the researchers. Coming to the safety in handling the organisms, except for the particular harmful strain (O157:H7), the normal organism from the flora of the gut is safe to handle under suitable microbiological environment. The first completely sequenced genome is an additional feather in the cap of E. coli making the bacteria easier to use in recombinant DNA technology which involves nothing but the ultimate expression of proteins. Also the competence of the E. coli bacteria as a host for foreign DNAs and simple laboratory procedure to cultivate and adaptability to both aerobic and anaerobic environment made the E. coli bacteria a pioneer in the field of biotechnology.

Industrial Applications of *E.coli*

Human Insulin

Human insulin was developed through the 1960s and 1970s and approved for pharmaceutical use in 1982. Before human insulin was developed animal insulin, usually a purified form of porcine (pork) insulin, was used. Human insulin in laboratory created by growing insulin proteins within *E.coli* bacteria (*Escherichia coli*).

Human insulin is produced in a very controlled and clean environment. Genetically-engineered bacteria are grown in large stainless steel fermentation vessels. The vessel contains all the nutrients needed for growth. When the fermentation is complete, the mixture containing the bacteria is harvested. The bacteria are filtered off and broken open to release the insulin they have produced. It is then purified and packaged into bottles for distribution. All the equipment is kept sterile so that contamination cannot get into the medicine. Regular checks make sure that all the processes are working properly and the insulin meets the required quality.

Human insulin is available in two forms, a short acting (regular) form and an intermediate acting (NPH) form. NPH (Neutral Protamine Hagedorn) insulin, also known as isophane insulin, is a suspension meaning that the insulin vial should be rolled or repeatedly turned upside down to ensure the solution is uniformly cloudy.

Some examples of Human Insulin

Regular (short acting): Humulin S, Actrapid, Insuman Rapid

NPH (intermediate acting): Humulin I, Insuman basal, Insulatard

Premixed human insulins: Humulin M2, M3 and M5, Insuman Comb 15, 25 and 50

Premixed insulins consist of a mix of regular and NPH insulin. The premixed insulins are available in a number of different ratios of mixing.

Threonine: Even before the application of the rDNA technology, the first industrial application of E. coli being the production of the amino acid threonine in the year 1961 just by exposing the organism to mutagens resulting in various mutants which were screened for the desired type of mutant enabling the synthesis of the amino acid threonine and those organisms were isolated and used for large scale production

rDNA Technology: The process of gene cloning in E.coli involves a series of steps like isolation of the desired DNA and ligasing it to a suitable vector resulting in the production recombinant molecules. These molecules are screened for the expression of the desired gene and then the selected molecules are passed on to the E.coli which express the desired gene. The types of vectors used may be either a plasmid or a cosmid or a phage and the various methods which allow the vector to enter the bacteria are transformation, transfection and transduction. Thus the genetically modified E. coli bacteria made its way into industrial biotechnology.

Human insulin: The genetically engineered *E.coli* bacteria were employed in the production of human insulin by successfully introducing the human gene responsible for insulin production into the gene sequence of the *E.coli* bacteria and cultivating the modified bacteria under suitable laboratory environment. Then the insulin is extracted from the cells and purified and used in humans. Also human growth hormone is produced using genetically modified *E.coli* bacteria.

Biofuel: There is evidence of biofuel production by using the genetically modified *E.coli*. The ability of the modified bacteria to convert the cellulose structure into sugars is the theory behind the production of biofuel using *E.coli*. The ideal character of genetically modified E. coli in producing hydrogen was discovered by a Texas scientist and he applied this principle in generating a fuel cell and proving *E.coli* as a house of power generation.

Biodiesel: *E.coli* are engineered to generate biodiesel as a potential means of generating renewable energy. The genetic makeup of *E.coli* cells are manipulated to produce biodiesel derived from fatty acids. One of the alternative ways is to alter the *E.coli* cells to make it overproduce fatty acids, which are utilized in the production of biodiesel.

Antibody molecules: The fully identified gene sequence and the ability to make the gene construction in the vectors directly and a very good transformation rate of *E.coli* are the salient features enabled scientists to develop specific antibody molecules which will be a promising field to humans on extension.

Tryptophan: In an effort to lower the production cost, genetically engineered E. coli were used as an alternative method in the production of the amino acid tryptophan with wide medicinal application.

Bio sensor: Scientists from Cambridge University are on their way in developing a bio sensor *E.coli* to detect the presence of toxic elements in water and air. Also by extending this research, they promise the use of genetically engineered *E.coli* (called as *E. chromi*) in identifying various diseases like cancer and stomach ulcer by 2039.

Hydrogen as an alternative fuel: The current significance on the variety of global energy sources, while minimizing the fossil fuel consumption, has sited new interest on hydrogen as an alternative fuel and its production through bioconversions that are mediated by microbes. *Escherichia coli* (strain ZF1) are currently being used in the production of hydrogen under anaerobic growth conditions.

Plants: Genetic engineering of plants also utilizes *Escherichia coli*. They are often used to generate numerous copies of a gene construct that is finally transferred into a plant.

Painting: Microbial colonies of *E. coli* are grown deliberately to form images as they are fast reproducing and generally harmless, that is images are made by simply painting a petri dish with *E. coli* and allowing it to grow called as microbial art. Scientists have also engineered the jelly fish DNA to *E. coli* making them glow and utilizing as a photo paper.

Bio-Computers: *E. coli* transcriptor has been developed by the researchers utilizing DNA and Enzymes. This is a potential step towards building working computers within living cells (Bio-Computers) that could be programmed to control gene expression in an organism.

Nanobots: *E. coli* are used to generate cancer-fighting drugs. One of the projects manipulated *E. coli* micro-organism to carry an enzyme that fights cancer. Researchers are also working on a method of nanobots that would contain *E. coli* programmed with instructions to attack cancer cells, so that when a nanobot finds a tumour, it is able to dispatch speedy bacteria to call the other nanobots to it.

Fermentation end products of *E.coli*:

- Ethanol
- Lactic acid
- Succinic acid
- Acetic acid
- CO_2 and H_2

12.9.2 Industrial Applications of Penicillium Species

1. *Penicillium notatum*:

- In 1928, Alexander fleming observed that the growth of the bacterium *Staphylococcus aureus* was inhibited in the area surrounding the colony of a mold that had contaminated a petri plate
- The mold was identified as *Penicillium notatum*, and its active compound, which was isolated a short time later, was named penicillin.

Medium requirements for the production of penicillin:

Penicillium species required the production medium which contains

Lactose	:	1%
$CaCO_3$	:	1%
Cornsteep liqor	:	8.5 %
Glucose	:	1%
Sodium hydrogen phosphate	:	0.4%
Phenyl acetic acid	:	0.5 gm
pH	:	5 - 6
Temperature for incubation	:	23 - 25 °C

Aeration and agitation are necessary

2. *Penicillium chrysogenum*:

- Penicillium chrysogenum is a mold that could inhibit the growth of a bacterium

- By using ultraviolet rays penicillin production by a mold *Penicillium chrysogenum* has been increased by about thousand fold greater to what was produced at Fleming's time.

Fungi	Antibiotic
Penicillium griseofulvum	Griseofulvin
Penicillium chrysogenum	Penicillin

Penicillins

Penicillins are a class of beta-lactam antibiotics. Penicillin was the first antibiotic discovered from the mold *Penicillium notatum* in 1928 by Alexander Fleming at St.Mary's Hospital in London, England.

The basic structure of penicillins is a nucleus consisting of a beta-lactam ring (4 membered cyclic amide) and a side chain. The beta-lactam ring is necessary for antibacterial activity, and the side chain determines the antibacterial spectrum and pharmacologic properties.

Beta-lactamases: (also called penicillinases) are enzymes that deactivate penicillins by destroying the beta-lactam ring via hydrolysis. Beta-lactamases allow bacteria to be resistant to penicillin.

Various penicillins differ mainly by the structure of the side chain. In addition to their structural differences, the penicillins differ in their antimicrobial spectrum, pattern of β-lactamase resistance (susceptibility to penicillinase), the ability to penetrate the outer membrane of gram-negative bacteria, stability to gastric acids, and their behavior within the body.

Organisms that are not actively multiplying or do not have a cell wall are NOT susceptable to penicillins.

Classification

The penicillins can be classified according to their antibacterial activity:

- Natural penicillins
- Antistaphylococcal penicillins
- Aminopenicillins
- Extended spectrum penicillins: carboxypenicillins and ureidopenicillins

Natural Penicillins

- Penicillin G (Benzylpenicillin)
- Penicillin V

Natural penicillins, the first agents in the penicillin family, are obtained directly from the *Penicillium* mold and do not require further modification.

Penicillin G is the prototype of the class and the most potent of all penicillins against susceptible gram-positive bacteria. It is sensitive to stomach acids and requires intravenous or intramuscular administration.

Penicillin G is short acting, but its salts, procaine and benzathine, have extended duration of action because they can distribute into storage tissues to be released slowly.

Probenecid blocks tubular secretion of penicillin and has been used to increase the serum concentration and prolong the half-life of penicillin G and other penicillins.

The natural penicillins are very susceptible to inactivation by beta-lactamases.

Spectrum: The natural penicillins are active against non β-lactamase–producing gram-positive cocci (*Pneumococci*, *Staphylococci*, *Streptococci*), few gram-negative cocci (*meningococci* and *gonococci*), gram-positive bacilli (*Bacillus anthracis*, *Bacillus perfringens*, *Bacillus diphtheriae*), anaerobes (*Clostridum perfringens*, *C. tetani*), and spirochetes (*Treponema pallidum*, *T. pertenue* and *Leptospira*).

Antistaphylococcal Penicillins

- Cloxacillin
- Dicloxacillin
- Oxacillin
- Nafcillin
- Methicillin

The antistaphylococcal penicillins (also called the "penicillinase-resistant penicillins") have bulky side chains that prevent their inactivation by the staphylococcal β-lactamases. These penicillins are useful in treating infections caused by *Staphylococcus aureus* and *Staphylococcus epidermidis*.

Methicillin was the first member of this group, followed by oxacillin, nafcillin, cloxacillin and dicloxacillin. Methicillin was the first penicillin developed through rational drug modification. Since then all bacteria which are resistant to any type of penicillin are designated as methicillin resistant (e.g., MRSA - methicillin-resistant S. aureus).

Due to the bulky side group, all of the antistaphylococcals have difficulty penetrating the cell membrane and have a poor range of activity compared to other penicillins.

Spectrum: Antistaphylococcals have a very narrow spectrum as they were developed solely for killing β-lactamase producing staphylococci. Their major clinical indications are susceptible *S. aureus* and *S. epidermidis* infections.

Note: Antistaphylococcals are the only penicillins that by themselves are resistant to penicillinases. Their rank order of resistance is methicillin > cloxacillin = dicloxacillin > oxacillin.

Aminopenicillins

- Ampicillin
- Amoxicillin
- Bacampicillin
- Cyclacillin
- Hetacillin

The aminopenicillins have a wider range of activity than natural or antistaphylococcal penicillins. However, they lack the bulky side groups and are susceptible to inactivation by beta-lactamases. Aminopenicillins have additional hydrophilic groups, allowing the drug to penetrate into Gram-negative bacteria via the porins.

Advantages of aminopenicillins include higher oral absorption, higher serum levels, and longer half-lives. Aminopenicillins are resistant to gastric acids so can be administered orally.

Bacampicillin is more expensive but it does not have any significant advantages over the other aminopenicillins.

***Spectrum*:** Aminopenicillins are similar to penicillin G in the activity against Gram-positive organisms but are slightly weaker than the latter. Aminopenicillins are more active against *enterococci* and *Listeria monocytogenes* compared to penicillin G.

Gram-negative spectrum includes *Haemophilus influenzae*, *Salmonella*, *Shigella, Escherichia coli*, *Proteus mirabilis*, *N. gonorrhoeae*, *N. meningitidis*.

Extended-Spectrum Penicillins (Antipseudomonals)

- Carbenicillin
- Ticarcillin
- Piperacillin
- Azlocillin
- Mezlocillin

Extended-spectrum penicillins (also called antipseudomonals) include both carboxypenicillins (carbenicillin and ticarcillin) and ureidopenicillins (piperacillin, azlocillin, and mezlocillin). Antipseudomonal penicillins are similar to the aminopenicillins in structure but have either a carboxyl group or urea group instead of the amine.

In general, the antipseudomonal penicillins have greater activity than do other penicillins against gram-negative bacteria (especially *Pseudomonas* and *Proteus*) due to enhanced penetration through the cell wall of these bacteria.

The major advantage of carboxypenicillins is their activity against *Pseudomonas aeruginosa* (one of the major pathogens responsible for nosocomial pneumonia) and certain indole-positive *Proteus* species that are resistant to aminopenicillins. Ticarcillin is stronger against *P. aeruginosa* and *Enterobacter* species than carbenicillin.

Against anaerobes and Gram-positive organisms, carboxypenicillins generally have the same spectrum of activity as penicillin G. However, they are substantially weaker in comparison with penicillin G.

Ureidopenicillins have greater activity against *P. aeruginosa* compared to carbenicillin and ticarcillin. Piperacillin is the most potent of the extended-spectrum penicillins against *Pseudomonas*. The spectrum of piperacillin and mezlocillin is extended to include *Klebsiella*, *Enterobacter*, *Citrobacter*.

All antipseudomonals are destroyed by β-lactamases.

The extended-spectrum penicillins are not used in the treatment of infections caused by Gram-positive bacteria because penicillin G and aminopenicillins are more potent against these organisms.

Antipseudomonals penicillins may be used in combination with Aminoglycosides.

ß-lactamase Inhibitors

- Clavulanic acid
- Sulbactam
- Tazobactam

The ß-lactamase inhibitors act as suicide inhibitors of the ß-lactamases. These compounds are very slowly released after attack of the penicillinase resulting in irreversible inhibition of the enzyme, i.e. the enzyme remains acylated. This protects the penicillins from degradation and expands their utility.)

Bacterial Susceptibility to Penicillins:

- The susceptibility of gram-positive bacteria to penicillin and sulfonamide is high
- The susceptibility of gram-negative bacteria to penicillin and sulfonamide is low

Mode of Action

- Penicillin interferes with the final linking of the peptidoglycan rows by peptide cross-bridges. As a result cell wall is greatly weakened and the cell undergoes lysis, destruction caused by rupture of the plasma membrane and the loss of cytoplasm.
- Eukaryotic cells do not contain peptidoglycan, the framework of the prokaryotic cell wall. This is significant medically because antibiotics, such as penicillins and cephalosporins, act against peptidoglycan and therefore do not affect human eukaryotic cells.
- Penicillin, is a group of several penicillin compounds, differ from one another in the side chain attached to its amino group.

- Most of these penicillins are 6-aminopenicillanic acid derivatives and all have β-lactam ring which is responsible for the antibiotic activity
- Penicillin acts against gram-positive bacteria and inhibit their cell wall synthesis. These are non-toxic to mammals except for certain allergic reactions.

1. ***Natural Penicillins*:** Penicillin extracted from cultures of the mold penicillium exists in several closely related forms. These are the so-called natural penicillins

   ***E.g.*,** Penicillin G and penicillin V

   - *Penicillin G*: It has narrow but useful spectrum of activity
   - Drug of choice against staphylococci, streptococci and several spirochetes.
   - When injected intramuscularly, penicillin G is rapidly excreted from the body in 3 to 6 hours
   - When taken orally, the acidity of the digestive fluids in the stomach diminishes its concentration
   - Procaine penicillin, a combination of the drugs procaine and penicillin G, is retained at detectable concentrations for up to 24 hours.
   - *Penicillin V*: It is stable in stomach acids and can be taken orally.

2. ***Semi synthetic penicillins*:** A large number of semi synthetic penicillins have been developed to overcome the disadvantages of natural penicillins

   - Scientists develop these penicillins in either of two ways: first, they can interrupt synthesis of the molecule by penicillium and obtain only the common penicillin nucleus for use
   - Second, they can remove the side chains from the completed natural molecules and then chemically add other side chains that make them more resistant to penicillinase

   e.g., Oxacillin, Ampicillin

3. Penicillinase-resistant penicillins: Methicillin, oxacillin, naficillin.
4. Extended spectrum penicillins: Amoxicillin, Ampicillin, Carbenicillin.
5. Penicillins plus β-lactamase inhibitors: Clavulanic acid
6. Carbapenems: Primaxin, a combination of imipenem and cilastin
7. Monobactams: Aztreonam

Table 12.9 Spectrum of Penicillins Semi Synthetic Penicillins

Drugs by Mode of Action	**Comments**
Inhibitors of cell wall synthesis	
Natural penicillins	Penicillins inhibit bacterial transpeptidage enzymes which are involved in the synthesis of the bacterial cell wall
Penicillin G	Against gram + ve bacteria, requires injection
Penicillin V	Against gram + ve bacteria, oral administration
Semisynthetic penicillins	
Oxacillin	Resistant to penicillinase
Ampicillin	Broad spectrum
Amoxicillin	Broad spectrum, combined with inhibitor of Penicillinase
Aztreonam	Monobactam, effective for gram – ve bacteria
Imipenem	A carbapenem, very broad spectrum

Units of Antibiotics

- The potency of antibiotics is normally expressed in terms of units/mL of solution or in 1 mg (U/mg).
- In most cases, the antibiotic vial shows the quantity expressed in terms of weight as well as activity for example 1 mg of penicillin G (benzyl penicillin) is equivalent to 1665 units.

Uses

- Penicillins are the safest antibiotics used against gram + ve infections
- Used in sexually transmitted diseases and coccal infections
- In case of GIT infections Ampicillin is used

12.9.3 Industrial Applications of Streptomyces species

- *Streptomyces* are filamentous branching, many of them produce antibiotics
- *Streptomyces* come under the class *Actinobacteria* (the high G + C Gram-positive bacteria) and order Actinomycetales
- The reproductive asexual spores of *streptomyces* are formed at the ends of aerial filaments
- If each spore lands on a suitable substrate, it is capable of germinating into a new colony
- These organisms are strict aerobes

- They often produce extracellular enzymes that enable them to utilize proteins, polysaccharides, such as starch, cellulose, and many other organic materials found in soil.
- *Streptomyces* characteristically produce a gaseous compound called **"geosmin"**, which gives fresh soil
- Species of *streptomyces* are valuable because they produce most of our commercial antibiotics shown in Table 12.10.

Table 12.10 List of Antibiotics produced by Streptomyces Species

Microorganism	Antibiotic
Actinomycetes	
Streptomyces nodosus	Amphotericin B
Streptomyces Venezulae	Chloramphenicol
Streptomyces aureofaciens	Chlortetracycline
Streptomyces fradiae	Neomycin
Streptomyces griseus	Streptomycin
Streptomyces aureofaciens	Tetracyclines

Susceptibility of bacteria to Streptomycin

- The susceptibility of Gram + ve bacteria to streptomycin is low
- The susceptibility of Gram – ve bacteria to streptomycin is high

Mode of action

- Several antibiotics work by inhibiting protein synthesis on prokaryotic ribosomes
- Antibiotics such as Streptomycin and Gentamicin attach to the 30s subunit and interfere with protein synthesis

Aminoglycosides

- Aminoglycosides are a group of antibiotics in which amino sugars are linked by glycoside bonds
- They were among the first antibiotics to have significant activity against gram – ve bacteria
- The best known Aminoglycoside is **Streptomycin**
- Streptomycin is still used as an alternative drug in the treatment of tuberculosis
- Aminoglycosides are bactericidal and inhibit protein synthesis
- Neomycin is present in many nonprescription topical preparations shown in Table 12.11.

Table 12.11 Antibiotics and their mechanism of Action

Drugs by mode of action	Comments
1 Penicillins	Inhibitors of protein synthesis
2. Chloramphenicol	Broad spectrum, potentially toxic
Aminoglycosides	
3. Streptomycin	Broad spectrum, including mycobacteria
4. Neomycin	Topical use, broad spectrum
Tetracyclines	
5. Tetracycline, (Oxytetracycline, Chlortetracycline)	Broad spectrum, including Chlamydias and Rickettsias, animal feed additives

Media composition for the production of Streptomycin

Soya bean meal	-	10 gm
Glucose	-	10 gm
Peptone	-	5 gm
Meat extract	-	5 gm
NaCl	-	5 gm
pH	-	7.6-8.0
Temperature	-	28 °C

Media composition for the production of Chlortetracycline:

Sugar	3%
Corn steep liquor	1%
$CaCO_3$	1%
$(NH_4)_2 SO_4$	0.2%
NH_4Cl	0.1%
pH	6-7

12.9.4 Tetracyclines

Tetracyclines

- Tetracyclines are a group of closely related broad spectrum antibiotics produced by *streptomyces* species *streptomyces aureofaciens*.
- They are not only effective against Gram + ve and Gram – ve bacteria but also penetrate body tissues well and especially valuable against the intracellular *Rickettsial* and *Chlamydial* infections.
- Three of the more commonly used tetracyclines are Oxytetracycline, Chlortetracycline and Tetracycline itself.

- Some semisynthetic tetracyclines such as Doxycycline and Minocycline are also available in the market.
- Tetracyclines are used to treat many urinary tract infections (UTI), and infections caused by micro-organisms like *Mycoplasmas, Pneumonia* and *Chlamydia* and *Rickettsia*.
- They are also frequently used as alternative drugs for sexually transmitted diseases such as syphilis and gonorrhea.

12.9.4.1 Chloramphenicol

- Chloramphenicol is a broad-spectrum antibiotic with serious toxicity problems.
- It is less expensive for the pharmaceutical industry to synthesize it chemically, than to isolate it from *Streptomyces species streptomyces venezulae.*
- It is relatively small molecular size promotes its diffusion into areas of the body that are normally inaccessible to many other drugs.

12.9.5 Saccharomyces Species

(i) *Saccharomyces cerevisiae*

- The yeasts *Saccharomyces cerevisiae* are used to make bread and wine.
- *Saccharomyces cerevisiae* are also genetically modified to produce a variety of proteins, including Hepatitis B vaccine.
- *Saccharomyces* are also used as a protein supplement for humans and cattle. Yeasts are capable of facultative anaerobic growth.
- Yeasts can use oxygen or an organic compound as the final electron acceptor.
- If given access to oxygen, yeasts perform aerobic respiration to metabolize carbohydrates to CO_2 and H_2O. If oxygen is denied, they ferment carbohydrates and produce ethanol and CO_2. This fermentation is used in brewing, wine-making and baking industries.
- *Saccharomyces* species produce ethanol in brewed beverages and CO_2 for leavening bread dough.

Saccharomyces cerevisiae industrial uses are given in Table 12.12. This is the most well characterized eukaryote, the preferred microbial cell factory for the largest industrial biotechnology product (bioethanol). *Saccharomyces cerevisiae* offers a strong commercially compatible skeleton to be exploited for diverse chemical production. **Succinic acid** is a highly sought after added-value chemical for which there is no native liability for production and accumulation in *S. cerevisiae*. The genetic reconstruction of *S. cerevisiae* by using an evolutionary programming method enabled the organism to couple biomass and succinate production.

Table 12.12 Industrial uses of *Saccharomyces cerevisiae*

Fermentation end product	Industrial use	Starting material	Microorganism
Glycerol	Pharmaceutical, industrial uses	Molasses	*Saccharomyces cerevisiae*
Ethanol	Beer	Malt extract	*Saccharomyces cerevisiae*
Ethanol	Wine	Grapes or other fruit juices	*Saccharomyces cerevisiae var ellipsoideus*

(ii) *Saccharomyces fragalis*

Invertase – (saccharase or sucrose): *Saccharomyces fragIlis*, *S.cerevisiae* and some other *saccharomyces* species are the richest source of enzyme Invertase.

- This enzyme splits sucrose into glucose and fructose. It is widely distributed in nature.
- Invertase is produced in industries from bakers or brewer's yeast

Production of Invertase: Industrially, enzyme invertase is produced by special strains of yeast which grow on bottom. The medium contains sucrose, ammonium salt, phosphate buffer and other minerals.

The pH is adjusted to 4.5; fermentation is carried out for about 8 hr at 28 - 30 °C

Recovery: The yeast cells are filtered off, compressed, plasmolysed and autolyzed. The invertase extracted may be dried or held in sucrose syrup. The enzyme can also be purified by dialysis.

Uses:

- Invertase is used in confectionery to make invert sugar for the preparation of ice-cream etc.
- Chocolate - coated candies are also prepared
- Used in the manufacture of artificial honey.

(iii) *Saccharomyces pyriformis*

Ginger beer is the beverage produced by *Saccharomyces pyriformis.* In this case the beverage is made by the fermentation of a sugar solutions flavored with ginger. The starter culture in the 'ginger-beer plant' in which yeast *Saccharomyces pyriformis* and *Lactobacillus vermiformis* are used.

(iv) *Saccharopolyspora erythraea*

Erythromycin antibiotic is produced by *Saccharopolyspora erythraea.*

12.9.6 Future Prospects

The basic knowledge of molecular biology and genetics accumulated during the past few decades is rapidly being translated into practical objectives and is revolutionizing industrial microbiology. More than 200 companies throughout the world built upon the new biotechnology have come into being during the last several years. Another future prospective is a large sector of industry is pursuing the studies in the genetic engineering of micro-organisms and other cells.

Essay Questions

1. Write a note on soil microbiology
2. Write a note on various fermentative methods
3. Explain the modes of actions of as peniciliins, tetracyclines
4. Write a note on microbiology of cheese

Multiple Choice Questions

1. Spontaneous generation theory is also known as
   (a) Biogenesis
   (b) Abiogenesis
   (c) Neobiogenesis
   (d) Microbiogenesis
2. Which among the following Fungi are lignin decomposers
   (a) Agaricus
   (b) Aspergillus
   (c) penicillium
   (d) fusarium
3. Spoilage of fresh meat is by which of the following micro-organism
   (a) Rhodotorula
   (b) Psuedomonas
   (c) Rhizopusnigrans
   (d) Alcaligens
4. Semi sythethetic penicillin among the following is
   (a) Oxacillin
   (b) penicillin V
   (c) penicillin G
   (d) aztreonam
5. Neomycin is produced by
   (a) Streptomyces fradiae
   (b) streptomyces griseus
   (c) streptomuces aurofaciens
   (d) Streptomyces nodosus
6. Saccharomyces crevice is used in the fermentation of
   (a) glycerol
   (b) ethanol
   (c) chocolate
   (d) rice bran

Answers

1. (a)	2. (d)	3. (a)
4. (a)	5. (a)	6. (b)

INDEX

C

D

E

F

G

M

N

O

P

Q

R

S

T

U

Ingram Content Group UK Ltd.
Milton Keynes UK
UKHW052145080623
423089UK00003B/36

9 789386 819666